Exploring Medical Language

A STUDENT-DIRECTED APPROACH 8th Edition

understand.

be understood.

Myrna LaFleur Brooks, RN, BEd
Founding President
National Association of Health Unit Coordinators
Faculty Emeritus
Maricopa County Community College District
Phoenix, Arizona

Danielle LaFleur Brooks, MEd, MATLA
Adjunct Faculty
Community Colleges of Vermont
Montpelier, Vermont

ELSEVIER
MOSBY

ELSEVIER
MOSBY

3251 Riverport Lane
St. Louis, Missouri 63043

EXPLORING MEDICAL LANGUAGE, A STUDENT-DIRECTED APPROACH, 8TH EDITION ISBN: 978-0-323-07308-0

Notices

Knowledge and best practice in this field are constantly changing. As new research and experience broaden our understanding, changes in research methods, professional practices, or medical treatment may become necessary.

Practitioners and researchers must always rely on their own experience and knowledge in evaluating and using any information, methods, compounds, or experiments described herein. In using such information or methods they should be mindful of their own safety and the safety of others, including parties for whom they have a professional responsibility.

With respect to any drug or pharmaceutical products identified, readers are advised to check the most current information provided (i) on procedures featured or (ii) by the manufacturer of each product to be administered, to verify the recommended dose or formula, the method and duration of administration, and contraindications. It is the responsibility of practitioners, relying on their own experience and knowledge of their patients, to make diagnoses, to determine dosages and the best treatment for each individual patient, and to take all appropriate safety precautions.

To the fullest extent of the law, neither the Publisher nor the authors, contributors, or editors, assume any liability for any injury and/or damage to persons or property as a matter of products liability, negligence or otherwise, or from any use or operation of any methods, products, instructions, or ideas contained in the material herein.

ISBN: 978-0-323-07308-0

Vice President and Publisher: Andrew Allen
Publisher: Jeanne Olson
Developmental Editor: Luke Held
Publishing Services Manager: Julie Eddy
Senior Project Manager: Andrea Campbell
Medical Illustrator: Jeanne Robertson
Design Direction: Jessica Williams

Printed in the United States

Last digit is the print number: 9 8 7 6 5 4 3 2 1

What advice would you give to students just starting to learn medical terminology?

I remember, as a young medical student, having a reaction to some of these big words... feeling that some of the medical language was just too fancy, highbrow, or unnecessary at times. However, as I progressed I came to realize I was learning a language—a very precise language that I needed to understand so that I could properly communicate my intentions. For example, "diaphoresis"... why not just say "sweating?" Well, diaphoresis means sweating without exertion—from vagal stimulation maybe. Very different from sweating from normal exercise. If you fall outside of this you [may] become discredited and cannot communicate [effectively] with others in the field. So, if you can accept that this is a highly precise language... learn it... break it down... you'll find it an immense tool.

From an interview with Peter Goth, MD, FACEP, conducted by Michaella Warren, student, as part of a medical terminology class assignment.

CONTENTS

PREFACE

TABLES

EVOLVE APPENDICES

Visit the Evolve website (*http://evolve.elsevier.com/*) to access the following appendices:

PREFACE

Welcome to the eighth edition of *Exploring Medical Language*. Medical terminology, like any living language, changes over time. The content of the eighth edition has been updated to reflect current use, ensuring the textbook remains an effective tool for preparing those entering medical professions, as well as those entering related fields, including software development, computer applications and support, insurance, law, equipment supply, pharmaceutical sales, and medical writing, all of whom need to both understand medical language and be understood.

Revising this edition has been especially exciting because it involved moving our popular and dynamic CD activities to the Elsevier Evolve website. Now a wide variety of multimedia learning tools is available in one place! Throughout each chapter, students are invited to reach beyond the textbook and expand their learning possibilities, visually by watching **animations**; actively by playing **games**; interactively by hearing, typing, and saying terms in the **spelling** and **pronunciation** exercises; and concretely by completing **medical vignettes** and reading **medical documents**.

In the past, many have recommended adding more anatomy and physiology to the textbook. We have been hesitant to do so, because the focus of *Exploring Medical Language* is on building a medical vocabulary. For this edition, we feel we have found a solution. Each body system chapter invites the student desiring more A & P to visit a new online program entitled **A & P Booster**, which is available on the Evolve website. This feature, which includes illustrations and animations, allows students to deepen their understanding as needed.

Of course we have kept the features that set our textbook apart from others: grouping terms in lists categorized by terms built from word parts and those not built from word parts, and further dividing them into disease and disorder terms, surgical terms, diagnostic terms, and complementary terms. Supporting these lists are the many and varied exercises for the student to learn to define, spell, and speak the terms. Many updated and new diagrams, tables, boxed information, and appendices are all also present to assist in understanding the language of medicine.

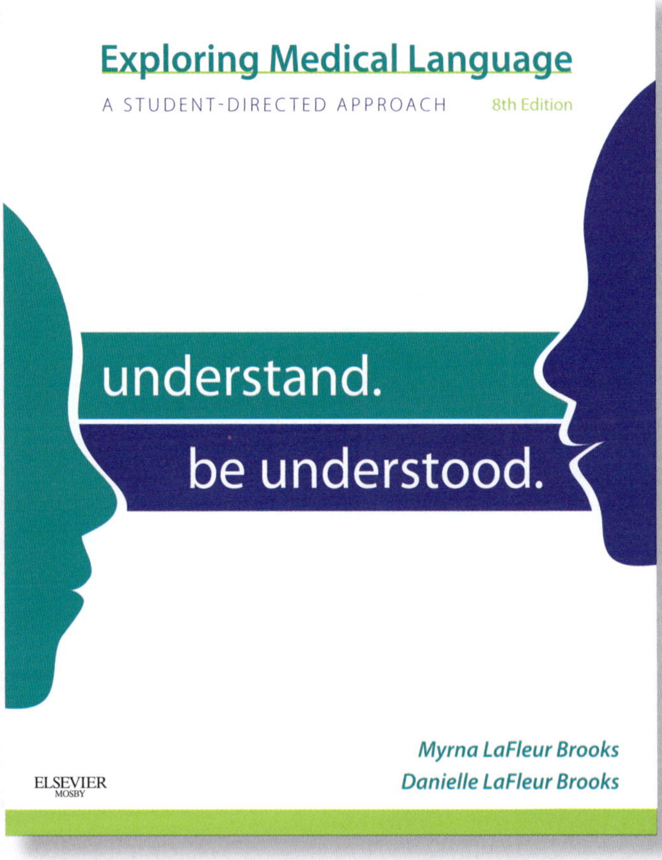

DISTINGUISHING FEATURES

- **Chapter Outlines**, providing easy navigation of topics, term lists, and tables
- **Objectives**, indicating what needs to be mastered to complete the chapter
- **Organized Term Lists**, grouping terms built from word parts and terms from modern language
- **Chapters Follow a Pattern**, moving the student through recognizable steps
- **Paced Content**, inviting the student to read, then do
- **Specific Term Lists**, including only the terms a beginning student needs to know
- **Focused on Medical Language**, developing writing and speaking skills above all else
- **Dedicated Pronunciation and Spelling Exercises**, including the ability to hear and spell the terms online
- **Medical Documents and Practical Application**, providing a view into the clinical setting
- **Student Choice**, placing multiple learning tools at their fingertips, such as flashcards, animations, games, and audio for spelling and pronunciation
- **Varied Ways for Students to Connect with Terms**, highlighting history, current use, integrative medicine, and images in margin boxes and tables
- **Online Learning Connected with Chapter Content**, appealing to all learning styles
- **Self-Assessment**, giving students immediate feedback on progress by providing answers at the end of each chapter and by self-testing in assessment mode of online practice activities
- **Multimedia Activities**, allowing students to see, hear, type, and play while building their skills
- **Figures**, illustrating anatomy, disease processes, and surgical and diagnostic procedures

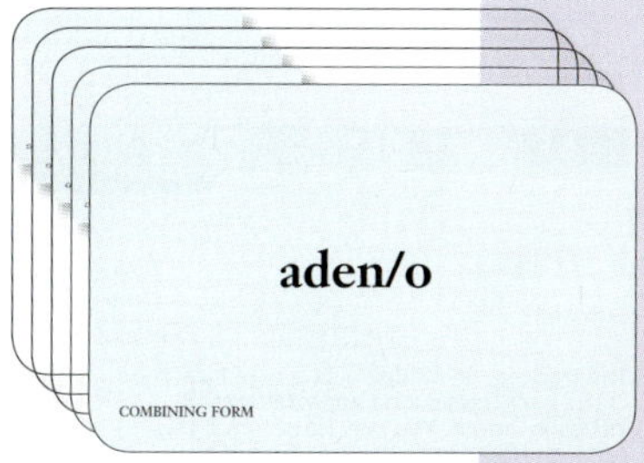

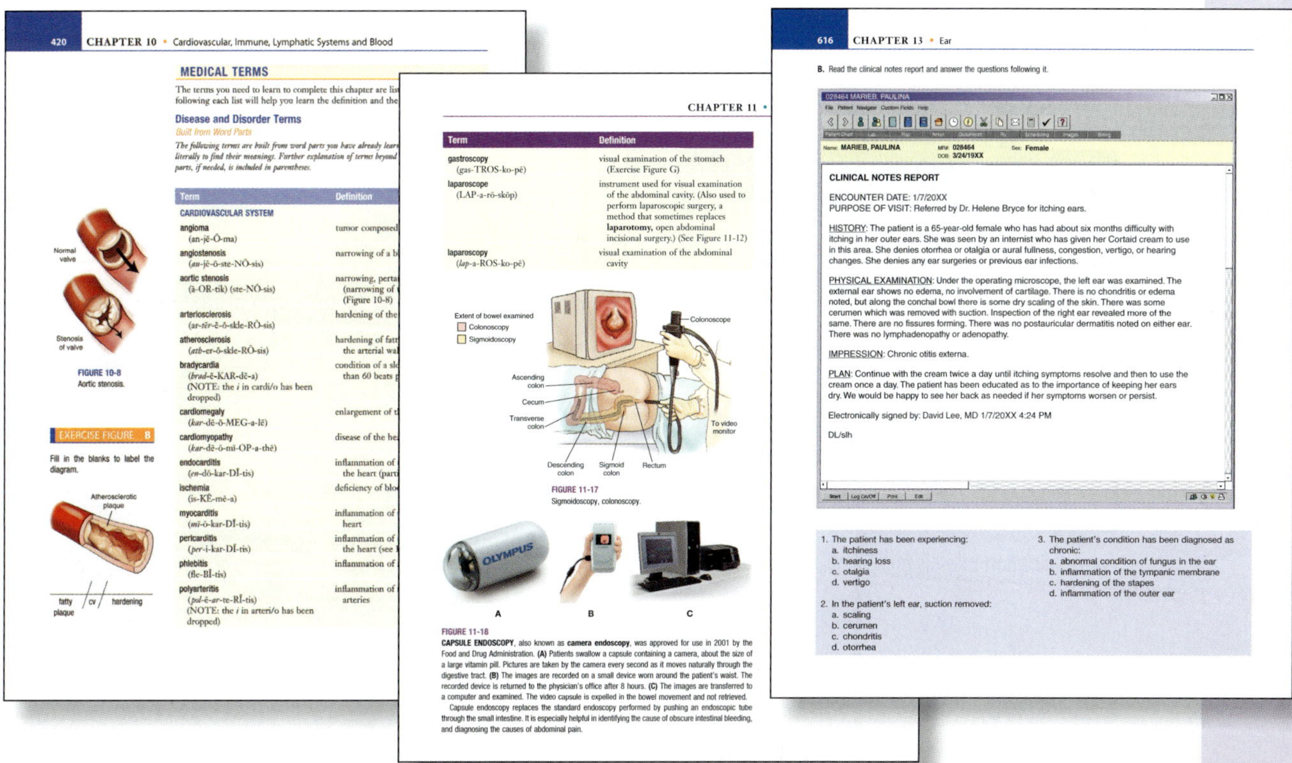

NEW FEATURES

A & P Boosters on the Evolve website allow students to deepen their understanding of anatomy and physiology beyond what is presented in the textbook. Terms are linked to an English/Spanish medical terminology glossary, including audio pronunciations and written definitions.

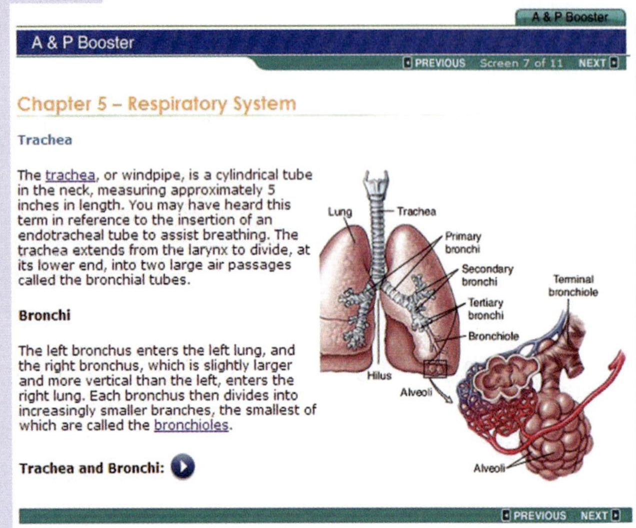

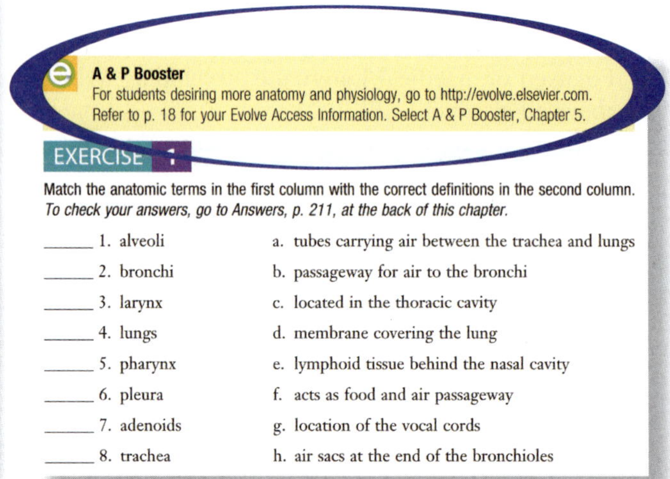

A & P Booster
For students desiring more anatomy and physiology, go to http://evolve.elsevier.com. Refer to p. 18 for your Evolve Access Information. Select A & P Booster, Chapter 5.

EXERCISE 1

Match the anatomic terms in the first column with the correct definitions in the second column. *To check your answers, go to Answers, p. 211, at the back of this chapter.*

_____ 1. alveoli	a. tubes carrying air between the trachea and lungs
_____ 2. bronchi	b. passageway for air to the bronchi
_____ 3. larynx	c. located in the thoracic cavity
_____ 4. lungs	d. membrane covering the lung
_____ 5. pharynx	e. lymphoid tissue behind the nasal cavity
_____ 6. pleura	f. acts as food and air passageway
_____ 7. adenoids	g. location of the vocal cords
_____ 8. trachea	h. air sacs at the end of the bronchioles

Wide variety of multimedia learning tools located in one place: the Evolve website allows students to see, hear, type and play while building their skills.

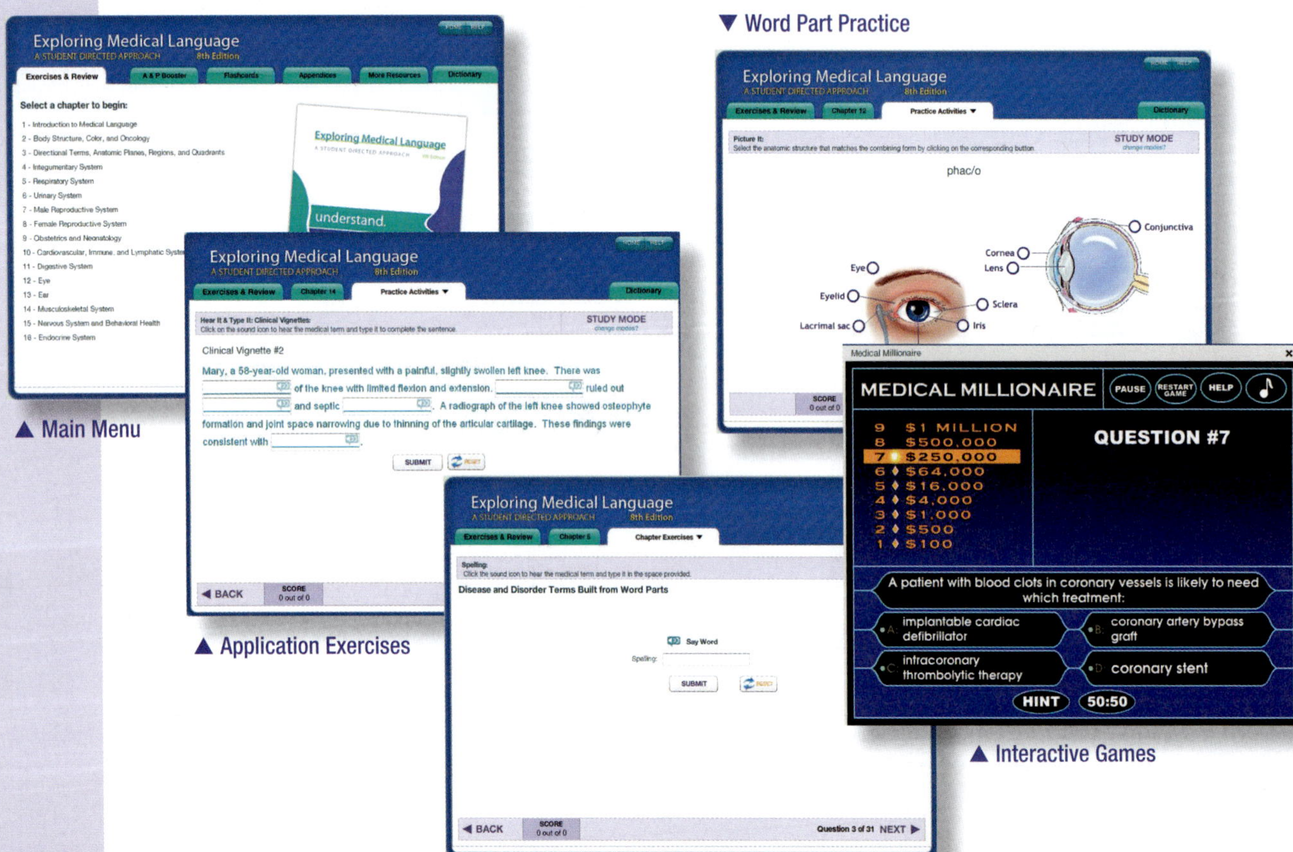

▼ Word Part Practice

▲ Main Menu

▲ Application Exercises

▲ Interactive Games

▲ Pronunciation and Spelling

New Illustrations give visual meaning to anatomic structure, disease process, and procedures

▼ Flow of Urine

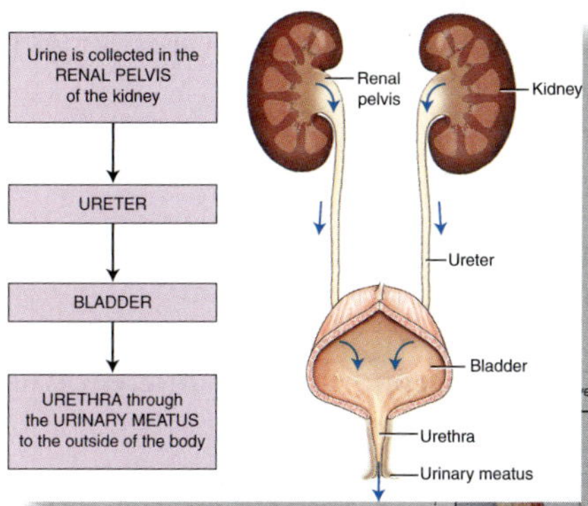

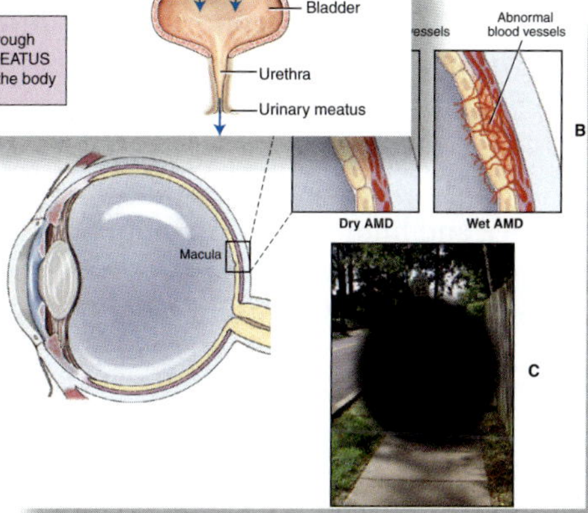

▲ Macular Degeneration

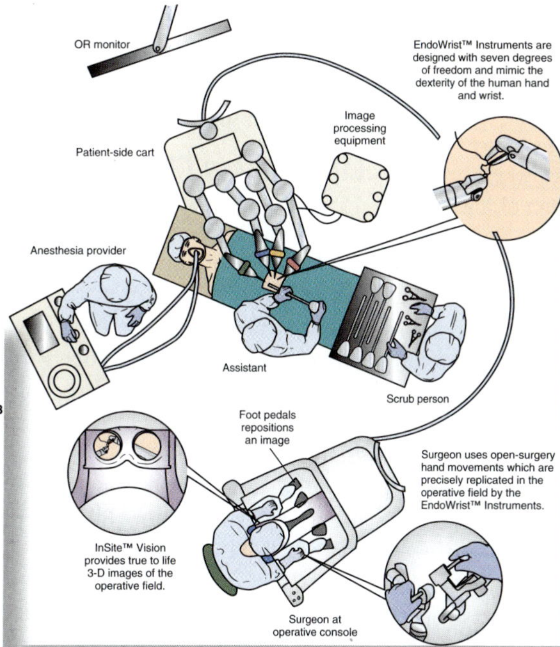

▲ Operating room set-up for robotic-assisted laparoscopic radical prostatectomy (RALRP) with a da Vinci robotic system

New and Updated Medical Documents provide interactive application opportunities

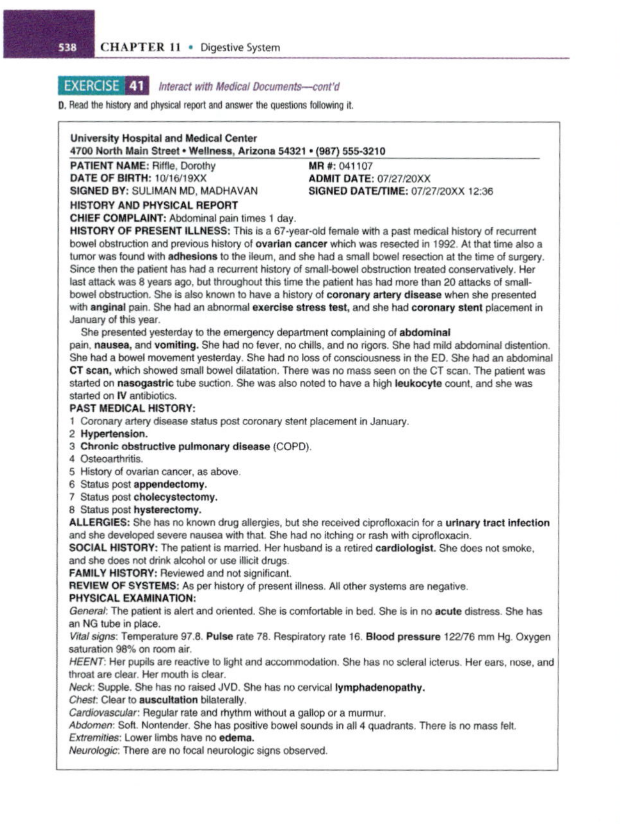

538 CHAPTER 11 • Digestive System

EXERCISE 41 *Interact with Medical Documents—cont'd*

D. Read the history and physical report and answer the questions following it.

University Hospital and Medical Center
4700 North Main Street • Wellness, Arizona 54321 • (987) 555-3210

PATIENT NAME: Riffle, Dorothy — **MR #:** 041107
DATE OF BIRTH: 10/16/19XX — **ADMIT DATE:** 07/27/20XX
SIGNED BY: SULIMAN MD, MADHAVAN — **SIGNED DATE/TIME:** 07/27/20XX 12:36

HISTORY AND PHYSICAL REPORT

CHIEF COMPLAINT: Abdominal pain times 1 day.

HISTORY OF PRESENT ILLNESS: This is a 67-year-old female with a past medical history of recurrent bowel obstruction and previous history of **ovarian cancer** which was resected in 1992. At that time also a tumor was found with **adhesions** to the ileum, and she had a small bowel resection at the time of surgery. Since then the patient has had a recurrent history of small-bowel obstruction treated conservatively. Her last attack was 8 years ago, but throughout this time the patient has had more than 20 attacks of small-bowel obstruction. She is also known to have a history of **coronary artery disease** when she presented with **anginal** pain. She had an abnormal **exercise stress test,** and she had **coronary stent** placement in January of this year.

She presented yesterday to the emergency department complaining of **abdominal** pain, **nausea,** and **vomiting.** She had no fever, no chills, and no rigors. She had mild abdominal distention. She had a bowel movement yesterday. She had no loss of consciousness in the ED. She had an abdominal **CT scan,** which showed small bowel dilatation. There was no mass seen on the CT scan. The patient was started on **nasogastric** tube suction. She was also noted to have a high **leukocyte** count, and she was started on **IV** antibiotics.

PAST MEDICAL HISTORY:
1 Coronary artery disease status post coronary stent placement in January.
2 **Hypertension.**
3 **Chronic obstructive pulmonary disease** (COPD).
4 Osteoarthritis.
5 History of ovarian cancer, as above.
6 Status post **appendectomy.**
7 Status post **cholecystectomy.**
8 Status post **hysterectomy.**

ALLERGIES: She has no known drug allergies, but she received ciprofloxacin for a **urinary tract infection** and she developed severe nausea with that. She had no itching or rash with ciprofloxacin.

SOCIAL HISTORY: The patient is married. Her husband is a retired **cardiologist.** She does not smoke, and she does not drink alcohol or use illicit drugs.

FAMILY HISTORY: Reviewed and not significant.

REVIEW OF SYSTEMS: As per history of present illness. All other systems are negative.

PHYSICAL EXAMINATION:
General: The patient is alert and oriented. She is comfortable in bed. She is in no **acute** distress. She has an NG tube in place.
Vital signs: Temperature 97.8. **Pulse** rate 78. Respiratory rate 16. **Blood pressure** 122/76 mm Hg. Oxygen saturation 98% on room air.
HEENT: Her pupils are reactive to light and accommodation. She has no scleral icterus. Her ears, nose, and throat are clear. Her mouth is clear.
Neck: Supple. She has no raised JVD. She has no cervical **lymphadenopathy.**
Chest: Clear to **auscultation** bilaterally.
Cardiovascular: Regular rate and rhythm without a gallop or a murmur.
Abdomen: Soft. Nontender. She has positive bowel sounds in all 4 quadrants. There is no mass felt.
Extremities: Lower limbs have no **edema.**
Neurologic: There are no focal neurologic signs observed.

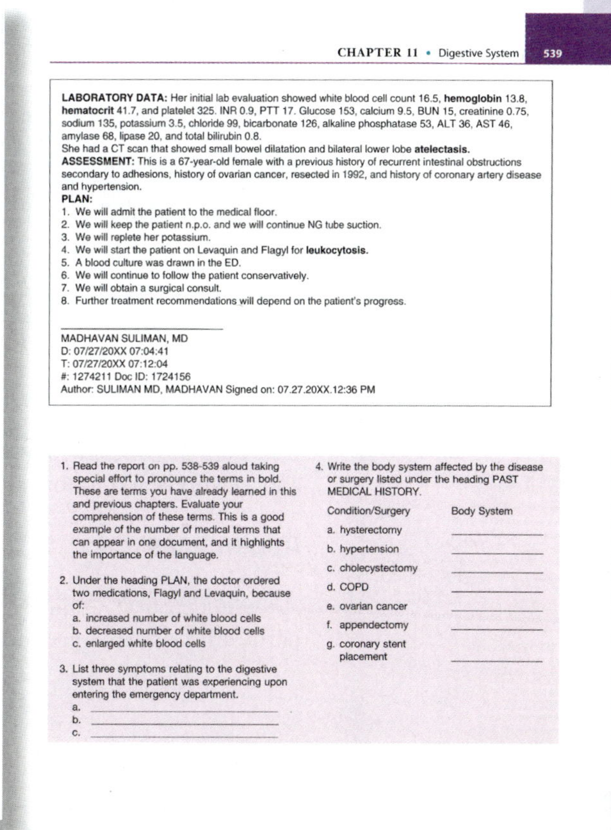

CHAPTER 11 • Digestive System 539

LABORATORY DATA: Her initial lab evaluation showed white blood cell count 16.5, **hemoglobin** 13.8, **hematocrit** 41.7, and platelet 325. INR 0.9, PTT 17. Glucose 153, calcium 9.5, BUN 15, creatinine 0.75, sodium 135, potassium 3.5, chloride 99, bicarbonate 126, alkaline phosphatase 53, ALT 36, AST 46, amylase 68, lipase 20, and total bilirubin 0.8.
She had a CT scan that showed small bowel dilatation and bilateral lower lobe **atelectasis.**

ASSESSMENT: This is a 67-year-old female with a previous history of recurrent intestinal obstructions secondary to adhesions, history of ovarian cancer, resected in 1992, and history of coronary artery disease and hypertension.

PLAN:
1. We will admit the patient to the medical floor.
2. We will keep the patient n.p.o. and we will continue NG tube suction.
3. We will replete her potassium.
4. We will start the patient on Levaquin and Flagyl for **leukocytosis.**
5. A blood culture was drawn in the ED.
6. We will continue to follow the patient conservatively.
7. We will obtain a surgical consult.
8. Further treatment recommendations will depend on the patient's progress.

____
MADHAVAN SULIMAN, MD
D: 07/27/20XX 07:04:41
T: 07/27/20XX 07:12:04
#: 1274211 Doc ID: 1724156
Author: SULIMAN MD, MADHAVAN Signed on: 07.27.20XX.12:36 PM

1. Read the report on pp. 538-539 aloud taking special effort to pronounce the terms in bold. These are terms you have already learned in this and previous chapters. Evaluate your comprehension of these terms. This is a good example of the number of medical terms that can appear in one document, and it highlights the importance of the language.

2. Under the heading PLAN, the doctor ordered two medications, Flagyl and Levaquin, because of:
   a. increased number of white blood cells
   b. decreased number of white blood cells
   c. enlarged white blood cells

3. List three symptoms relating to the digestive system that the patient was experiencing upon entering the emergency department.
   a. ______
   b. ______
   c. ______

4. Write the body system affected by the disease or surgery listed under the heading PAST MEDICAL HISTORY.

Condition/Surgery	Body System
a. hysterectomy	______
b. hypertension	______
c. cholecystectomy	______
d. COPD	______
e. ovarian cancer	______
f. appendectomy	______
g. coronary stent placement	______

USING MEDICAL TERMS

Using medical terms to communicate allows for quick, concise communication. For example, using the medical term **osteoarthritis,** which means **inflammation of the bone and joint,** offers clear and concise written or verbal communication using one word instead of six.

EXERCISE FIGURE E

Fill in the blanks to label the diagram.

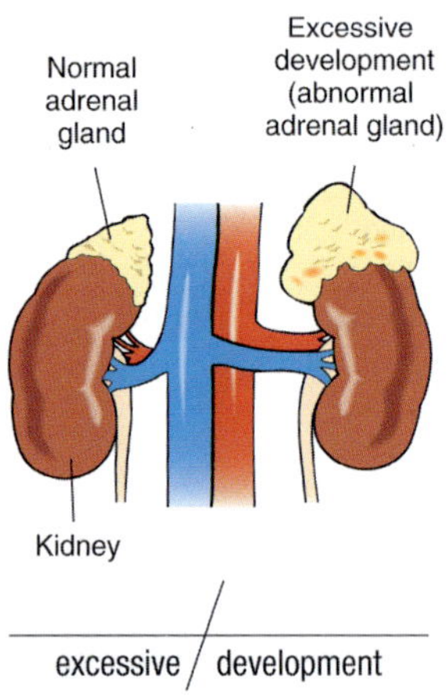

ORGANIZATION OF THE TEXTBOOK

Chapters 1 through 3 are introductory chapters, providing a foundation for building medical vocabulary. Chapters 5 through 16 are body systems chapters, presenting related word parts, terms, and abbreviations. The textbook concludes with a series of appendices designed to extend student learning as desired.

Introductory Chapters

Chapter 1 ... may be the most important chapter in the text, because you will apply the knowledge you acquire here in the rest of the chapters to learn terms in an easy, quick fashion. You are introduced to the two **categories of terms**—those built from word parts and those which are not; each category is accompanied by different types of exercises. Also introduced in this chapter are **the four word parts**—word root, suffix, prefix, and combining vowel, which are the basis of terms built from word parts category.

Chapter 2 ... introduces **body structure** and immediately provides practice in recognizing the two categories of terms along with corresponding exercises for each. You will likely be surprised at how fast you will learn the meaning and spelling of many medical terms.

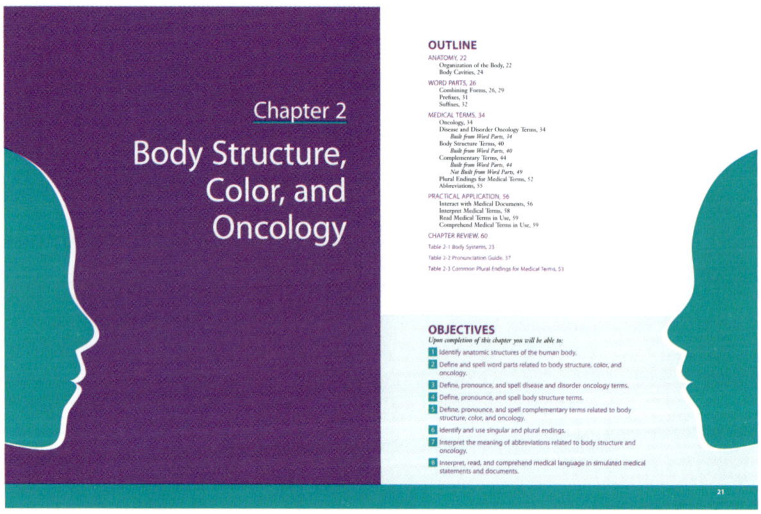
Chapter 2

Body Structure, Color, and Oncology

OUTLINE

OBJECTIVES

Chapter 3 ... covers directional terms, planes, positioning, regions, and quadrants, providing a framework for understanding the body systems and their related terms.

Body System Chapters

Chapters 4-16 ... introduce specific body systems with related word parts, terms, and abbreviations and follow a consistent format.

Appendices

Appendices A-D ... appear in the textbook and provide a comprehensive lists of word parts, a list of error-prone abbreviations, and pharmacology terms.

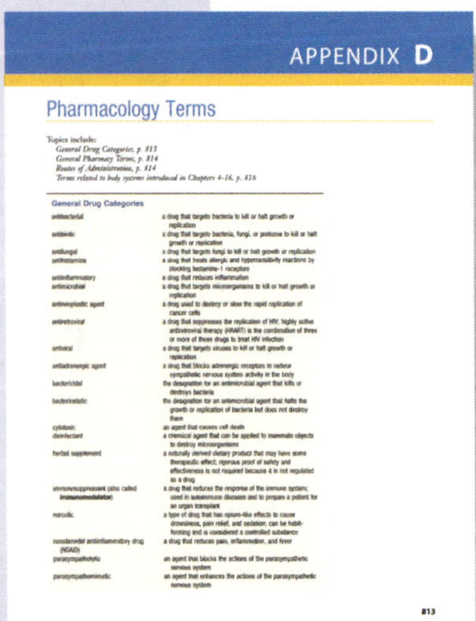
APPENDIX D

Pharmacology Terms

General Drug Categories

ANATOMY OF A CHAPTER

It can be difficult to determine, at a glance, all that is included in a chapter, so let's take a closer look at a typical body system chapter: Chapter 5, Respiratory System, pp. 148-215.

OUTLINE, p. 149

OBJECTIVES, p. 149

ANATOMY

- Function, p. 150
- Organs of the Respiratory System, p. 150-152

WORD PARTS

- Combining Forms of the Respiratory System, p. 153
- Combining Forms Commonly Used with the Respiratory System Terms, p. 156
- Prefixes, p. 157
- Suffixes, p. 158

MEDICAL TERMS

- Disease and Disorder Terms
  - Built from word parts, p. 160
  - Not built from word parts, p. 167
- Surgical Terms
  - Built from word parts, p. 173
- Diagnostic Terms
  - Built from word parts, p. 179
  - Not built from word parts, p. 187
- Complementary Terms
  - Built from word parts, p. 191
  - Not built from word parts, p. 196
- Abbreviations, p. 201

PRACTICAL APPLICATION

- Interact with Medical Documents, p. 203
- Interpret Medical Terms, p. 206
- Read Medical Terms In Use, p. 207
- Comprehend Medical Terms, p. 207

CHAPTER REVIEW

- Online Chapter Review, p. 208
  - Chapter Exercises
  - Practice Activities, study mode & assessment mode
  - Animations
  - Games
- Review of Word Parts, p 208
- Review of Terms, p. 209

ANSWERS, p. 211

HOW WILL I LEARN MEDICAL TERMS USING *EXPLORING MEDICAL LANGUAGE?*

You will learn medical terms by completing the many and varied exercises, activities, and games, using all learning styles. Upon completion, you will be able to speak and write the language of medicine, preparing you to understand and be understood in a medical setting.

Let's travel through Chapter 5, Respiratory System, and explore how you will acquire this new language.

Anatomy

If you have not previously studied anatomy, this section is for you. You will learn the content by:

- Reading content, example p. 150
- Studying diagrams, example p. 151
- Completing exercises and checking answers, example, p. 152, p. 211
- Using the **online** A & P Booster, example box p. 152

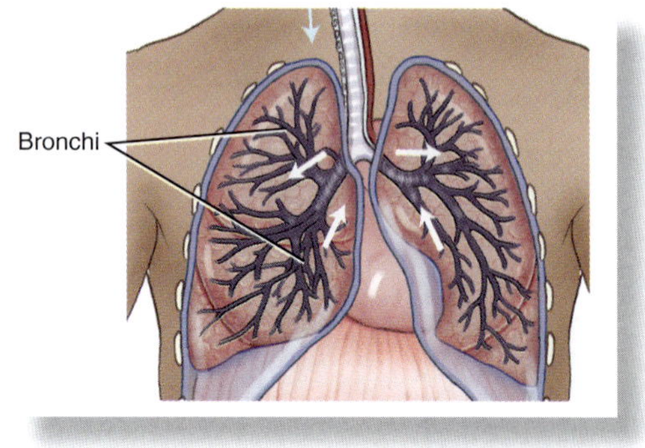

Word Parts

Many medical terms are made up of Greek and Latin word parts. By learning their meaning and spelling, you will be able to define the many terms built from word parts included in this text and many more.

You will learn the meaning and spelling of word parts by:

- Reading each word part and its definition, example p. 153
- Labeling anatomic diagrams with word parts, example p. 154
- Completing exercises and checking answers, example p. 155, p. 211
- Using paper or **online** flashcards

endo-
trache/o
-al

Medical Terms Built from Word Parts

Medical terms built from word parts are constructed from word parts learned in the word part section mentioned above. You will apply this newfound knowledge in learning the meaning and spelling of these terms.

You will learn to speak and write medical terms built from word parts by:

- Reading each of the terms and its definition, example p. 160
- Referring to diagrams demonstrating disease processes, surgery, or diagnostic studies, example p. 162
- Referring to tables and boxes on use of terms, historical and clinical contexts, and tips to navigate the material, example p. 162
- Filling in word parts to label the Exercise Figures, example p. 163
- Pronouncing each of the terms and hearing them **online**, example box p. 163
- Completing analyzing and defining exercises and checking answers, example p. 163, p. 212
- Completing word-building exercises and checking answers, example p. 164
- Completing spelling exercises by in-person or **online** dictation, example p. 166

endo/trache/al

Medical Terms Not Built from Word Parts

Terms appearing in the "Not Built from Word Parts" lists may indeed contain recognizable word parts; however, they cannot be easily defined through the meanings of the word parts. Memorization is the method used to learning these terms.

You will learn to speak and write these terms not built from word parts by:

chronic obstructive pulmonary disease

- Reading each of the terms and its definition, example, p. 167
- Referring to tables and boxes on use of terms, historical and clinical contexts, and tips to navigate the material, examples p. 167
- Referring to diagrams demonstrating disease processes, surgery, or diagnostic studies, example p. 168
- Pronouncing each of the terms and hearing them **online**, example, p. 170
- Completing fill-in-the-blank and matching exercises, and checking answers, example pp. 171-172, p. 213
- Completing the spelling exercises by in-person or **online** dictation, example p. 173, p. 213

Abbreviations

COPD

Abbreviations are frequently used in healthcare settings.

You will learn abbreviations by:

- Reading each abbreviation and its definition, example p. 201
- Completing the exercises and checking answers, example p. 201, p. 215

Practical Application

Practical application offers an opportunity for you to apply your newfound knowledge in clinical situations and with medical documents.

You will apply what you have learned by:

- Interacting with medical documents, example p. 203
- Interpreting medical terms, example p. 206
- Reading medical terms in use, in the text and **online**, p. 207
- Comprehending medical terms, p. 207

EXERCISE 47 *Read Medical Terms in Use*

Practice pronunciation of terms by reading the following document. Use the pronunciation key following the medical term to assist you in saying the word.

To hear these terms, go to http://evolve.elsevier.com. Refer to p. 18 for your Evolve Access Information. Select Exercises & Review, Chapter 15, Chapter Exercises, Read Medical Terms in Use.

A 78-year-old right-handed male presented to the Emergency Department with a right **hemiparesis** (*hem*-ē-pa-RĒ-sis), expressive **aphasia** (a-FĀ-zha), and no apparent **cognitive** (COG-ni-tiv) decline. He has a history of hypertension and 2 years ago had a **transient ischemic** (is-KĒ-mik) **attack.** A **computed tomography** (tō-MOG-ra-fē) **scan of the brain** was negative for an **intracerebral** (in-tra-SER-e-bral) hemorrhage. A **neurologist** (nū-ROL-o-jist) was consulted. She confirmed the diagnosis of an **ischemic stroke** (strōk) after **magnetic resonance imaging** (mag-NET-ik) (REZ-ō-nans) (IM-a-jing) **of the brain** demonstrated an ischemic area of the left **cerebral** (se-RĒ-bral) cortex caused by a **cerebral embolism** (se-RĒ-bral) (EM-bō-lizm).

Chapter Review

Online and Textbook chapter review provides you the opportunity to evaluate and practice your newfound knowledge, example pp. 208-210.

CHAPTER REVIEW

ONLINE CHAPTER REVIEW

To access the Evolve website, go to http://evolve.elsevier.com. Refer to p. 18 for your Evolve Access Information. Select Exercises & Review, Chapter 5, then select Chapter Exercises, Practice Activities, Animations, or Games. Place a check mark in the box when you have completed an exercise or activity, watched an animation, or played a game. Have fun!

Chapter Exercises

Exercises in this section of your Evolve resources correlate to exercises in your textbook. You may have completed them as you worked through the chapter.

- ☐ Pronunciation
- ☐ Spelling
- ☐ Read Medical Terms in Use

Practice Activities

Practice in study mode, then test your learning in assessment mode. Keep track of your scores from assessment mode if you wish.

	SCORE
☐ Picture It	_____
☐ Define Word Parts	_____
☐ Build Medical Terms	_____
☐ Word Shop	_____
☐ Define Medical Terms	_____
☐ Use It	_____
☐ Hear It and Type It: Clinical Vignettes	_____

Animations

- ☐ Atelectasis
- ☐ Asthma
- ☐ Pneumonia
- ☐ Pneumothorax
- ☐ Pulse oximeter
- ☐ Tuberculosis

Games

- ☐ Name that Word Part
- ☐ Term Storm
- ☐ Term Explorer
- ☐ Termbusters
- ☐ Medical Millionaire
- ☐ Crossword Puzzle

TO THE INSTRUCTOR

If you are new to teaching medical terminology, we offer a wide variety of teaching resources you can use to prepare for classes, including lesson plans, handouts, PowerPoint presentations, and lecture outlines. These resources are chapter objective–based and can be used as is, or may be altered to suit your teaching needs.

If you are a veteran instructor and have your classroom materials developed, you might choose to add the Tournament of Terminology game, which can be played by the whole class to prepare for exams, or weave illustrations from the image collection into your PowerPoint presentations. All resources are easily accessible on the Evolve website for *Exploring Medical Language* (EML).

Available on the Evolve website (see pp. 16 and 18 for login instructions to Evolve), **TEACH is the primary instructional resource for EML**, providing one place to view all of the teaching materials, available by chapter objective. For each objective, TEACH identifies the page numbers of chapter content, specific chapter exercises, figures, online activities, handouts, and PowerPoint slides, as well as suggestions for class activities and discussion questions to meet the objective. Using TEACH can save time, plus give new and creative ideas to promote student learning. Supplemental teaching and course management tools are also available on the Evolve website.

We are dedicated to supporting your teaching efforts and look forward to hearing from you. We welcome your comments and questions by e-mail. Danielle currently teaches medical terminology online and is happy to share teaching ideas and materials suited for the online learning environment. We can be reached at the following addresses:

myrnabrooks@comcast.net
danielle.lafleurbrooks@ccv.edu.

Thank you for choosing *Exploring Medical Language*.

Myrna and Danielle

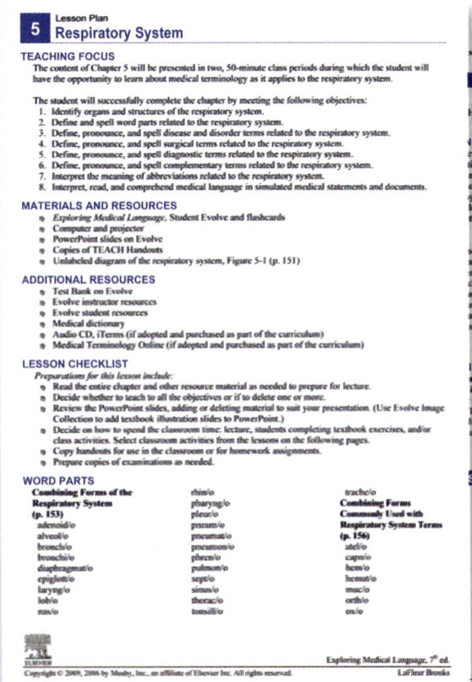

Lesson Plan
5 Respiratory System

TEACHING FOCUS

The content of Chapter 5 will be presented in two, 50-minute class periods during which the student will have the opportunity to learn about medical terminology as it applies to the respiratory system.

The student will successfully complete the chapter by meeting the following objectives:

1. Identify organs and structures of the respiratory system.
2. Define and spell word parts related to the respiratory system.
3. Define, pronounce, and spell disease and disorder terms related to the respiratory system.
4. Define, pronounce, and spell surgical terms related to the respiratory system.
5. Define, pronounce, and spell diagnostic terms related to the respiratory system.
6. Define, pronounce, and spell complementary terms related to the respiratory system.
7. Interpret the meaning of abbreviations related to the respiratory system.
8. Interpret, read, and comprehend medical language in simulated medical statements and documents.

MATERIALS AND RESOURCES

- *Exploring Medical Language*, Student Evolve and flashcards
- Computer and projector
- PowerPoint slides on Evolve
- Copies of TEACH Handouts
- Unlabeled diagram of the respiratory system, Figure 5-1 (p. 151)

ADDITIONAL RESOURCES

- Test Bank on Evolve
- Evolve instructor resources
- Evolve student resources
- Medical dictionary
- Audio CD, iTerms (if adopted and purchased as part of the curriculum)
- Medical Terminology Online (if adopted and purchased as part of the curriculum)

LESSON CHECKLIST

Preparations for this lesson include:

- Read the entire chapter and other resource material as needed to prepare for lecture.
- Decide whether to teach to all the objectives or if to delete one or more.
- Review the PowerPoint slides, adding or deleting material to suit your presentation. (Use Evolve Image Collection to add textbook illustration slides to PowerPoint.)
- Decide on how to spend the classroom time: lecture, students completing textbook exercises, and/or class activities. Select classroom activities from the lessons on the following pages.
- Copy handouts for use in the classroom or for homework assignments.
- Prepare copies of examinations as needed.

WORD PARTS

Combining Forms of the Respiratory System (p. 153)		
adenoid/o	rhin/o	trache/o
alveol/o	pharyng/o	**Combining Forms Commonly Used with Respiratory System Terms (p. 156)**
bronch/o	pleur/o	atel/o
bronchi/o	pneum/o	capn/o
diaphragmat/o	pneumat/o	hem/o
epiglott/o	pneumon/o	hemat/o
laryng/o	phren/o	muc/o
lob/o	pulmon/o	orth/o
nas/o	sept/o	ox/o
	sinus/o	
	thorac/o	
	tonsill/o	

Exploring Medical Language, 7th ed. LaFleur Brooks

Copyright © 2009, 2006 by Mosby, Inc., an affiliate of Elsevier Inc. All rights reserved.

▲ TEACH Lesson Plan

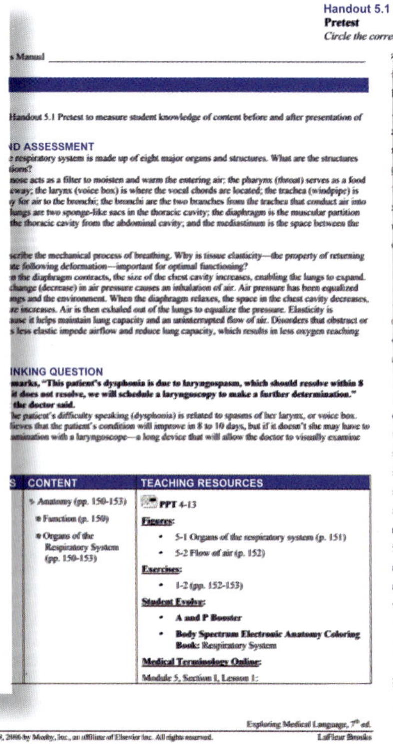

▲ TEACH Critical Assessment

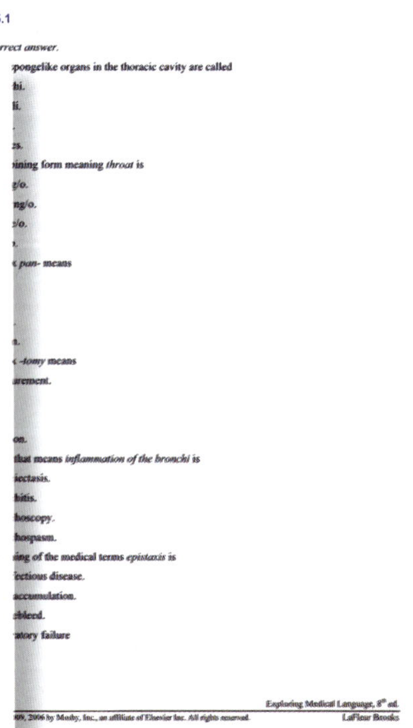

Handout 5.1
Pretest
Circle the correct answer.

▲ TEACH Handout

Evolve for Instructors, online teaching resources

- **Chapter Pretests** for measuring pre- and post-chapter knowledge
- **Materials and Resources Lists** for classroom preparation
- **Assessment and Critical Thinking Questions** to use as an introduction to lectures
- **Lesson Plans** that correlate chapter objectives with textbook content and teaching resources
- **Lecture Outlines** that feature PowerPoint slides with talking points and clicker questions
- **Classroom Handouts, Discussion Questions, and Suggested Classroom Activities** organized by chapter objective
- **PowerPoint presentations** for each chapter for use as lecture aids
- **Performance Evaluation** plan for monitoring and evaluating student progress

Teaching Tools:

- **ExamView Test Bank** with objective-based questions for each chapter (also available as RTF files)
- **Image Collection** from the textbook to download for use in the classroom
- **Tournament of Terminology**, a Jeopardy-like game for exam preparation by reviewing chapter content
- **Electronic Flashcards** for classroom use, accessible through the Student site
- **Spanish/English glossary**, accessible through the Student site

Course Management Tools:

- **Online discussion boards**
- **Online calendar**
- **Outline of course syllabus, outlines, and lecture notes**
- **Sample course outline and syllabus**
- **Web links**

ALSO AVAILABLE

Mosby's Medical Terminology Online

Mosby's Medical Terminology Online to accompany *Exploring Medical Language* is a great resource to supplement your textbook. This web-delivered course supplement provides a range of visual, auditory, and interactive elements to reinforce your learning and synthesize concepts presented in the text. Objective-based quizzes at the end of each section and an end-of-module exam provide you with self-testing tools. In addition, related Internet resources may be accessed by links provided throughout the program. This online course supplement may be accessed if you have purchased the PIN code packaged with your book. If you did not purchase the PIN code, ask your instructor for information or visit http://evolve.elsevier.com/LaFleur/Exploring/ to purchase it.

Instructors interested in *Mosby's Medical Terminology Online*, please contact your sales rep, call Faculty Support at 1-800-222-9570, or visit http://evolve.elsevier.com/LaFleur/Exploring/ for more information.

Audio CDs and iTerms

The audio CDs that accompany *Exploring Medical Language* include pronunciations and definitions. Because the CDs include definitions, they are an additional tool for learning and reviewing terms. The CDs are especially helpful when using your book is impractical, such as when you are driving in a car, walking, or doing daily chores. You may purchase the audio CDs separately or packaged with the book for a small additional cost. This audio product is available for download for MP3 players and is called *iTerms for Exploring Medical Language, ed 8.*

CONTRIBUTORS

Catherine J. Cerulli, MEd
Director
Interwoven Healing Arts
Montpelier, Vermont
Appendix G-Complementary and Alternative Medicine Therapies (Evolve website)

Carolyn Ehrlich, MSN Psy, NP
Private Practice, Psychiatry
Phoenix, Arizona
Appendix H-Behavioral Health Terms (Evolve website)

Elaine A. Gillingham, AAS, BA
Program Director, Health Unit Coordinator Program (1993-2005)
GateWay Community College
Phoenix, Arizona
Appendix A-Combining Forms, Prefixes, and Suffixes Alphabetized According to Word Part
Appendix B-Combining Forms, Prefixes, and Suffixes Alphabetized According to Definition
Appendix C-Abbreviations
Appendix E-Additional Combining Forms, Prefixes, and Suffixes (Evolve website)

Cynthia Heiss, PhD, RD
Professor
Department of Healthcare Professions
Metropolitan State College of Denver
Denver, Colorado
Appendix J-Nutritional Terms (Evolve website)

Marjorie "Meg" A. Holloway, RN, MS, ARNP
Nurse Navigator
The Center for Women's Health & Breast Center, Shawnee Mission Medical Center
Shawnee Mission, Kansas
Chapter 8-Female Reproductive System
Chapter 9-Obstetrics and Neonatology
Chapter 10-Cardiovascular, Immune, and Lymphatic Systems and Blood
Chapter 14-Musculoskeletal System
Chapter 15-Nervous System and Behavioral Health

Erinn Kao, PharmD
GE Medical
St. Louis, Missouri
Appendix D-Pharmacology Terms

Sharon Tompkins Luczu, RN, MA, MBA
Program Director
Health Services Management
Gateway Community College
Phoenix, Arizona
Appendix F-Health Care Delivery Terms (Evolve website)

Linda Mottle, MSM-HSA, RN, CCRP
Director Center for Health Innovation & Clinical Trials
Director Clinical Research Management Graduate Programs
Associate Clinical Professor
Arizona State University
College of Nursing & Health Innovation
Phoenix, Arizona
Appendix I-Clinical Research Terms (Evolve website)

REVIEWERS AND ADVISORS

William W. Bohnert, MD, FACS
Urologist
Arizona Urologic Specialists
Scottsdale, Arizona

Richard K. Brooks, MD, FACP, FACG
Internal Medicine and Gastroenterology
Mayo Clinic, retired
Scottsdale, Arizona

Christine Costa, GCM, HUC
Geriatric Care Manager
Rise Services, Inc.
Glendale, Arizona

Peter M. Dixon, PA-C
Otolarygology Department
Dartmouth Hitchcock Medical Center
Lebanon, New Hampshire

Patricia Faur, MAed, BA
Phoenix, Arizona

Robert L. Fortune, MD
Cardiovascular Surgery, retired
Scottsdale, Arizona

Elaine A. Gillingham, AAS, BA
Program Director, Health Unit Coordinator Program (1993-2005)
GateWay Community College
Phoenix, Arizona

Marjorie "Meg" A. Holloway, RN, MS, ARNP
Nurse Navigator
The Center for Women's Health & Breast Center, Shawnee Mission Medical Center
Shawnee Mission, Kansas

John P. Lampignano, MEd, RT(R)(CT)
Director, Center for Teaching and Learning
Gateway Community College
Phoenix, Arizona

Stephen M. Picca, MD
Instructor
Mandl School, The College of Allied Health
New York, New York

Maynard D. Poland, MD
Internal Medicine Board-certified
Retired:
Medical Director Milwaukee Medical Clinic & Columbia—St. Mary's Hospitals, Milwaukee, Wisconsin
Asst. Clinical Professor, Medical College of Wisconsin
Adjunct Faculty Edison State College, Fort Myers, Florida

Toni L. Rodriguez, EdD, RRT
Program Director, Respiratory Care
Gateway Community College
Phoenix, Arizona

Stanley R. Shorb, MD
Ophthalmologist
St. Joseph's Hospital
Phoenix, Arizona

ACKNOWLEDGMENTS

We depend on so many to assist us in keeping the textbook and electronic content current and accurate, in incorporating the latest learning styles and technologies, and in having the printed pages and electronic screens appeal to the learner. We are indebted to the following:

Luke Held, developmental editor, who guided us through the revision process, all the while demonstrating exceptional patience, follow-through, and dedication.

Jessica Williams, designer, who worked with us to create an attractive and engaging book.

Andrea Campbell, project manager, who seemed to effortlessly bring our vision of the print pages to fruition.

Jeanne Olson, publisher, who continues to provide exceptional support, resources, and know-how as needed.

Contributors listed on page xvii and **Reviewers and Advisors** listed on page xviii who shared with us their expertise, knowledge, and precious time.

Meg Holloway, who joined us as a contributor and skillfully applied her knowledge and clinical resources to revising Chapters 8, 9, 10, 14, and 15.

Chris Costa, who assisted with the revision of the Evolve student activities and games as well as spending many hours adroitly searching through the manuscript with a tireless concern for the accuracy of the printed word.

Elaine Gillingham, for applying her knowledge gained from years of teaching to adeptly revise the test bank, flashcards, and PowerPoint slides.

Carolyn Kruse, for using her linguistic knowledge and pleasing voice for updating pronunciation, both in print and audio.

Richard K. Brooks, MD, my husband, who reviewed and assisted with revisions for all content in the text and who was willing to be there for us every step of the way.

Danielle LaFleur Brooks, my daughter, who has joined me as an author bringing with her the everyday experiences of an online medical terminology instructor as well as an irrefutable integrity for the written word.

Winifred K. Starr (1921-1993), who was my first coauthor and whose creative contributions remain in the text today.

Faculty, who have adopted the text to use in their classrooms, and have used their valuable time to give us feedback.

Students, who over the years have worn thin the pages of previous editions to acquire their own language of medicine.

Each page of the 8th Edition is better because of your collective contributions. Thank you.

TO THE STUDENT

For more than 28 years, students have turned to *Exploring Medical Language* as a starting point for learning medical language. Often as they begin to work through the text, students have told us there are just too many exercises. Usually by the time chapter 4 is completed, the refrain changes significantly, and we hear about how valuable the textbook and exercises are! We hear that the repetition and variety of exercises are the keys to remembering the terms. Time and time again, students are astonished at how much they learn over a relatively short period of time, including how to define, use, spell, and speak the terms. Student success both encourages us to continue the work and convinces us that our learning system is unique and effective.

We hope you find the exercises, one of the strongest features of the book, useful as well. Upon completing one chapter, you will feel confident and eager to move on to the next. We wish you the best as you begin your discovery of the language of medicine.

We would like to hear from you. We can be reached at the following e-mail addresses:

myrnabrooks@comcast.net
danielle.lafleurbrooks@ccv.edu.

Myrna and Danielle

Exploring Medical Language

A STUDENT-DIRECTED APPROACH

Chapter 1

Introduction to Medical Language

OUTLINE

OBJECTIVES

Upon completion of this chapter you will be able to:

1. Describe four origins of medical language.
2. Define two categories of medical terms.
3. Identify and define the four word parts and the combining form.
4. Analyze and define medical terms.
5. Build medical terms for given definitions.
6. Create an account and register on the Evolve website.

USING MEDICAL TERMS

Using medical terms to communicate allows for quick, concise communication. For example, using the medical term **osteoarthritis,** which means **inflammation of the bone and joint,** offers clear and concise written or verbal communication using one word instead of six.

ORIGINS OF MEDICAL LANGUAGE

Medicine has a language of its own, and its vocabulary includes terms built from **Greek and Latin word parts, eponyms, acronyms,** and **modern language** (Figure 1-1). Like a language of a people, medical language is dynamic and develops over time. As clinical settings, current practice, technology, and medical knowledge evolve with scientific advancement, medical language changes. Some words are discarded, the meanings of others are altered, and new words are added.

The majority of medical terms in use today are composed of **Greek and Latin word parts,** some of which were used by Hippocrates and Aristotle more than 2400 years ago. Many can be translated literally to find their meaning. In *Exploring Medical Language*, these terms are taught through a step-by-step word-building process that includes learning the meanings of word parts and how they fit together to form medical terms. Acquiring this skill will enable you to learn scores of medical terms quickly, and it will give you the tools you need to understand new terms you encounter in school or on the job.

Medical terms that are **eponyms, acronyms,** or **based on modern language** need to be learned by memorization. Medical terms composed of Greek and Latin word parts that cannot be literally translated through the meanings of their word parts will also be learned by memorization. Illustrations, notes on current use, historical information, and learning tips will be presented with these terms to help you become familiar with their meanings as easily as possible. Although it takes effort, memorization is a fundamental step that allows you to create a foundation of knowledge. You will find that *Exploring Medical Language* creates multiple opportunities for you to practice, and practice itself will help you internalize the meanings and use of medical terms.

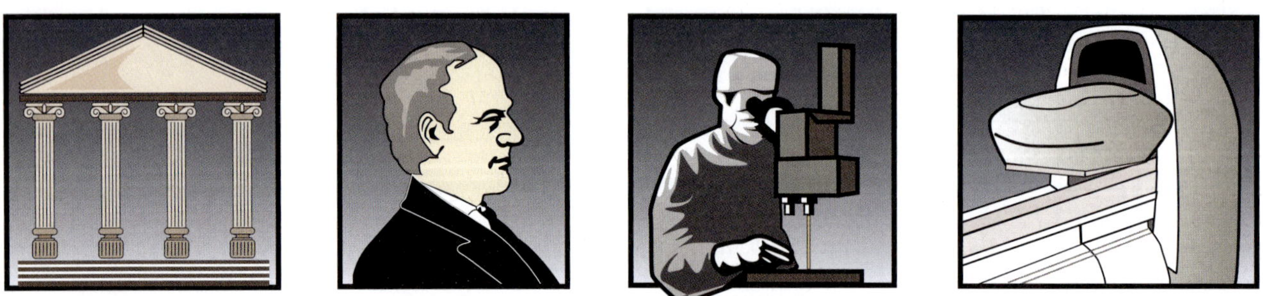

Greek and Latin
Terms built from Greek and Latin word parts such as ***arthritis***

Eponyms
Terms derived from the name of a person, often a physician or scientist who was the first to identify a condition or technique such as ***Alzheimer disease***

Acronyms
Terms formed from the first letters of the words in a phrase that can be spoken as a whole word and usually contain a vowel, such as ***laser*** (light amplification by stimulated emission of radiation)

Modern language
Terms derived from the English language such as ***nuclear medicine scanner***

FIGURE 1-1
Origins of medical language.

EXERCISE 1

Place the letter from the first column to identify the origin of the term in the second column. You may use an answer more than once. *To check your answers to the exercises in this chapter, go to Answers, p. 19, at the end of the chapter.*

a. components of Greek and Latin word parts
b. eponym
c. acronym
d. modern language

_____ 1. Parkinson disease
_____ 2. hepatitis
_____ 3. MRSA (methicillin-resistant *Staphylococcus aureus*)
_____ 4. posttraumatic stress disorder
_____ 5. arthritis
_____ 6. nuclear medicine scanner
_____ 7. AIDS (acquired immunodeficiency syndrome)
_____ 8. Alzheimer disease

CATEGORIES OF MEDICAL TERMS

All medical terms in the text are divided into two categories (Table 1-1):

1. terms built from word parts
2. terms not built from word parts

Terms are arranged in these categories according to the learning strategy for each. Terms built from word parts can be translated literally to find their meaning, whereas terms not built from word parts cannot. Each category of terms is learned by using different types of exercises.

TABLE 1-1
Categories of Medical Terms

Category	Origin	Example
Terms Built from Word Parts (can be translated literally to find their meaning)	1. Word parts of Greek and Latin origin put together to form words that can be translated literally to find their meanings	arthr/itis
Terms not Built from Word Parts (cannot be easily translated literally to find their meaning)	1. Eponyms, terms derived from the name of a person	Alzheimer disease
	2. Acronyms, terms formed from the first letters of a phrase that can be spoken as a whole word and usually contains a vowel	MRSA (methicillin-resistant *Staphylococcus aureus*)
	3. Modern language, terms derived from the English language	complete blood count and differential
	4. Terms of Greek and Latin word parts that cannot be easily translated to find their meanings	orthopedics

EXERCISE 2

Complete the following:

Medical terms built from word parts can be translated literally to find their meaning, whereas medical terms not built from word parts cannot be easily translated literally to find their meaning.

MEDICAL TERMS BUILT FROM WORD PARTS

Terms built from word parts are composed of Greek and Latin word roots, prefixes, and suffixes and can be translated literally to find their meanings. A combining vowel is often added to ease pronunciation. Techniques to learn these terms are **analyzing, defining**, and **building** medical terms.

Four Word Parts

Most medical terms built from word parts consist of some or all of the following components:

1. Word root
2. Prefix
3. Suffix
4. Combining form

Word Root

The word root is the word part that is the core of the word. The word root contains the fundamental meaning of the word.

EXAMPLES:

In the word	play/er, *play* is the word root.
In the medical term	arthr/itis, *arthr* (which means *joint*) is the word root.
In the medical term	hepat/itis, *hepat* (which means *liver*) is the word root.

The word root is the core of the word; therefore, each medical term contains one or more word roots.

EXERCISE 3

Complete the following: A word root is the word part that is the core of the word

Suffix

The suffix is a word part attached to the end of the word root to modify its meaning.

EXAMPLES:

In the word	play/er, *-er* is the suffix.
In the medical term	hepat/ic, *-ic* (which means *pertaining to*) is the suffix. *Hepat* is the word root for *liver;* therefore, *hepatic* means *pertaining to the liver.*
In the medical term	hepat/itis, *-itis* (which means *inflammation*) is the suffix. The medical term *hepatitis* means *inflammation of the liver.*

SUFFIXES

frequently indicate:
- *procedures,* such as **-scopy**, meaning visual examination, or **-tomy**, meaning incision
- *conditions,* such as **-itis**, meaning inflammation
- *diseases,* such as **-oma**, meaning tumor.

The suffix is used to modify the meaning of a word. Most medical terms have a suffix.

EXERCISE 4

Complete the following: The suffix is a word part attached to the end of the word root to modify its meaning.

Prefix

The prefix is a word part attached to the beginning of a word root to modify its meaning.

EXAMPLES:

In the word	re/play, *re-* is the prefix.
In the medical term	sub/hepat/ic, *sub-* (which means *under*) is the prefix. *Hepat* is the word root for *liver,* and *-ic* is the suffix for *pertaining to.* The medical term *subhepatic* means *pertaining to under the liver.*
In the medical term	intra/ven/ous, *intra-* (which means *within*) is the prefix, *ven* (which means *vein*) is the word root, and *-ous* (which means *pertaining to*) is the suffix. The medical term *intravenous* means *pertaining to within the vein.*

PREFIXES

often indicate:
- *number* such as **bi-,** meaning two
- *position,* such as **sub-,** meaning under
- *direction,* such as **intra-,** meaning within
- *time,* such as **brady-,** meaning slow
- *negation,* such as **a-,** meaning without

A prefix can be used to modify the meaning of a word. Many medical terms do not have a prefix.

EXERCISE 5

Complete the following: The prefix is ____

Combining Vowel

The combining vowel is a word part, usually an *o*, used to ease pronunciation (Table 1-2).

The combining vowel is:

- Placed to connect two word roots
- Placed to connect a word root and a suffix
- **Not** placed to connect a prefix and a word root

EXAMPLES:

In the medical term	oste/**o**/arthr/itis *o* is the combining vowel used between two word roots *oste* (which means bone) and *arthr* (which means joint).
In the medical term	arthr/**o**/pathy, *o* is the combining vowel used between the word root *arthr* and the suffix *-pathy* (which means *disease*).
In the medical term	sub/hepat/ic, the combining vowel is **not** used between the prefix *sub-* and the word root *hepat.*

VOWELS

are speech sounds represented by the letters *a, e, i, o, u,* and sometimes *y.*

Four Guidelines for Using Combining Vowels

Learning the four guidelines for using combining vowels will assist you in correctly spelling medical terms built from word parts. Refer to Table 1-2, p. 9, as you build terms in the following chapters until the guidelines are a part of your memory.

Guideline One

When connecting a word root and a suffix, a combining vowel is used if the suffix does not begin with a vowel (Table 1-2).

EXAMPLE:

In the medical term	arthr/o/pathy, the suffix *-pathy* does not begin with a vowel; therefore, a combining vowel is used.

Guideline Two

When connecting a word root and a suffix, a combining vowel is usually not used if the suffix begins with a vowel.

EXAMPLE:

In the medical term hepat/ic,
the suffix *-ic* begins with the vowel *i;* therefore, a combining vowel is not used.

Guideline Three

When connecting two word roots, a combining vowel is usually used even if vowels are present at the junction.

EXAMPLE:

In the medical term oste/o/arthr/itis,
o is the combining vowel used, even though the word root *oste* ends with the vowel *e*, and the word root *arthr* begins with the vowel *a*.

Guideline Four

When connecting a prefix and a word root, a combining vowel is **not** used.

EXAMPLE:

In the medical term sub/hepat/ic,
the combining vowel is **not** used between the prefix *sub-* and the word root *hepat*.

The combining vowel is used to ease pronunciation; therefore *not all medical terms have combining vowels.* Medical terms introduced throughout the text that have combining vowels other than *o* are highlighted at their introduction.

TABLE 1-2

Guidelines for Using Combining Vowels

Combining Vowel Guideline	Example
1. When connecting a word root and a suffix, a **combining vowel *Is Used* if the suffix *Does Not Begin* with a vowel.**	arthr/**o**/pathy
2. When connecting a word root and a suffix, a **combining vowel *Is Usually Not Used* if the suffix *Begins* with a vowel.**	hepat/ic
3. When connecting two word roots, a **combining vowel *Is Usually Used* even if vowels are present at the junction.**	oste/**o**/arthr/itis
4. When connecting a prefix and a word root, **a combining vowel is *Not Used*.**	sub/hepat/ic

EXERCISE 6

Complete the following:

1. A combining vowel is ______________________________
____
2. When connecting a word root and a suffix, a combining vowel is ______________ if the suffix does not begin with a vowel.
3. When connecting a word root and a suffix, a combining vowel is usually not used if the suffix begins with a ______________.
4. When connecting two ______________ ______________, a combining vowel is usually used, even if vowels are present at the junction.
5. When connecting a prefix and a word root, a combining vowel is ______________ used.

Combining Form

A combining form is a word root with the combining vowel attached, separated by a vertical slash (Table 1-3).

Examples: arthr/o
oste/o
ven/o

The combining form is not a word part per se; rather it is the word root and the combining vowel. *For learning purposes, word roots are presented together with their combining vowels as* ***combining forms*** *throughout the text.*

EXERCISE 7

Complete the following: A combining form is ______________________________
____
____

Word roots are presented as combining forms throughout the text.

TABLE 1-3

Word Parts and Combining Form

Word root	The core of the word	**hepat**/itis
Suffix	Attached at the end of a word root to modify its meaning	hepat/**itis**
Prefix	Attached at the beginning of a word root to modify its meaning	**sub**/hepatic
Combining vowel	Usually an "o" used to ease pronunciation	hepat/**o**/megaly
Combining form	Word root with a combining vowel attached, separated by a slash	**hepat/o**

EXERCISE 8

Match the phrases in the first column with the correct terms in the second column.

______ 1. attached at the beginning		a. combining vowel
______ 2. usually an *o*		b. prefix
______ 3. all medical terms contain at least one		c. combining form
______ 4. attached at the end of a word root		d. word root
______ 5. word root with combining vowel attached		e. suffix

EXERCISE 9

Answer *T* for true and *F* for false.

______ 1. There are always prefixes at the beginning of medical terms.

______ 2. A combining vowel is always used when connecting a word root and a suffix that begins with the letter *o*.

______ 3. A prefix modifies the meaning of the word.

______ 4. A combining vowel is used to ease pronunciation.

______ 5. *I* is the most commonly used combining vowel.

______ 6. The word root is the core of a medical term.

______ 7. A combining vowel is used between a prefix and a word root.

______ 8. A combining form is a word part.

______ 9. A combining vowel is used when connecting a word root and a suffix if the suffix begins with the letter *g*.

TECHNIQUES FOR LEARNING MEDICAL TERMS BUILT FROM WORD PARTS

Analyzing, defining, and **building** medical terms are used in this text to learn medical terms built from word parts. You will use them many times to complete exercises in the following chapters. Refer to Table 1-4, p. 15, as often as needed until you become familiar with these techniques.

Analyzing Medical Terms

To analyze medical terms, divide them into word parts and label each word part and each combining form (Table 1-4 on p. 15). Follow the procedure below:

1. **Divide the term** into word parts with vertical slashes.

   Example: oste / o / arthr / o / pathy

2. **Label each word part** by using the following abbreviations.

WR	Word Root
P	Prefix
S	Suffix
CV	Combining Vowel

   WR CV WR CV S
   Example: oste / o / arthr / o / pathy

3. **Label each combining form.**

   WR CV WR CV S
   Example: oste / o / arthr / o / pathy
   CF CF

EXERCISE 10

Analyze the following medical term. Use the word part list below as a reference:

o s t e o p a t h y

EXERCISE 11

Complete the following. Three steps to analyze medical terms are:

1. ______________________________
2. ______________________________
3. ______________________________

Defining Medical Terms

To define medical terms, apply the meaning of each word part contained in the term.

EXERCISE 12

Define the medical term:

oste/o/arthr/o/pathy

Use the Word Part List below as a reference.

1. Begin by defining the suffix, *-pathy*. Write the definition on the line below.
2. Move to the beginning of the term, define the word roots *oste* and *arthr*. Write the definitions on the line below, continuing the definition of the term.

oste/o/arthr/o/pathy means ________ of the ________ and ________
-pathy oste arthr

Most medical terms built from word parts can be defined by beginning with the meaning of the suffix; however, this does not always apply.

Word Part List

Word Roots	Definition	Suffixes	Definition
arthr	joint	-itis	inflammation
hepat	liver	-ic	pertaining to
ven	vein	-ous	pertaining to
oste	bone	-pathy	disease
		-megaly	enlargement
Prefixes		**Combining Vowel**	
intra-	within	o	
sub-	under		

EXERCISE 13

Complete the following: To define medical terms built from word parts, apply the meaning of each word part contained in the term

EXERCISE 14

Using the Word Part List on p. 12 to identify the word parts and their meanings, analyze and define the following terms.

Example: oste / o / arthr / o / pathy (WR CV WR CV S; CF CF) disease of the bone and joint

1. arthritis arthr/itis inflammation of the joint
2. hepatitis hepat/itis inflammation of the liver
3. subhepatic sub/hepat/ic pertaining to under the liver
4. intravenous intra/ven/ous pertaining to within the vein
5. arthropathy arthr/o/pathy disease of the joint
6. osteitis oste/itis inflammation of the bone
7. hepatomegaly hepat/o/megaly enlargement of the liver

Building Medical Terms

To build medical terms, place word parts together to form words.

EXERCISE 15

Build the medical term for

disease of a joint

Use the Word Part List on p. 12 as a reference.

1. Find the word part for *disease*. Write the word part in the correct space below.
2. Find the word part for *joint*. Write the word part in the correct space below.
3. The suffix does not begin with a vowel.

Insert the combining vowel *o* in the correct space below. (*A combining vowel is needed because the suffix does not begin with a vowel.*)

arthr / o / pathy
WR / CV / S

EXERCISE 16

Complete the following: To build medical terms means place word parts together to form words

Keep in mind that the beginning of the definition usually indicates the suffix.

EXERCISE 17

Using the Word Part List on p. 12 as a reference, build medical terms for the following definitions.

Example: disease of a joint — arthr / o / pathy (WR / CV / S)

1. inflammation of a joint — arthr / itis (WR / S)
2. pertaining to the liver — hepat / ic (WR / S)
3. pertaining to under the liver — sub / hepat / ic (P / WR / S)
4. pertaining to within the vein — intra / ven / ous (P / WR / S)
5. inflammation of the bone — oste / itis (WR / S)
6. inflammation of the liver — hepat / itis (WR / S)
7. disease of the bone and joint — oste / o / arthr / o / pathy (WR / CV / WR / CV / S)
8. enlargement of the liver — hepat / o / megaly (WR / CV / S)

EXERCISE FIGURE A

Fill in the blanks to complete labeling of the diagram. *To check your answers, go to p. 19.*

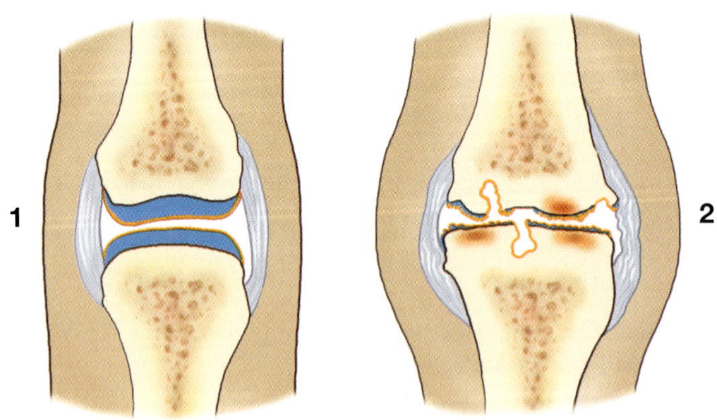

1. Normal knee joint

2. Knee joint showing oste / o / arthr / istis (bone / cv / joint / inflammation)

At this time, do not be concerned about which word root goes first when building a term that contains two word roots. The order is usually dictated by common practice; for surgical or diagnostic terms, word roots are sometimes arranged by the order of function or by the order in which an instrument may encounter a structure. As you practice and learn, you will become accustomed to the accepted order.

TABLE 1-4

Techniques to Learn Medical Terms Built from Word Parts

Technique	Step	Example
• Analyzing	1. Divide medical terms into word parts	oste / o / arthr / o / pathy
	2. Label each word part	**WR CV WR CV S** oste / o / arthr / o / pathy
	3. Label each combining form	WR CV WR CV S oste / o / arthr / o / pathy **CF** (oste/o) **CF** (arthr/o)
• Defining	1. Apply the meaning of each word part contained in the term (*begin by defining the suffix, then move to the beginning of the term*) **oste** / o / **arthr** / o / **pathy** WR WR S	***disease*** *of the* ***bone*** *and* ***joint***
• Building	1. Place word parts together to form terms (*the beginning of the definition usually indicates the suffix*)	
	disease of the **bone** and **joint**	***oste*** */ /* ***arthr*** */ /* ***pathy*** WR WR S
	2. Add **combining vowels** as needed	oste / **o** / arthr / **o** / pathy WR CV WR CV S

MEDICAL TERMS NOT BUILT FROM WORD PARTS

Medical terms not built from word parts are terms that cannot be easily translated to find their meanings. Many exercises using memorization are presented in each chapter to assist in learning these terms. Origins of terms not built from word parts are:

1. **eponyms,** terms derived from the name of a person, such as Alzheimer disease
2. **acronyms,** terms formed from the first letter of words in a phrase that can be spoken as a whole word and usually contains a vowel, such as MRSA (methicillin-resistant *Staphylococcus aureus*)
3. **modern language**, terms derived from the English language such as complete blood count and differential
4. **terms made up of Greek and Latin word parts that cannot be easily translated to find their meaning**, such as orthopedic. Orth/o/ped/ic is made up of three word parts: orth/o meaning straight, ped/o meaning child or foot, and -ic meaning pertaining to. Translated literally, **orthopedic** means **pertaining to a straight child or foot,** whereas its meaning as used today is **a branch of medicine dealing with the study and treatment of diseases and abnormalities of the musculoskeletal system**. As you can see, the term *orthopedic* cannot be translated literally to find its meaning.

EXERCISE 18

Place a check mark in the space provided to identify terms not built from word parts. This may be the first time you have seen some of these terms. Apply your newly acquired knowledge and see how you do.

1. ______ arthritis
2. ______ upper respiratory infection
3. ______ Lyme disease
4. ______ AIDS
5. ______ macular degeneration
6. ______ hepatitis
7. ______ nuclear medicine scanner
8. ______ malignant
9. ______ osteopathy
10. ______ Alzheimer disease

ONLINE LEARNING

Evolve is the website that accompanies the textbook, providing multimedia learning activities and resources. This Evolve icon seen throughout the text directs you to online experiences such as **spelling, pronunciation, practice activities, games, animations,** and **exercises to help you prepare for examinations,** and solidify your learning. These online learning activities provide many ways to see and hear the chapter content. Exercises and activities provide immediate feedback on your performance, allowing you to focus your studies. The audio and video features allow you to see and hear the terms, as well as provide information about related medical concepts. Table 1-5 shows all of the available chapter activities and additional resources.

Create an Account and Register

Let's get started by connecting to the Evolve website, creating an account, and registering.

For problem solving go to http://evolve.elsevier.com/studentresources or call 1-800-401-9962.

EXERCISE 19

Place a check mark next to the step once you have completed it.

_____ 1. Go to http://evolve.elsevier.com

_____ 2. Select **STUDENT Site**

_____ 3. Select **Join Evolve Communities**. Follow the steps to create a password. Use upper and lowercase letters and numbers such as "Mugsi123". Record your password for future reference.

Password: ____________________

You will be issued a username. Record your username for future reference.

Username: ____________________

_____ 4. Select **Jump Right In**

_____ 5. Type **Exploring Medical Language** in the search box at the top of the screen and follow the links to the 8th edition.

_____ 6. Select **Exploring Medical Language 8th Edition**

_____ 7. Select **Register**

_____ 8. Select **Register** again and follow the steps. Although a "shopping cart" may appear on screen, there is no purchase necessary.

_____ 9. Sign the **Registered User Agreement** by clicking in the box at the end of the form.

_____ 10. Select **Get Started,** on the lower left of the screen

_____ 11. Select **Resources** listed below My Content

_____ 12. Select **LaFleur Brooks: Exploring Medical Language, 8th Edition**

_____ 13. Select **Course Documents**

_____ 14. Select **Resources**

Congratulations! You are now registered with the Evolve website for Exploring Medical Language. You are also logged onto the website. If you wish, you may proceed to **ONLINE CHAPTER REVIEW**, p. 18 to complete **Practice Activities** and/or play the **Medical Millionaire Game.** If you choose to log out at this time, log back in by following the steps listed under **Evolve Access Information,** p. 18.

TABLE 1-5
Online Learning Activities and Resources on the Evolve Website

Chapter Exercises	Practice Activities	Animations	Games
Textbook exercises allow you to hear the terms: Pronunciation Spelling Read Medical Terms in Use	*Additional practice and assessments test your learning:* Picture It Define Word Parts Analyze Medical Terms Build Medical Terms Define Medical Terms Use It Hear It & Type It: Clinical Vignettes	*Videos depicting disease and disorders and/or procedures related to chapter content*	Name that Word Part Term Storm Term Explorer Termbusters Medical Millionaire Crossword Puzzles

Additional Resources

A&P Booster	Answers to Chapter Exercises	Evolve Appendices	Flashcards
More information about body systems, organs, and how they work	*All in one place and ready to print so you can have them on hand to check your answers immediately*	**E**—Additonal Combining Forms, Prefixes, and Suffixes **F**—Health Care Delivery Terms **G**—Complementary and Alternative Medicine Therapies **H**—Behavioral Health Terms **I**—Clinical Research Terms **J**—Nutritional Terms	*Practice with electronic flashcards for word parts presented in each chapter*

SUMMARY

Categories of Medical Terms

Terms built from word parts—can be translated literally to find their meaning
Terms not built from word parts—cannot be translated literally to find their meaning

Medical Terms Built from Word Parts

Word Parts and Combining Form

Word root—core of a word; example, **hepat**
Suffix—attached at the end of a word root to modify its meaning; example, **-ic**
Prefix—attached at the beginning of a word to modify its meaning; example, **sub-**
Combining vowel—usually an **o** used between two word roots or a word root and suffix to ease pronunciation; example, hepat **o** pathy
Combining form—word root plus combining vowel separated by a vertical slash; example, **hepat/o**

Techniques for Learning Medical Terms Built from Word Parts

Analyzing—dividing medical terms into word parts, then labeling each word part and combining form
Defining—applying the meaning of each word part contained in the medical term to derive its meaning
Building—placing word parts together to form words

Medical Terms Not Built from Word Parts

Eponyms—name of a person; example, **Alzheimer disease**
Acronyms—from first letter of words, example, **MRSA**
Modern Language—terms derived from the English language, example, **complete blood count**
Terms not easily translated from word parts—example, **orthopedic**

CHAPTER REVIEW

To complete this chapter successfully, you do not need to know what the word parts, such as *arthr*, mean. You will learn these in subsequent chapters. **It is important that you have met these objectives:**

1. Can you describe four origins of medical language? yes ☐ no ☐
2. Can you define two categories of medical terms? yes ☐ no ☐
3. Can you identify and define the four word parts and combining form? yes ☐ no ☐
4. Can you use word parts to analyze and define medical terms? yes ☐ no ☐
5. Can you use word parts to build medical terms for a given definition? yes ☐ no ☐
6. Have you created an account and registered on the Evolve website? yes ☐ no ☐

If you answered yes to these questions, you need no further practice because you will be using these concepts repeatedly as you work your way through this text. Refer to this chapter to refresh your memory as needed. Move on to Chapter 2 and begin to build your medical vocabulary so that you will be better prepared than Grimm in Figure 1-2 to understand and use the language of medicine.

EVOLVE ACCESS INFORMATION

Use the following steps to access the Evolve website to complete learning activities designated by (e), appearing throughout each textbook chapter.

For problem solving, go to http://evolve.elsevier.com/studentresources or call 1-800-401-9962.

Steps to login to Evolve:

1. Go to http://evolve.elsevier.com
2. Select **STUDENT Site**
3. Login in with your user name and password. For future reference, record in the spaces below your username and password from Exercise 19, page 16.

   Username: ______________________________

   Password: ______________________________
4. Select **Resources** listed below My Content on the left side of the screen
5. Select **LaFleur Brooks: Exploring Medical Language, 8th Edition**
6. Select **Course Documents**
7. Select **Resources**

ONLINE CHAPTER REVIEW

Place a check mark next to the step once it is completed.

______ 1. If not already logged on, use the steps listed above in the Evolve Access Information section to login.

______ 2. Select **Chapter 1**

______ 3. Select **Practice Activities**

______ 4. Select **Define Word Parts**

______ 5. Select **Study Mode** and follow instructions.

Congratulations: you should see your first **Practice Activity** on the screen. Follow the instructions and have fun.

______ 6. Complete the remaining **Practice Activities** and play the **Medical Millionaire Game.**

Practice Activities

Practice in study mode and then test your learning in assessment mode. Keep track of your scores from Assessment mode if you wish.

	Score
☐ Define Word Parts	______
☐ Analyze Medical Terms	______
☐ Build Medical Terms	______
☐ Define Medical Terms	______

Games

☐ Medical Millionaire

Exercise Figure
Exercise Figure
A. oste/o/arthr/itis

Exercise 1

1. b
2. a
3. c
4. d
5. a
6. d
7. c
8. b

Exercise 2
built from word parts; not built from word parts

Exercise 3
a word part that is the core of the word

Exercise 4
a word part attached to the end of the word root to modify its meaning

Exercise 5
a word part attached at the beginning of a word root to modify its meaning

Exercise 6

1. a word part, usually an o, used to ease pronunciation
2. used
3. vowel
4. word roots
5. not

Exercise 7
a word root with the combining vowel attached, separated by a vertical slash

Exercise 8
1. b 2. a 3. d 4. e 5. c

Exercise 9

1. *F*, a medical term may begin with the word root and have no prefix.
2. *F*, if the suffix begins with a vowel, the combining vowel is usually not used.
3. *T*
4. *T*
5. *F*, *o* is the combining vowel most often used.
6. *T*
7. *F*, a combining vowel is used between two word roots or between a word root and a suffix to ease pronunciation.
8. *F*, a combining form is a word root with a combining vowel attached and is not one of the four word parts.
9. *T*

Exercise 10
WR CV S
oste/o/pathy
CF

Exercise 11
(1) divide the term into word parts; (2) label each word part; and (3) label each combining form

Exercise 12
disease of the bone and joint

Exercise 13
apply the meaning of each word part contained in the term

Exercise 14

1. WR S
   arthr/itis
   inflammation of a joint
2. WR S
   hepat/itis
   inflammation of the liver
3. P WR S
   sub/hepat/ic
   pertaining to under the liver
4. P WR S
   intra/ven/ous
   pertaining to within the vein
5. WR CV S
   arthr/o/pathy
   CF
   disease of a joint
6. WR S
   oste/itis
   inflammation of the bone
7. WR CV S
   hepat/o/megaly
   CF
   enlargement of the liver

Exercise 15
arthr/o/pathy

Exercise 16
to place word parts together to form words

Exercise 17

1. arthr/itis
2. hepat/ic
3. sub/hepat/ic
4. intra/ven/ous
5. oste/itis
6. hepat/itis
7. oste/o/arthr/o/pathy
8. hepat/o/megaly

Exercise 18
Check marks for numbers 2, 3, 4, 5, 7, 8, 10

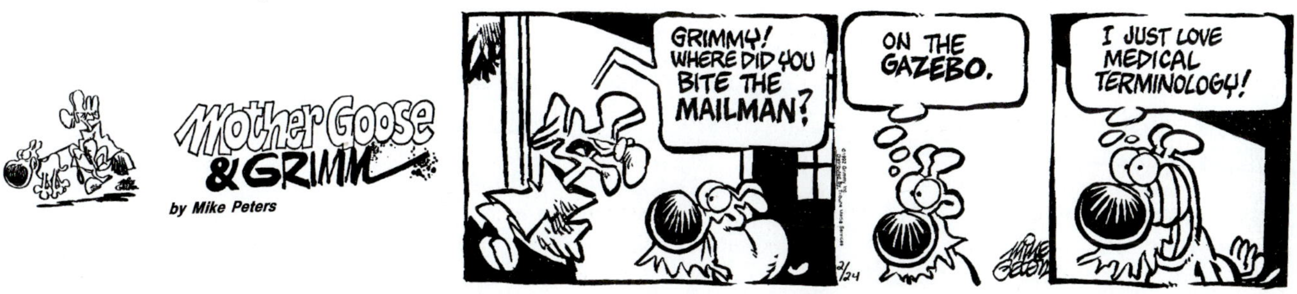
Mother Goose & GRIMM
by Mike Peters
GRIMMY! WHERE DID YOU BITE THE MAILMAN?
ON THE GAZEBO.
I JUST LOVE MEDICAL TERMINOLOGY!

FIGURE 1-2
Reprinted by permission of Tribune Media Services.

Chapter 2

Body Structure, Color, and Oncology

OUTLINE

OBJECTIVES

Upon completion of this chapter you will be able to:

1. Identify anatomic structures of the human body.
2. Define and spell word parts related to body structure, color, and oncology.
3. Define, pronounce, and spell disease and disorder oncology terms.
4. Define, pronounce, and spell body structure terms.
5. Define, pronounce, and spell complementary terms related to body structure, color, and oncology.
6. Identify and use singular and plural endings.
7. Interpret the meaning of abbreviations related to body structure and oncology.
8. Interpret, read, and comprehend medical language in simulated medical statements and documents.

ANATOMY

Organization of the Body

The structure of the human body falls into the following four categories: cells, tissues, organs, and systems. Each structure is a highly organized unit of smaller structures (Exercise Figure A).

Term	Definition
cell	basic unit of all living things (Figure 2-1). The human body is composed of trillions of cells, which vary in size and shape according to function.
cell membrane	forms the boundary of the cell
cytoplasm	gel-like fluid inside the cell
nucleus	largest structure within the cell, usually spherical and centrally located. It contains chromosomes for cellular reproduction and is the control center of the cell.
chromosomes	located in the nucleus of the cell. There are 46 chromosomes in all normal human cells, with the exception of mature sex cells, which have 23.
genes	regions within the chromosome. Each chromosome has several thousand genes that determine hereditary characteristics.
DNA (deoxyribonucleic acid)	comprises each gene; is a genetic material that regulates the activities of the cell
tissue	group of similar cells that performs a specific function (see Exercise Figure B)
muscle tissue	composed of cells that have a special ability to contract, usually producing movement
nervous tissue	found in the nerves, spinal cord, and brain. It is responsible for coordinating and controlling body activities.
connective tissue	connects, supports, penetrates, and encases various body structures. Adipose (fat), osseous (bone) tissues, and blood are types of connective tissue.
epithelial tissue	the major covering of the external surface of the body; forms membranes that line body cavities and organs and is the major tissue in glands
organ	two or more kinds of tissues that together perform special body functions. For example, the skin is an organ composed of epithelial, connective, muscle, and nerve tissue.
system	group of organs that work together to perform complex body functions. For example, the cardiovascular system consists of the heart, blood vessels, and blood. Its function is to transport nutrients and oxygen to the cells and remove carbon dioxide and other waste products. (see Table 2-1)

MEDICAL GENOMICS

A **genome** is the complete set of genes in a chromosome of each cell of a specific organism. **Genomics** is the study of the genome and its products and interactions.

Medical genomics is the study of the genome and how it can be used in the cause, treatment, and prevention of disease. It is thought that it will alter twenty-first century medicine.

Gene therapy is any therapeutic procedure in which genes are intentionally introduced into human body cells to achieve gene repair, gene suppression, or gene addition. Gene therapy is still in its infancy. The first human gene transfer was performed on a patient with malignant melanoma in 1989.

CHROMOSOME

is derived from the Greek ***chromos***, meaning ***color***, and ***soma***, meaning ***body***. German anatomist Waldeyer first used the term in 1888.

For clinical research terms, go to http://evolve.elsevier.com. Refer to p. 18 for your Evolve Access Information. Select **Appendices, Appendix I, Clinical Research Terms.**

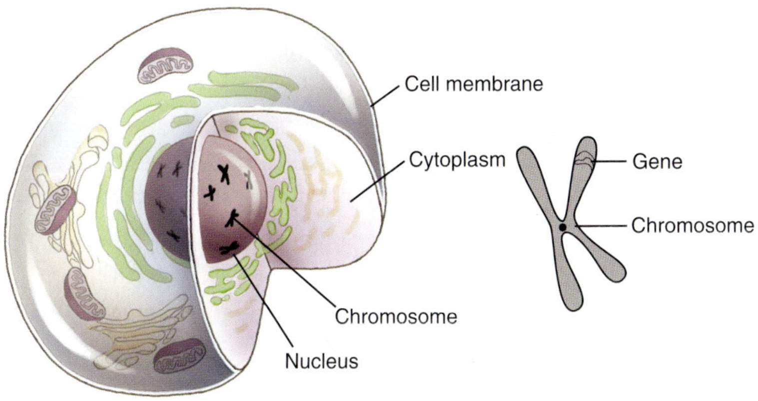

FIGURE 2-1
Body cell.

TABLE 2-1
Body Systems

Body Systems	Organs and Function
Integumentary System	Composed of skin, nails, and glands. Forms a protective covering for the body, regulates body temperature, and helps manufacture vitamin D.
Respiratory System	Composed of nose, pharynx (throat), larynx (voice box), trachea (windpipe), bronchial tubes, and lungs. Performs respiration which provides for the exchange of oxygen and carbon dioxide within the body.
Urinary System	Composed of kidneys, ureters, bladder, and urethra. Removes waste material (urine) from the body, regulates fluid volume, and maintains electrolyte concentration.
Reproductive System	Female reproductive system is composed of ovaries, uterine tubes, uterus, vagina, and mammary glands. Male reproductive system is composed of testes, urethra, penis, prostate gland, and associated tubes. Responsible for heredity and reproduction.
Cardiovascular System	Composed of the heart and blood vessels. Pumps and transports blood throughout the body.
Lymphatic System	Composed of a network of vessels, ducts, nodes, and organs. Provides defense against infection.
Digestive System	Composed of the gastrointestinal tract which includes the esophagus, stomach, large and small intestine plus accessory organs, liver, gallbladder, and pancreas. Prepares food for use by the body cells and eliminates waste.
Musculoskeletal System	Composed of muscle, bones, and joints. Provides movement and framework for the body, protects vital organs such as the brain, stores calcium, and produces red blood cells.
Nervous System	Composed of the brain, spinal cord, and nerves. Regulates body activities by sending and receiving messages.
Endocrine System	Composed of glands that secrete hormones. Hormones regulate many body activities.

STEM CELLS

Hematopoietic stem cells are immature cells found in the bone marrow and peripheral blood. They have the potential to develop into mature cells of any type of body tissue or form mature blood cells. Hematopoietic stem cells for transplantation may be obtained from the patient (**autologous**), from an identical twin (**synergetic**), or from a sibling or other individual (**allogenic**).

Embryonic stem cells are derived from the earliest stage of development of the embryo and have the potential to develop into mature body cells.

Stem cell transplantation is used to treat **leukemia** (cancer involving the white blood cells), **aplastic anemia** (disease in which there is inadequate production of blood cells), **multiple myeloma** (cancer that forms tumors in the bone marrow), **lymphoma** (cancer involving lymphoid cells), and **immune deficiency disorders**.

Body Cavities

The body is not a solid structure as it appears on the outside, but has five cavities (Figure 2-2), each containing an orderly arrangement of the internal organs.

Term	Definition
cranial cavity	space inside the skull (cranium) containing the brain
spinal cavity	space inside the spinal column containing the spinal cord
thoracic, or chest, cavity	space containing the heart, aorta, lungs, esophagus, trachea, and bronchi
abdominal cavity	space containing the stomach, intestines, kidneys, liver, gallbladder, pancreas, spleen, and ureters
pelvic cavity	space containing the urinary bladder, certain reproductive organs, parts of the small and large intestine, and the rectum
abdominopelvic cavity	both the pelvic and abdominal cavities

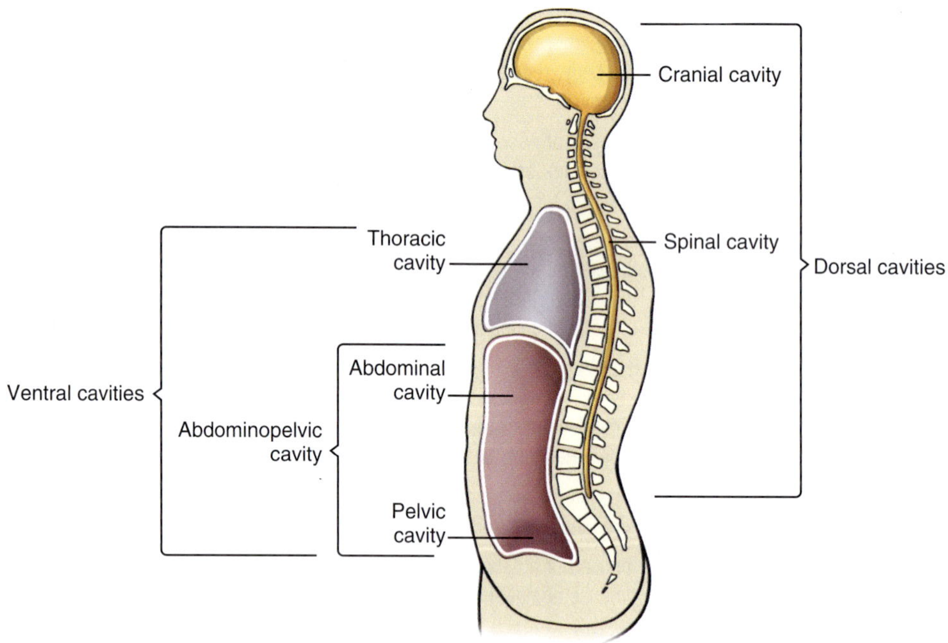

FIGURE 2-2
Body cavities.

A & P Booster
For students desiring more anatomy and physiology, go to http://evolve.elsevier.com. Refer to p. 18 for your Evolve Access information. Select A & P Booster, Chapter 2.

EXERCISE 1

Match the anatomic terms in the first column with the correct definitions in the second column. *To check your answers to the exercises in this chapter, go to Answers, p. 62, at the back of the chapter.*

_____ 1. chromosomes
_____ 2. nucleus
_____ 3. cytoplasm
_____ 4. cell
_____ 5. muscle tissue
_____ 6. nerve tissue
_____ 7. epithelial tissue
_____ 8. bone
_____ 9. genes
_____ 10. DNA

a. type of connective tissue
b. regions within the chromosome
c. covers external body surface, lines body cavities and organs
d. gel-like fluid inside the cell
e. contains chromosomes
f. coordinates body activities
g. usually produces movement
h. contain genes
i. chest cavity
j. a genetic material that regulates the activities of the cell
k. basic unit of all living things

EXERCISE 2

Match the anatomic terms in the first column with the correct definitions in the second column.

_____ 1. spinal cavity
_____ 2. thoracic cavity
_____ 3. organ
_____ 4. cranial cavity
_____ 5. pelvic cavity
_____ 6. system
_____ 7. abdominal cavity

a. group of organs functioning together
b. chest cavity
c. composed of two or more tissues
d. found in the skin
e. space inside the skull
f. contains the stomach
g. contains the urinary bladder
h. contains the spinal cord

WORD PARTS

Begin building your medical vocabulary by learning the word parts listed next. The list may appear long to you; however, the many exercises that follow are designed to help you understand and remember the word parts.

Use the flashcards accompanying this text or electronic flashcards to assist you in memorizing the word parts for this chapter.

To use electronic flashcards, go to http://evolve.elsevier.com. Refer to p. 18 for your Evolve Access Information. Select Flashcards, Chapter 2.

Combining Forms of Body Structure

Reminder: the word root is the core of the word. The combining form is the word root with the combining vowel attached, separated by a vertical slash.

EPITHELIUM

originally meant **surface over the nipple. Epi** means **upon,** and **thela** means **nipple** (or projecting surfaces of many kinds).

Combining Form	Definition
aden/o	gland
cyt/o	cell
epitheli/o	epithelium
fibr/o	fiber
hist/o	tissue
kary/o	nucleus
lip/o	fat
my/o	muscle
neur/o	nerve
organ/o	organ
sarc/o	flesh, connective tissue
system/o	system
viscer/o	internal organs

EXERCISE FIGURE A

Fill in the blanks with combining forms in this diagram of the organization of the body. *To check your answers, go to p. 62.*

2. Tissue

CF: histo

1. Cell

CF: cyto

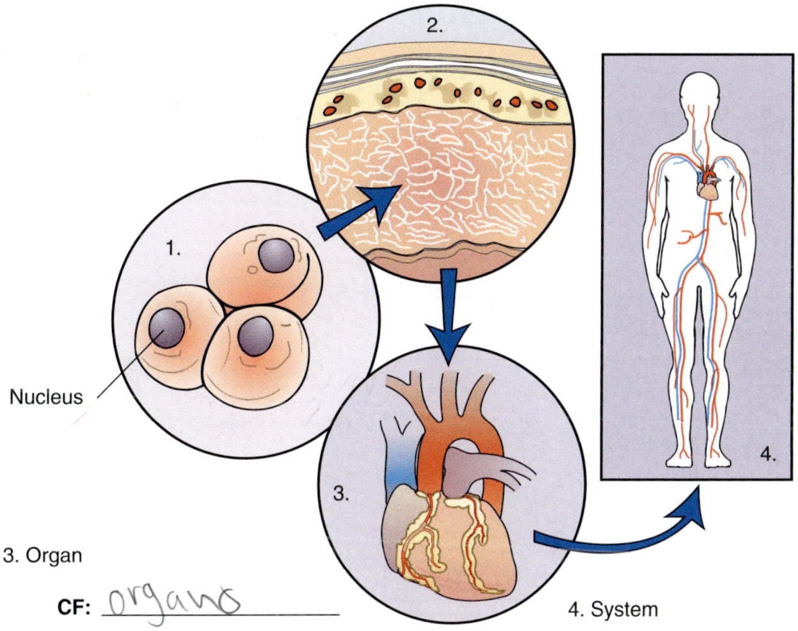

3. Organ

CF: organo

4. System

CF: systemo

EXERCISE 3

Write the definitions of the following combining forms.

1. sarc/o flesh, connective tissue
2. lip/o fat
3. kary/o nucleus
4. viscer/o internal organs
5. cyt/o cell
6. hist/o tissue
7. my/o muscle
8. neur/o nerve
9. organ/o organo
10. system/o system
11. epitheli/o epithelium
12. fibr/o fiber
13. aden/o gland

EXERCISE FIGURE B

Fill in the blanks with combining forms in this diagram of types of tissues.

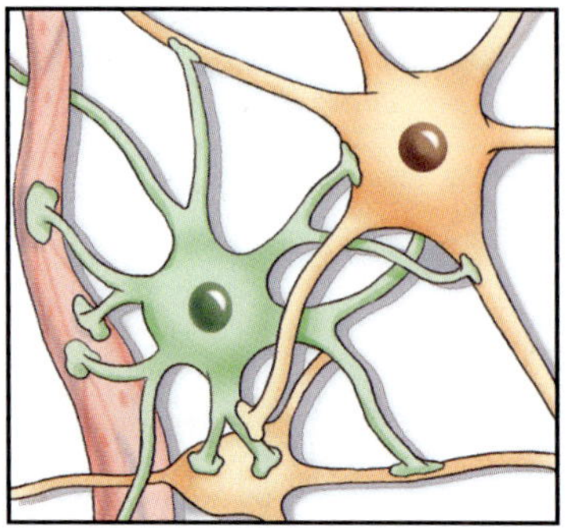

1. Nerve

CF: neuro

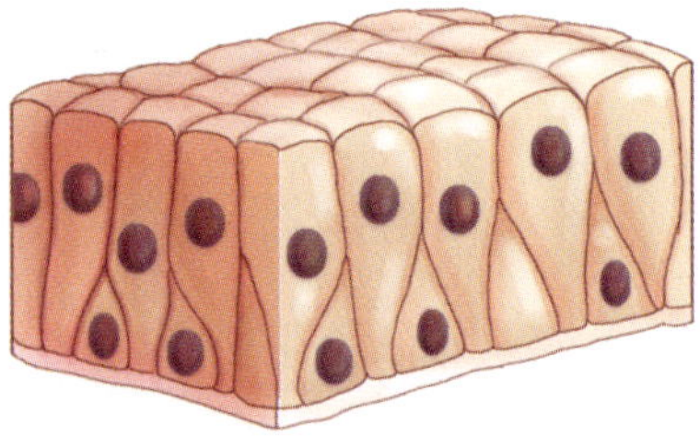

2. Epithelium

CF: epithelio

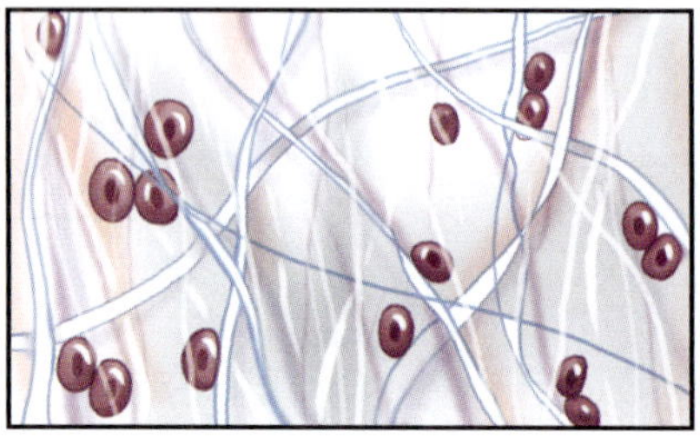

3. Connective

CF: sacro

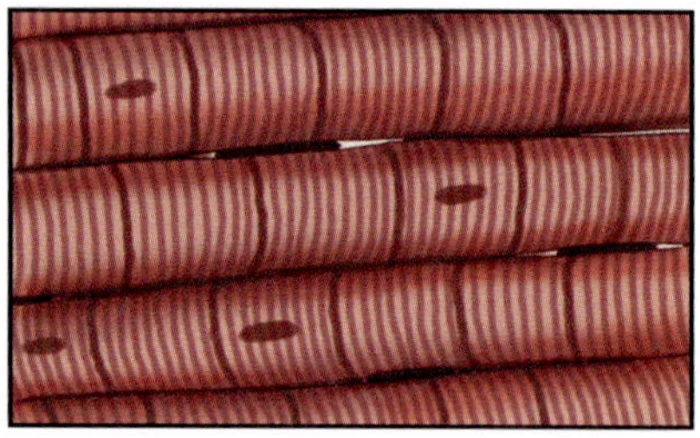

4. Muscle

CF: myo

EXERCISE 4

Write the combining form for each of the following.

1. internal organs vicero
2. epithelium epithelio
3. organ organo
4. nucleus karyo
5. cell cyto
6. tissue histo
7. nerve neuro
8. muscle myo
9. fat lipo
10. system systemo
11. flesh, connective tissue sarcro
12. fiber fibro
13. gland adeno

Combining Forms Commonly Used with Body Structure Terms

Combining Form	Definition
cancer/o, carcin/o	cancer (a disease characterized by the unregulated, abnormal growth of new cells)
eti/o	cause (of disease)
gno/o	knowledge
iatr/o	physician, medicine (also means treatment)
lei/o	smooth
onc/o	tumor, mass
path/o	disease
rhabd/o	rod-shaped, striated
somat/o	body

CANCER

Carcin and ***cancer*** are derived from Latin and Greek words meaning ***crab***. They originated before the nature of malignant growth was understood. One explanation was that the swollen veins around the diseased area looked like the claws of a crab.

EXERCISE 5

Write the definitions of the following combining forms.

1. onc/o tumer, mass
2. carcin/o cancer
3. eti/o cause (of disease)
4. path/o disease
5. somat/o body
6. cancer/o cancer
7. rhabd/o rod-shaped, striated
8. lei/o smooth
9. gno/o knowledge
10. iatr/o physician, medicine

EXERCISE 6

Write the combining form for each of the following.

1. disease patho
2. tumor, mass onco
3. cause (of disease) etio
4. cancer a. cancero b. carcino
5. body somato
6. smooth leio
7. rod-shaped, striated rhabdo
8. knowledge gnoo
9. physician, medicine iatro

ERYTHRO

Aristotle noted "two colors of blood" and applied the term ***erythro*** to the dark red blood.

Combining Forms that Describe Color

Combining Form	Definition
chlor/o	green
chrom/o	color
cyan/o	blue
erythr/o	red
leuk/o	white
melan/o	black
xanth/o	yellow

EXERCISE 7

Write the definitions of the following combining forms.

1. cyan/o blue
2. erythr/o red
3. leuk/o white
4. xanth/o yellow
5. chrom/o color
6. melan/o black
7. chlor/o green

EXERCISE 8

Write the combining form for each of the following.

1. blue cyano
2. red erythro
3. white leuko
4. black melano
5. yellow xantho
6. color chromo
7. green chloro

Prefixes

Reminder: prefixes are placed at the beginning of word roots to modify their meanings.

Prefix	Definition
dia-	through, complete
dys-	painful, abnormal, difficult, labored
hyper-	above, excessive
hypo-	below, incomplete, deficient
meta-	after, beyond, change
neo-	new
pro-	before

EXERCISE 9

Write the definitions of the following prefixes.

1. neo- ____________________
2. hyper- ____________________
3. meta- ____________________
4. hypo- ____________________
5. dys- ____________________
6. dia- ____________________
7. pro- ____________________

EXERCISE 10

Write the prefix for each of the following.

1. new ____________________
2. above, excessive ____________________
3. below, incomplete, deficient ____________________
4. after, beyond, change ____________________
5. abnormal, painful, labored, difficult ____________________
6. through, complete ____________________
7. before ____________________

Suffixes

Reminder: suffixes are placed at the end of word roots to modify their meanings.

Suffix	Definition
-al, -ic, -ous	pertaining to
-cyte (NOTE: the combining form for cell is *cyt/o*; the suffix for cell is *-cyte*, ending with an *e*.)	cell
-gen	substance or agent that produces or causes
-genic	producing, originating, causing
-logist	one who studies and treats (specialist, physician)
-logy	study of
-oid	resembling
-oma	tumor, swelling
-osis	abnormal condition (means **increase** when used with blood cell word roots)
-pathy	disease
-plasia	condition of formation, development, growth
-plasm	growth, substance, formation
-sarcoma	malignant tumor
-sis	state of
-stasis	control, stop, standing

INCIDENTALOMA

refers to a mass lesion involving an organ that is discovered unexpectedly by the use of ultrasound, computed tomography scan, or magnetic resonance imaging and has nothing to do with the patient's symptoms or primary diagnosis.

Some suffixes are made of a word root plus a suffix; they are presented as suffixes for ease of learning. For example, **-pathy** is made up of the word root **path** and the suffix **-y.** When analyzing a medical term, divide the suffixes as learned. For example, **somatopathy** should be divided somat/o/pathy and **not** somat/o/path/y.

Refer to **Appendix A** and **Appendix B** for alphabetized lists of word parts and their meanings.

EXERCISE 11

Match the suffixes in the first column with their correct definitions in the second column.

_____	1. -logy	a. producing, originating, causing
_____	2. -osis	b. cell
_____	3. -pathy	c. specialist, physician
_____	4. -plasm	d. new
_____	5. -al, -ic, -ous	e. disease
_____	6. -stasis	f. growth, substance, formation
_____	7. -oid	g. pertaining to
_____	8. -cyte	h. resembling
_____	9. -logist	i. study of
_____	10. -oma	j. control, stop, standing
_____	11. -gen	k. substance that produces
_____	12. -sarcoma	l. abnormal condition
_____	13. -plasia	m. condition of formation, development, growth
_____	14. -genic	n. tumor, swelling
_____	15. -sis	o. state of
		p. malignant tumor

SARCOMA

has been used since the time of ancient Greece to describe any fleshy tumor. Since the introduction of cellular pathology, the meaning was restricted to mean a **malignant connective tissue tumor.**

Often, an additional word root is used to denote the type of tissue involved, such as ***oste*** in ***osteosarcoma***, which refers to a malignant tumor of the bone.

EXERCISE 12

Write the definitions of the following suffixes.

1. -logist _______________
2. -pathy _______________
3. -logy _______________
4. -ic _______________
5. -stasis _______________
6. -cyte _______________
7. -osis _______________
8. -ous _______________
9. -plasm _______________
10. -al _______________
11. -plasia _______________
12. -oid _______________
13. -gen _______________

> Practice two things in your dealings with disease: either help or do not harm the patient.
> —**Hippocrates** 460–375 BC

14. -genic producing, originating, causing
15. -oma tumor, swelling
16. -sarcoma malignant tumor
17. -sis state of

MEDICAL TERMS

Oncology

Oncology is the study of tumors. Tumors develop from excessive growth of cells from a body part. Tumors, or masses, are benign (noncancerous) or malignant (cancerous). The names of tumors are often made of the word root for the body part and the suffix **-oma,** as in the term *my/oma*, which means "tumor composed of muscle."

Oncology terms are introduced in this chapter because of their relation to cells and cell abnormalities. This is an introductory list only. **More oncology terms appear in subsequent chapters and are presented with the introduction of the related body systems.**

Disease and Disorder Oncology Terms

> Medical terms built from word parts can be translated literally to find their meanings. The terms are learned by completing all of the analyzing, defining, and word-building exercises.

TNM STAGING SYSTEM OF CANCER

AJCC (American Joint Commission on Cancer) has devised a classification widely used to stage certain types of cancer properly.

T refers to size and the extent of the primary tumor (ranked 0-4).

N denotes the involvement of the lymph nodes (ranked 0-4).

M defines whether there is metastasis (0 = none; 1 = present).

For example, T_2 N_1 M_0

T_2 refers to the primary tumor of 2 cm.

N_1 means spread of tumor to ipsilateral (same side) lymph nodes.

M_0 means no distant metastasis.

This system helps communicate the extent of cancer and is frequently cited by oncologists, surgeons, and radiation oncologists.

Built from Word Parts

The following terms are built from word parts you have already learned and can be translated literally to find their meanings. Further explanation of terms beyond the definition of their word parts, if needed, is included in parentheses. At first the list of terms may seem long to you; however, many of the word parts are repeated in many of the words. You will soon find that knowing parts of the terms makes learning the words easy. **Analyzing, defining,** and **word building exercises** are used to learn these terms and their meanings.

Term	Definition
adenocarcinoma (*ad*-e-nō-*kar*-si-NŌ-ma)	cancerous tumor of glandular tissue
adenoma (ad-e-NŌ-ma)	tumor composed of glandular tissue (benign)
carcinoma (CA) (*kar*-si-NŌ-ma)	cancerous tumor (malignant) (Exercise Figure C)
chloroma (klo-RŌ-ma)	tumor of green color (malignant, arising from myeloid tissue)
epithelioma (*ep*-i-*thē*-lē-Ō-ma)	tumor composed of epithelium (may be benign or malignant)
fibroma (fī-BRŌ-ma)	tumor composed of fiber (fibrous tissue) (benign)

Term	Definition
fibrosarcoma (fī-brō-sar-KŌ-ma)	malignant tumor composed of fiber (fibrous tissue)
leiomyoma (*lī*-ō-mī-Ō-ma)	tumor composed of smooth muscle (benign)
leiomyosarcoma (*lī*-ō-*mī*-ō-sar-KŌ-ma)	malignant tumor of smooth muscle
lipoma (li-PŌ-ma)	tumor composed of fat (benign tumor)
liposarcoma (*lip*-ō-sar-KŌ-ma)	malignant tumor of fat
melanocarcinoma (*mel*-a-nō-*kar*-si-NŌ-ma)	cancerous black tumor (malignant)
melanoma (mel-a-NŌ-ma)	black tumor (primarily of the skin) (Exercise Figure C)
myoma (mī-Ō-ma)	tumor composed of muscle (benign)
neoplasm (NĒ-ō-plazm)	new growth (of abnormal tissue or tumor)
neuroma (nū-RŌ-ma)	tumor composed of nerve (benign)
rhabdomyoma (*rab*-dō-mī-Ō-ma)	tumor composed of striated muscle (benign)
rhabdomyosarcoma (*rab*-dō-*mī*-ō-sar-KŌ-ma)	malignant tumor of striated muscle (Exercise Figure C)
sarcoma (sar-KŌ-ma) (NOTE: sarc/o also is presented in this chapter as a word root.)	tumor of connective tissue (such as bone or cartilage) (highly malignant) (Exercise Figure C)

EXERCISE 13

Practice saying aloud each of the disease and disorder oncology terms built from word parts on these two pages. Use Table 2-2, p. 37, for explanation of the pronunciation key.

To hear the terms, go to http://evolve.elsevier.com. Refer to p. 18 for your Evolve Access information. Select Exercises & Review, Chapter 2, Chapter Exercises, Pronunciation.

☐ Place a check mark in the box when you have completed this exercise.

EXERCISE FIGURE C

Fill in the blanks to complete labeling of these diagrams of types of cancers.

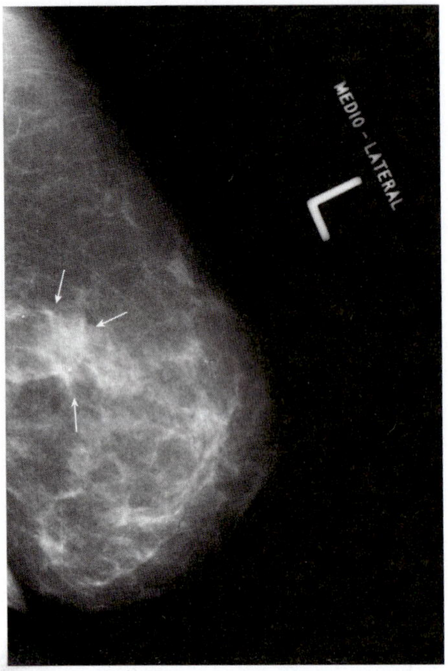

1. carcino / onco of the breast
   cancer / tumor

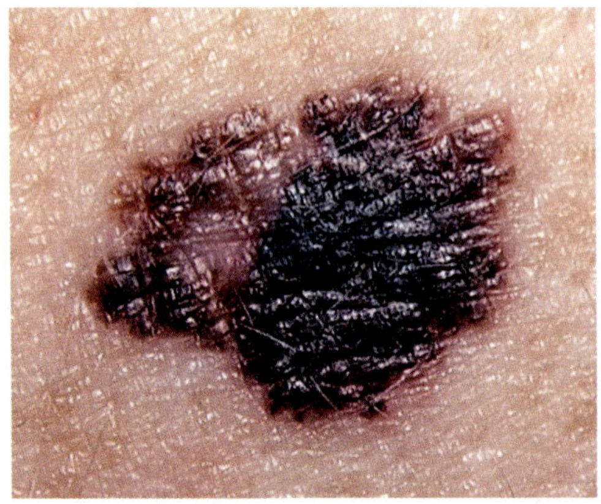

2. melano / onco
   black / tumor

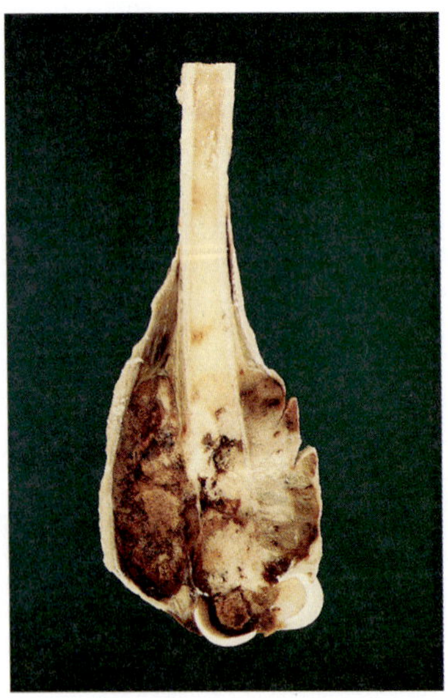

3. _______ / onco of the femur
   connective tissue / tumor

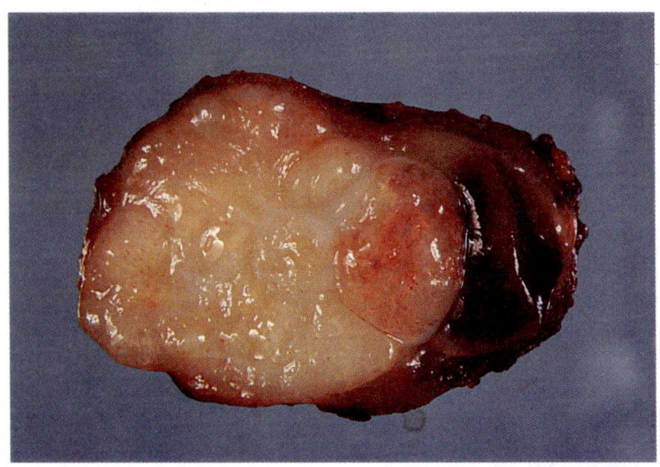

4. _______ / _____ / _______ / _____ / _______
   striated / cv / muscle / cv / malignant tumor

TABLE 2-2

Pronunciation Guide

Use the following guide for practicing pronunciation of the medical terms. The pronunciations are only approximate and there may be geographical variations in pronunciations.

In respelling for pronunciation, words are minimally distorted to indicate phonetic sound.

Example: doctor (dok-tor)
gastric (gas-trik)

A special mark called the macron (¯) is used to indicate the long vowel sounds.

Example: donate (dō-nāt)
hepatoma (hep-a-tō-ma)
ā as in *ate, say*
ē as in *eat, beet, see*
ī as in I, *mine, sky*
ō as in *oats, so*
ū as in *unit, mute*

Vowels with no markings have the short sound.

Example: discuss (dis-kus)
medical (med-i-kal)
a as in *at, lad*
e as in *edge, bet*
i as in *itch, wish*
o as in *ox, top*
u as in *sun, come*

An accent mark indicates the stress on a certain syllable. The primary accent is indicated by capital letters, and the secondary accent (which is stressed, but not as strongly as the primary accent) is indicated by italics.

Example: altogether (*all*-tū-GETH-er)
pancreatitis (*pan*-krē-a-TĪ-tis)

EXERCISE 14

Analyze and define the following disease and disorder oncology terms. Refer to Chapter 1, pp. 11-12, to review analyzing and defining techniques. **This is an important exercise; do not skip any portion of it.**

WR CV WR CV S
Example: lei / o / my / o / sarcoma <u>malignant tumor of smooth muscle</u>
CF CF

1. sarcoma sarc/oma
2. melanoma melan/oma
3. epithelioma epitheli/oma
4. lipoma lip/oma
5. neoplasm neo/plasm
6. myoma my/oma
7. neuroma neur/oma
8. carcinoma carcin/oma
9. melanocarcinoma melon/o/ carcin/oma
10. rhabdomyosarcoma rhabd/o/myo/sarcoma
11. leiomyoma lei/o/my/oma
12. rhabdomyoma rhabd/o/myo/ma
13. fibroma fibr/oma
14. liposarcoma lip/o/sarc/oma

15. fibrosarcoma fibr/o/sarcoma
16. adenoma aden/oma
17. adenocarcinoma aden/o/carcin/oma
18. chloroma chlor/oma

EXERCISE 15

Build medical disease and disorder oncology terms for the following definitions by using the word parts you have learned. If you need help, refer to p. 13 to review medical term building techniques. **Once again, this is an integral part of the learning process; do not skip any part of this exercise.**

Example: a tumor composed of fat lip / oma (WR / S)

1. black tumor melano / oma (WR / S)
2. cancerous tumor carcin / oma (WR / S)
3. new growth neo / genesis (P / S(WR))

When analyzing medical terms that have a suffix containing a word root, it may appear, as in the word **neoplasm,** that the term is composed of only a prefix and a suffix. Keep in mind that the word root is embedded in the suffix and is indicated in the *Building Medical Terms* exercises by S(WR).

4. tumor composed of epithelium epitheli / oma (WR / S)
5. tumor of connective tissue sarc / oma (WR / S)
6. cancerous black tumor melan / o / carcin / oma (WR / CV / WR / S)
7. tumor composed of nerve neur / oma (WR / S)
8. tumor composed of muscle my / oma (WR / S)
9. malignant tumor of striated muscle rhabd / o / my / o / sarcoma (WR / CV / WR / CV / S)
10. tumor composed of smooth muscle lei / o / my / oma (WR / CV / WR / S)
11. tumor composed of striated muscle rhabd / o / my / oma (WR / CV / WR / S)

12. malignant tumor of smooth muscle lei / o / my / o / sarcoma
WR / CV / WR / CV / S

13. malignant tumor of fat lip / o / sarcoma
WR / CV / S

14. tumor composed of fiber (fibrous tissue) fibr / oma
WR / S

15. malignant tumor of fiber (fibrous tissue) fibr / o / sarcoma
WR / CV / S

16. tumor composed of glandular tissue aden / oma
WR / S

17. cancerous tumor of glandular tissue aden / o / carcin / oma
WR / CV / WR / S

18. tumor of green color chlor / oma
WR / S

EXERCISE 16

Spell each of the disease and disorder oncology terms built from word parts on pp. 34-35 by having someone dictate them to you.

To hear and spell the terms, go to http://evolve.elsevier.com. Refer to p. 18 for your Evolve Access Information. Select Exercises & Review, Chapter 2, Chapter Exercises, Spelling.

☐ Place a check mark in the box if you have completed this exercise online.

You may type the terms on the screen or write them below in the spaces provided.

1.	______	11.	______
2.	______	12.	______
3.	______	13.	______
4.	______	14.	______
5.	______	15.	______
6.	______	16.	______
7.	______	17.	______
8.	______	18.	______
9.	______	19.	______
10.	______		

EXERCISE FIGURE D

Fill in the blanks to label this diagram of blood cells.

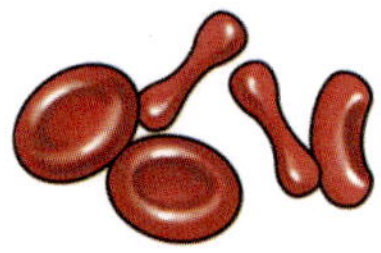

1. ______ red / cv / cell(s)

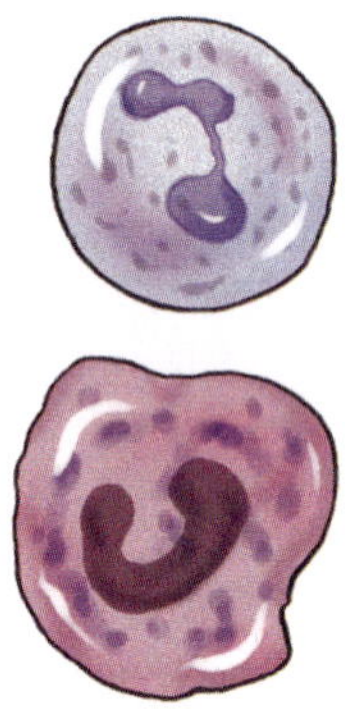

2. ______ white / cv / cell(s)

EXERCISE FIGURE E

Fill in the blanks to label the diagram.

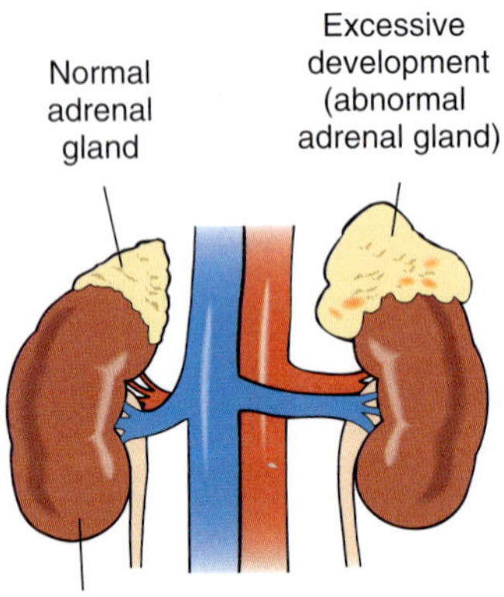

______ excessive / development

Body Structure Terms

Built from Word Parts

The following terms are built from word parts you have already learned and can be translated literally to find their meanings. Further explanation of terms beyond the definition of their word parts, if needed, is included in parentheses. By analyzing, defining, and building the terms in the exercises that follow, you will come to know the terms.

Term	Definition
cytogenic (*sī*-tō-JEN-ik)	producing cells
cytoid (SĪ-toid)	resembling a cell
cytology (*sī*-TOL-o-jē)	study of cells
cytoplasm (SĪ-tō-plazm)	cell substance
dysplasia (dis-PLĀ-zha)	abnormal development (see Figure 2-6, p. 50)
epithelial (*ep*-i-THĒ-lē-al)	pertaining to epithelium
erythrocyte (RBC) (e-RITH-rō-sīt)	red (blood) cell (Exercise Figure D)
erythrocytosis (e-*rith*-rō-sī-TŌ-sis)	increase in the number of red (blood) cells
histology (his-TOL-o-jē)	study of tissue
hyperplasia (*hī*-per-PLĀ-zha)	excessive development (number of cells) (Exercise Figure E) (see Figure 2-6, p. 50)
hypoplasia (hī-pō-PLĀ-zha)	incomplete development (of an organ or tissues)
karyocyte (KĀR-ē-ō-sīt)	cell with a nucleus
karyoplasm (KĀR-ē-ō-*plazm*)	substance of a nucleus
leukocyte (WBC) (LŪ-kō-sīt)	white (blood) cell (Exercise Figure D)
leukocytosis (*lū*-kō-sī-TŌ-sis)	increase in the number of white (blood) cells
lipoid (LIP-oid)	resembling fat

Ellipsis is the practice of omitting an essential part of a word by common consent. Note this practice in the terms **erythrocyte** (red **blood** cell) and **leukocyte** (white **blood** cell). The word root for blood is omitted.

Term	Definition
myopathy (mī-OP-a-thē)	disease of the muscle
neuroid (NŪ-rōyd)	resembling a nerve
somatic (sō-MAT-ik)	pertaining to the body
somatogenic (sō-ma-tō-JEN-ik)	originating in the body (organic as opposed to psychologic)
somatopathy (sō-ma-TOP-a-thē)	disease of the body
somatoplasm (sō-MAT-ō-plazm)	body substance
systemic (sis-TEM-ik)	pertaining to a (body) system (or the body as a whole)
visceral (VIS-er-al)	pertaining to the internal organs

COMPLEMENTARY AND ALTERNATIVE MEDICINE (CAM)

According to the National Institutes of Health, **CAM** is defined as "a group of diverse medical and healthcare systems, practices, and products that are not presently considered to be a part of conventional medicine."

Complementary medicine is used in conjunction with conventional medicine.

Alternative medicine is used in place of conventional medicine.

Integrative medicine is the combination of mainstream medical therapies and evidence-based CAM therapies. Use of CAM has increased dramatically in recent years as healthcare consumers search for a multitude of ways to treat illness and promote wellness.

CAM terms

Look for the CAM terms appearing throughout the text.

For a complete list of CAM terms, go to http:evolve.elsevier.com. Refer to p. 18 for your Evolve Access Information. Select **Appendices, Appendix G, Complementary and Alternative Medical Therapies.**

EXERCISE 17

Practice saying aloud each of the body structure terms built from word parts on pp. 40-41.

To hear the terms, go to http://evolve.elsevier.com. Refer to p. 18 for your Evolve Access Information. Select Exercises & Review, Chapter 2, Chapter Exercises, Pronunciation.

☐ Place a check mark in the box when you have completed this exercise.

EXERCISE 18

Analyze and define the following body structure terms.

Example: cyt / o / genic (WR CV S; cyt/o = CF) producing cells

1. cytology cyt/o/logy study of cells
2. histology hist/o/logy study of tissue
3. visceral vis/ceral pertaining to the internal organs
4. karyocyte kary/o/cyte cell with a neucleus
5. karyoplasm kary/o/plasm substance of a nucleus
6. systemic system/ic pertaining to a (body) system
7. cytoplasm cyt/o/plasm cell substance

8. somatic Somat/ic pertaining to the body
9. somatogenic Somat/o/genic originating in the body
10. somatoplasm Somat/o/plasm body substance
11. somatopathy Somat/o/pathy disease of the body
12. neuroid neur/oid resembling a nerve
13. myopathy my/o/pathy disease of the muscle
14. erythrocyte erythr/o/cyte red blood cell
15. leukocyte leuk/o/cyte white blood cell
16. epithelial epitheli/al pertaining to epithelium
17. lipoid lip/oid resembling fat
18. hyperplasia hyper/plasia excessive development
19. erythrocytosis erythr/o/cyt/o/sis increase the # of red blood cells
20. leukocytosis leuk/o/cyt/o/sis increase the # of white blood cells
21. hypoplasia hypo/plasia incomplete development
22. cytoid cyt/oid resembling a cell
23. dysplasia dys/plasia abnormal development

EXERCISE 19

Build medical terms for the following body structure definitions by using the word parts you have learned.

Example: producing cells cyt / o / genic (WR / CV / S)

1. cell substance Cyt / o / plasm (WR / CV / S)
2. substance of a nucleus kary / o / plasm (WR / CV / S)
3. pertaining to the body Somat / ic (WR / S)
4. disease of the muscle my / o / pathy (WR / CV / S)
5. body substance Somat / o / plasm (WR / CV / S)
6. pertaining to the internal organs viscer / al (WR / S)

7. originating in the body somat / o / genic
WR /CV/ S

8. disease of the body somat / o / pathy
WR /CV/ S

9. red (blood) cell erythr / o / cyte
WR /CV/ S

10. resembling a nerve cyt / oid
WR / S

11. pertaining to a (body) system systom / ic
WR / S

12. white (blood) cell leuk / o / cyte
WR /CV/ S

13. cell with a nucleus kary / o / cyte
WR /CV/ S

14. resembling fat lip / oid
WR / S

15. study of cells cyt / o / logy
WR /CV/ S

16. excessive development (of cells) hyper / plasia
P / S(WR)

17. resembling a cell cyt / oid
WR / S

18. pertaining to epithelium epitheli / al
WR / S

19. study of tissue hist / o / logy
WR /CV/ S

20. increase in the number of red (blood) cells erythr / o / cyt / osis
WR /CV/ WR / S

21. incomplete development (of an organ or tissue) hypo / plasia
P / S(WR)

22. increase in the number of white (blood) cells leuk / o / cyt / osis
WR /CV/ WR / S

23. abnormal development dys / plasia
P / S(WR)

EXERCISE 20

Spell each of the body structure terms built from word parts on pp. 40-41 by having someone dictate them to you.

To hear and spell the terms, go to http://evolve.elsevier.com. Refer to p. 18 for your Evolve Access Informatiion. Select Exercises & Review, Chapter 2, Chapter Exercises, Spelling.
☐ Place a check mark in the box if you have completed this exercise online.

1.	____________	13.	____________
2.	____________	14.	____________
3.	____________	15.	____________
4.	____________	16.	____________
5.	____________	17.	____________
6.	____________	18.	____________
7.	____________	19.	____________
8.	____________	20.	____________
9.	____________	21.	____________
10.	____________	22.	____________
11.	____________	23.	____________
12.	____________	24.	____________

Complementary Terms

Complementary terms complete the vocabulary presented in the chapter by describing **signs, symptoms, medical specialties, specialists,** and **related words.**

Built from Word Parts

The following terms are built from word parts you have already learned and can be translated literally to find their meanings. Further explanation of terms beyond the definition of their word parts, if needed, is included in parentheses.

SIGNS AND SYMPTOMS

A **sign** is objective information and is detected on physical examination such as observation that the patient has **cyanosis of the nail beds.**

A **symptom** is subjective information; it is what patients say about themselves such as stating the feeling of **pain in their chest while walking.**

Term	Definition
cancerous (KAN-ser-us)	pertaining to cancer
carcinogen (kar-SIN-o-jen)	substance that causes cancer
carcinogenic (*kar*-sin-ō-JEN-ik)	producing cancer
cyanosis (*sī*-a-NŌ-sis)	abnormal condition of blue (bluish discoloration of the skin caused by inadequate supply of oxygen in the blood) (Figure 2-3)

Term	Definition
diagnosis (Dx) (*dī*-ag-NŌ-sis)	state of complete knowledge (identifying a disease)
etiology (*ē*-tē-OL-o-jē)	study of causes (of diseases)
iatrogenic (ī-*at*-rō-JEN-ik)	produced by a physician (the unexpected results from a treatment prescribed by a physician)
iatrology (*ī*-a-TROL-o-jē)	study of medicine
metastasis (mets) **(*pl.* metastases)** (me-TAS-ta-sis) (me-TAS-ta-sēz)	beyond control (spread of disease from one organ to another, as in the transfer of malignant tumors) (Figure 2-4)
neopathy (nē-OP-a-thē)	new disease
oncogenic (*ong*-kō-JEN-ik)	causing tumors
oncologist (ong-KOL-o-jist)	a physician who studies and treats tumors
oncology (ong-KOL-o-jē)	study of tumors (a branch of medicine concerned with the study of malignant tumors)
organic (or-GAN-ik)	pertaining to an organ
organoid (OR-ga-noid)	resembling an organ
pathogenic (path-ō-JEN-ik)	producing disease
pathologist (pa-THOL-o-jist)	a physician who studies diseases (examines biopsies and performs autopsies to determine the cause of disease or death)
pathology (pa-THOL-o-jē)	study of disease (a branch of medicine dealing with the study of the causes of disease and death)
prognosis (Px) (prog-NŌ-sis)	state of before knowledge (prediction of the outcome of disease)
xanthochromic (*zan*-thō-KRŌ-mik)	pertaining to yellow color
xanthosis (zan-THŌ-sis)	abnormal condition of yellow (discoloration)

ONCOLOGY AND ONCOLOGIC

are used to name the medical specialty and healthcare nursing units devoted to the treatment and care of cancer patients.

PROGNOSIS

was used by Hippocrates to mean the same then as now: ***to foretell the course of a disease.***

The suffix **-logist** many indicate a specialist such as in **psychologist who is not a physician** or a specialist such as in **oncologist who is physician.** For learning purposes in the text, if the specialist is a physician, it will be indicated in the definition such as **oncologist . . . a physician who studies and treats tumors.**

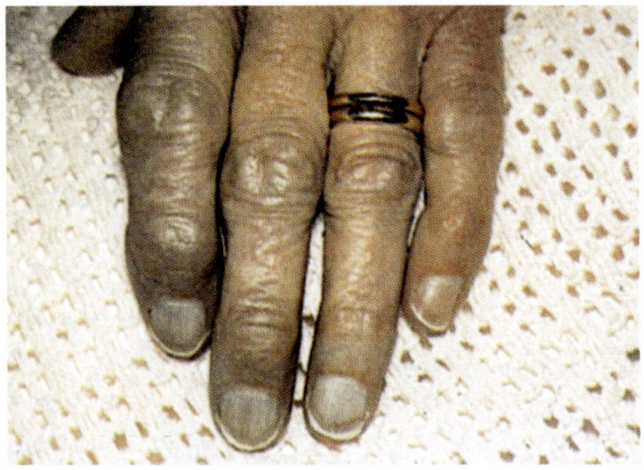

FIGURE 2-3
Cyanosis in an elderly patient.

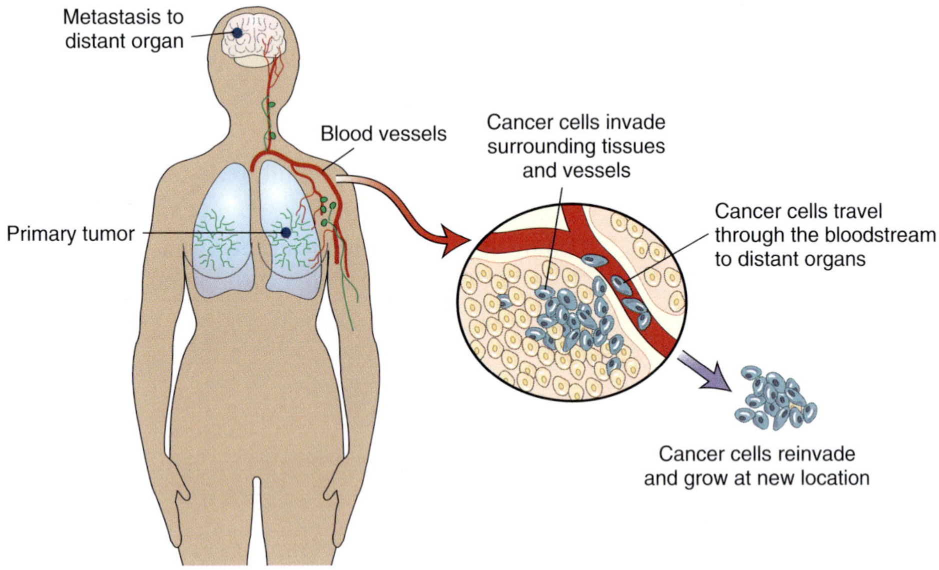

FIGURE 2-4
Metastasis.

EXERCISE 21

Practice saying aloud each of the complementary terms built from word parts on pp. 44-45.

To hear the terms, go to http://evolve.elsevier.com. Refer to p. 18 for your Evolve Access Information. Select Exercises & Review, Chapter 2, Chapter Exercises, Pronunciation.

☐ Place a check mark in the box when you have completed this exercise.

EXERCISE 22

Analyze and define the following complementary terms.

Example: path / o / genic (WR CV S; path/o = CF) *producing disease*

1. pathology ______________________
2. pathologist ______________________

3. metastasis ______________________________
4. oncogenic ______________________________
5. oncology ______________________________
6. neopathy ______________________________
7. cancerous ______________________________
8. carcinogenic ______________________________
9. cyanosis ______________________________
10. etiology ______________________________
11. xanthosis ______________________________
12. xanthochromic ______________________________
13. carcinogen ______________________________
14. oncologist ______________________________
15. prognosis ______________________________
16. organic ______________________________
17. diagnosis ______________________________
18. iatrogenic ______________________________
19. iatrology ______________________________
20. organoid ______________________________

EXERCISE 23

Build medical terms for the following definitions of complementary terms by using the word parts you have learned.

Example: producing disease path / o / genic
WR / CV / S

1. pertaining to yellow color ______ / ______ / ______ / ______
WR / CV / WR / S

2. beyond control ______ / ______
P / S(WR)

3. new disease ______ / ______
P / S(WR)

4. study of the cause (of disease) ______ / ______ / ______
WR / CV / S

5. study of tumors ______ / ______ / ______
WR / CV / S

6. study of diseases ______ / ______ / ______
WR / CV / S

7. a physician who studies diseases ______ / ______ / ______
WR / CV / S

8. abnormal condition of yellow ______ / ______
WR / S

9. causing tumors ______ / ______ / ______
WR / CV / S

10. pertaining to cancer ______ / ______
WR / S

11. abnormal condition of blue ______ / ______
WR / S

12. producing cancer ______ / ______ / ______
WR / CV / S

13. substance that causes cancer ______ / ______ / ______
WR / CV / S

14. physician who studies and treats tumors ______ / ______ / ______
WR / CV / S

15. study of medicine ______ / ______ / ______
WR / CV / S

16. pertaining to an organ ______ / ______
WR / S

17. state of complete knowledge ______ / ______ / ______
P / WR / S

18. produced by a physician ______ / ______ / ______
WR / CV / S

19. state of before knowledge ______ / ______ / ______
P / WR / S

20. resembling an organ ______ / ______
WR / S

EXERCISE 24

Spell each of the complementary terms built from word parts on pp. 44-45 by having someone dictate them to you.

To hear and spell the terms, go to http://evolve.elsevier.com. Refer to p. 18 for your Evolve Access Information. Select Exercises & Review, Chapter 2, Chapter Exercises, Spelling.

☐ Place a check mark in the box if you have completed this exercise online.

1. ______
2. ______
3. ______
4. ______
5. ______
6. ______
7. ______
8. ______
9. ______
10. ______
11. ______
12. ______
13. ______
14. ______
15. ______
16. ______
17. ______
18. ______
19. ______
20. ______

Complementary Terms
Not Built from Word Parts

Medical terms not built from word parts cannot be translated literally to find their meanings. ***The terms are learned by memorizing the whole word*** by using recall and spelling exercises.

The terms in this list are not built from word parts. The terms are commonly used in the medical world and you will need to know them. *In some of the words, you may recognize a word part; however, these terms cannot be literally translated to find the meaning.* New knowledge may have changed the meanings of the terms since they were coined; some terms are eponyms, some are acronyms, and some have no apparent explanation for their names. Memorization is used in the following exercises to learn the terms.

Term	Definition
benign (be-NĪN)	not malignant, nonrecurrent, favorable for recovery (Figure 2-5)
carcinoma in situ (kar-si-NŌ-ma) (in SĪ-too)	cancer in the early stage before invading surrounding tissue (Figure 2-6)
chemotherapy (chemo) (kē-mō-THER-a-pē)	treatment of cancer with drugs (Figure 2-7)
encapsulated (en-KAP-sū-lā-ted)	enclosed in a capsule, as with benign tumors (Figure 2-8)
exacerbation (eg-*zas*-er-BĀ-shun)	increase in the severity of a disease or its symptoms
idiopathic (*id*-ē-ō-PATH-ik)	pertaining to disease of unknown origin
inflammation (in-fla-MĀ-shun)	response to injury or destruction of tissue characterized by redness, swelling, heat, and pain
in vitro (in) (VĒ-trō)	within a glass, observable within a test tube
in vivo (in) (VĒ-vō)	within the living body
malignant (ma-LIG-nant)	tending to become progressively worse and to cause death, as in cancer (Figure 2-5)
radiation therapy (XRT) (*rā*-dē-Ā-shun) (THER-a-pē)	treatment of cancer with a radioactive substance, x-ray, or radiation (also called **radiation oncology** and **radiotherapy**) (Figure 2-9)
remission (rē-MISH-un)	improvement or absence of signs of disease

Inflammatory and **inflammation** are spelled with two *m's. Inflame* and *inflamed* have one *m.*

CANCER THERAPIES

Neoadjuvant therapy is a cancer treatment that precedes other treatment, such as administering chemotherapy or radiation therapy to a patient before surgery.

Adjuvant chemotherapy is the use of chemotherapy after or in combination with another form of cancer treatment such as administering chemotherapy after surgery or with radiation therapy.

Brachytherapy is the use of radiotherapy in which the source of radiation is placed within or close to the area being treated, such as implantation of radiation sources into the breast to treat cancer.

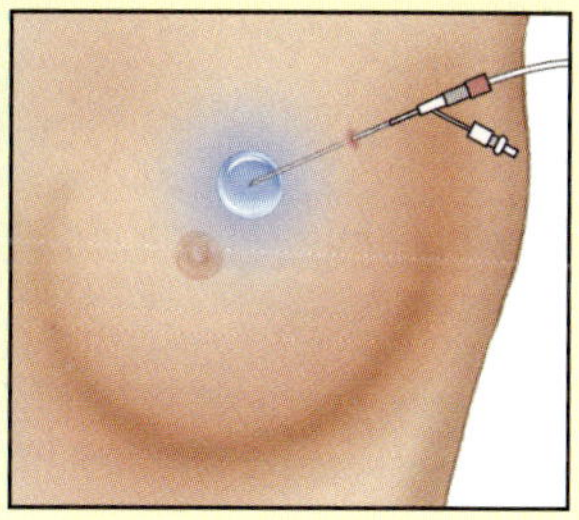

IDIOPATHIC

is derived from the Greek word **idios** meaning ***one's own*** and **path** or ***disease***. The term probably originated from the idea that disease of unknown origin comes from within oneself and is not acquired from without.

MALIGNANT

is derived from the Latin word root **mal** meaning ***bad***, as used in **malicious**, **malaise**, **malady**, and **malign**.

BENIGN

is derived from the Latin word root **bene,** meaning **well** or **good,** as used in **benefit** or **benefactor.**

SITU

is from the Latin term **situs,** which means **position** or **place.** Think of **in situ** as meaning "in place" or "not wandering around."

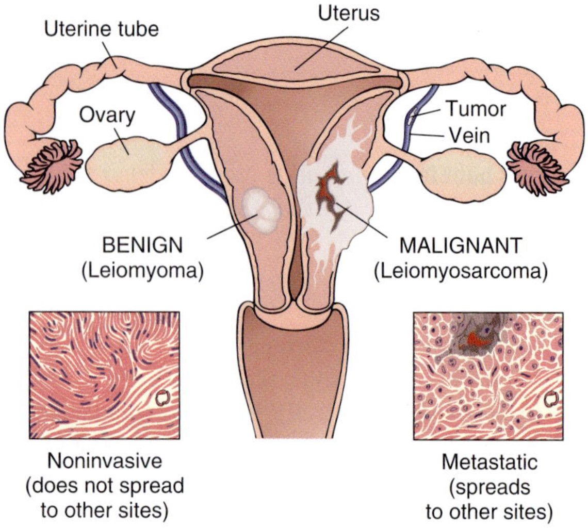

FIGURE 2-5
Examples of benign and malignant tumors.

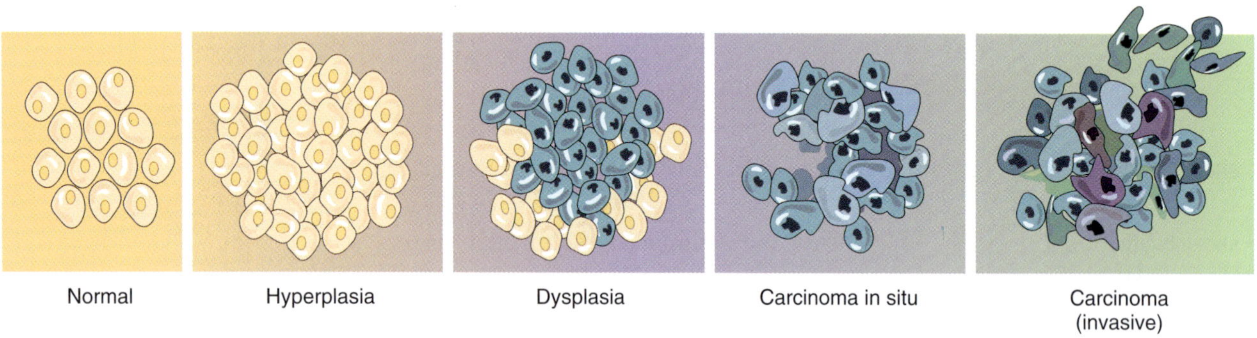

FIGURE 2-6
Progression of cell growth.

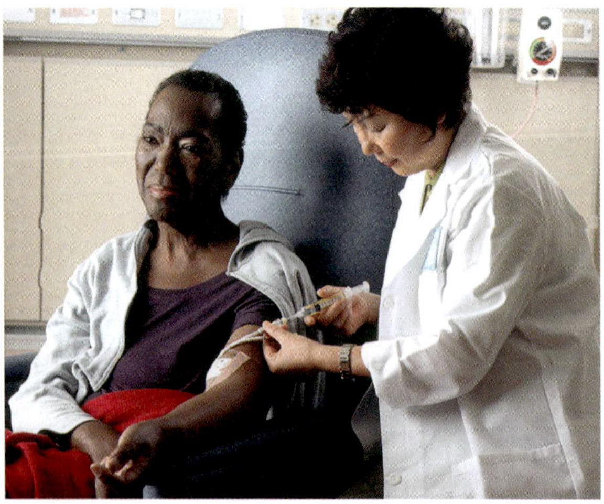

FIGURE 2-7
A patient receiving intravenous chemotherapy. Chemotherapy may also be administered orally in pill form.

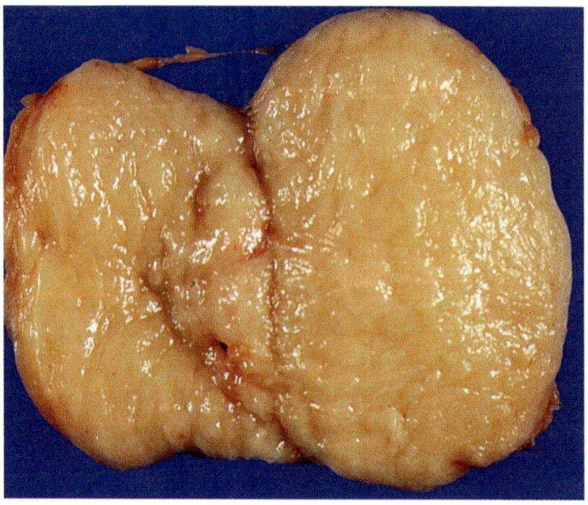

FIGURE 2-8
An encapsulated benign tumor.

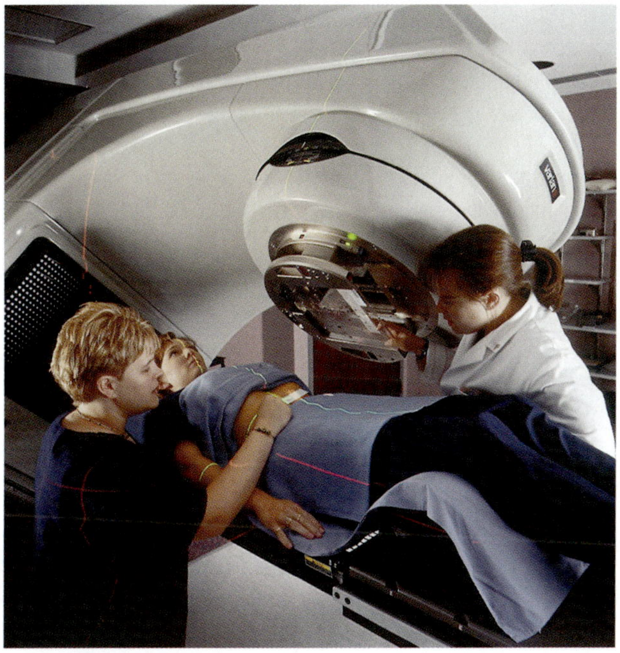

FIGURE 2-9
Radiation therapist preparing the patient for radiation therapy.

EXERCISE 25

Practice saying aloud each of the complementary terms not built from word parts on p. 49.

To hear the terms, go to http://evolve.elsevier.com. Refer to p. 18 for your Evolve Access Information. Select Exercises & Review, Chapter 2, Chapter Exercises, Pronunciation.

☐ Place a check mark in the box when you have completed this exercise.

EXERCISE 26

Write the definitions for the following terms.

1. benign __________
2. malignant __________
3. remission __________
4. idiopathic __________
5. inflammation __________
6. chemotherapy __________
7. radiation therapy __________
8. encapsulated __________
9. in vitro __________
10. in vivo __________
11. carcinoma in situ __________
12. exacerbation __________

EXERCISE 27

Spell each of the complementary terms not built from word parts on p. 49 by having someone dictate them to you.

To hear and spell the terms, go to http://evolve.elsevier.com. Refer to p. 18 for your Evolve Access Information. Select Exercises & Review, Chapter 2, Chapter Exercises, Spelling.

☐ Place a check mark in the box if you have completed this exercise online.

1. ______________________
2. ______________________
3. ______________________
4. ______________________
5. ______________________
6. ______________________
7. ______________________
8. ______________________
9. ______________________
10. ______________________
11. ______________________
12. ______________________

Refer to **Appendix D** for pharmacology terms related to oncology.

Plural Endings for Medical Terms

Most medical terms originate from Greek and Latin; therefore, plural endings differ from those used in English. Table 2-3, Common Plural Endings, lists the most common singular and plural endings used in medical terminology. When appropriate, both singular and plural endings are included in the word lists throughout the text, such as metastasis/metastases on p. 45.

TABLE 2-3
Common Plural Endings for Medical Terms

Singular Endings	Singular Form	Plural Formation	Plural Form
-a	vertebr**a** 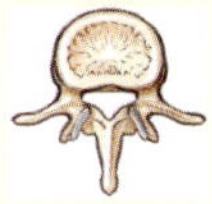	-ae	vertebr**ae** 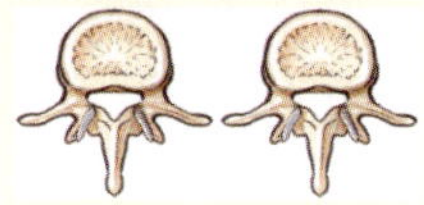
-ax	thor**ax** 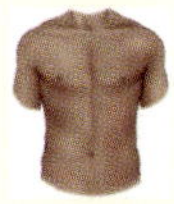	-aces	thor**aces** 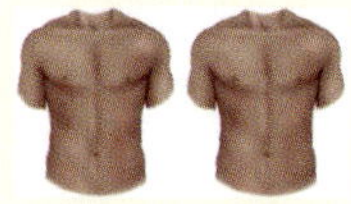
-is	test**is** 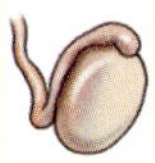	-es	test**es** 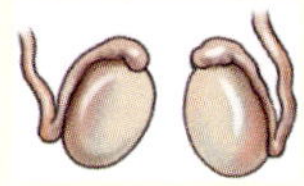
-ix	append**ix** 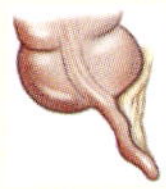	-ices	append**ices** 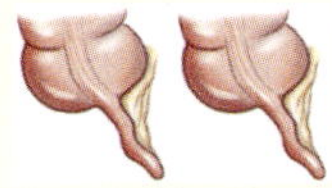
-ma	carcino**ma** 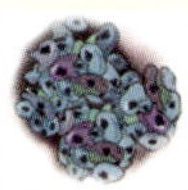	-mata	carcino**mata** 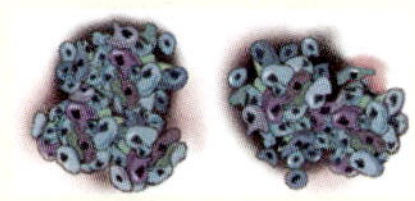
-on	gangli**on** 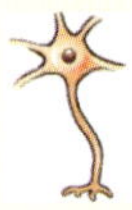	-a	gangli**a** 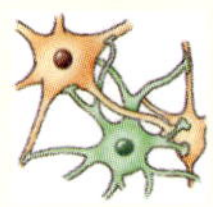
-sis	metasta**sis** 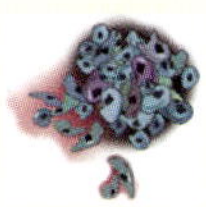	-ses	metasta**ses** 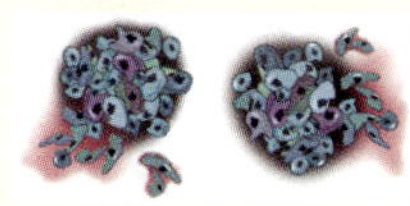
-um	ov**um** 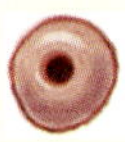	-a	ov**a** 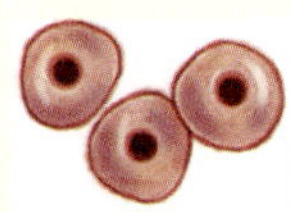
-us	fung**us** 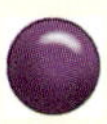	-i	fung**i** 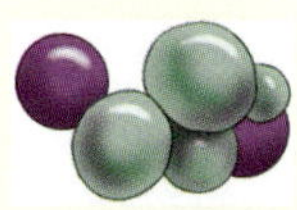
-nx	lary**nx** 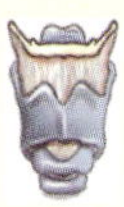	-nges	lary**nges** 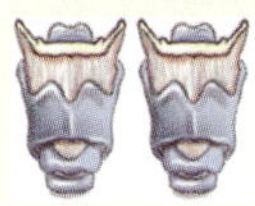
-y	biops**y** 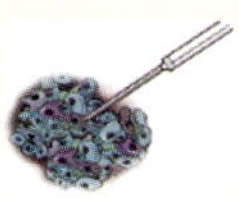	-ies	biops**ies** 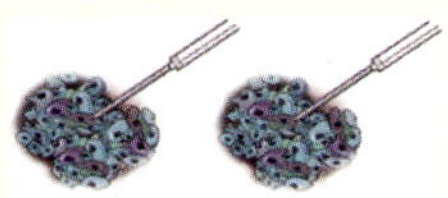

Complete the following exercises to become familiar with how plurals are formed. Do not be concerned about the meaning of these terms; concentrate only on the plural endings.

EXERCISE 28

Convert each of the following terms from singular to plural. Refer to Table 2-3, Plural Endings, on p. 53 for guidance.

1. etiology ______
2. *Staphylococcus* ______
3. cyanosis ______
4. bacterium ______
5. nucleus ______
6. pharynx ______
7. sarcoma ______
8. carcinoma ______
9. anastomosis ______
10. pubis ______
11. prognosis ______
12. spermatozoon ______
13. fimbria ______
14. thorax ______
15. appendix ______

EXERCISE 29

Circle the correct singular or plural form in each sentence.

1. During a colonoscopy the gastroenterologist noted that the patient had several (**diverticula, diverticulum**) in his transverse colon.
2. Bronchogenic carcinoma was diagnosed in the patient's left (**bronchus, bronchi**).
3. Bilateral (two sides) orchiditis is inflammation of the (**testes, testis**).
4. The light brown mole with notched borders turned out to be a (**melanomata, melanoma**).
5. Multiple (**embolus, emboli**) were observed on the lung scan.

6. Many (**diagnosis, diagnoses**) of benign tumors are picked up during whole-body scanning.
7. Diagnostic studies have shown (**metastasis, metastases**) of the patient's carcinoma of the breast to both her lungs and brain.

Abbreviations

Abbreviations are frequently used verbally and in writing to communicate in the medical and healthcare setting. Abbreviations of the terms included in the chapter are listed below.

CA	carcinoma
chemo	chemotherapy
Dx	diagnosis
mets	metastasis
Px	prognosis
RBC	red blood cell
XRT	radiation therapy
WBC	white blood cell

Abbreviations that are easily misinterpreted and may lead to medication errors are reported to the **Institute for Safe Medication Practice.** A list of these abbreviations is in **Appendix C** along with The Joint Commission's "do not use" list of abbreviations.

Refer to **Appendix C** for a complete list of abbreviations.

EXERCISE 30

Write the term for each of the abbreviations in the following paragraph.

A 55-year-old white woman was admitted to the oncology unit with a **Dx** _____________ of **CA** _____________ of the breast, **mets** _____________ to the lung. Her **Px** _____________ was guarded. Laboratory tests, including **RBC** _____________ _____________ _____________ and **WBC** _____________ _____________ _____________ counts, were ordered. She will receive both **chemo** _____________________________________ and **XRT** _____________ _____________.

PRACTICAL APPLICATION

EXERCISE 31 *Interact with Medical Documents*

A. Below is a physician's progress note. Complete the record by writing the medical terms in the blanks that correspond to the numbered definitions.

University Hospital and Medical Center
4700 North Main Street • Wellness, Arizona 54321 • (987) 555-3210

PATIENT NAME: Morris Greeley **CASE NUMBER:** 830293-ONC
DATE OF BIRTH: 08/03/19XX **DATE:** 02/12/20XX

PROGRESS NOTE

SUBJECTIVE: Mr. Greeley arrives today for a 1. ____________________ treatment for 2. ____________________ of the sigmoid colon.

He had an anterior sigmoid resection in October. 3. ____________________ study revealed 4. ____________________ tumor cells in two of six lymph nodes.

The 5FU/Leucovorin protocol is being administered weekly for 6 weeks. Today is his sixth infusion. We plan to start 5. ____________________ ____________________ after a 2-week hiatus from the chemotherapy.

The patient continues to do well and is receiving significant support from his family. He has had no hair loss, oral ulcerations, abdominal pain, nausea, or diarrhea.

OBJECTIVE: Vital signs show a temperature of 98. Pulse is 60. Respirations 20. Blood pressure is 152/65 mm Hg. His current weight is 183 pounds. HEENT: Tongue and pharynx are normal. PULMONARY: Clear to auscultation. HEART: Regular rate and rhythm without a murmur, rub, or gallop. ABDOMEN: Soft and nontender. No masses or organomegaly. EXTREMITIES: No edema or 6. ____________________.

ASSESSMENT:
1. Adenocarcinoma of the sigmoid colon with 7. ____________________ to regional lymph nodes.

PLAN:
1. 5FU/Leucovorin protocol as outlined above, treatment six of six today, followed by radiation therapy after 2-week period of rest.

____
Brian Smith, MD

BS/mcm

1. treatment of cancer by using drugs
2. cancerous tumor of glandular tissue
3. study of disease
4. tending to become progressively worse
5. treatment of cancer by using radioactive substance, x-rays, or radiation
6. abnormal condition of blue
7. beyond control

EXERCISE 31 *Interact with Medical Documents—cont'd*

B. Read the office visit report and answer the following questions.

49920 THATCH, MARTIN R.

File Patient Navigate Custom Fields Help

Patient Chart | Lab | Rad | Notes | Documents | Rx | Scheduling | Images | Billing

Name: **THATCH, MARTIN R.** MR#: **49920** Sex: **M**
DOB: **5/12/19XX**

POSTOPERATIVE OFFICE VISIT

ENCOUNTER DATE: 10/21/20XX

The patient is a 45-year-old white male who underwent removal of a 2.5 cm firm mass of the lateral portion of the proximal right thigh one week ago. Inspection of operative site shows a normal healing wound. Preoperative lab work showed a normal erythrocyte and leukocyte count. Histology of the surgical specimen revealed an encapsulated lipoma. The etiology of the lipoma is unknown, but it is definitely a benign lesion. His prognosis is excellent.

Electronically signed by: Ronald Bryan, MD 10/21/20XX 11:15 AM

Start | Log On/Off | Print | Edit

1. The firm mass was confirmed as a lipoma from the surgical specimen in which area of study?
   a. cell
   b. tissue
   c. blood
   d. plasma

2. The lipoma was
   a. spreading.
   b. enclosed in a capsule.
   c. inflamed.
   d. blue in color.

3. *Erythr* and *leuk* refer to the ____________ of cells.
   a. size
   b. shape
   c. amount
   d. color

4. Write the plural form of
   a. prognosis ____________________
   b. lipoma ____________________
   c. histology ____________________

EXERCISE 32 *Interpret Medical Terms*

To test your understanding of the terms introduced in this chapter, circle the words that correctly complete each sentence. The italicized words refer to the correct answer.

1. Mr. Roberts was diagnosed as having a cancerous *tumor of connective tissue*, or (**sarcoma, melanoma, lipoma**). The doctor said the tumor was *becoming progressively worse*; that is, it was (**benign, malignant, pathogenic**).
2. The blood test showed an *increased amount of red blood cells*, or (**erythrocytosis, leukocytosis, cyanosis**).
3. (**Organic, Visceral, Systemic**) means *pertaining to internal organs.*
4. A *tumor composed of fat*, or (**neuroma, carcinoma, lipoma**), is benign, or (**recurrent, nonrecurrent, cancerous**).
5. Many substances are thought to be *cancer producing*, or (**carcinogenic, carcinogen, cancerous**).
6. *Etiology* is the study of (**the causes of disease, tissue disease, the causes of tumors**).
7. A *tumor* may be called a (**cytoplasm, neoplasm, karyoplasm**).
8. The pain *originated in the body*, or was (**somatogenic, oncogenic, pathogenic**).
9. Any *disease of a muscle* is called (**myoma, myopathy, somatopathy**).
10. The term for *abnormal development* is (**hypoplasia, dysplasia, hyperplasia**).
11. The term that means *produced by a physician* is (**diagnosis, iatrogenic, prognosis**).
12. The incidence of malignant *black tumor* (**fibrosarcoma, fibroma, melanoma**) is increasing in the white population. One *study of disease* (**pathology, pathogenic, liposarcoma**) finding influencing *state of before knowledge* (**cancer in situ, in vitro, prognosis**) may be tumor thickness.
13. The term that means *within the living organism* is (**in vitro, in vivo, encapsulated**).
14. A (**liposarcoma, fibroma, myoma**) is a *malignant tumor.*
15. (**DNA, RBC, WBC**) regulates the *activities of a cell.*

EXERCISE 33 *Read Medical Terms in Use*

Practice pronunciation of terms by reading aloud the following medical document.

Use the pronunciation key after each medical term to assist you in saying the words. The script contains medical terms not yet presented. Treat them as information only; you will learn more about them as you continue to study. Or, if desired, look for their meanings in your medical dictionary.

To hear these terms go to http://evolve.elsevier.com. Refer to p. 18 for your Evolve Access Information. Select Exercises & Review, Chapter 2, Chapter Exercises, Read Medical Terms in Use.

A 54-year-old woman presented to the office with a 3-week history of bloody diarrhea. She had been diagnosed with ulcerative colitis at age 25 years. She was referred for a colonoscopy. The examination revealed a suspicious lesion in the transverse colon. A biopsy was performed and a **cytology** (sī-TOL-o-jē) specimen was obtained. The **pathologist** (pa-THOL-o-jist) made a **diagnosis** (dī-ag-NŌ-sis) of **carcinoma** (kar-si-NŌ-ma) of the colon. Advanced **dysplasia** (dis-PLĀ-zha) and **inflammation** (in-fla-MĀ-shun) existed in the specimen. The patient underwent surgery and was found to have no evidence of **metastasis** (me-TAS-ta-sis). Her entire colon was removed because of a high risk for developing a **malignant** (ma-LIG-nant) lesion in the remaining colon. She made an uneventful recovery and was referred to an **oncologist** (ong-KOL-o-jist) for consideration of **chemotherapy** (kē-mō-THER-a-pē). Her **prognosis** (prog-NŌ-sis) is generally positive. **Radiation therapy** (rā-dē-Ā-shun) (THER-a-pē) is not indicated in this case.

EXERCISE 34 *Comprehend Medical Terms in Use*

Test your comprehension of terms in the previous medical document by answering *T* for true and *F* for false.

______ 1. The cancer has spread from the colon to other surrounding organs.

______ 2. The specimen is described as having abnormal development.

______ 3. The patient's prognosis is carcinoma of the colon.

______ 4. The patient's colon was removed to avoid development of a malignant lesion in the remaining colon.

______ 5. The patient was referred to a pathologist for consideration of treatment for the cancer with drugs.

WEB LINK

For additional information on cancer visit the **National Cancer Institute** at *http://www.nci.nih.gov.*

CHAPTER REVIEW

ONLINE CHAPTER REVIEW

To access the Evolve website, go to http://evolve.elsevier.com. Refer to p. 18 for your Evolve Access Information. Select Exercises & Review, Chapter 2, then select Chapter Exercises, Practice Activities, Animations, or Games. Place a check mark in the box when you have completed an exercise or activity, watched an animation, or played a game. Have fun!

Chapter Exercises

Exercises in this section of your Evolve resources correlate to exercises in your textbook. You may have completed them as you worked through the chapter.

- ☐ Pronunciation
- ☐ Spelling
- ☐ Read Medical Terms in Use

Practice Activities

Practice in study mode, then test your learning in assessment mode. Keep track of your scores from assessment mode if you wish.

	SCORE
☐ Define Word Parts	______
☐ Plural Endings	______
☐ Analyze Medical Terms	______
☐ Build Medical Terms	______
☐ Define Medical Terms	______
☐ Use It	______
☐ Hear It and Type It: Clinical Vignettes	______

Animations

- ☐ Breast Cancer Metastasis
- ☐ Chemotherapy
- ☐ Neoplasms
- ☐ Radiation Therapy

Games

- ☐ Name that Word Part
- ☐ Term Storm
- ☐ Termbusters
- ☐ Medical Millionaire
- ☐ Crossword puzzle

REVIEW OF WORD PARTS

Can you define and spell the following word parts?

Combining Forms

aden/o	erythr/o	leuk/o	rhabd/o
cancer/o	eti/o	lip/o	sarc/o
carcin/o	fibr/o	melan/o	somat/o
chlor/o	gno/o	my/o	system/o
chrom/o	hist/o	neur/o	viscer/o
cyan/o	iatr/o	onc/o	xanth/o
cyt/o	kary/o	organ/o	
epitheli/o	lei/o	path/o	

Prefixes	Suffixes		
dia-	-al	-logist	-pathy
dys-	-cyte	-logy	-plasia
hyper-	-gen	-oid	-plasm
hypo-	-genic	-oma	-sarcoma
meta-	-ic	-osis	-sis
neo-		-ous	-stasis
pro-			

REVIEW OF TERMS

Can you define, spell, and pronounce the following terms *built from word parts?*

Oncology	Body Structure	Complementary
adenocarcinoma	cytogenic	cancerous
adenoma	cytoid	carcinogen
carcinoma (CA)	cytology	carcinogenic
chloroma	cytoplasm	cyanosis
epithelioma	dysplasia	diagnosis (Dx)
fibroma	epithelial	etiology
fibrosarcoma	erythrocyte (RBC)	iatrogenic
leiomyoma	erythrocytosis	iatrology
leiomyosarcoma	histology	metastasis (mets)
lipoma	hyperplasia	neopathy
liposarcoma	hypoplasia	oncogenic
melanocarcinoma	karyocyte	oncologist
melanoma	karyoplasm	oncology
myoma	leukocyte (WBC)	organic
neoplasm	leukocytosis	organoid
neuroma	lipoid	pathogenic
rhabdomyoma	myopathy	pathologist
rhabdomyosarcoma	neuroid	pathology
sarcoma	somatic	prognosis (Px)
	somatogenic	xanthochromic
	somatopathy	xanthosis
	somatoplasm	
	systemic	
	visceral	

Can you define, pronounce, and spell the following terms *not built from word parts?*

Complementary

benign
carcinoma in situ
chemotherapy (chemo)
encapsulated
exacerbation
idiopathic
inflammation
in vitro
in vivo
malignant
radiation therapy (XRT)
remission

ANSWERS

Exercise Figures

Exercise Figure

A. 1. cell: cyt/o
2. tissue: hist/o
3. organ: organ/o
4. system: system/o

Exercise Figure

B. 1. neur/o
2. epitheli/o
3. sarc/o
4. my/o

Exercise Figure

C. 1. carcin/oma
2. melan/oma
3. sarc/oma
4. rhabd/o/my/o/sarcoma

Exercise Figure

D. 1. erythr/o/cyte
2. leuk/o/cyte

Exercise Figure

E. hyper/plasia

Exercise 1

1. h
2. e
3. d
4. k
5. g
6. f
7. c
8. a
9. b
10. j

Exercise 2

1. h
2. b
3. c
4. e
5. g
6. a
7. f

Exercise 3

1. flesh, connective tissue
2. fat
3. nucleus
4. internal organs
5. cell
6. tissue
7. muscle
8. nerve
9. organ
10. system
11. epithelium
12. fiber
13. gland

Exercise 4

1. viscer/o
2. epitheli/o
3. organ/o
4. kary/o
5. cyt/o
6. hist/o
7. neur/o
8. my/o
9. lip/o
10. system/o
11. sarc/o
12. fibr/o
13. aden/o

Exercise 5

1. tumor, mass
2. cancer
3. cause (of disease)
4. disease
5. body
6. cancer
7. rod-shaped, striated
8. smooth
9. knowledge
10. physician, medicine

Exercise 6

1. path/o
2. onc/o
3. eti/o
4. a. cancer/o
   b. carcin/o
5. somat/o
6. lei/o
7. rhabd/o
8. gno/o
9. iatr/o

Exercise 7

1. blue
2. red
3. white
4. yellow
5. color
6. black
7. green

Exercise 8

1. cyan/o
2. erythr/o
3. leuk/o
4. melan/o
5. xanth/o
6. chrom/o
7. chlor/o

Exercise 9

1. new
2. above, excessive
3. after, beyond, change
4. below, incomplete, deficient
5. painful, abnormal, difficult, labored
6. through, complete
7. before

Exercise 10

1. neo-
2. hyper-
3. hypo-
4. meta-
5. dys-
6. dia-
7. pro-

Exercise 11

1. i
2. l
3. e
4. f
5. g
6. j
7. h
8. b
9. c
10. n
11. k
12. p
13. m
14. a
15. o

Exercise 12

1. one who studies and treats (specialist, physician)
2. disease
3. study of
4. pertaining to
5. control, stop, standing
6. cell
7. abnormal condition
8. pertaining to
9. growth, substance, formation
10. pertaining to
11. condition of formation, development, growth
12. resembling
13. substance or agent that produces or causes
14. producing, originating, causing
15. tumor, swelling
16. malignant tumor
17. state of

Exercise 13

Pronunciation Exercise

Exercise 14

1. WR S
   sarc/oma
   tumor composed of connective tissue
2. WR S
   melan/oma
   black tumor
3. WR S
   epitheli/oma
   tumor composed of epithelium
4. WR S
   lip/oma
   tumor composed of fat
5. P S(WR)
   neo/plasm
   new growth
6. WR S
   my/oma
   tumor composed of muscle
7. WR S
   neur/oma
   tumor composed of nerve
8. WR S
   carcin/oma
   cancerous tumor
9. WR CV WR S
   melan/o/carcin/oma
   CF
   cancerous black tumor

10. WR CV WR CV S
rhabd/o/my/o/sarcoma
CF CF
malignant tumor of striated muscle

11. WRCVWR S
lei/o/my/oma
CF
tumor composed of smooth muscle

12. WR CV WR S
rhabd/o/my/oma
CF
tumor composed of striated muscle

13. WR S
fibr/oma
tumor composed of fiber (fibrous tissue)

14. WR CV S
lip/o/sarcoma
CF
malignant tumor of fat

15. WR CV S
fibr/o/sarcoma
CF
malignant tumor of fiber (fibrous tissue)

16. WR S
aden/oma
tumor composed of glandular tissue

17. WR CV WR S
aden/o/carcin/oma
CF
cancerous tumor composed of glandular tissue

18. WR S
chlor/oma
tumor of green color

Exercise 15

1. melan/oma
2. carcin/oma
3. neo/plasm
4. epitheli/oma
5. sarc/oma
6. melan/o/carcin/oma
7. neur/oma
8. my/oma
9. rhabd/o/my/o/sarcoma
10. lei/o/my/oma
11. rhabd/o/my/oma
12. lei/o/my/o/sarcoma
13. lip/o/sarcoma
14. fibr/oma
15. fibr/o/sarcoma
16. aden/oma
17. aden/o/carcin/oma
18. chlor/oma

Exercise 16

Spelling Exercise; see text p. 39.

Exercise 17

Pronunciation Exercise

Exercise 18

1. WR CV S
cyt/o/logy
CF
study of cells

2. WR CV S
hist/o/logy
CF
study of tissue

3. WR S
viscer/al
pertaining to internal organs

4. WR CV S
kary/o/cyte
CF
cell with a nucleus

5. WR CV S
kary/o/plasm
CF
substance of a nucleus

6. WR S
system/ic
pertaining to a (body) system

7. WR CV S
cyt/o/plasm
CF
cell substance

8. WR S
somat/ic
pertaining to the body

9. WR CV S
somat/o/genic
CF
originating in the body

10. WR CV S
somat/o/plasm
CF
body substance

11. WR CV S
somat/o/pathy
CF
disease of the body

12. WR S
neur/oid
resembling a nerve

13. WR CV S
my/o/pathy
CF
disease of the muscle

14. WR CV S
erythr/o/cyte
CF
red (blood) cell

15. WR CV S
leuk/o/cyte
CF
white (blood) cell

16. WR S
epitheli/al
pertaining to epithelium

17. WR S
lip/oid
resembling fat

18. P S(WR)
hyper/plasia
excessive development (of cells)

19. WR CV WR S
erythr/o/cyt/osis
CF
increase in the number of red (blood) cells

20. WR CV WR S
leuk/o/cyt/osis
CF
increase in the number of white (blood) cells

21. P S(WR)
hypo/plasia
incomplete development (of an organ or tissue)

22. WR S
cyt/oid
resembling a cell

23. P S(WR)
dys/plasia
abnormal development

Exercise 19

1. cyt/o/plasm
2. kary/o/plasm
3. somat/ic
4. my/o/pathy
5. somat/o/plasm
6. viscer/al
7. somat/o/genic
8. somat/o/pathy
9. erythr/o/cyte
10. neur/oid
11. system/ic
12. leuk/o/cyte
13. kary/o/cyte
14. lip/oid
15. cyt/o/logy
16. hyper/plasia
17. cyt/oid
18. epitheli/al
19. hist/o/logy
20. erythr/o/cyt/osis

21. hypo/plasia
22. leuk/o/cyt/osis
23. dys/plasia

Exercise 20

Spelling Exercise; see text pp. 40-41.

Exercise 21

Pronunciation Exercise

Exercise 22

1. WR CV S
   path/o/logy
   CF
   study of disease
2. WR CV S
   path/o/logist
   CF
   a physician who studies diseases
3. P S(WR)
   meta/stasis
   beyond control (transfer of disease)
4. WR CV S
   onc/o/genic
   CF
   causing tumors
5. WR CV S
   onc/o/logy
   CF
   study of tumors
6. P S(WR)
   neo/pathy
   new disease
7. WR S
   cancer/ous
   pertaining to cancer
8. WR CV S
   carcin/o/genic
   CF
   producing cancer
9. WR S
   cyan/osis
   abnormal condition of blue (bluish discoloration of the skin)
10. WR CV S
    eti/o/logy
    CF
    study of causes (of disease)
11. WR S
    xanth/osis
    abnormal condition of yellow
12. WR CV WR S
    xanth/o/chrom/ic
    CF
    pertaining to yellow color
13. WR CV S
    carcin/o/gen
    CF
    substance that causes cancer
14. WR CV S
    onc/o/logist
    CF
    physician who studies and treats tumors
15. P WR S
    pro/gno/sis
    state of before knowledge
16. WR S
    organ/ic
    pertaining to an organ
17. P WR S
    dia/gno/sis
    state of complete knowledge
18. WR CV S
    iatr/o/genic
    CF
    produced by a physician
19. WR CV S
    iatr/o/logy
    CF
    study of medicine
20. WR S
    organ/oid
    resembling an organ

Exercise 23

1. xanth/o/chrom/ic
2. meta/stasis
3. neo/pathy
4. eti/o/logy
5. onc/o/logy
6. path/o/logy
7. path/o/logist
8. xanth/osis
9. onc/o/genic
10. cancer/ous
11. cyan/osis
12. carcin/o/genic
13. carcin/o/gen
14. onc/o/logist
15. iatr/o/logy
16. organ/ic
17. dia/gno/sis
18. iatr/o/genic
19. pro/gno/sis
20. organ/oid

Exercise 24

Spelling Exercise; see text pp. 44-45.

Exercise 25

Pronunciation Exercise

Exercise 26

1. not malignant, nonrecurrent, favorable for recovery
2. tending to become progressively worse and to cause death, as in cancer
3. improvement or absence of signs of disease
4. pertaining to disease of unknown origin
5. response to injury or destruction of tissue; signs are redness, swelling, heat, and pain
6. treatment of cancer with drugs
7. treatment of cancer with radioactive substance, such as x-ray or radiation
8. enclosed in a capsule, as in benign tumors
9. within a glass, observable within a test tube
10. within the living body
11. cancer in the early stage before invading the surrounding tissue
12. increase in the severity of a disease or its symptoms

Exercise 27

Spelling Exercise; see text p. 49.

Exercise 28

1. etiologies
2. staphylococci
3. cyanoses
4. bacteria
5. nuclei
6. pharynges
7. sarcomata
8. carcinomata
9. anastomoses
10. pubes
11. prognoses
12. spermatozoa
13. fimbriae
14. thoraces
15. appendices

Exercise 29

1. diverticula
2. bronchus
3. testes
4. melanoma
5. emboli
6. diagnoses
7. metastases

Exercise 30

diagnosis; carcinoma; metastasis; prognosis; red blood cell; white blood cell; chemotherapy; radiation therapy

Exercise 31

A. 1. chemotherapy
2. adenocarcinoma
3. pathology
4. malignant
5. radiation therapy
6. cyanosis
7. metastasis

Exercise 31

B. 1. b
2. b
3. d
4. a. prognoses
b. lipomata
c. histologies

Exercise 32

1. sarcoma, malignant
2. erythrocytosis
3. visceral
4. lipoma, nonrecurrent
5. carcinogenic
6. causes of disease
7. neoplasm
8. somatogenic
9. myopathy
10. dysplasia
11. iatrogenic
12. melanoma, pathology, prognosis
13. in vivo
14. liposarcoma
15. DNA

Exercise 33

Reading Exercise

Exercise 34

1. *F,* "no evidence of metastasis" (transfer of disease from one organ to another) means the cancer has not spread to surrounding organs.
2. *T*
3. *F,* prognosis means "prediction of the outcome of disease"; diagnosis means "identifying a disease."
4. *T*
5. *F,* an oncologist treats patients with cancer; a pathologist studies body changes caused by disease usually from a specimen in a laboratory setting.

Chapter 3

Directional Terms, Planes, Positions, Regions, and Quadrants

OUTLINE

OBJECTIVES

Upon completion of this chapter you will be able to:

1. Define and spell word parts related to directional terms.
2. Define, pronounce, and spell terms used to describe directions with respect to the body.
3. Define, pronounce, and spell terms used to describe anatomic planes.
4. Define, pronounce, and spell terms used to describe body positions.
5. Define, pronounce, and spell terms used to describe abdominopelvic regions.
6. Identify and spell the four abdominopelvic quadrants.
7. Interpret the meaning of abbreviations presented in this chapter.
8. Interpret, read, and comprehend medical language in simulated medical statements and documents.

Types of body movement are presented in Chapter 14, Musculoskeletal System, on page 634. Terms related to body movement are: *abduction*, *adduction*, *inversion*, *eversion*, *extension*, *flexion*, *pronation*, *supination*, and *rotation*.

ANATOMIC POSITION

In the description and use of body directions and planes, the body is assumed to be in the standard, neutral position of reference called the *anatomic position.* In this position, the body is viewed as standing erect, arms at the side, palms of the hands facing forward, and feet placed side by side (Figure 3-1).

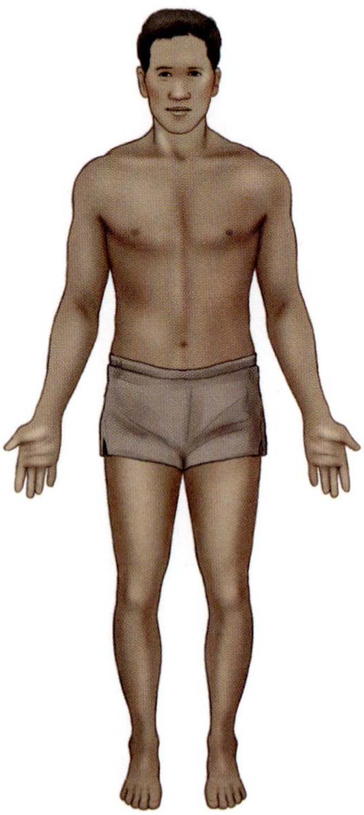

FIGURE 3-1
Anatomic position.

WORD PARTS

Combining Forms of Directional Terms

Word parts you need to learn to complete this chapter are listed on the following pages. The exercises at the end of each list will help you learn their definitions and spelling.

Use the flashcards accompanying this text or electronic flashcards to assist you in memorizing the word parts for this chapter.

To use electronic flashcards, go to http://evolve.elsevier.com. Refer to p. 18 for your Evolve Access Information. Select Flashcards, Chapter 3.

Combining Form	Definition
anter/o	front
caud/o	tail (downward)
cephal/o	head (upward)
dist/o	away (from the point of attachment of a body part)
dors/o	back
infer/o	below
later/o	side
medi/o	middle
poster/o	back, behind
proxim/o	near (the point of attachment of a body part)
super/o	above
ventr/o	belly (front)

EXERCISE 1

Write the definitions for the following combining forms. *To check your answers to the exercises in this chapter, go to Answers, p. 93, at the end of the chapter.*

1. ventr/o ____________
2. cephal/o ____________
3. later/o ____________
4. medi/o ____________
5. infer/o ____________
6. proxim/o ____________
7. super/o ____________
8. dist/o ____________
9. dors/o ____________
10. caud/o ____________
11. anter/o ____________
12. poster/o ____________

EXERCISE FIGURE A

Fill in the blanks with directional combining forms. *To check your answers, go to p. 93.*

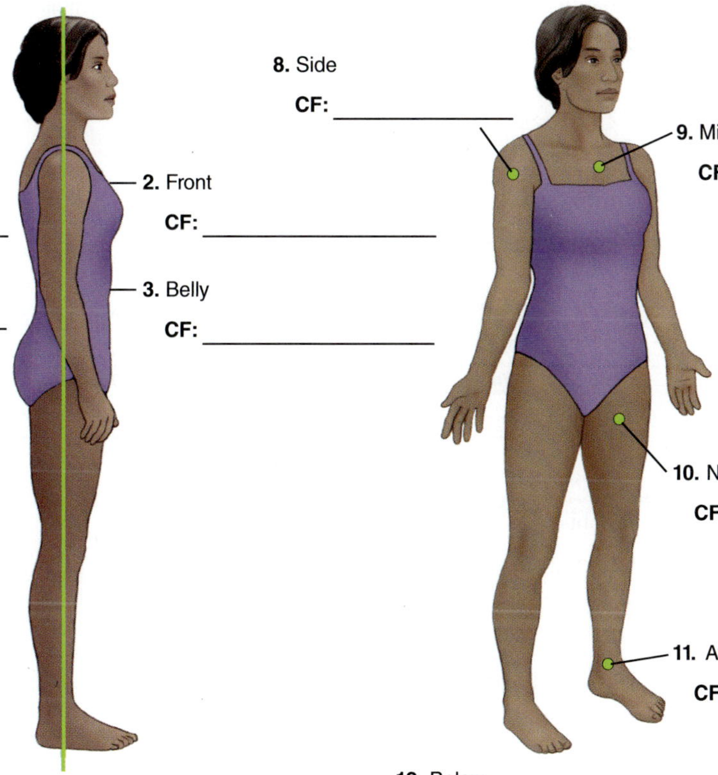

Prefixes

Prefix	Definition
bi-	two
uni-	one

Suffixes

Suffix	Definition
-ad	toward
-ior	pertaining to

Refer to **Appendix A** and **Appendix B** for alphabetized lists of word parts and their meanings.

Many suffixes mean **pertaining to.** You have already learned three of them in Chapter 2: **-al, -ic,** and **-ous.** You will learn more in subsequent chapters. With practice, you will learn which suffix is most commonly used with a particular word root or combining form.

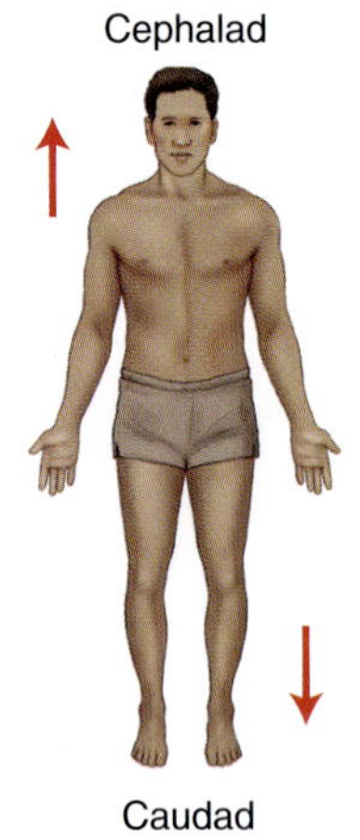

FIGURE 3-2
Caudad and cephalad.

EXERCISE 2

Match the prefixes and suffixes in the first column with their correct definitions in the second column.

_____ 1. -ad	a. one
_____ 2. -ior	b. pertaining to
_____ 3. bi-	c. toward
_____ 4. uni-	d. two

EXERCISE 3

Write the definitions of the following prefixes and suffixes.

1. -ior ____________________
2. -ad ____________________
3. bi- ____________________
4. uni- ____________________

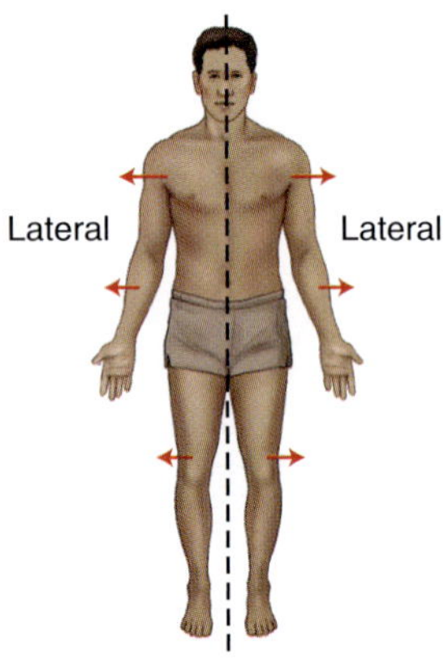

FIGURE 3-3
Lateral.

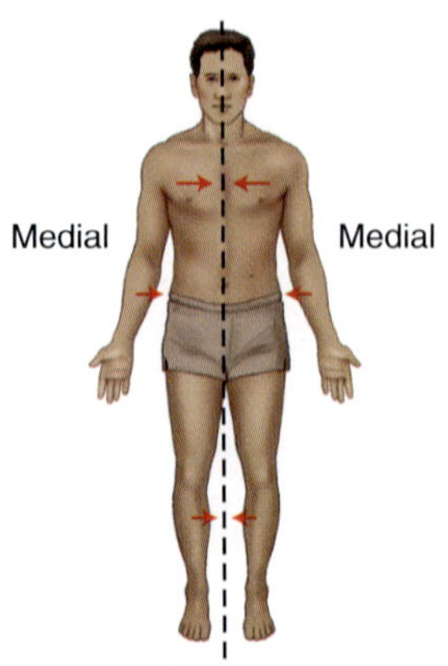

FIGURE 3-4
Medial.

MEDICAL TERMS

Directional Terms

The following terms are built from word parts you have already learned and can be translated literally to find their meanings. Further explanation of terms beyond the definition of their word parts, if needed, is included in parentheses.

Term	Definition
caudad (KAW-dad)	toward the tail (downward) (Figure 3-2)
cephalad (SEF-a-lad)	toward the head (upward) (Figure 3-2)
lateral (lat) (LAT-er-al)	pertaining to a side (Figure 3-3)
medial (med) (MĒ-dē-al)	pertaining to the middle (Figure 3-4)
unilateral (ū-ni-LAT-er-al)	pertaining to one side (only)
bilateral (bī-LAT-er-al)	pertaining to two sides
mediolateral (*mē*-dē-ō-LAT-er-al)	pertaining to the middle and to the side
distal (DIS-tal)	pertaining to away (from the point of attachment of a body part) (Figure 3-5)

EXERCISE 6

Build directional terms for the following definitions by using the word parts you have learned.

1. toward the head (upward) ______ / ______ (WR / S)
2. pertaining to the head ______ / ______ (WR / S)
3. pertaining to the tail ______ / ______ (WR / S)
4. pertaining to the front ______ / ______ (WR / S)
5. pertaining to the back ______ / ______ (WR / S)
   ______ / ______ (WR / S)
6. pertaining to above ______ / ______ (WR / S)
7. pertaining to below ______ / ______ (WR / S)
8. pertaining to near ______ / ______ (WR / S)
9. pertaining to away ______ / ______ (WR / S)
10. pertaining to a side ______ / ______ (WR / S)
11. pertaining to the middle ______ / ______ (WR / S)
12. toward the tail (downward) ______ / ______ (WR / S)
13. pertaining to the belly ______ / ______ (WR / S)
14. pertaining to the back and to the front ______ /CV/ ______ / ______ (WR / CV / WR / S)
15. pertaining to the middle and to the side ______ /CV/ ______ / ______ (WR / CV / WR / S)
16. pertaining to one side (only) ______ / ______ / ______ (P / WR / S)
17. pertaining to the front and to the back ______ /CV/ ______ / ______ (WR / CV / WR / S)
18. pertaining to two sides ______ / ______ / ______ (P / WR / S)

EXERCISE FIGURE C

Fill in the blanks to label the diagram.

1 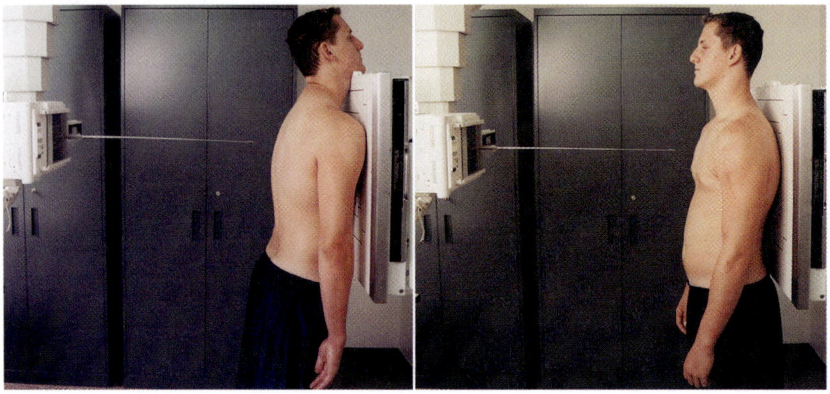 2

1. ______ / cv / ______ / ______ projection
back / cv / front / pertaining to

2. ______ / cv / ______ / ______ projection
front / cv / back / pertaining to

EXERCISE 7

Spell each of the directional terms on pp. 70-71 by having someone dictate them to you.

To hear and spell the terms, go to http://evolve.elsevier.com. Refer to p. 18 for your Evolve Access Information. Select Exercises & Review, Chapter 3, Chapter Exercises, Spelling.

☐ Place a check mark in the box if you have completed this exercise online.

1. ______
2. ______
3. ______
4. ______
5. ______
6. ______
7. ______
8. ______
9. ______
10. ______
11. ______
12. ______
13. ______
14. ______
15. ______
16. ______
17. ______
18. ______
19. ______

Anatomic Planes

Planes are imaginary flat fields used as points of reference to identify or view the location of organs and anatomical structures. Anatomic planes are frequently used in diagnostic imaging and surgery. The body is assumed to be in the anatomic position unless specified otherwise. (Table 3-1).

Term	Definition
frontal or coronal (FRON-tal) (ko-RŌN-al)	vertical field passing through the body from side to side, dividing the body into anterior and posterior portions (Figure 3-7)
midsagittal (mid-SAJ-i-tal)	vertical field running through the body from front to back at the midline, dividing the body equally into right and left halves (Figure 3-7)
parasagittal (*par*-a-SAJ-i-tal)	vertical field running through the body from front to back, dividing the body into unequal left and right sides
sagittal (SAJ-i-tal)	vertical field running through the body from front to back, dividing the body into right and left sides (any plane parallel to the midsagittal plane)
transverse (trans-VERS)	horizontal field dividing the body into superior and inferior portions (Figure 3-7)

MIDLINE

is an imaginary line that separates the body, or body parts, into halves. In medical language, midline is used as a common reference point.

Sagittal describes vertical planes dividing the body into right and left sides. **Midsagittal** and **parasagittal** planes are both sagittal planes with the midsagittal plane dividing the body equally into halves and the parasagittal plane dividing the body into unequal sides.

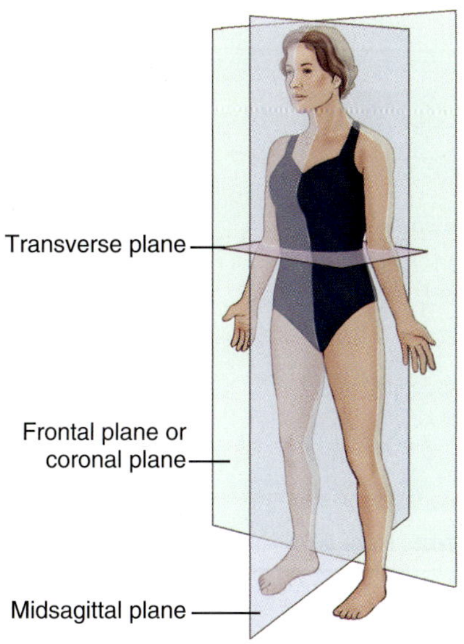

FIGURE 3-7
Anatomic planes.

EXERCISE 8

Practice saying aloud each of the anatomic planes on p. 75.

To hear the terms, go to http://evolve.elsevier.com. Refer to p. 18 for your Evolve Access Information. Select Exercises & Review, Chapter 3, Chapter Exercises, Pronunciation.

☐ Place a check mark in the box when you have completed this exercise.

TABLE 3-1

Anatomic Planes and Diagnostic Images

Coronal or Frontal	Midsagittal	Transverse
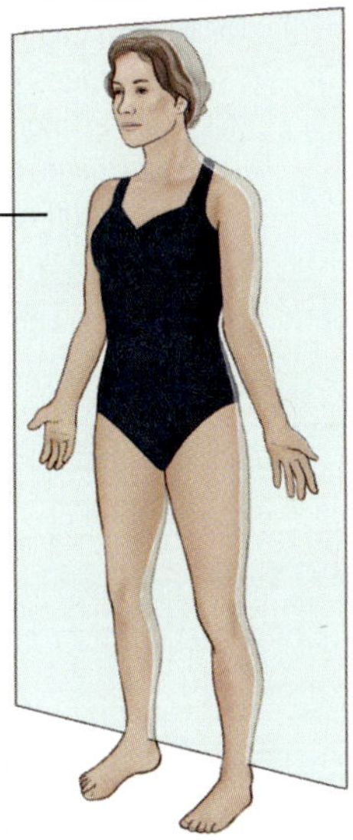	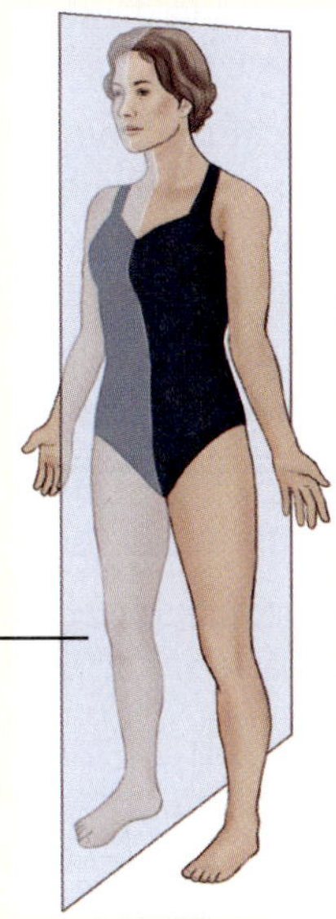	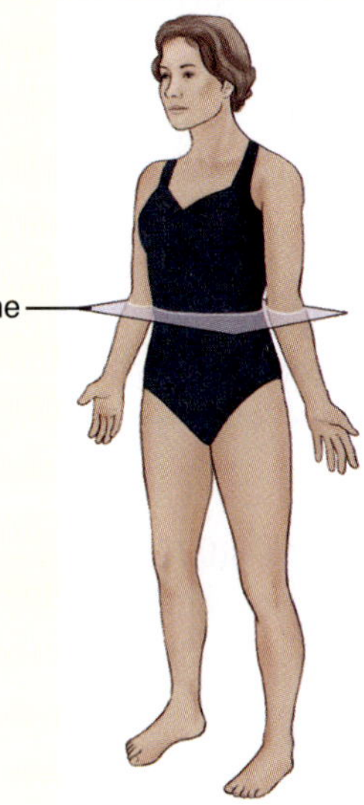
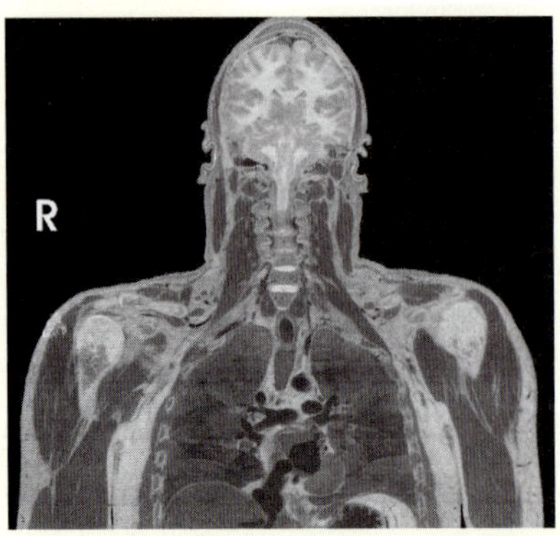 Frontal or coronal diagnostic image (MRI)	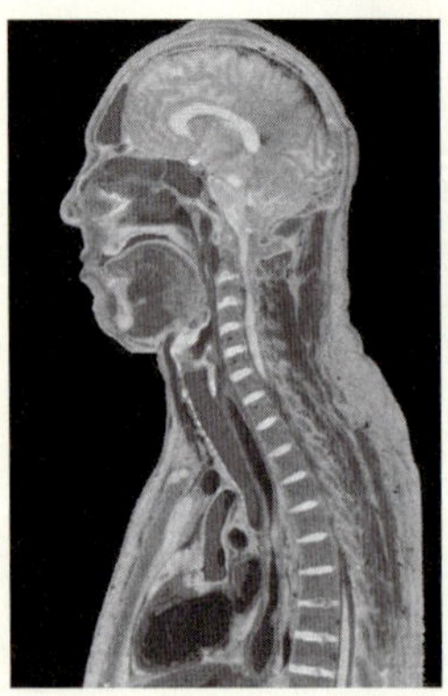 Midsagittal diagnostic image (MRI)	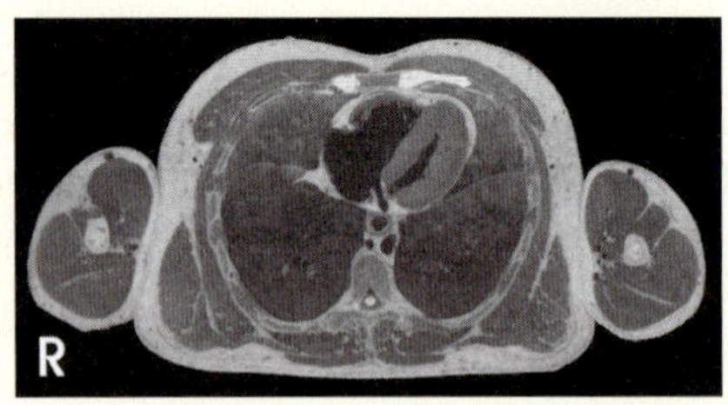 Transverse diagnostic image (MRI)

EXERCISE 9

Fill in the blanks with the correct terms.

1. The plane that divides the body into superior and inferior portions is the ________________ plane.
2. The plane that divides the body **equally** into right and left halves is the ________________ plane.
3. The plane that divides the body into anterior and posterior portions is referred to as ________________ or ________________ plane.
4. Any plane that divides the body into right and left sides is referred to as a(n) ________________ plane.
5. The plane that divides the body into **unequal** right and left sides is the ________________ plane.

EXERCISE FIGURE D

Fill in the blanks with anatomic planes.

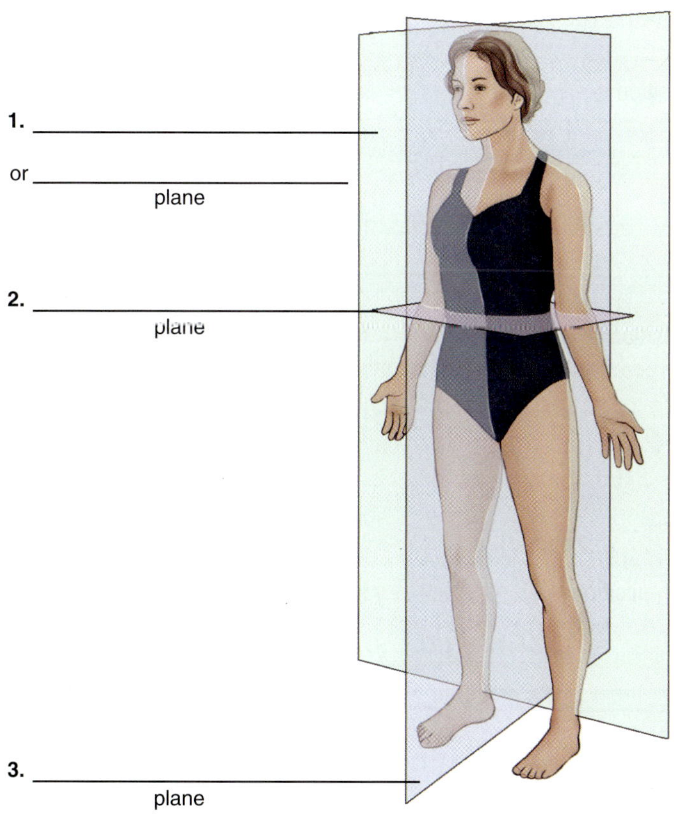

EXERCISE 10

Spell each of the anatomic plane terms on p. 75 by having someone dictate them to you.

To hear and spell the terms, go to http://evolve.elsevier.com. Refer to p. 18 for your Evolve Access Information. Select Exercises & Review, Chapter 3, Chapter Exercises, Spelling.

☐ Place a check mark in the box if you have completed this exercise online.

1. ______________________ 4. ______________________
2. ______________________ 5. ______________________
3. ______________________ 6. ______________________

Body Positions

Position terms are used in health care settings to communicate how the patient's body is placed for physical examination, diagnostic procedures, surgery, treatment, and recovery.

Term	Definition
Fowler position (FOW-ler) (pe-ZISH-en)	semi-sitting position with slight elevation of the knees (Exercise Figure F)
lithotomy position (lith-OT-o-mē) (pe-ZISH-en)	lying on back with legs raised and feet in stirrups (Exercise Figure G)
orthopnea position (or-THOP-nē-a) (pe-ZISH-en)	sitting erect in a chair or sitting upright in bed supported by pillows behind the head and chest (also called **orthopneic position**)
prone position (prōn) (pe-ZISH-en)	lying on abdomen, facing downward (head may be turned to one side) (Exercise Figure E)
recumbent position (rē-KUM-bent) (pe-ZISH-en)	lying down in any position
Sims position (simz) (pe-ZISH-en)	lying on left side with right knee drawn up and with left arm drawn behind, parallel to the back (Exercise Figure G)
supine position (SOO-pine) (pe-ZISH-en)	lying on back, facing upward (Exercise Figure E)
Trendelenburg position (tren-DEL-en-berg) (pe-ZISH-en)	lying on back with body tilted so that the head is lower than the feet (Exercise Figure F)

FOWLER POSITION

indicates the patient is in a sitting position with the head of the bed raised between 30° and 90°. Variations in the angle are denoted by **high Fowler**, indicating an upright position at approximately 90°, **Fowler** indicating an angle between 45° and 60°, **semi-Fowler**, 30° to 45°, and **low Fowler**, where the head is slightly elevated.

EXERCISE 11

Practice saying aloud each of the body position terms on p. 78.

To hear the terms, go to http://evolve.elsevier.com. Refer to p. 18 for your Evolve Access Information. Select Exercises & Review, Chapter 3, Chapter Exercises, Pronunciation.

☐ Place a check mark in the box when you have completed this exercise.

EXERCISE 12

Match the body position terms in the first column with their correct definitions in the second column.

_____ 1. orthopnea position
_____ 2. Fowler position
_____ 3. lithotomy position
_____ 4. prone position
_____ 5. supine position
_____ 6. recumbent position
_____ 7. Sims position
_____ 8. Trendelenburg position

a. lying on back with legs raised and feet in stirrups
b. lying down in any position
c. lying on back, facing upward
d. lying on back with body tilted so that the head is lower than the feet
e. sitting erect in a chair or sitting upright in bed supported by pillows behind the head and chest
f. lying on left side with right knee drawn up and with left arm drawn behind, parallel to the back
g. semi-sitting position with slight elevation of the knees
h. lying on abdomen, facing downward (head may be turned to one side)

EXERCISE FIGURE E

Label the following diagrams by writing the term for the corresponding definition.

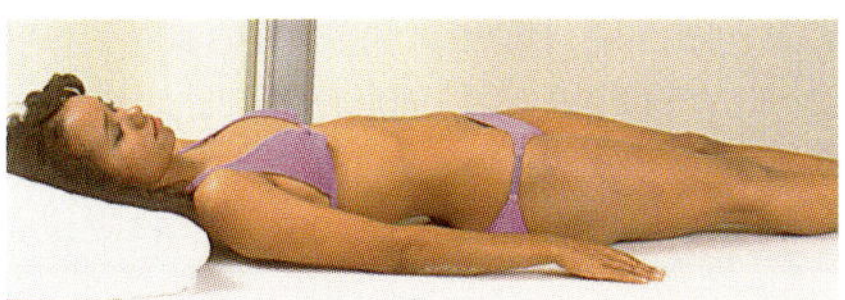
1

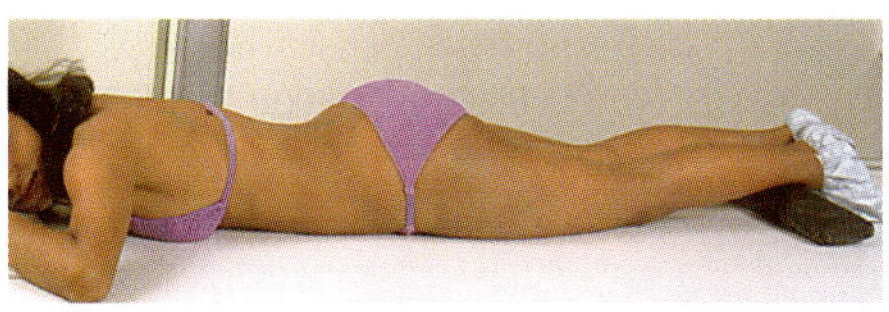
2

1) __________ __________, lying on back, facing upward

2) __________ __________, lying on abdomen, facing downward

EXERCISE FIGURE F

Label the following diagrams by writing the term for the corresponding definition.

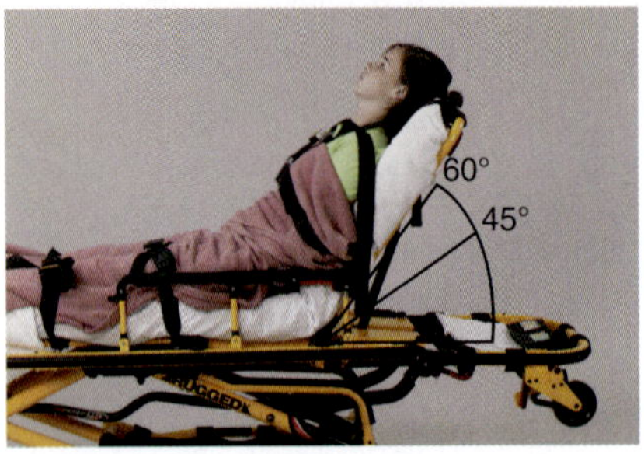

1

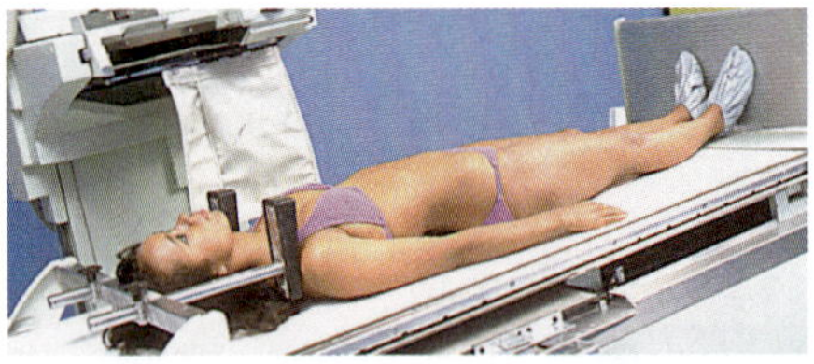

2

1) ____________ ____________, semi-sitting position with slight elevation of the knees

2) ____________ ____________, lying on back with body tilted so that the head is lower than the feet

EXERCISE FIGURE G

Label the following diagrams by writing the term for the corresponding definition.

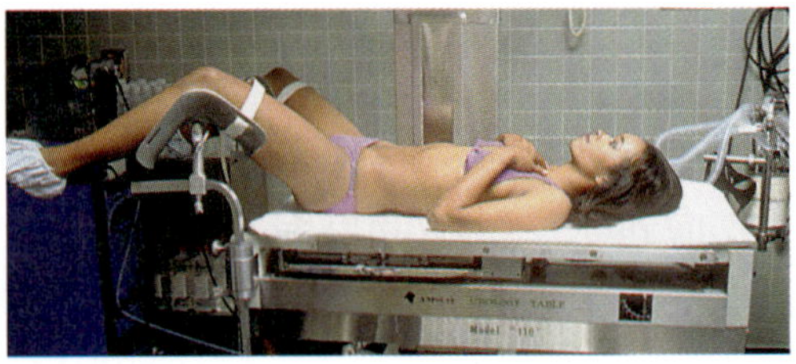

1

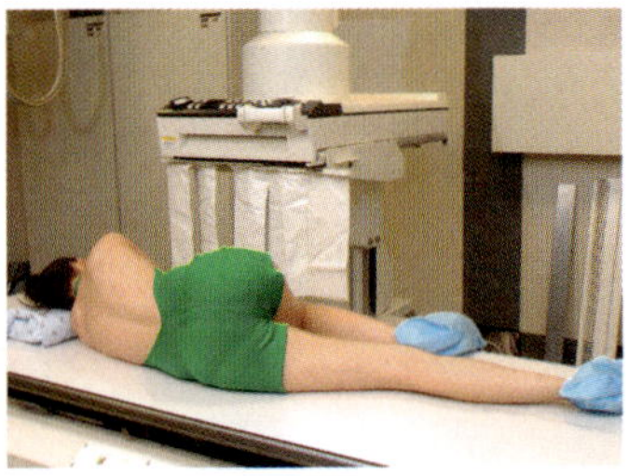

2

1) Modified ____________ ____________, lying on back with legs raised (notice legs are supported under the knees rather than by stirrups)

2) Modified ____________ ____________, lying on left side with right knee drawn up (notice the arm is placed in front, rather than behind the body)

EXERCISE 13

Spell each of the body position terms on p. 78 by having someone dictate them to you.

To hear and spell the terms, go to http://evolve.elsevier.com. Refer to p. 18 for your Evolve Access Information. Select Exercises & Review, Chapter 3, Chapter Exercises, Spelling.

☐ Place a check mark in the box if you have completed this exercise online.

1. ____________________
2. ____________________
3. ____________________
4. ____________________
5. ____________________
6. ____________________
7. ____________________
8. ____________________

Abdominopelvic Regions

To assist in locating medical problems with greater accuracy and for identification purposes, the abdomen and pelvis are divided into nine regions (Figure 3-8). Abdominopelvic regions are often used in relation to physical examination and medical history to describe signs and symptoms. The number in parentheses indicates the number of regions.

Term	Definition
umbilical region (1) (um-BIL-i-kal) (RĒ-jun)	around the navel (umbilicus)
lumbar regions (2) (LUM-bar) (RĒ-junz)	to the right and left of the umbilical region, near the waist
epigastric region (1) (*ep*-i-GAS-trik) (RĒ-jun)	superior to the umbilical region, generally above the stomach
hypochondriac regions (2) (*hī*-pō-KON-drē-ak) (RĒ-junz)	to the right and left of the epigastric region
hypogastric region (1) (*hī*-pō-GAS-trik) (RĒ-jun)	inferior to the umbilical region
iliac regions (2) (IL-ē-ak) (RĒ-junz)	to the right and left of the hypogastric region, near the groin (also called *inguinal regions*)

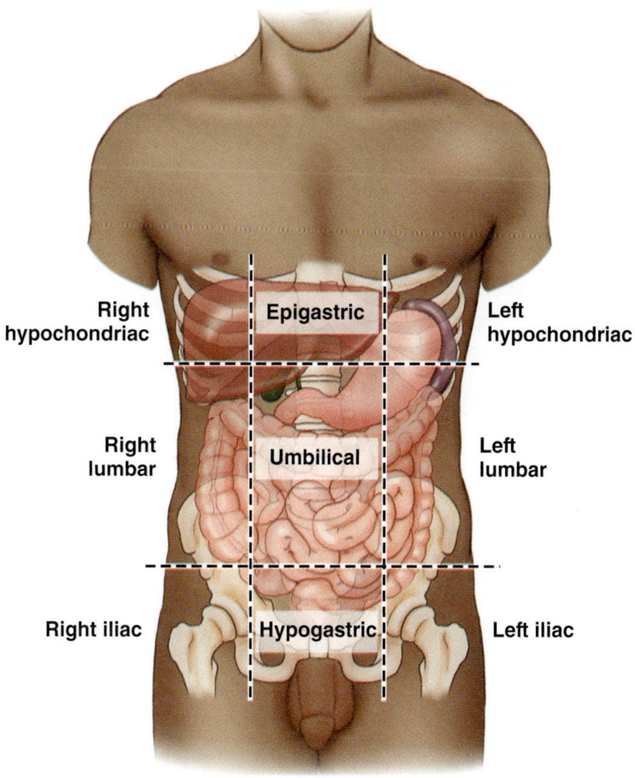

FIGURE 3-8
Abdominopelvic regions.

UMBILICUS

is a term derived from the Latin **umbo,** which denoted the boss, or protuberant part, of a shield. Around the first century the term was used to designate either a raised or a depressed spot in the middle of anything.

HYPOCHONDRIAC

is derived from the Greek **hypo,** meaning **under,** and **chondros,** meaning **cartilage.** This ancient term was used by Hippocrates to refer to the region just below the cartilages of the ribs. In 1765, the term was first used to refer to people who experienced discomfort or painful sensations in this area but had no organic findings. Now, a person who falsely believes he or she has an illness is referred to as a **hypochondriac.**

CYBERCHONDRIA

emerged in 2000 as a term describing a pattern of using Internet research to self-diagnose symptoms, fueling health anxiety and worry.

EXERCISE 14

Practice saying aloud each of the abdominopelvic region terms on p. 81.

To hear the terms, go to http://evolve.elsevier.com. Refer to p. 18 for your Evolve Access Information. Select Exercises & Review, Chapter 3, Chapter Exercises, Pronunciation.

☐ Place a check mark in the box when you have completed this exercise.

EXERCISE FIGURE H

Fill in the blanks with abdominopelvic regions.

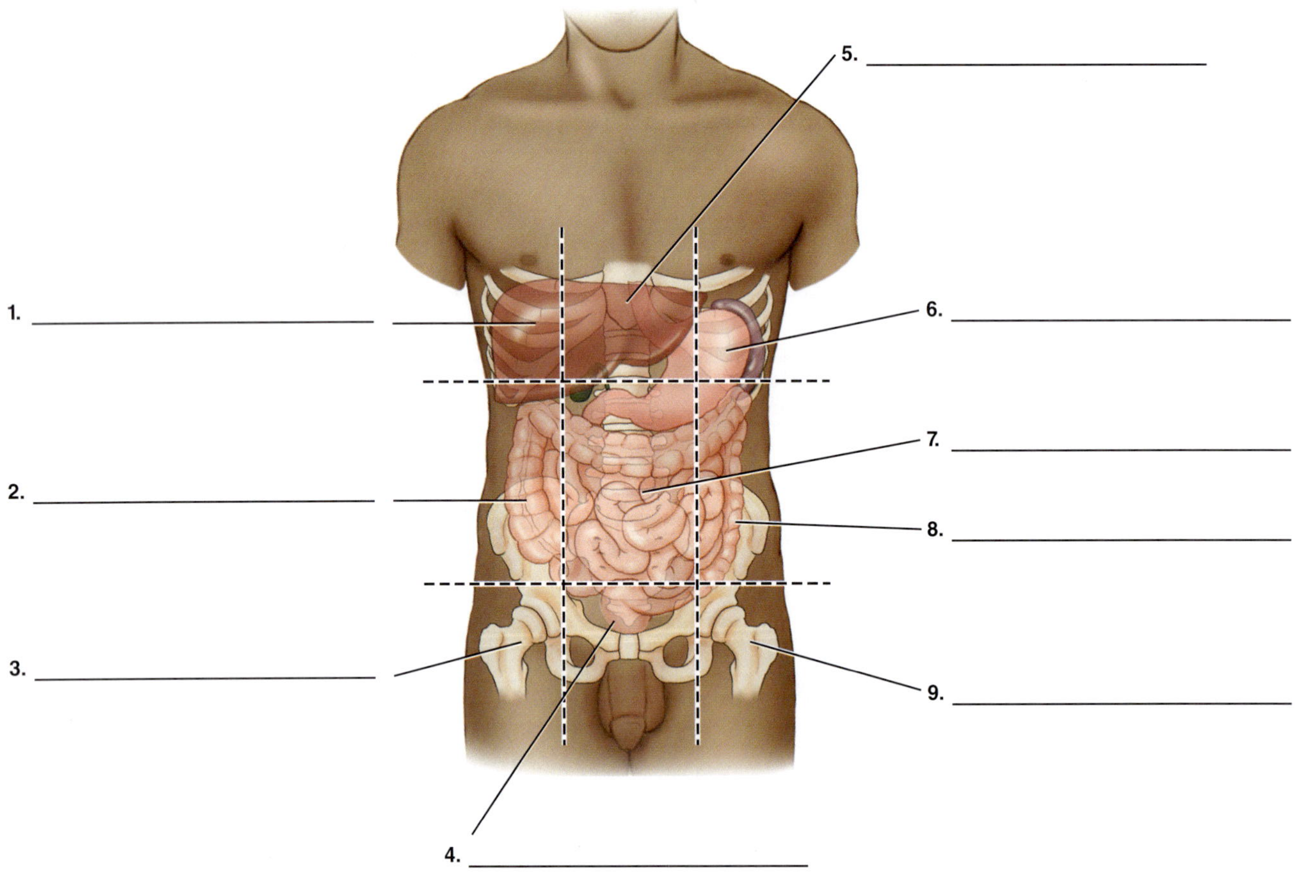

1. ______________________________
2. ______________________________
3. ______________________________
4. ______________________________
5. ______________________________
6. ______________________________
7. ______________________________
8. ______________________________
9. ______________________________

EXERCISE 15

Fill in the blanks with the correct terms.

1. The regions to the right and left of the hypogastric region, near the groin, are the ____________________ regions.
2. The ____________________ region is superior to the umbilical region, generally above the stomach.
3. Inferior to the umbilical region is the ____________________ region.
4. The ____________________ are the regions to the right and left of the epigastric region.
5. Superior to the hypogastric region is the ____________________ region.
6. To the right and the left of the umbilical region, near the waist, are the ____________________ regions.

EXERCISE 16

Match the terms in the first column with the correct definitions in the second column.

_____ 1. epigastric	a. inferior to the umbilical region
_____ 2. hypochondriac	b. superior to the umbilical region, generally above the stomach
_____ 3. hypogastric	c. right and left of the umbilical region, near the waist
_____ 4. iliac	d. right and left of the epigastric region
_____ 5. lumbar	e. right and left of the hypogastric region, near the groin
_____ 6. umbilical	f. inferior to the hypogastric region
	g. inferior to the epigastric region

EXERCISE 17

Spell each of the abdominopelvic region terms on p. 81 by having someone dictate them to you.

To hear and spell the terms, go to http://evolve.elsevier.com. Refer to p. 18 for your Evolve Access Information. Select Exercises & Review, Chapter 3, Chapter Exercises, Spelling.

☐ Place a check mark in the box if you have completed this exercise online.

1. ____________________ 4. ____________________
2. ____________________ 5. ____________________
3. ____________________ 6. ____________________

Abdominopelvic Quadrants

The abdominopelvic area can also be divided into four quadrants by using imaginary vertical and horizontal lines that intersect at the umbilicus. These divisions are used by health professionals to specify an anatomic position and to describe pain, incisions, markings, lesions, and so forth. The quadrants provide a more general denotation than the abdominopelvic regions, and they are used in describing signs and symptoms from the physical examination and medical history (Figure 3-9).

Term	Definition
right upper quadrant (RUQ) (KWOD-rant)	refers to the area encompassing the right lobe of the liver, the gallbladder, part of the pancreas, and portions of the small and large intestines
left upper quadrant (LUQ) (KWOD-rant)	refers to the area encompassing the left lobe of the liver, the stomach, the spleen, part of the pancreas, and portions of the small and large intestines
right lower quadrant (RLQ) (KWOD-rant)	refers to the area encompassing portions of the small and large intestines, the appendix, the right ureter, and the right ovary and uterine tube in women or the right spermatic duct in men
left lower quadrant (LLQ) (KWOD-rant)	refers to the area encompassing portions of the small and large intestines, the left ureter, and the left ovary and uterine tube in women or the left spermatic duct in men

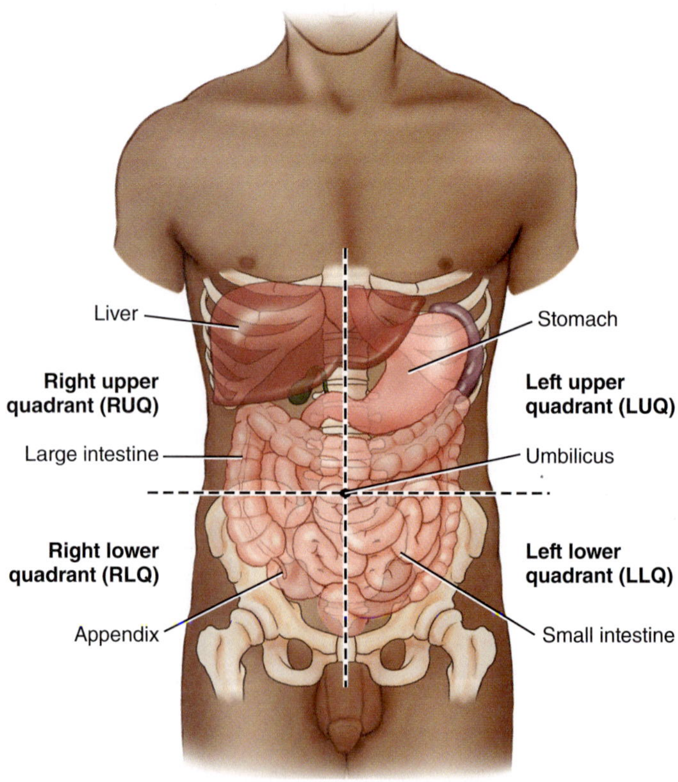

FIGURE 3-9
Abdominopelvic quadrants.

EXERCISE 18

Write the abbreviation for the abdominopelvic quadrant associated with the following organs.

______ 1. appendix

______ 2. right lobe of the liver

______ 3. left spermatic duct in men

______ 4. the stomach and the spleen

______ 5. right ovary and uterine tube in women

______ 6. gallbladder

______ 7. right ureter

EXERCISE FIGURE I

Fill in the blanks with abdominopelvic quadrants and the abbreviations for each.

(1) ______________________

____

____

Abbrev. ______________

(2) ______________________

____

____

Abbrev. ______________

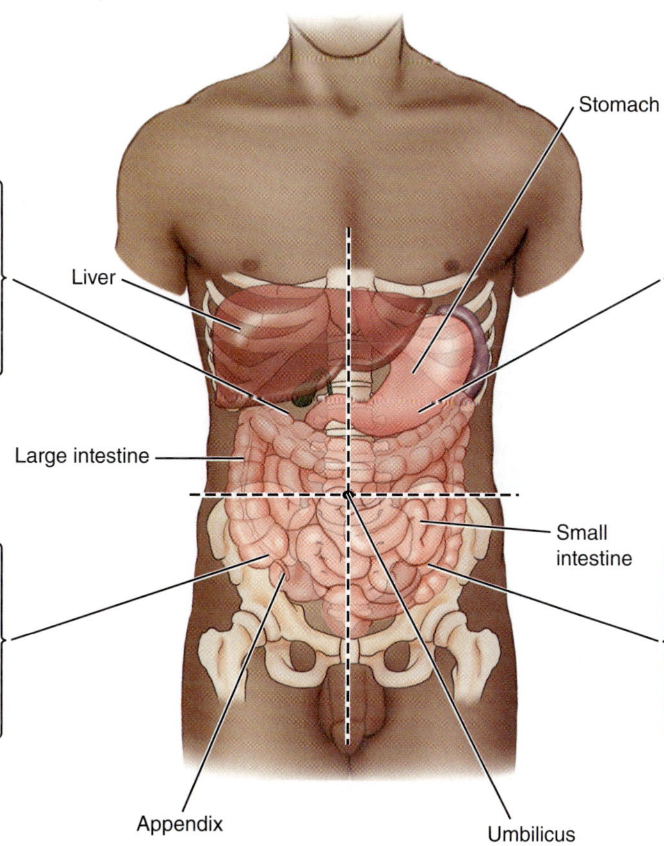

(3) ______________________

____

____

Abbrev. ______________

(4) ______________________

____

____

Abbrev. ______________

EXERCISE 19

Spell each of the abdominopelvic quadrant terms on p. 84 by having someone dictate them to you.

To hear and spell the terms, go to http://evolve.elsevier.com. Refer to p. 18 for your Evolve Access Information. Select Exercises & Review, Chapter 3, Chapter Exercises, Spelling.
☐ Place a check mark in the box if you have completed this exercise online.

1. ____________________ 3. ____________________
2. ____________________ 4. ____________________

Abbreviations

ant	anterior
AP	anteroposterior
inf	inferior
lat	lateral
LLQ	left lower quadrant
LUQ	left upper quadrant
med	medial
PA	posteroanterior
RLQ	right lower quadrant
RUQ	right upper quadrant
sup	superior

Refer to **Appendix C** for a complete list of abbreviations.

EXERCISE 20

Write the meaning of each abbreviation in the space provided.

1. sup ____________________
2. ant ____________________
3. inf ____________________
4. PA ____________________
5. AP ____________________
6. med ____________________
7. lat ____________________

PRACTICAL APPLICATION

EXERCISE 21 *Interact with Medical Documents*

A. Complete the physician's progress note by writing the medical terms in the blanks. Use the list of definitions with corresponding numbers following the document.

University Hospital and Medical Center
4700 North Main Street • Wellness, Arizona 54321 • (987) 555-3210

PATIENT NAME: Zoe Parker **CASE NUMBER:** 817254-DPQ
DATE OF BIRTH: 03/27/19XX **DATE:** 11/24/20XX

PROGRESS NOTE

Mrs. Parker is here today for follow-up for degenerative joint disease of both knees. She arrived ambulatory with the assistance of a cane, walking slowly with a fairly steady gait.

On examination of the knees, there is marked crepitus that is palpable with pressure applied to the patellae with the knees flexed and extended, right greater than left. She has a range of motion from 10 degrees to 110 degrees in the right knee. Pain is evident at the end of extension at 10 degrees. The right knee is stable when stressed in an 1. ________________________________, valgus, and varus manner.

On examination of the right ankle, there is some mild tenderness on palpation above the right ankle. The right ankle moves from 0 degrees of dorsiflexion to 25 degrees of plantar flexion. From the 2. ________________ joint line at the knee to the malleolus at the ankle, the right tib/fib is 1.5 cm shorter than the left. There is pigment change mainly on the 3. ________________ and 4. ________________ aspect of the right lower leg. There is a slight bony deformity over the 5. ________________ aspect of the mid-tibial area.

IMPRESSION:
1. Degenerative joint disease of both knees and ankle, stable.

PLAN:
1. Patient is to continue on current medications unchanged.

____
Robert Means, MD

RM/mcm

1. pertaining to the front and to the back
2. pertaining to the side
3. pertaining to the back
4. pertaining to the middle
5. pertaining to the front

EXERCISE 21 *Interact with Medical Documents—cont'd*

B. Read the procedure for palpating arterial pulses and answer the questions following it.

PROCEDURE FOR PALPATING ARTERIAL PULSES

Palpate arteries with the distal pads of the first two fingers. The fingertips are used because they are the most sensitive parts of the hand. Unless contraindicated, simultaneous palpation is preferred.

Temporal: Palpate over the temporal bone on each side of the head lateral to each eyebrow.

Carotid: Palpate the anterior edge of the sternocleidomastoid muscle, just medial and inferior to the angle of the jaw. To avoid reduction of blood flow, do not palpate right and left carotid pulses simultaneously.

Brachial: Palpate in the groove between the biceps and triceps, just medial to the biceps tendon.

Radial: Palpate lateral and anterior side of wrist, proximal to the first metacarpal phalangeal joint.

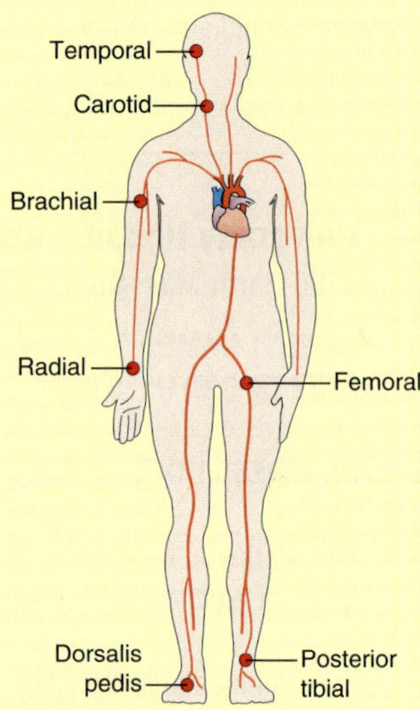

FIGURE 3-10 Location of the pulse points on the body.

Femoral: This pulse is inferior to the inguinal ligament; if the patient is obese, the pulse is found midway between anterior superior iliac spine and pubic tubercle.

Dorsalis pedis: Lightly palpate the dorsal surface of the foot, with the foot slightly dorsiflexed.

Posterior tibial: This pulse is found posterior and slightly inferior to the medial malleolus of the ankle.

1. The **temporal pulse** is palpated
   a. just above the eyebrow.
   b. to the side of the eyebrow.
   c. below the eyebrow.
   d. to the middle of the eyebrow.

2. The **radial pulse** is palpated on the
   a. lateral and front of the wrist.
   b. lateral and back of the wrist.
   c. medial and back of the wrist.
   d. medial and front of the wrist.

3. The **femoral pulse** is located
   a. below the inguinal ligament.
   b. above the inguinal ligament.
   c. to the front of the inguinal ligament.
   d. to the back of the inguinal ligament.

4. When used with the foot, the directional term ***dorsal*** has a slightly different meaning. With the use of your medical dictionary, describe the dorsal surface of the foot. Hint: try *dorsum* and *dorsal pedis* as search terms.

   The dorsal surface of the foot is ______________

   ______________________________________.

EXERCISE 22 *Interpret Medical Terms*

To test your understanding of the terms introduced in this chapter, complete the sentence by filling in the blank with the term that corresponds to the definition provided.

1. The ________________ plane is a general term specifying the vertical field running through the body from front to back. (**dividing the body into right and left sides**) The terms ________________ plane and ________________ plane more specifically describe the sagittal plane by indicating whether the body is divided in half or in unequal portions. (**dividing the body equally into halves**) (**dividing the body into unequal sides**)
2. A polyp was found in the colon ________________ to the splenic flexure. (**pertaining to away from the point of attachment of a body part**)
3. The drainage catheter is placed over the right ________________ pelvis. (**pertaining to the front**)
4. The incision was made at the ________________ pole of the lesion. (**pertaining to above**)
5. A(n) ________________ chest radiograph is taken in the ________________ plane. (**pertaining to the front and to the back**) (**dividing the body into anterior and posterior portions**)
6. The patient complained of ________________ pain. (**superior to umbilical region, generally above the stomach**)
7. A ________________ chest radiograph displays the anatomy in the ________________ plane. (**pertaining to a side**) (**divides the body into right and left sides**)
8. The patient was scheduled for an ultrasound-guided ________________ thoracentesis. (**pertaining to two [both] sides**)
9. The doctor's order indicated that the patient with dyspnea was to be placed in the ________________ position to facilitate breathing. (**sitting erect or upright**)
10. The patient being treated for cardiovascular shock was placed in the ________________ position. (**lying on back with the head lower than the feet**)
11. Gallbladder pain is likely to be in the ________________ ________________ ________________. (**abbreviated as RUQ**)
12. ________________ is often used to describe the back of the hand or upper surface of the foot. (**pertaining to the back**)
13. Just before birth, the fetus shifted to a ________________ presentation. (**pertaining to the head**)
14. ________________ epidural steriod injection may be performed to relieve chronic low back pain. (**pertaining to the tail**)

15. The pathology report for the patient with a palpable right breast lump included the following sections:

   a. Right axillary sentinel lymph node, biopsy;

   b. Right breast, ________________ margin biopsy (**pertaining to above**);

   c. Right breast, ________________ margin, biopsy (**pertaining to below**);

   d. Right breast, deep margin, biopsy;

   e. Right breast, ________________ margin, biopsy (**pertaining to the middle**); and

   f. Right breast, ________________ margin, biopsy (**pertaining to a side**).

EXERCISE 23 *Read Medical Terms in Use*

Practice pronunciation of terms by reading aloud the following medical document. Use the pronunciation key following the medical term to assist you in saying the word. The script contains medical terms not yet presented. Treat them as information only; you will learn more about them as you continue to study. Or, if desired, look for their meanings in your medical dictionary.

To hear these terms, go to http://evolve.elsevier.com. Refer to p.18 for your Evolve Access Information. Select Exercises & Review, Chapter 3, Chapter Exercises, Read Medical Terms in Use.

The patient presented to her physician with pain in the right **lumbar** (LUM-bar) **region** and right **unilateral** (ū -ni-LAT-er-al) leg pain. The pain was felt in the **posterior** (pos-TĒR-ē -or) portion of the leg and radiated to the **distal** (DIS-tal) **lateral** (LAT-er-al) portion of the extremity. There was some **proximal** (PROK-si-mal) muscle weakness reported of the affected leg. A lumbar spine radiograph was normal. If the pain does not respond to antiinflammatory medication, she will be referred to an orthopedist.

EXERCISE 24 *Comprehend Medical Terms in Use*

Test your comprehension of terms in the previous medical document by answering *T* for true and *F* for false.

______ 1. The patient had pain on both sides of her leg and to the right of the hypogastric region.

______ 2. The pain was felt at the back of the leg and radiated away from this point to the side of the extremity.

______ 3. The muscle weakness was felt near the point of attachment.

CHAPTER REVIEW

ONLINE CHAPTER REVIEW

To access the Evolve website, go to http://evolve.elsevier.com. Refer to p. 18 for your Evolve Access Information. Select Exercises & Review, Chapter 3, then select Chapter Exercises, Practice Activities, Animations, or Games. Place a check mark in the box when you have completed an exercise or activity, watched an animation, or played a game. Have fun!

Chapter Exercises

Exercises in this section of your Evolve resources correlate to exercises in your textbook. You may have completed them as you worked through the chapter.

- ☐ Pronunciation
- ☐ Spelling
- ☐ Read Medical Terms in Use

Practice Activities

Practice in study mode, then test your learning in assessment mode. Keep track of your scores from assessment mode if you wish.

	SCORE
☐ Picture It	_______
☐ Define Word Parts	_______
☐ Analyze Medical Terms	_______
☐ Build Medical Terms	_______
☐ Define Medical Terms	_______
☐ Use It	_______
☐ Hear It and Type It: Clinical Vignettes	_______

Animations

- ☐ Directions of the Body
- ☐ Quadrants of the Body
- ☐ LLQ Pain
- ☐ LUQ Pain
- ☐ RLQ Pain
- ☐ RUQ Pain
- ☐ Epigastric Pain

Games

- ☐ Name that Word Part
- ☐ Medical Millionaire
- ☐ Crossword Puzzle

REVIEW OF WORD PARTS

Can you define and spell the following word parts?

Combining Forms

anter/o
caud/o
cephal/o
dist/o
dors/o
infer/o
later/o
medi/o
poster/o
proxim/o
super/o
ventr/o

Prefixes

bi-
uni-

Suffixes

-ad
-ior

REVIEW OF TERMS

Can you define, pronounce, and spell the following terms?

Body Directional Terms

anterior (ant)
anteroposterior (AP)
bilateral
caudad
caudal
cephalad
cephalic
distal
dorsal
inferior (inf)
lateral (lat)
medial (med)
mediolateral
posterior
posteroanterior (PA)
proximal
superior (sup)
unilateral
ventral

Anatomic Planes

frontal or coronal
midsagittal
parasagittal
sagittal
transverse

Body Positions

Fowler position
lithotomy position
orthopnea position
prone position
recumbent position
Sims position
supine position
Trendelenburg position

Abdominopelvic Regions

epigastric region
hypochondriac regions
hypogastric region
iliac regions
lumbar regions
umbilical region

Abdominopelvic Quadrants

left lower quadrant (LLQ)
left upper quadrant (LUQ)
right lower quadrant (RLQ)
right upper quadrant (RUQ)

Types of body movement are presented in Chapter 14, Musculoskeletal System, on page 634. Terms related to body movement are: *abduction*, *adduction*, *inversion*, *eversion*, *extension*, *flexion*, *pronation*, *supination*, and *rotation*.

ANSWERS

Exercise Figures

Exercise Figure

A. 1. head: cephal/o
2. front: anter/o
3. belly: ventr/o
4. back: dors/o
5. back, behind: poster/o
6. tail: caud/o
7. above: super/o
8. side: later/o
9. middle: medi/o
10. near: proxim/o
11. away: dist/o
12. below: infer/o

Exercise Figure

B. 1. super/ior
2. cephal/ic
3. cephal/ad
4. poster/ior, dors/al
5. infer/ior
6. caud/al
7. caud/ad
8. anter/ior
9. ventr/al

Exercise Figure

C. 1. poster/o/anter/ior
2. anter/o/poster/ior

Exercise Figure

D. 1. coronal or frontal plane
2. transverse plane
3. midsagittal plane

Exercise Figure

E. 1. supine position
2. prone position

Exercise Figure

F. 1. Fowler position
2. Trendelenburg position

Exercise Figure

G. 1. lithotomy position
2. Sims position

Exercise Figure

H. 1. right hypochondriac
2. right lumbar
3. right iliac
4. left hypogastric
5. left epigastric
6. left hypochondriac
7. umbilical
8. lumbar
9. iliac

Exercise Figure

I. 1. right upper quadrant (RUQ)
2. left upper quadrant (LUQ)
3. right lower quadrant (RLQ)
4. left lower quadrant (LLQ)

Exercise 1

1. belly (front)
2. head (upward)
3. side
4. middle
5. below
6. near (point of attachment of a body part)
7. above
8. away (from the point of attachment of a body part)
9. back
10. tail (downward)
11. front
12. back, behind

Exercise 2

1. c
2. b
3. d
4. a

Exercise 3

1. pertaining to
2. toward
3. two
4. one

Exercise 4

Pronunciation Exercise

Exercise 5

1. WR S
cephal/ad
toward the head
2. WR S
cephal/ic
pertaining to the head
3. WR S
caud/ad
toward the tail
4. WR S
caud/al
pertaining to the tail
5. WR S
anter/ior
pertaining to the front
6. WR S
poster/ior
pertaining to the back
7. WR S
dors/al
pertaining to the back
8. WR S
super/ior
pertaining to above
9. WR S
infer/ior
pertaining to below
10. WR S
proxim/al
pertaining to near
11. WR S
dist/al
pertaining to away
12. WR S
later/al
pertaining to a side
13. WR S
medi/al
pertaining to the middle
14. WR S
ventr/al
pertaining to the belly (front)
15. WR CV WR S
poster/o/anter/ior
CF
pertaining to the back and to the front
16. P WR S
uni/later/al
pertaining to one side
17. WR CV WR S
medi/o/later/al
CF
pertaining to the middle and to the side
18. WR CV WR S
anter/o/poster/ior
CF
pertaining to the front and to the back
19. P WR S
bi/later/al
pertaining to two sides

Exercise 6

1. cephal/ad
2. cephal/ic
3. caud/al
4. anter/ior
5. poster/ior, dors/al
6. super/ior
7. infer/ior
8. proxim/al
9. dist/al
10. later/al
11. medi/al
12. caud/ad
13. ventr/al
14. poster/o/anter/ior
15. medi/o/later/al
16. uni/later/al
17. anter/o/poster/ior
18. bi/later/al

Exercise 7

Spelling Exercise; see text pp. 70-71.

Exercise 8

Pronunciation Exercise

Exercise 9

1. transverse
2. midsagittal
3. coronal or frontal
4. sagittal
5. parasagittal

Exercise 10

Spelling Exercise; see text p. 75.

Exercise 11

Pronunciation Exercise

Exercise 12

1. e
2. g
3. a
4. h
5. c
6. b
7. f
8. d

Exercise 13

Spelling Exercise; see text p. 78.

Exercise 14

Pronunciation Exercise

Exercise 15

1. iliac
2. epigastric
3. hypogastric
4. hypochondriac
5. umbilical
6. lumbar

Exercise 16

1. b
2. d
3. a
4. e
5. c
6. g

Exercise 17

Spelling Exercise; see text p. 81.

Exercise 18

1. RLQ
2. RUQ
3. LLQ
4. LUQ
5. RLQ
6. RUQ
7. RLQ

Exercise 19

Spelling Exercise; see text p. 84.

Exercise 20

1. superior
2. anterior
3. inferior
4. posteroanterior
5. anteroposterior
6. medial
7. lateral

Exercise 21

A. 1. anteroposterior
2. lateral
3. posterior or dorsal
4. medial
5. anterior

B. 1. b
2. a
3. a
4. answers may vary: the upper surface of the foot; the surface opposite the sole

Exercise 22

1. sagittal, midsagittal, parasagittal
2. distal
3. anterior
4. superior
5. anteroposterior; frontal (or coronal)
6. epigastric
7. lateral; sagittal
8. bilateral
9. orthopnea
10. Trendelenburg
11. right upper quadrant
12. dorsal
13. cephalic
14. caudal
15. a. no answer, b. superior, c. inferior, d. medial, e. lateral

Exercise 23

Reading Exercise

Exercise 24

1. *F*, "unilateral" means one side; "bilateral" means two sides. The right lumbar region is to the right of the umbilical region.
2. *T*
3. *T*

NOTES

Chapter 4

Integumentary System

OUTLINE

The remaining chapters are organized according to body systems; therefore, they present material in a consistent format. The better you understand the format, the quicker and easier you will learn the material. Take time now to review How I Will Learn Medical Terms using *Exploring Medical Language*, pp. xii-xiii in the Front Matter to reacquaint yourself with the finer points of using this textbook to its ultimate potential.

OBJECTIVES

Upon completion of this chapter you will be able to:

1. Identify organs and structures of the integumentary system.
2. Define and spell word parts related to the integumentary system.
3. Define, pronounce, and spell disease and disorder terms related to the integumentary system.
4. Define, pronounce, and spell surgical terms related to the integumentary system.
5. Define, pronounce, and spell complementary terms related to the integumentary system.
6. Interpret the meaning of abbreviations related to the integumentary system.
7. Interpret, read, and comprehend medical language in simulated medical statements and documents.

ANATOMY

The integumentary system is composed of the skin, nails, and glands.

Function

The skin forms a protective covering for the body that, when unbroken, prevents entry of bacteria and other invading organisms. The skin also protects the body from water loss and the damaging effects of ultraviolet light. Other functions include regulation of body temperature and synthesis of vitamin D (Figure 4-1).

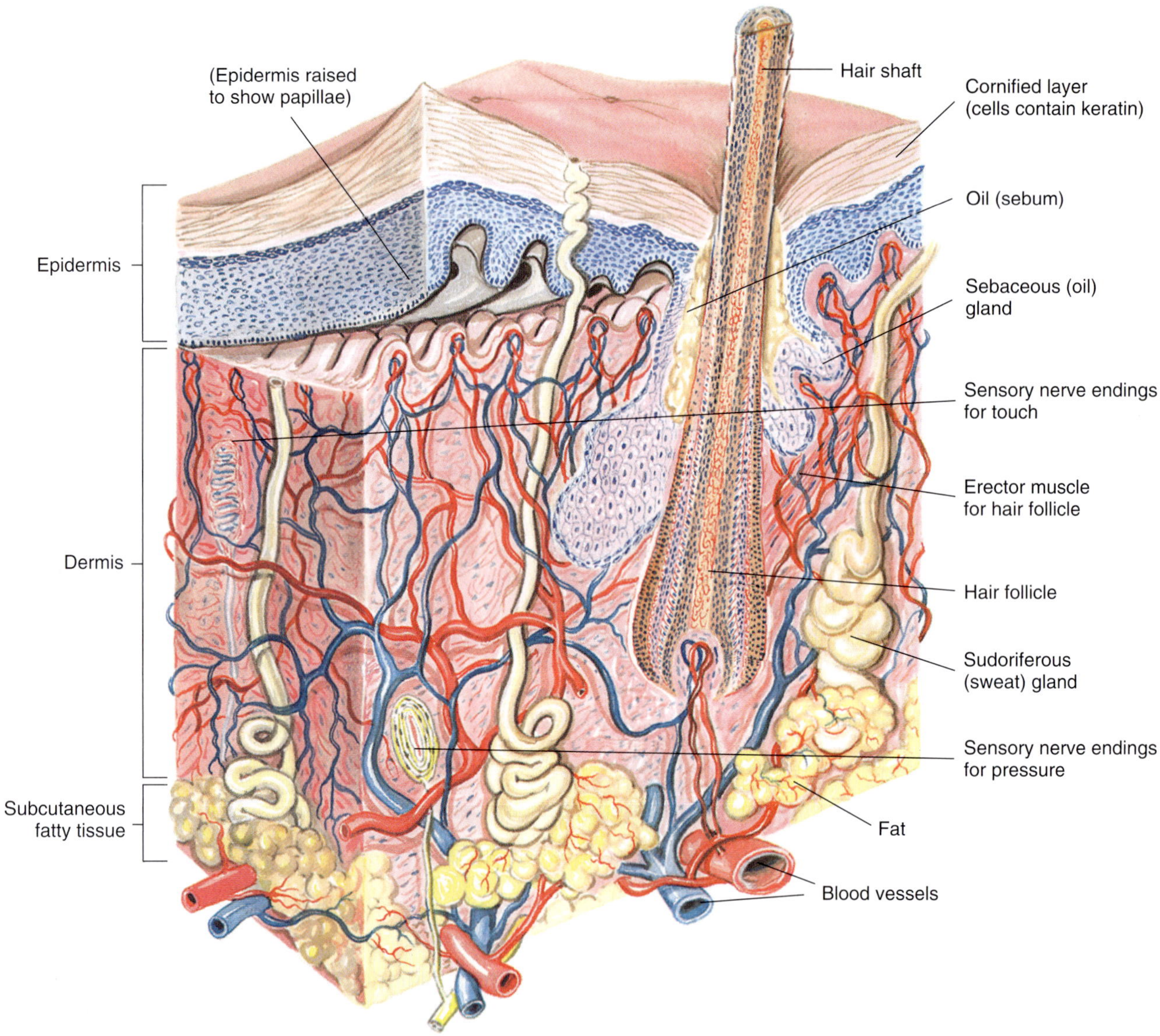

Figure 4-1
Structure of the skin.

The Skin

Term	Definition
epidermis	outer layer of skin
keratin	horny, or cornified, layer composed of protein. It is contained in the hair, skin, and nails.
melanin	color, or pigmentation, of the skin
dermis	inner layer of skin (also called the true skin)
sudoriferous (sweat) glands	tiny, coiled, tubular structures that emerge through pores on the skin's surface and secrete sweat
sebaceous glands	secrete sebum (oil) into the hair follicles where the hair shafts pass through the dermis

INTEGUMENTARY
is derived from the Latin word ***teqere***, meaning ***to cover***.

Accessory Structures of the Skin

Term	Definition
hair	compressed, keratinized cells that arise from hair follicles, the sacs that enclose the hair fibers
nails	originate in the epidermis. Nails are found on the upper surface of the ends of the fingers and toes. The white area at the base of the nail is called the **lunula**, or **moon**.

A & P Booster
For students desiring more anatomy and physiology, go to http://evolve.elsevier.com. Refer to p. 18 for your Evolve Access Information. Select A & P Booster, Chapter 4.

EXERCISE 1

Match the terms in the first column with the correct definitions in the second column. *To check your answers to the exercises in this chapter, go to Answers, p. 144, at the end of the chapter.*

______ 1.	dermis	a. secrete sweat
______ 2.	epidermis	b. responsible for skin color
______ 3.	hair	c. true skin
______ 4.	melanin	d. outermost layer of the skin
______ 5.	nail	e. white area at the nail's base
______ 6.	sebaceous glands	f. originates in the epidermis
______ 7.	sudoriferous glands	g. composed of compressed, keratinized cells
		h. secrete sebum

WORD PARTS

Word parts you need to learn to complete this chapter are listed on the following pages. The exercises at the end of each list will help you learn their definitions and spelling.

Use the flashcards accompanying this text or electronic flashcards to assist you in memorizing the word parts for this chapter.

To use electronic flashcards, go to http://evolve.elsevier.com. Refer to p. 18 for your Evolve Access Information. Select Flashcards, Chapter 4.

Combining Forms of the Integumentary System

Combining Form	Definition
cutane/o, derm/o, dermat/o	skin
hidr/o	sweat
kerat/o (NOTE: *kerat/o* is also used to refer to the cornea of the eye; see Chapter 12.)	horny tissue, hard
onych/o, ungu/o	nail
seb/o	sebum (oil)
trich/o	hair

Do not be concerned about which **combining form** to use for **skin** or **nail**. As you continue to study and use medical terms, you will become familiar with common usage of each word part.

EXERCISE FIGURE A

Fill in the blanks with combining forms in this diagram of a cross section of the skin. *To check your answers, go to p. 144.*

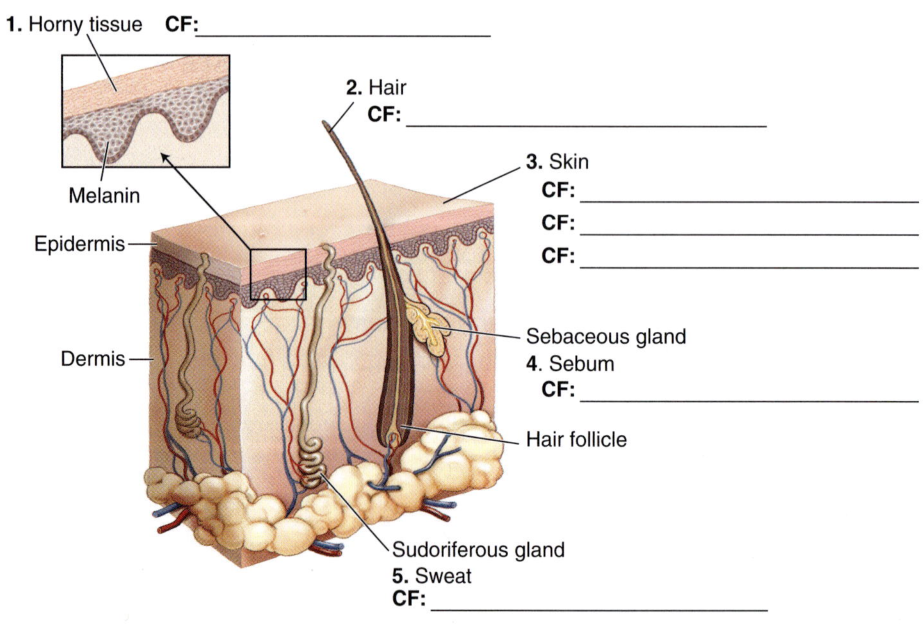

EXERCISE FIGURE B

Fill in the blanks with combining forms in this cross section of the finger with nail.

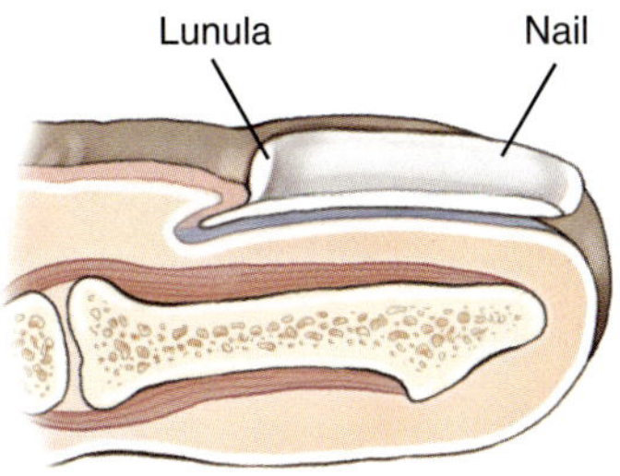

CF: ______________________

CF: ______________________

EXERCISE 2

Write the definitions of the following combining forms.

1. hidr/o ______________
2. derm/o ______________
3. onych/o ______________
4. trich/o ______________
5. kerat/o ______________
6. dermat/o ______________
7. seb/o ______________
8. ungu/o ______________
9. cutane/o ______________

EXERCISE 3

Write the combining form for each of the following.

1. hair ______________
2. sweat ______________
3. nail
   a. ______________
   b. ______________
4. sebum ______________
5. skin
   a. ______________
   b. ______________
   c. ______________
6. horny tissue, hard ______________

Combining Forms Commonly Used with Integumentary System Terms

Combining Form	Definition
aut/o	self
bi/o	life
coni/o	dust
crypt/o	hidden
heter/o	other
myc/o	fungus
necr/o	death (cells, body)
pachy/o	thick
rhytid/o	wrinkles
staphyl/o	grapelike clusters
strept/o	twisted chains
xer/o	dry

The prefix **bi-,** which means **two**, was presented in Chapter 3. The word root **bi** means **life.**

EXERCISE 4

Write the definitions of the following combining forms.

1. necr/o ______________
2. staphyl/o ______________
3. crypt/o ______________
4. pachy/o ______________
5. coni/o ______________
6. myc/o ______________
7. bi/o ______________
8. heter/o ______________
9. strept/o ______________
10. xer/o ______________
11. aut/o ______________
12. rhytid/o ______________

EXERCISE 5

Write the combining form for each of the following.

1. fungus ______
2. death (cells, body) ______
3. other ______
4. dry ______
5. thick ______
6. twisted chains ______
7. wrinkles ______
8. grapelike clusters ______
9. self ______
10. hidden ______
11. dust ______
12. life ______

Prefixes

Prefix	Definition
epi-	on, upon, over
intra-	within
para-	beside, beyond, around, abnormal
per-	through
sub-	under, below
trans-	through, across, beyond

EXERCISE 6

Write the definitions of the following prefixes.

1. sub- ______
2. para- ______
3. epi- ______
4. intra- ______
5. per- ______
6. trans- ______

EXERCISE 7

Write the prefix for each of the following.

1. within ______
2. under, below ______
3. on, upon, over ______
4. beside, beyond, around, abnormal ______
5. through ______
6. through, across, beyond ______

Suffixes

Suffix	Definition
-a	noun suffix, no meaning
-coccus (*pl.* -cocci)	berry-shaped (form of bacterium)
-ectomy	excision or surgical removal
-ia	diseased or abnormal state, condition of
-itis	inflammation
-malacia	softening
-opsy	view of, viewing
-phagia	eating or swallowing
-plasty	surgical repair
-rrhea	flow, discharge
-tome	instrument used to cut

Refer to **Appendix A** and **Appendix B** for alphabetical lists of word parts and their meanings.

EXERCISE 8

Match the suffixes in the first column with the correct definitions in the second column.

______	1. -coccus	a.	inflammation
______	2. -ectomy	b.	surgical repair
______	3. -itis	c.	berry-shaped
______	4. -malacia	d.	eating or swallowing
______	5. -opsy	e.	excision or surgical removal
______	6. -rrhea	f.	instrument used to cut
______	7. -phagia	g.	thick
______	8. -plasty	h.	flow, discharge
______	9. -tome	i.	view of, viewing
______	10. -ia	j.	softening
______	11. -a	k.	diseased or abnormal state, condition of
		l.	noun suffix, no meaning

EXERCISE 9

Write the definitions of the following suffixes.

1. -plasty ____________________
2. -ectomy ____________________
3. -malacia ____________________
4. -itis ____________________
5. -tome ____________________
6. -phagia ____________________
7. -rrhea ____________________
8. -coccus ____________________
9. -opsy ____________________
10. -ia ____________________
11. -a ____________________

MEDICAL TERMS

The terms you need to learn to complete this chapter are listed on the following pages. The exercises at the end of each list will help you learn each word well enough to add it to your vocabulary.

Disease and Disorder Terms

Built from Word Parts

The following terms are built from word parts you have already learned and can be translated literally to find their meanings. Further explanation of terms beyond the definition of their word parts, if needed, is included in parentheses.

Term	Definition
dermatitis (*der*-ma-TĪ-tis)	inflammation of the skin (Figures 4-2 and 4-3)
dermatoconiosis (*der*-ma-tō-*kō*-nē-Ō-sis)	abnormal condition of the skin caused by dust
dermatofibroma (*der*-ma-tō-fī-BRŌ-ma)	fibrous tumor of the skin
hidradenitis (*hī*-drad-e-NĪ-tis)	inflammation of a sweat gland
leiodermia (*lī*-ō-DER-mē-a)	condition of smooth skin
leukoderma (*lū*-kō-DER-ma)	white skin (white patches caused by depigmentation)
onychocryptosis (*on*-i-kō-krip-TŌ-sis)	abnormal condition of a hidden nail (also called **ingrown nail**)
onychomalacia (*on*-i-kō-ma-LĀ-sha)	softening of the nails

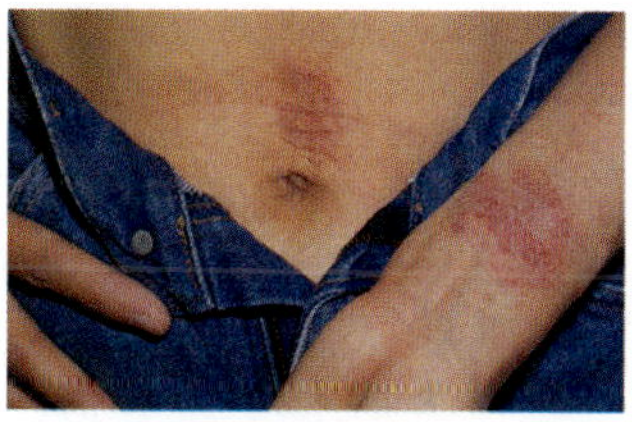

Figure 4-2
Contact dermatitis.

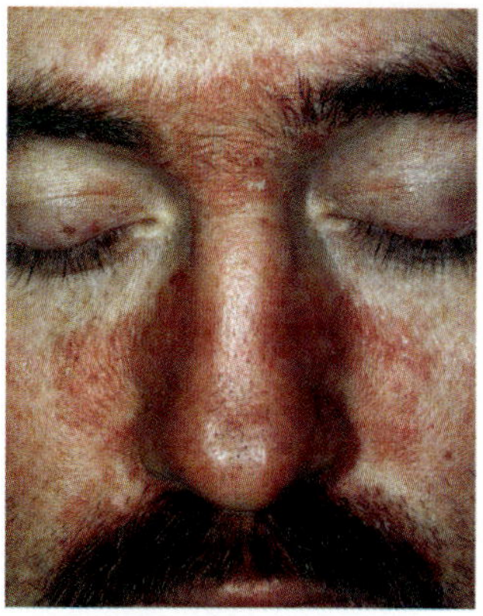

Figure 4-3
Seborrheic dermatitis.

Disease and Disorder Terms—*cont'd*

Built from Word Parts

Term	Definition
onychomycosis (*on*-i-kō-mī-KŌ-sis)	abnormal condition of a fungus in the nails (Exercise Figure C)
onychophagia (*on*-i-kō-FĀ-ja)	eating the nails (nail biting)
pachyderma (*pak*-i-DER-ma)	thickening of the skin
paronychia (*par*-ō-NIK-ē-a) (NOTE: the *a* from para- has been dropped. The final vowel in a prefix may be dropped when the word to which it is added begins with a vowel.)	diseased state around the nail (Exercise Figure C)
seborrhea (seb-o-RĒ-a)	discharge of sebum (excessive)
trichomycosis (*trik*-ō-mī-KŌ-sis)	abnormal condition of a fungus in the hair
xeroderma (*zē*-rō-DER-ma)	dry skin (a mild form of a cutaneous disorder characterized by keratinization and noninflammatory scaling)

CAM TERM

Light therapy is the therapeutic use of ultraviolet, colored, and laser lights to reestablish the body's natural rhythm, reduce pain and depression, and improve other health conditions. Numerous studies have investigated and found clinical efficacy in the use of a variety of light therapies to **rejuvenate damaged skin**.

EXERCISE FIGURE C

Fill in the blanks to label the diagrams.

1
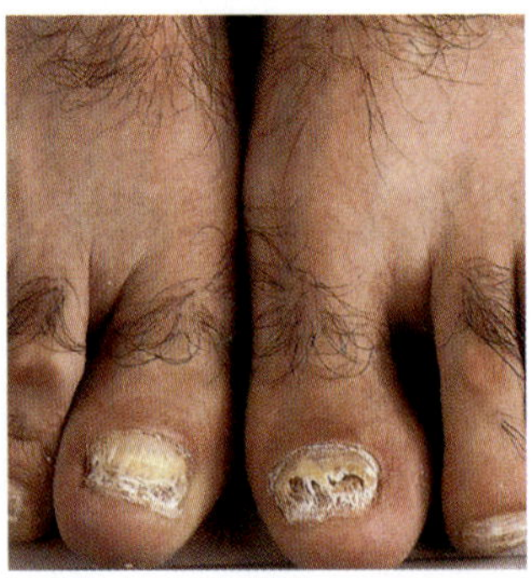

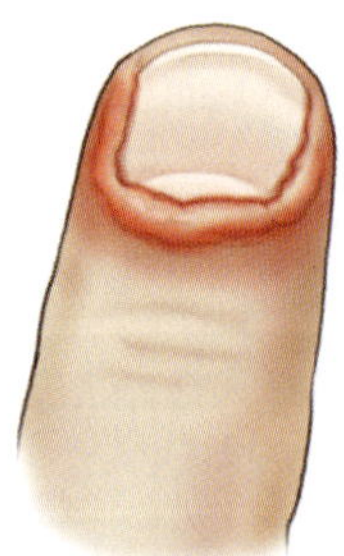
2

1. ______ / ______ / ______ / ______
   nail / cv / fungus / abnormal condition

2. ______ / ______ / ______
   around / nail / diseased state

EXERCISE 10

Practice saying aloud each of the disease and disorder terms built from word parts on pp. 105-106.

To hear the terms, go to http://evolve.elsevier.com. Refer to p. 18 for your Evolve Access Information. Select Exercises & Review, Chapter 4, Chapter Exercises, Pronunciation.

☐ Place a check mark in the box when you have completed this exercise.

EXERCISE 11

Analyze and define the following disease and disorder terms built from word parts. If needed, refer to pp. 11-12 to review analyzing and defining techniques.

WR CV WR S

Example: onych / o / myc / osis abnormal condition of a fungus in the nails

CF

1. dermatoconiosis ____________________
2. hidradenitis ____________________
3. dermatitis ____________________
4. pachyderma ____________________
5. onychomalacia ____________________
6. trichomycosis ____________________
7. dermatofibroma ____________________
8. paronychia ____________________
9. onychocryptosis ____________________
10. seborrhea ____________________
11. onychophagia ____________________
12. xeroderma ____________________
13. leiodermia ____________________
14. leukoderma ____________________

EXERCISE 12

Build disease and disorder terms for the following definitions by using the word parts you have learned. If you need help, refer to p. 13 to review word-building techniques.

Example: abnormal condition of a fungus in the hair trich / o / myc / osis
WR / CV / WR / S

1. thickening of the skin ________ / ________ / ________
   WR / WR / S
2. abnormal condition of a fungus in the nails ________ / ___ / ________ / ________
   WR / CV / WR / S
3. discharge of sebum (excessive) ________ / ___ / ________
   WR / CV / S
4. inflammation of the skin ________ / ________
   WR / S
5. fibrous tumor of the skin ________ / ___ / ________ / ________
   WR / CV / WR / S
6. softening of the nails ________ / ___ / ________
   WR / CV / S
7. inflammation of a sweat gland ________ / ________ / ________
   WR / WR / S
8. abnormal condition of a hidden nail ________ / ___ / ________ / ________
   WR / CV / WR / S
9. abnormal condition of the skin caused by dust ________ / ___ / ________ / ________
   WR / CV / WR / S
10. eating the nails ________ / ___ / ________
    WR / CV / S
11. diseased state around the nail ________ / ________ / ________
    P / WR / S
12. dry skin ________ / ___ / ________ / ________
    WR / CV / WR / S
13. condition of smooth skin ________ / ___ / ________ / ________
    WR / CV / WR / S
14. white skin ________ / ___ / ________ / ________
    WR / CV / WR / S

EXERCISE 13

Spell each of the disease and disorder terms built from word parts on pp. 105-106 by having someone dictate them to you.

To hear and spell the terms, go to http://evolve.elsevier.com. Refer to p. 18 for your Evolve Access Information. Select Exercises & Review, Chapter 4, Chapter Exercises, Spelling.

☐ Place a check mark in the box if you have completed this exercise online.

1. ______________________
2. ______________________
3. ______________________
4. ______________________
5. ______________________
6. ______________________
7. ______________________
8. ______________________
9. ______________________
10. ______________________
11. ______________________
12. ______________________
13. ______________________
14. ______________________
15. ______________________

Disease and Disorder Terms

Not Built from Word Parts

In some of the following terms, you may recognize word parts you have already learned; however, the full meaning of the terms cannot be discerned by the definition of their word parts.

Term	Definition
abrasion (a-BRĀ-zhun)	scraping away of the skin by mechanical process or injury
abscess (AB-ses)	localized collection of pus
acne (AK-nē)	inflammatory disease of the skin involving the sebaceous glands and hair follicles
actinic keratosis (ack-TIN-ik) (*ker*-a-TŌ-sis)	a precancerous skin condition of horny tissue formation that results from excessive exposure to sunlight (Figure 4-4, *A*). It may evolve into a squamous cell carcinoma.
albinism (AL-bi-niz-um)	congenital hereditary condition characterized by partial or total lack of pigment in the skin, hair, and eyes
basal cell carcinoma (BCC) (BĀ-sal) (sel) (*kar*-si-NŌ-ma)	epithelial tumor arising from the epidermis. It seldom metastasizes but invades local tissue (Figure 4-4, *C*). Common in individuals who have had excessive sun exposure.

ABSCESS

is derived from the Latin ***ab***, meaning ***from***, and ***cedo***, meaning ***to go***. The tissue dies and goes away, with the pus replacing it.

ALBINISM

Alb is Latin word root meaning **white. Leuk** is the Greek word root meaning **white**.

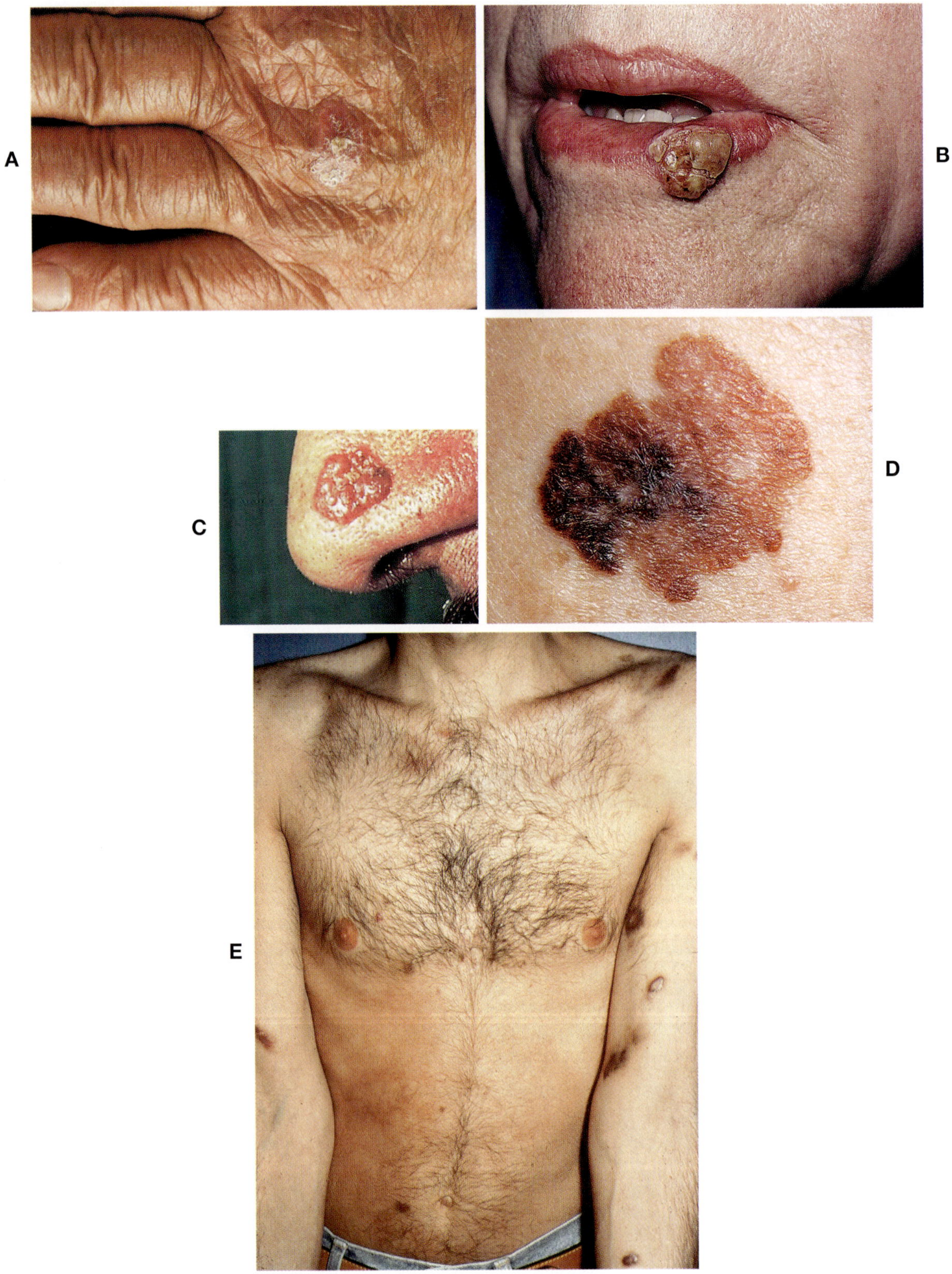

Figure 4-4
Percutaneous lesion and cancers of the skin. **A,** Actinic keratosis; **B,** squamous cell carcinoma; **C,** basal cell carcinoma; **D,** melanoma (covered in Chapter 2); **E,** Kaposi sarcoma.

Disease and Disorder Terms—*cont'd*

Not Built from Word Parts

Term	Definition
candidiasis (*kan*-di-DĪ-a-sis)	an infection of the skin, mouth (also called **thrush**), or vagina caused by the yeast-type fungus *Candida albicans. Candida* is normally present in the mucous membranes; overgrowth causes an infection. Esophageal candidiasis is often seen in patients with AIDS (acquired immunodeficiency syndrome).
carbuncle (KAR-bung-kl)	skin infection composed of a cluster of boils caused by staphylococcal bacteria
cellulitis (*sel*-ū-LĪ-tis)	inflammation of the skin and subcutaneous tissue caused by infection, leading to redness, swelling, and fever
contusion (kon-TŪ-zhun)	injury with no break in the skin, characterized by pain, swelling, and discoloration (also called a **bruise**)
eczema (EK-ze-ma)	noninfectious, inflammatory skin disease characterized by redness, blisters, scabs, and itching
fissure (FISH-ur)	slit or cracklike sore in the skin
furuncle (FER-ung-kl)	painful skin node caused by staphylococcal bacteria in a hair follicle (also called a **boil**) (Figure 4-5)
gangrene (GANG-grēn)	death of tissue caused by loss of blood supply followed by bacterial invasion (a form of necrosis)
herpes (HER-pēz)	inflammatory skin disease caused by herpes virus characterized by small blisters in clusters. Many types of herpes exist. *Herpes simplex*, for example, causes fever blisters; *herpes zoster*, also called shingles, is characterized by painful skin eruptions that follow nerves inflamed by the virus (see Table 4-1, p. 112).
impetigo (*im*-pe-TĪ-gō)	superficial skin infection characterized by pustules and caused by either staphylococci or streptococci (see Table 4-1, p. 112)
infection (in-FEK-shun)	the invasion of pathogens in body tissue. An infection may remain localized if the body's defense mechanisms are effective. If the infection persists, it may become acute, subacute, or chronic. A systemic infection occurs when the pathogen causing a local infection gains access to the vascular or lymphatic system and becomes disseminated throughout the body.

CANDIDA

comes from the Latin **candidus**, meaning **gleaming white; albicans** is from the Latin verb **albicare**, meaning **to make white**. The growth of the fungus is white, and the infection produces a white discharge.

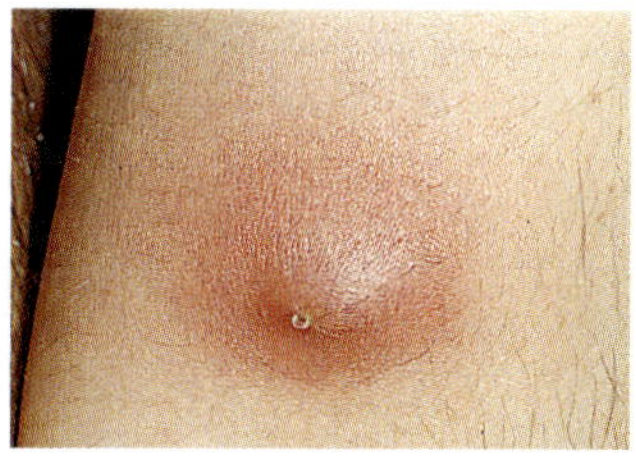

Figure 4-5
Furuncle resulting from a *Staphylococcus aureus* infection.

HERPES

is derived from the Greek **herpo**, meaning to **creep along**. It is descriptive of the course and type of skin lesion.

TYPES OF INFECTIONS

Infections may be caused by bacteria, fungus, parasite, or virus. Examples of common skin infections are:

Bacterial infections—carbuncle, cellulitis, furuncle, impetigo, MRSA infection, and paronychia

Fungal infections—candidiasis, tinea, and trichomycosis

Parasitic infections—scabies and pediculosis

Viral infections—fever blister (*herpes simplex*) and shingles (*herpes zoster*)

TABLE 4-1
Common Skin Disorders

Disorder	Examples	
Impetigo	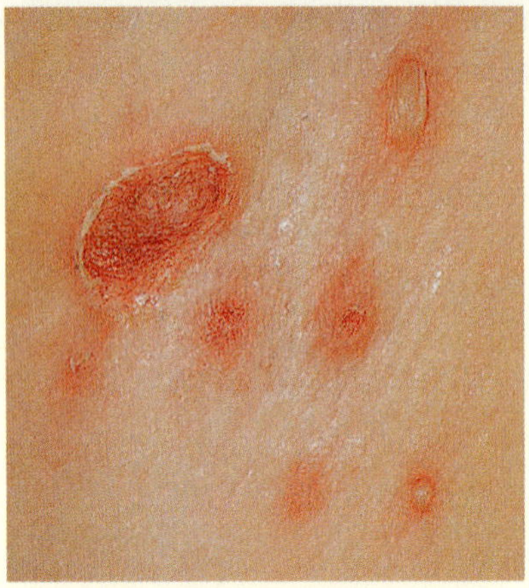	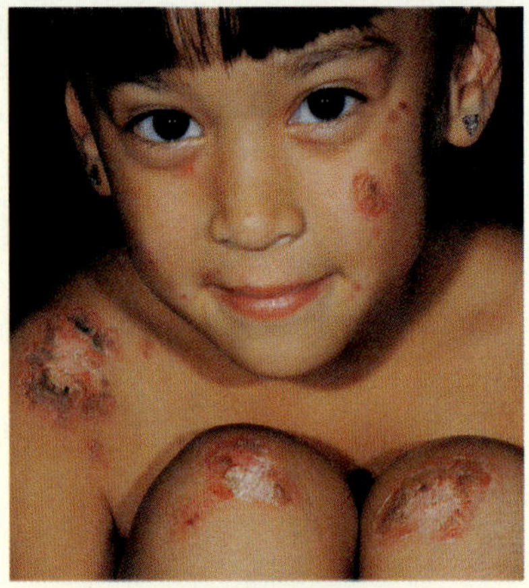
Tinea	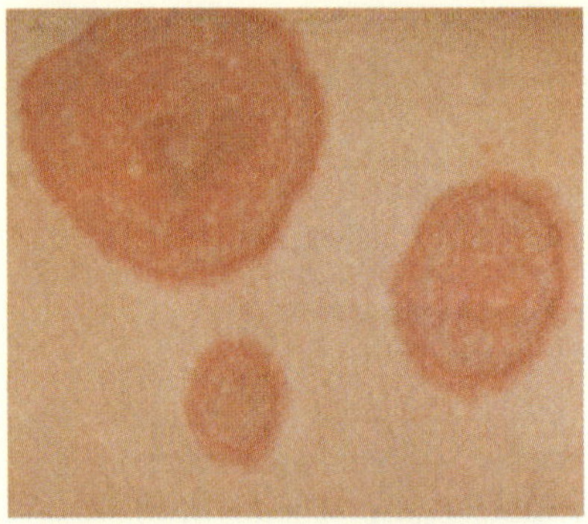 Tinea corporis (also called **ringworm**)	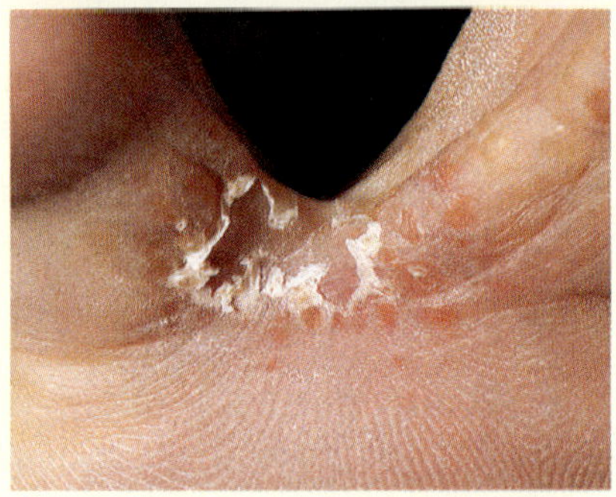 Tinea pedis (also called **athlete's foot**)
Scabies	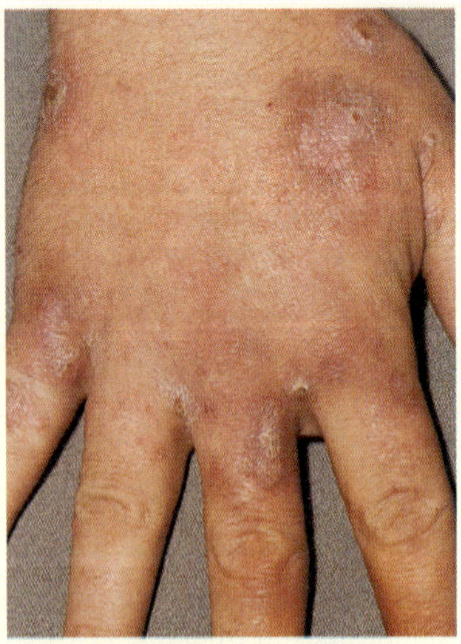	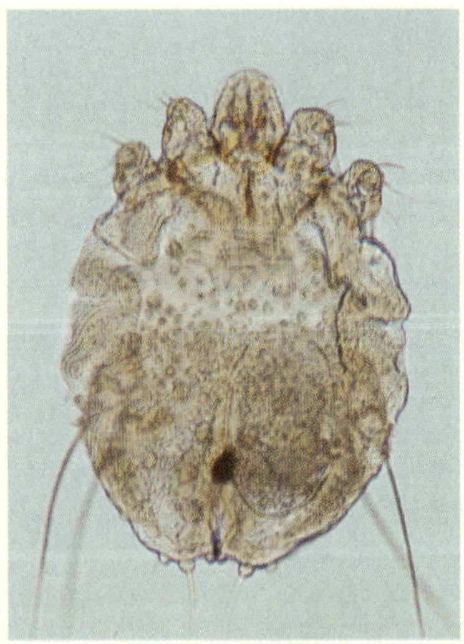 Scabies mite
Herpes zoster (also called shingles)	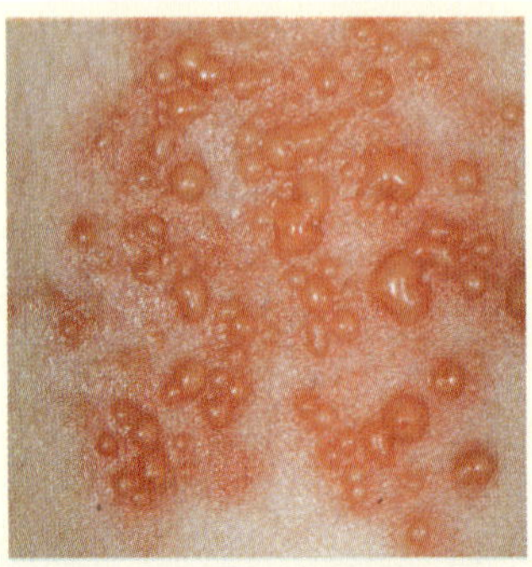	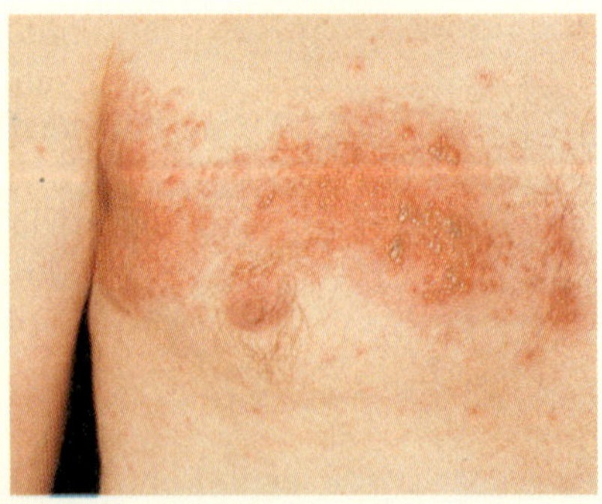

Disease and Disorder Terms—*cont'd*

Not Built from Word Parts

Term	Definition
Kaposi sarcoma (KAP-ō-sē) (sar-KŌ-ma)	a cancerous condition starting as purple or brown papules on the lower extremities that spreads through the skin to the lymph nodes and internal organs. Frequently seen with AIDS (Figure 4-4, *E*).
laceration (*las*-er-Ā-shun)	torn, ragged-edged wound
lesion (LĒ-zhun)	any visible change in tissue resulting from injury or disease. It is a broad term that includes sores, wounds, ulcers, and tumors.
MRSA infection (mer-SAH) (in-FEK-shun)	invasion of body tissue by methicillin-resistant *Staphylococcus aureus*, a strain of common bacteria that has developed resistance to penicillin and other antibiotics. It can produce skin and soft tissue infections and sometimes bloodstream infections and pneumonia, which can be fatal if not treated. MRSA is quite common in hospitals and long-term care facilities but is increasingly emerging as an important infection in the general population.
pediculosis (pe-*dik*-ū-LŌ-sis)	invasion into the skin and hair by lice
psoriasis (so-RĪ-a-sis)	chronic skin condition producing red lesions covered with silvery scales
rosacea (ro-ZĀ-shē-a)	chronic disorder of the skin that produces erythema, papules, pustules, and broken blood vessels, usually occurring on the central area of the face in people older than 30 years (Figure 4-6) (also called **acne rosacea**)
scabies (SKĀ-bēz)	skin infection caused by the itch mite, characterized by papule eruptions that are caused by the female burrowing into the outer layer of the skin and laying eggs. This condition is accompanied by severe itching (See Table 4-1, p. 112).
scleroderma (*skle*-rō-DER-ma)	a disease characterized by chronic hardening (induration) of the connective tissue of the skin and other body organs
squamous cell carcinoma (SqCCA) (SQWĀ-mus) (sel) (*kar*-si-NŌ-ma)	a malignant growth that develops from scalelike epithelial tissue. Unlike basal cell carcinoma, there is a significant potential for metastasis. The most frequent cause is chronic exposure to sunlight (Figure 4-4, B).

TYPES OF SKIN LESIONS

Primary lesions are physical changes of the skin of pathological origin. **Secondary lesions** may result from changes in primary lesions or may be caused by injury or infection. **Vascular lesions** are related to blood vessels and include the escape of blood into the tissues (hemorrhage). Examples of types of skin lesions include:

Primary lesions—macule, papule, nodule, wheal, vesicle, pustule, and cyst

Secondary lesions—cicatrix, keloid, and ulcer

Vascular lesions—petechia, purpura, and ecchymosis.

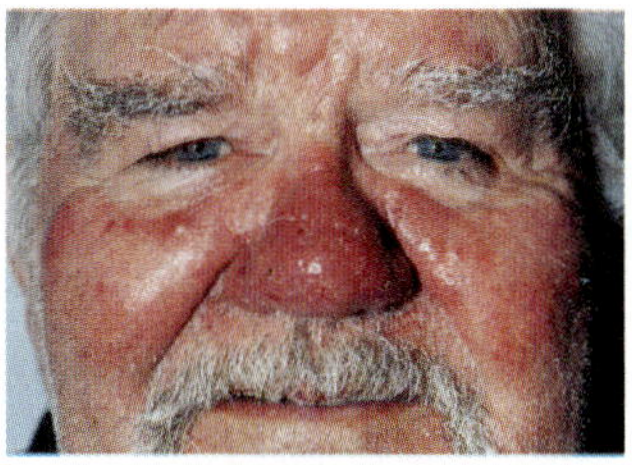

Figure 4-6
Rosacea.

Disease and Disorder Terms—*cont'd*

Not Built from Word Parts

Term	Definition
systemic lupus erythematosus (SLE) (sis-TEM-ik) (LŪ-pus) (*e*-ri-*thē*-*ma*-TŌ-sus)	a chronic inflammatory disease involving the skin, joints, kidneys, and nervous system. This autoimmune disease is characterized by periods of remission and exacerbations. It also may affect other organs.
tinea (TIN-ē-a)	fungal infection of the skin. The fungi may infect keratin of the skin, hair, and nails. Infections are classified by body regions such as *tinea capitis* (scalp), *tinea corporis* (body), and *tinea pedis* (foot). Tinea in general is also called **ringworm**, and tinea pedis specifically is also called **athlete's foot** (See Table 4-1, p. 112).
urticaria (*ur*-ti-KAR-ē-a)	an itching skin eruption composed of wheals of varying size and shape, which usually resolves in a short period of time. While often idiopathic, urticaria is sometimes associated with infections and with allergic reactions to food, medicine, or other agents. Other causes include internal disease, physical stimuli, and genetic disorders (also called **hives**) (See Table 4-2, p. 131).
vitiligo (*vit*-i-LĪ-gō)	white patches on the skin caused by the destruction of melanocytes associated with autoimmune disorders (Figure 4-7)

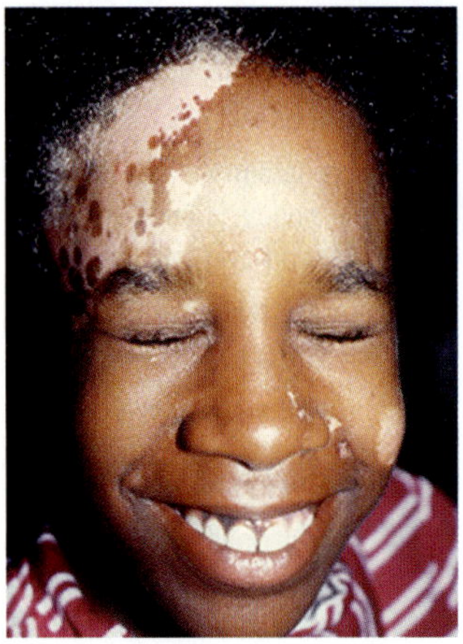

Figure 4-7
Vitiligo.

EXERCISE 14

Practice saying aloud each of the disease and disorder terms not built from word parts on pp. 109-114.

To hear the terms, go to http://evolve.elsevier.com. Refer to p. 18 for your Evolve Access Information. Select Exercises & Review, Chapter 4, Chapter Exercises, Pronunciation.

☐ Place a check mark in the box when you have completed this exercise.

EXERCISE 15

Fill in the blanks with the correct disease and disorder terms.

1. A chronic inflammatory disease affecting the skin, joints, and other organs is ________________ ________________ ________________.
2. A(n) ________________ is a localized collection of pus.
3. A cracklike sore in the skin is called a(n) ________________.
4. The scraping away of the skin by mechanical process or injury is called a(n) ________________.
5. ________________ is a chronic skin condition characterized by red lesions covered with silvery scales.
6. An inflammatory skin disease caused by a virus and characterized by small blisters in clusters is called ________________.
7. ________________ is the name given to the invasion of the skin and hair by lice.
8. A fungal infection of the skin, also known as *ringworm*, is called ________________.
9. An injury with no break in the skin and characterized by pain, swelling, and discoloration is called a(n) ________________.
10. ________________ is the name given to tissue death caused by a loss of blood supply followed by bacterial invasion.
11. Any visible change in tissue resulting from injury or disease is called a ________________.
12. ________________ ________________ is a cancerous condition starting as purple or brown papules on the lower extremities.
13. A horny tissue formation that results from excessive exposure to sunlight and is precancerous is called ________________ ________________.
14. A cluster of boils caused by staphylococcal bacteria is a ________________.
15. An inflammatory skin disease that involves the oil glands and hair follicles is called ________________.
16. ________________ is the name given to a torn, ragged-edged wound.
17. A painful skin node caused by staphylococcal bacteria in a hair follicle is called a(n) ________________.

18. A malignant growth that develops from scalelike epithelial tissue is known as ________________ ________________ carcinoma.

19. Inflammation of the skin and subcutaneous tissue caused by infection and creating redness, swelling, and fever is called ________________.

20. ________________ is the name given to a superficial skin infection characterized by pustules and caused by either staphylococci or streptococci.

21. ________________ is a noninfectious inflammatory skin disease characterized by redness, blisters, scabs, and itching.

22. A skin inflammation caused by the itch mite is called ________________.

23. ________________ is an itching skin eruption composed of wheals.

24. An epithelial tumor commonly found on the face of individuals who have had excessive sun exposure is ________________ ________________ carcinoma.

25. ________________ is a disease characterized by induration of the connective tissue.

26. ________________ is an infection of the mouth, skin, or vagina caused by *Candida albicans*.

27. An invasion of pathogens in body tissues is called ________________.

28. ________________ is a chronic disorder of the skin that produces erythema, papules, pustules, and broken blood vessels.

29. A congenital hereditary condition characterized by partial or total lack of pigment in the skin, hair, and eyes is ________________.

30. ________________ ________________ is an invasion of methicillin-resistant *Staphylococcus aureus* in the body tissue.

31. White patches on the skin caused by the destruction of melanocytes is called ________________.

EXERCISE 16

Match the words in the first column with their correct definitions in the second column.

______ 1. abrasion	a. death of tissue caused by loss of blood supply and entry of bacteria
______ 2. abscess	b. cracklike sore in the skin
______ 3. acne	c. cluster of boils
______ 4. actinic keratosis	d. induration of connective tissue
______ 5. basal cell carcinoma	e. noninfectious inflammatory skin disease having redness, blisters, scabs, and itching
______ 6. carbuncle	f. scraped-away skin
______ 7. cellulitis	g. involves sebaceous glands and hair follicles
______ 8. contusion	h. painful skin node caused by staphylococci in a hair follicle
______ 9. eczema	i. inflammation of skin and subcutaneous tissue with redness, swelling, and fever
______ 10. fissure	j. localized collection of pus
______ 11. furuncle	k. injury characterized by pain, swelling, and discoloration
______ 12. gangrene	l. precancerous skin condition caused by excessive exposure to sunlight
______ 13. scleroderma	m. usually occurring in the central area of the face in people older than 30 years
______ 14. rosacea	n. epithelial tumor commonly found in individuals who have had excessive sun exposure
______ 15. MRSA infection	o. red lesions with silvery scales
	p. potentially serious infection caused by methicillin-resistant *Staphylococcus aureus*

EXERCISE 17

Match the words in the first column with the correct definitions in the second column.

_____ 1. herpes
_____ 2. impetigo
_____ 3. Kaposi sarcoma
_____ 4. laceration
_____ 5. lesion
_____ 6. pediculosis
_____ 7. psoriasis
_____ 8. scabies
_____ 9. squamous cell carcinoma
_____ 10. systemic lupus erythematosus
_____ 11. tinea
_____ 12. urticaria
_____ 13. candidiasis
_____ 14. infection
_____ 15. albinism
_____ 16. vitiligo

a. skin inflammation caused by the itch mite
b. fungal infection of the skin, hair, and nails
c. red lesions covered by silvery scales
d. inflammatory skin disease having clusters of blisters and caused by a virus
e. chronic inflammatory disease involving the skin, joints, kidney, and nervous system
f. a cancerous condition that starts as brown or purple papules on the lower extremities
g. composed of wheals
h. torn, ragged-edged wound
i. superficial skin condition having pustules and caused by staphylococci or streptococci
j. characterized by lack of pigment in the skin, hair, and eyes
k. infection of the skin, mouth, or vagina caused by a yeast-type fungus
l. invasion of the hair and skin by lice
m. visible change in tissue resulting from injury or disease
n. a malignant growth that develops from scalelike epithelial tissue
o. invasion of body tissues by pathogens
p. cracklike sore in the skin
q. white patches on the skin caused by the destruction of melanocytes

EXERCISE 18

Spell each of the disease and disorder terms not built from word parts on pp. 109-114 by having someone dictate them to you.

To hear and spell the terms, go to http://evolve.elsevier.com. Refer to p. 18 for your Evolve Access Information. Select Exercises & Review, Chapter 4, Chapter Exercises, Spelling.
☐ Place a check mark in the box if you have completed this exercise online.

1. ______________________
2. ______________________
3. ______________________
4. ______________________
5. ______________________
6. ______________________
7. ______________________
8. ______________________

9. ______________________
10. ______________________
11. ______________________
12. ______________________
13. ______________________
14. ______________________
15. ______________________
16. ______________________
17. ______________________
18. ______________________
19. ______________________
20. ______________________
21. ______________________
22. ______________________
23. ______________________
24. ______________________
25. ______________________
26. ______________________
27. ______________________
28. ______________________
29. ______________________
30. ______________________
31. ______________________

Surgical Terms

Built from Word Parts

The following terms are built from word parts you have already learned and can be translated literally to find their meanings. Further explanation of terms beyond the definition of their word parts, if needed, is included in parentheses.

Term	Definition
biopsy (bx) (BĪ-op-sē)	view of life (the removal of living tissue from the body to be viewed under the microscope) (Figure 4-8)
dermatoautoplasty (*der*-ma-tō-AW-tō-*plas*-te)	surgical repair using one's own skin (skin graft) (also called **autograft**)
dermatoheteroplasty (*der*-ma-tō-HET-er-ō *plas*-tē)	surgical repair using skin from others (skin graft) (also called **allograft**)
dermatome (DER-ma-tōm) NOTE: when two consonants of the same letter come together, one is sometimes dropped.	instrument used to cut skin (in thin slices for skin grafts)
dermatoplasty (DER-ma-tō-*plas*-tē)	surgical repair of the skin
onychectomy (*on*-i-KEK-to-mē)	excision of a nail
rhytidectomy (*rit*-i-DEK-to-mē)	excision of wrinkles (also called **facelift**)
rhytidoplasty (RIT-i-dō-*plas*-tē)	surgical repair of wrinkles

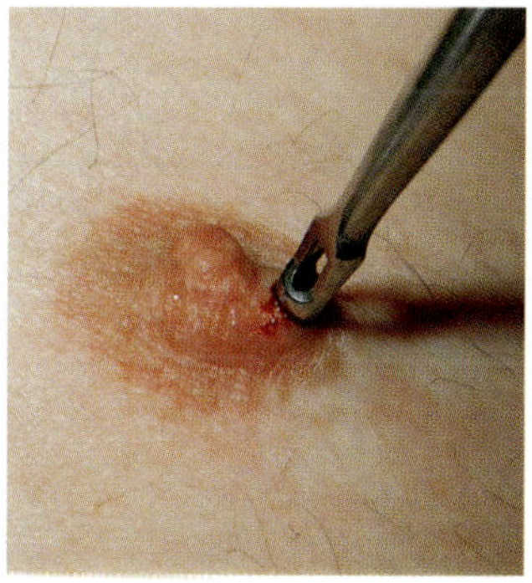

Figure 4-8
Punch biopsy.

BIOPSY OF THE SKIN

may be performed by the dermatologist during an office visit. Common techniques include:

- **excisional biopsy** removes the entire lesion along with a margin of surrounding tissue
- **punch biopsy** removes a cylindrical portion of tissue with a specifically designed round knife (see Figure 4-8)
- **shave biopsy** removes a sample of tissue with a cut parallel to the surrounding skin

DERMATOME

also refers to the **dermatomic area,** the area of skin supplied by a specific sensory nerve root.

EXERCISE 19

Practice saying aloud each of the surgical terms built from word parts on p. 119.

To hear the terms, go to http://evolve.elsevier.com. Refer to p. 18 for your Evolve Access Information. Select Exercises & Review, Chapter 4, Chapter Exercises, Pronunciation.

☐ Place a check mark in the box when you have completed this exercise.

EXERCISE 20

Analyze and define the following surgical terms.

Example: dermat / o / plasty (WR / CV / S; dermat/o = CF) — surgical repair of the skin

1. rhytidectomy ______
2. biopsy ______
3. dermatoautoplasty ______
4. onychectomy ______
5. rhytidoplasty ______
6. dermatoheteroplasty ______
7. dermatome ______

EXERCISE 21

Build surgical terms for the following definitions by using the word parts you have learned.

Example: surgical repair using one's own skin — dermat / o / aut / o / plasty (WR / CV / WR / CV / S)

1. excision of wrinkles ______ / ______ (WR / S)
2. view of life (removal of living tissue from the body) ______ / ______ (WR / S)
3. surgical repair using skin from others ______ / ______ / ______ / ______ / ______ (WR / CV / WR / CV / S)
4. excision of a nail ______ / ______ (WR / S)
5. surgical repair of wrinkles ______ / ______ / ______ (WR / CV / S)
6. surgical repair of the skin ______ / ______ / ______ (WR / CV / S)
7. instrument used to cut skin ______ / ______ (WR / S)

EXERCISE 22

Spell each of the surgical terms built from word parts on p. 119 by having someone dictate them to you.

To hear and spell the terms, go to http://evolve.elsevier.com. Refer to p. 18 for your Evolve Access Information. Select Exercises & Review, Chapter 4, Chapter Exercises, Spelling.

☐ Place a check mark in the box if you have completed this exercise online.

1. ______________________
2. ______________________
3. ______________________
4. ______________________
5. ______________________
6. ______________________
7. ______________________
8. ______________________

Surgical Terms

Not Built from Word Parts

In some of the following terms, you may recognize word parts you have already learned; however, the full meaning of the terms cannot be discerned by the definition of their word parts.

Term	Definition
cauterization (*kaw*-tur-ī-ZĀ-shun)	destruction of tissue with a hot or cold instrument, electric current, or caustic substance (also called **cautery**)
cryosurgery (*krī*-ō-SER-jer-ē)	destruction of tissue by using extreme cold, often by using liquid nitrogen (Figure 4-9)
débridement (dā-brēd-MA)	removal of contaminated or dead tissue and foreign matter from an open wound
dermabrasion (*derm*-a-BRĀ-zhun)	procedure to remove skin scars with abrasive material, such as sandpaper
excision (ek-SIZH-en)	removal by cutting
incision (in-SIZH-en)	surgical cut or wound produced by a sharp instrument
incision and drainage (I&D) (in-SIZH-en) and (DRĀ-nij)	surgical cut made to allow the free flow or withdrawal of fluids from a lesion, wound, or cavity
laser surgery (LĀ-zer) (SER-jer-ē)	procedure using an instrument that emits a high-powered beam of light used to cut, burn, vaporize, or destroy tissue
Mohs surgery (mōz) (SER-jer-ē)	technique of microscopically controlled serial excisions of skin cancers
suturing (SOO-cher-ing)	to stitch edges of a wound surgically (Figure 4-10)

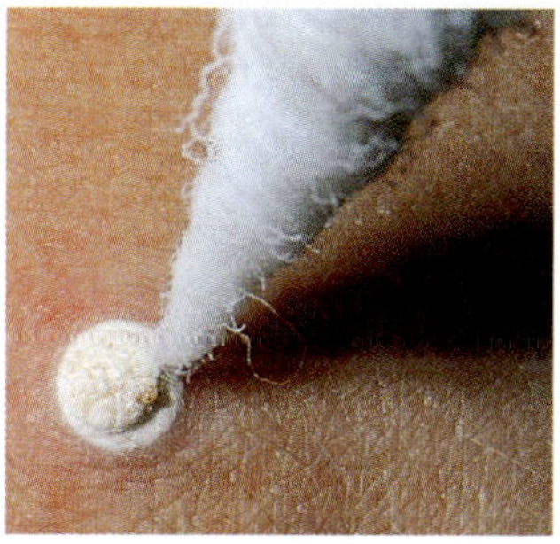

Figure 4-9
Cryosurgery performed with a nitrogen-soaked, cotton-tipped applicator.

MOHS SURGERY

allows for complete tumor removal while sparing surrounding normal tissue. It includes removing layers of tissue and examining them for tumor cells. If found, more tissue is removed until the margins are cancer free. It is used to treat recurrent skin cancers, especially lesions on the nose and ears, or areas that need tissue sparing. It is named after Dr. Frederic E. Mohs, Wisconsin, who first used the concept in 1936. The technique has evolved since that time.

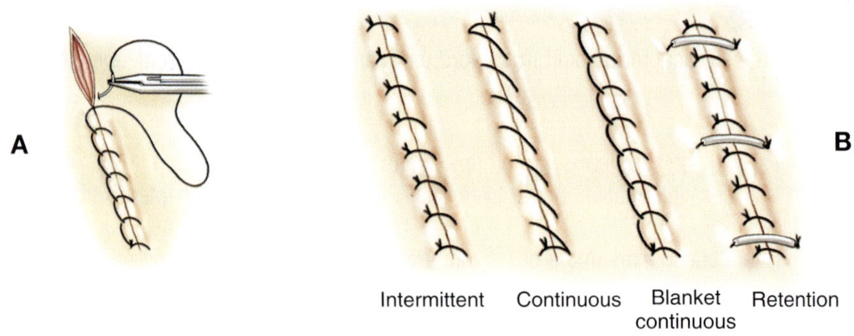

Figure 4-10
A, Suturing; **B,** types of sutures.

EXERCISE 23

Practice saying aloud each of the surgical terms not built from word parts on p. 121.

To hear the terms, go to http://evolve.elsevier.com. Refer to p. 18 for your Evolve Access Information. Select Exercises & Review, Chapter 4, Chapter Exercises, Pronunciation.

☐ Place a check mark in the box when you have completed this exercise.

EXERCISE 24

Fill in the blank with the correct surgical term.

1. ________________ ________________ is a technique of microscopically controlled serial excisions used for treatment of skin cancers.
2. A surgical cut or wound produced by a sharp instrument is called a(n) ________________.
3. Destruction of tissue with a hot or cold instrument, electric current, or caustic substance is called ________________.
4. ________________ is to stitch the edges of a wound surgically.
5. A surgical cut made to allow the free flow or withdrawal of fluids from a lesion, wound, or cavity is called ________________ ________________ ________________.
6. ________________ is the removal of contaminated or dead tissue and foreign matter from an open wound.
7. Removal by cutting is known as ________________.
8. ________________ ________________ is a procedure using an instrument that emits a high-powered beam of light used to cut, burn, vaporize, or destroy tissue.
9. The destruction of tissue by using extreme cold, often by using liquid nitrogen, is called ________________.
10. ________________ is a procedure to remove skin scars with abrasive material.

EXERCISE 25

Match the terms in the first column with their correct definitions in the second column.

_____ 1. suturing
_____ 2. dermabrasion
_____ 3. laser surgery
_____ 4. incision and drainage
_____ 5. cauterization
_____ 6. excision
_____ 7. Mohs surgery
_____ 8. débridement
_____ 9. cryosurgery
_____ 10. incision

a. destruction of tissue with a hot or cold instrument, electric current, or caustic substance
b. technique of microscopically controlled serial excisions of skin cancers
c. surgical cut or wound produced by a sharp instrument
d. surgical cut made to allow the free flow or withdrawal of fluids from a lesion, wound, or cavity
e. removal by cutting
f. removal of contaminated or dead tissue and foreign matter from an open wound
g. procedure using an instrument that emits a high-powered beam of light used to cut, burn, vaporize, or destroy tissue
h. procedure to remove skin scars with abrasive material, such as sandpaper
i. to stitch edges of a wound surgically
j. destruction of tissue by using extreme cold, often by using liquid nitrogen

EXERCISE 26

Spell each of the surgical terms not built from word parts on p. 121 by having someone dictate them to you.

To hear and spell the terms, go to http://evolve.elsevier.com. Refer to p. 18 for your Evolve Access Information. Select Exercises & Review, Chapter 4, Chapter Exercises, Spelling.
☐ Place a check mark in the box if you have completed this exercise online.

1. ____________________ 6. ____________________
2. ____________________ 7. ____________________
3. ____________________ 8. ____________________
4. ____________________ 9. ____________________
5. ____________________ 10. ____________________

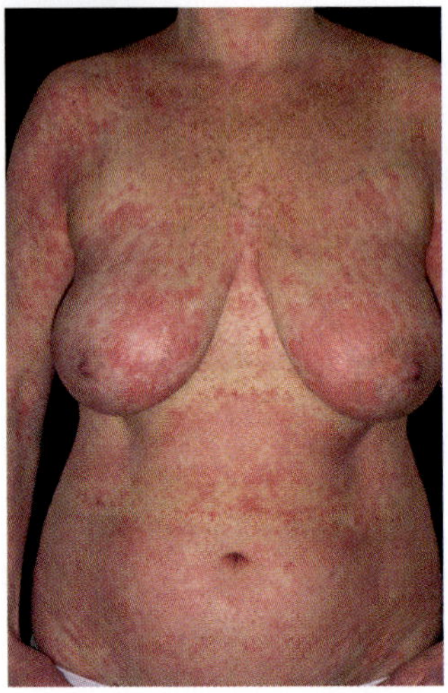

Figure 4-11
Exfoliative erythroderma. Erythroderma (red skin) may be caused by drugs, malignancy, psoriasis, and other conditions.

Complementary Terms

Built from Word Parts

The following terms are built from word parts you have already learned and can be translated literally to find their meanings. Further explanation of terms beyond the definition of their word parts, if needed, is included in parentheses.

Term	Definition
dermatologist (*der*-ma-TOL-o-jist)	a physician who studies and treats skin (diseases)
dermatology (derm) (der-ma-TOL-o-jē)	study of the skin (a branch of medicine that deals with the diagnosis and treatment of skin diseases)
epidermal (*ep*-i-DER-mal)	pertaining to upon the skin
erythroderma (e-rith-rō-DER-ma)	red skin (abnormal redness of the skin) (Figure 4-11)
hypodermic (*hī*-pō-DER-mik)	pertaining to under the skin (Exercise Figure D)
intradermal (ID) (*in*-tra-DER-mal)	pertaining to within the skin (Exercise Figure D)
keratogenic (*ker*-a-tō-JEN-ik)	originating in horny tissue
necrosis (ne-KRŌ-sis)	abnormal condition of death (cells and tissue die because of disease)
percutaneous (*per*-kū-TĀ-nē-us)	pertaining to through the skin
Staphylococcus **(*pl.* staphylococci) (staph)** (*staf*-il-ō-KOK-us) (*staf*-il-ō-KOK-sī)	berry-shaped (bacterium) in grapelike clusters (these bacteria cause many skin diseases) (Exercise Figure E)
streptococcus (pl. streptococci) (strep) (*strep*-tō-KOK-us) (*strep*-tō-KOK-sī)	berry-shaped (bacterium) in twisted chains (Exercise Figure E)
subcutaneous (subcut) (*sub*-kū-TĀ-nē-us)	pertaining to under the skin (Exercise Figure D)
transdermal (TD) (trans-DER-mel)	pertaining to through the skin (Exercise Figure D)
ungual (UNG-gwal)	pertaining to the nail
xanthoderma (*zan*-thō-DER-ma)	yellow skin (also called **jaundice**)

TRANSDERMAL

usually means entering through the skin and refers to the administration of a drug applied to the skin in ointment or patch form. **Percutaneous** usually means performed through the skin, as in the insertion of a needle, catheter, or probe. See **percutaneous endoscopic gastrostomy** highlighted in Chapter 11. (Figure 11-13)

EXERCISE FIGURE D

Fill in the blanks to build terms, related to the routes of administration pictured below.

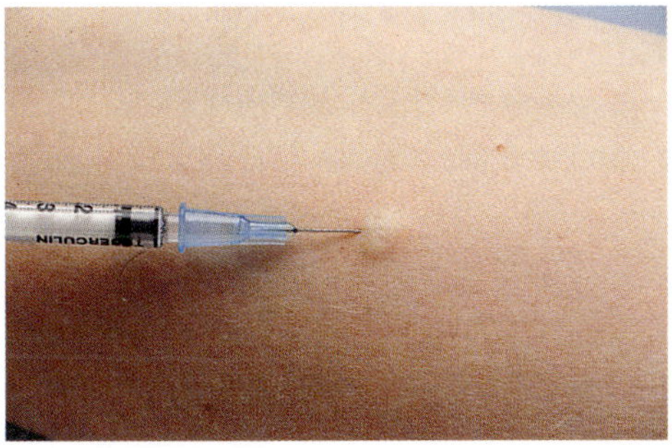

1. ______ / ______ / ______ injection
within / skin / pertaining to

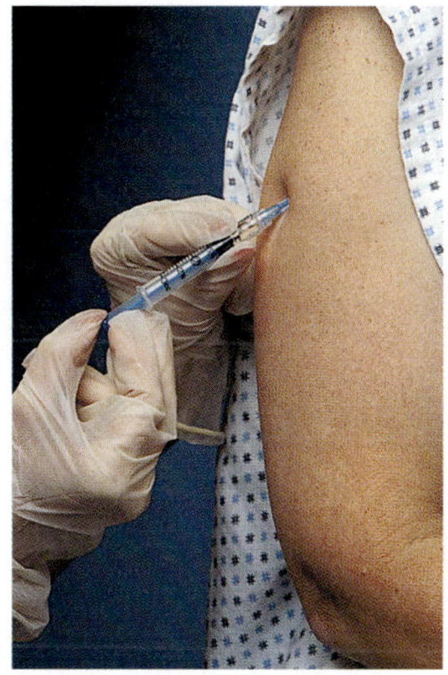

2. ______ / ______ / ______ injection
under / skin / pertaining to

using a ______ / ______ / ______ needle
under / skin / pertaining to

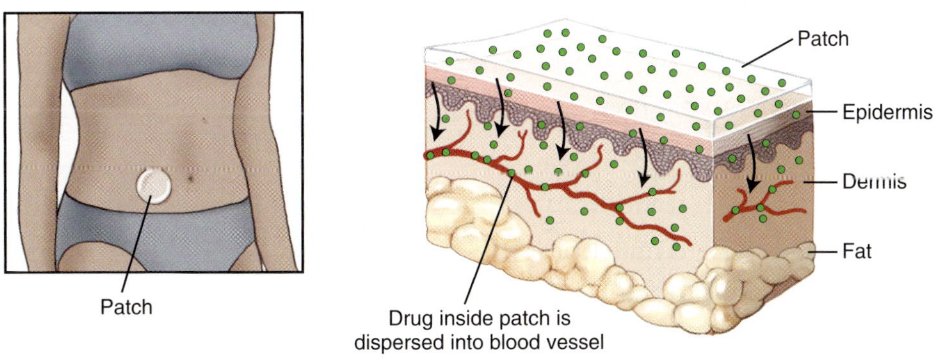

3. ______ / ______ / ______ patch
through / skin / pertaining to

EXERCISE FIGURE E

Fill in the blanks to label the diagrams.

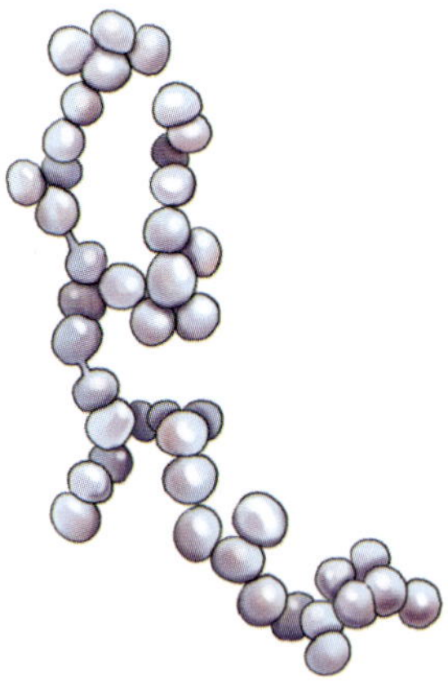

1. ______ / ______ / ______
grapelike clusters / cv / berry-shaped (plural)

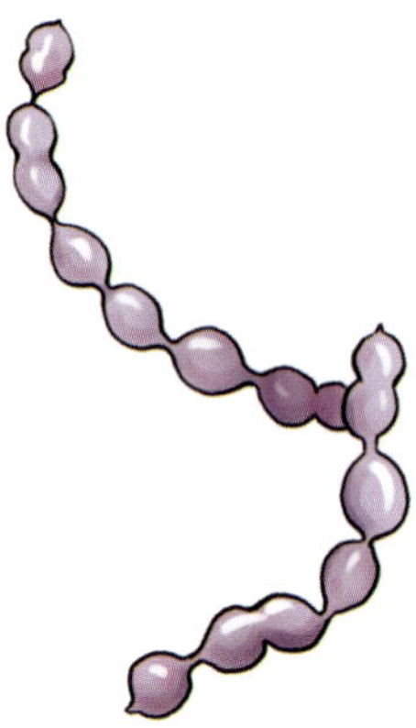

2. ______ / ______ / ______
twisted chains / CV / berry-shaped (plural)

EXERCISE 27

Practice saying aloud each of the complementary terms built from word parts on p. 124.

To hear the terms, go to http://evolve.elsevier.com. Refer to p. 18 for your Evolve Access Information. Select Exercises & Review, Chapter 4, Chapter Exercises, Pronunciation.

☐ Place a check mark in the box when you have completed this exercise.

EXERCISE 28

Analyze and define the following complementary terms.

Example: intra (P) / derm (WR) / al (S) *pertaining to within the skin*

1. ungual ______
2. transdermal ______
3. streptococcus ______
4. hypodermic ______
5. dermatology ______
6. subcutaneous ______
7. staphylococcus ______
8. keratogenic ______
9. dermatologist ______
10. necrosis ______
11. epidermal ______
12. xanthoderma ______
13. erythroderma ______
14. percutaneous ______

EXERCISE 29

Build complementary terms for the integumentary system by using the word parts you have learned.

Example: pertaining to under the skin hypo / derm / ic
P / WR / S

1. study of the skin ______ / ___ / ______
WR / CV / S

2. abnormal condition of death (of cells and tissue) ______ / ______
WR / S

3. pertaining to the nail ______ / ______
WR / S

4. berry-shaped bacterium in grapelike clusters (singular) ______ / ___ / ______
WR / CV / S

5. a physician who studies and treats skin (diseases) ______ / ___ / ______
WR / CV / S

6. pertaining to within the skin ______ / ______ / ______
P / WR / S

7. pertaining to upon the skin ______ / ______ / ______
P / WR / S

8. pertaining to under the skin ______ / ______ / ______
P / WR / S
______ / ______ / ______
P / WR / S

9. berry-shaped bacterium in twisted chains (singular) ______ / ___ / ______
WR / CV / S

10. originating in the horny tissue ______ / ___ / ______
WR / CV / S

11. red skin

_____ / _____ / _____ / _____
WR / CV / WR / S

12. yellow skin

_____ / _____ / _____ / _____
WR / CV / WR / S

13. pertaining to through the skin

_____ / _____ / _____
P / WR / S

_____ / _____ / _____
P / WR / S

EXERCISE 30

Spell each of the complementary terms built from word parts on p. 124 by having someone dictate them to you.

To hear and spell the terms, go to http://evolve.elsevier.com. Refer to p. 18 for your Evolve Access Information. Select Exercises & Review, Chapter 4, Chapter Exercises, Spelling.

☐ Place a check mark in the box if you have completed this exercise online.

1. _______________
2. _______________
3. _______________
4. _______________
5. _______________
6. _______________
7. _______________
8. _______________
9. _______________
10. _______________
11. _______________
12. _______________
13. _______________
14. _______________
15. _______________

Complementary Terms

Not Built from Word Parts

In some of the following terms, you may recognize word parts you have already learned; however, the full meaning of the terms cannot be discerned by the definition of their word parts.

Term	Definition
alopecia (*al*-ō-PĒ-sha)	loss of hair (Figure 4-12)
bacteria (s. bacterium) (bak-TĒR-ē-a) (bak-TĒR-ē-um)	single-celled microorganisms that reproduce by cell division and may cause infection by invading body tissue
cicatrix (SIK-a-triks)	scar
cyst (sist)	a closed sac containing fluid or semisolid material (Table 4-2, p. 131)
cytomegalovirus (CMV) (*sī*-to-MEG-a-lō-*vī*-rus)	a herpes-type virus that usually causes disease when the immune system is compromised
diaphoresis (*dī*-a-fo-RĒ-sis)	profuse sweating
ecchymosis (*pl.* ecchymoses) (*ek*-i-MŌ-sis) (*ek*-i-MŌ-sēz)	escape of blood into the skin (or mucous membrane), causing a small, flat, purple, or blue discoloration, as may occur when blood is withdrawn by a needle and syringe from an arm vein
edema (e-DĒ-ma)	puffy swelling of tissue from the accumulation of fluid
erythema (*er*-i-THĒ-ma)	redness
fungus (*pl.* fungi) (FUN-gus) (FUN-jī)	organism that feeds by absorbing organic molecules from its surroundings and may cause infection by invading body tissue; single-celled fungi (yeast) reproduce by budding; multicelled fungi (mold) reproduce by spore formation

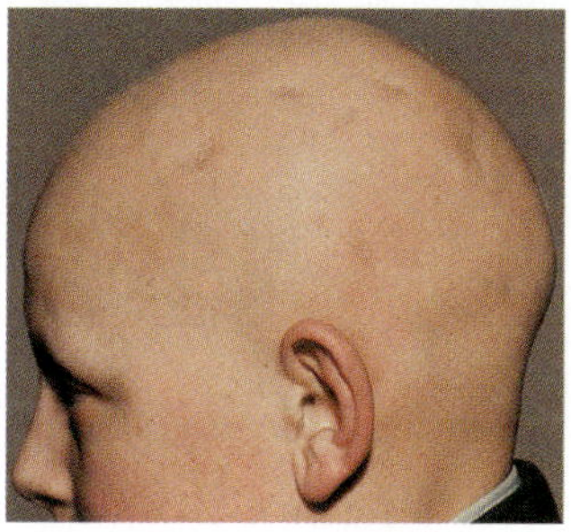

Figure 4-12
Alopecia totalis (loss of hair from the scalp) with absence of eyelashes.

ALOPECIA

is derived from the Greek **alopex**, meaning **fox.** One was thought to bald like a mangy fox.

DIAPHORESIS

is derived from Greek **dia**, meaning **through**, and **phoreo**, meaning **I carry.** Translated, it means the carrying through of perspiration.

ECCHYMOSIS, PETECHIA, AND PURPURA

are vascular lesions that are related to blood vessels and the escape of blood into the skin and mucous membrane (hemorrhage). They vary in size, with petechia being the smallest in size, up to .5 cm; purpura being the next largest, up to 1 cm; and ecchymosis being the largest, between 1 and 2 cm.

Complementary Terms—*cont'd*

Not Built from Word Parts

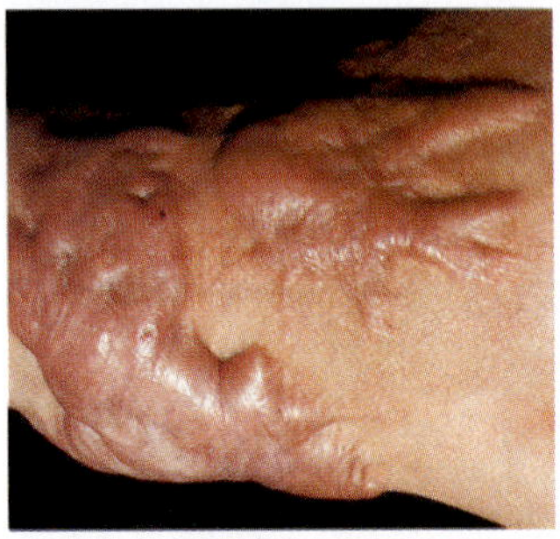

Figure 4-13
Burn keloid.

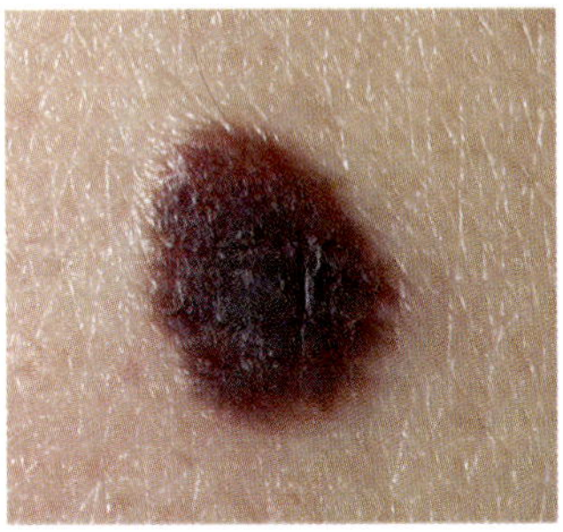

Figure 4-14
Nevus (also called **mole**).

MACULE

is probably derived from the ancient Sanskrit word **mala,** meaning **dirt.**

PETECHIA

is originally from the Italian **petechio,** meaning **flea bite.** The small hemorrhagic spot resembles the mark made by a flea.

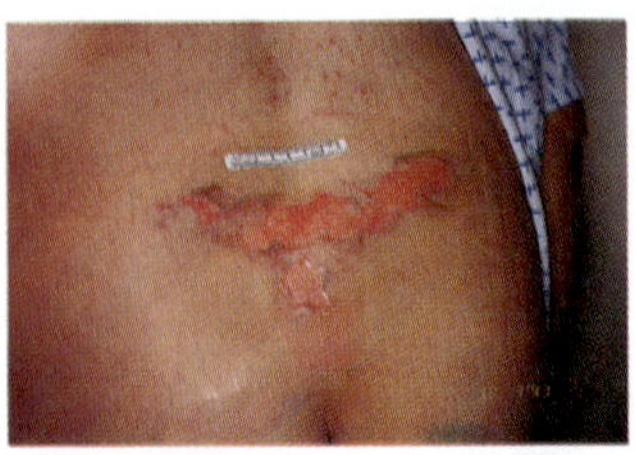

Figure 4-15
Stage 2 pressure ulcer (also called **decubitus ulcer** or **bed sore**).

Term	Definition
induration (*in*-dū-RĀ-shun)	abnormal hard spot(s)
jaundice (JAWN-dis)	condition characterized by a yellow tinge to the skin (also called **xanthoderma**)
keloid (KĒ-loyd)	overgrowth of scar tissue (Figure 4-13)
leukoplakia (*lū*-kō-PLĀ-kē-a)	condition characterized by white spots or patches on mucous membrane, which may be precancerous
macule (MAK-ūl)	flat, colored spot on the skin (see Table 4-2)
nevus (*pl.* nevi) (NĒ-vus) (NĒ-vī)	circumscribed malformation of the skin, usually brown, black, or flesh colored. A congenital nevus is present at birth and is referred to as a birthmark (Figure 4-14) (also called a **mole**).
nodule (NOD-ūl)	a small, knotlike mass that can be felt by touch (Table 4-2)
pallor (PAL-or)	paleness
papule (PAP-ūl)	small, solid skin elevation (Table 4-2)
petechia (*pl.* petechiae) (pe-TĒ-kē-a) (pe-TĒ-kē-ē)	a pinpoint skin hemorrhage
pressure ulcer (decub) (PRESH-ur) (UL-sir)	erosion of the skin caused by prolonged pressure, often occurring in bedridden patients (Figure 4-15) (also called **decubitus ulcer** or **bed sore**)
pruritus (prū-RĪ-tus)	severe itching
purpura (PER-pū-ra)	small hemorrhages in the skin (or mucous membrane), giving a purple-red discoloration; associated with blood disorders or vascular abnormalities
pustule (PUS-tūl)	elevation of skin containing pus (Table 4-2)
ulcer (UL-ser)	erosion of the skin or mucous membrane (Figure 4-15)

TABLE 4-2
Common Skin Lesions

Lesion	Definition	Cutaway Sections	Example
Macule	flat, colored spot on the skin	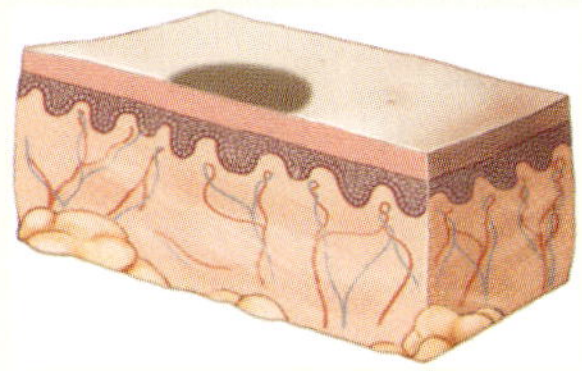	freckle
Papule	small, solid skin elevation	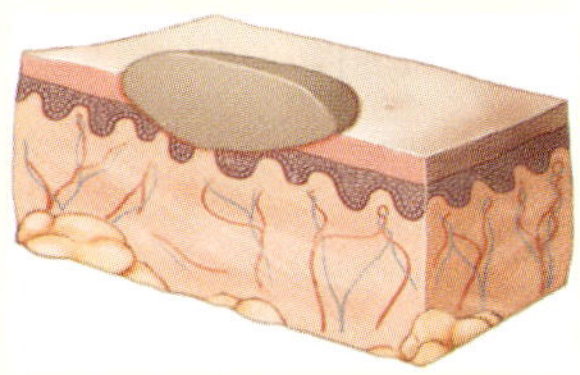	skin tag basal cell carcinoma
Nodule	a small, knotlike mass	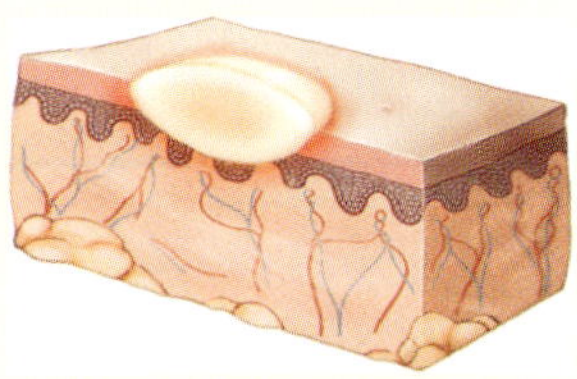	lipoma metastatic carcinoma rheumatoid nodule
Wheal	round, itchy elevation of the skin	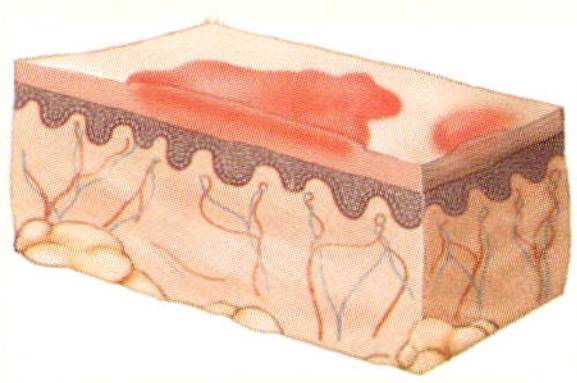	urticaria (hive)
Vesicle	small elevation of epidermis containing liquid	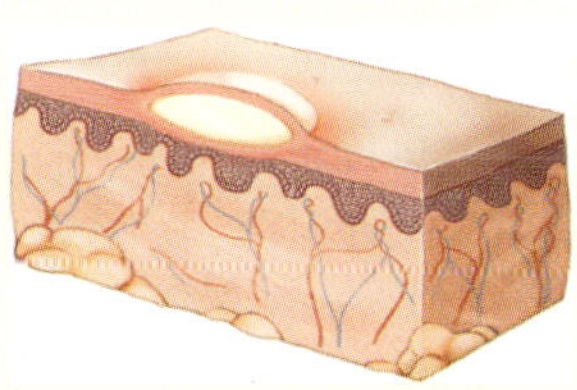	herpes zoster (shingles) herpes simplex contact dermatitis
Pustule	elevation of the skin containing pus	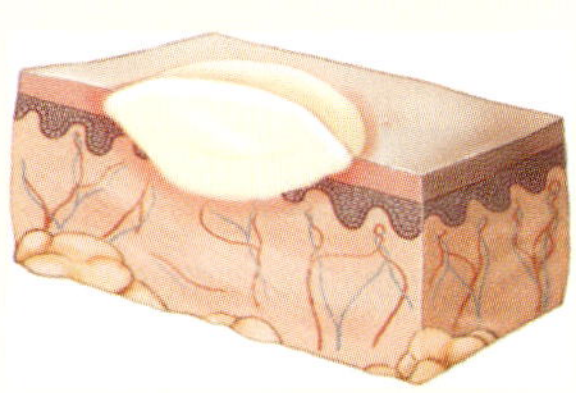	impetigo acne
Cyst	a closed sac containing fluid or semisolid material	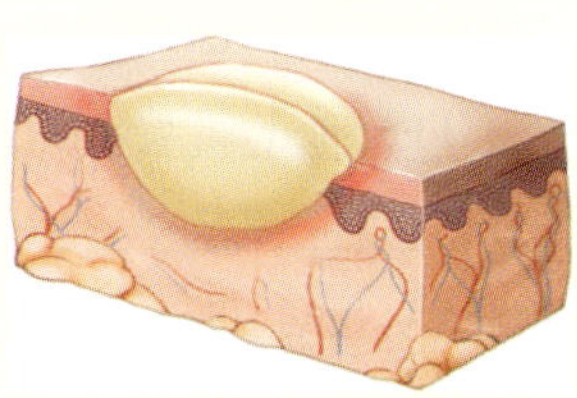	acne

Complementary Terms—*cont'd*

Not Built from Word Parts

Term	Definition
verruca (ver-RŪ-ka)	circumscribed cutaneous elevation caused by a virus (Figure 4-16) (also called **wart**)
vesicle (VES-i-kl)	small elevation of the epidermis containing liquid (See Table 4-2, p. 131) (also called **blister**)
virus (VĪ-ras)	minute microorganism, much smaller than a bacterium, characterized by a lack of independent metabolism and the ability to replicate only within living host cells; may cause infection by invading body tissue
wheal (hwēl)	transitory, itchy elevation of the skin with a white center and a red surrounding area; a wheal is an individual urticaria (hive) lesion (See Table 4-2, p. 131)

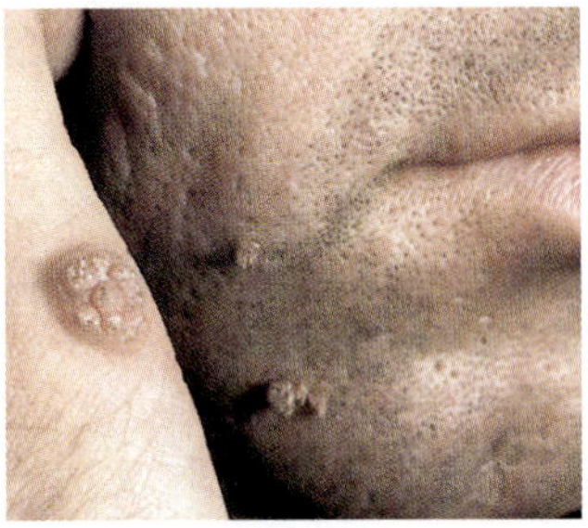

Figure 4-16
Verruca (also called **wart**)

DERMATOLOGY, OR GIVE ME A MAN WHO CALLS A SPADE A GEOTOME

I wish the *dermatologist*
Were less a firm apologist
For all the terminology
That's used in *dermatology*

Something you or I would
deem a
Redness he calls *erythema*;
If it's blistered, raw and warm
he
Has to call it multiforme
Things to him are never
simple;
Papule is his word for pimple
What's a macule, clearly
stated?
Just a spot that's over-rated!
Over the skin that looks unwell
He chants Latin like a spell;
What he's labeled and
obscured
Looks to him as good as
cured.

Reprinted with permission from *The New England Journal of Medicine*, 1977; 297(12):660.

Refer to **Appendix D** for pharmacology terms related to the integumentary system.

EXERCISE 31

Practice saying aloud each of the complementary terms not built from word parts on pp. 129-132.

To hear the terms, go to http://evolve.elsevier.com. Refer to p. 18 for your Evolve Access Information. Select Exercises & Review, Chapter 4, Chapter Exercises, Pronunciation.

☐ Place a check mark in the box when you have completed this exercise.

EXERCISE 32

Fill in the blanks with the correct terms.

1. Another name for scar is ____________________.
2. Profuse sweating is called ____________________.
3. The medical term for wart is ____________________.
4. ______________ is the name for a flat, colored skin spot.
5. A yellow skin condition is known as ____________________.
6. The condition of white spots or patches on mucous membrane is called ____________________.
7. ______________ is a pinpoint hemorrhage of the skin.

8. An erosion of the skin or mucous membrane is called a(n) ______________________.

9. A(n) ______________________ is an overgrowth of scar tissue.

10. Another name for paleness is ______________________.

11. Small, flat, purple or blue skin discoloration caused by hemorrhage, as seen after blood has been withdrawn by needle and syringe, is referred to as ______________________.

12. An erosion of the skin caused by prolonged pressure is a(n) ______________________ ______________________.

13. A small knotlike mass that can be felt by touch is called a(n) ______________________.

14. A closed sac containing fluid or semisolid material is called a(n) ______________________.

15. Severe itching is called ______________________.

16. Another name for redness is ______________________.

17. Small hemorrhages in the skin, showing a purple-red discoloration and associated with blood disorders or vascular abnormalities, is known as ______________________.

18. ______________________ is another name for mole.

19. Single-celled microorganisms that reproduce by cell division and may cause infection by invading body tissue are called ______________________.

20. The term for loss of hair is ______________________.

21. A small, solid skin elevation is called a(n) ______________________.

22. A transitory skin elevation with a white center and a red surrounding area is a(n) ______________________.

23. A(n) ______________________ is a skin elevation containing pus.

24. A blister is also called a(n) ______________________.

25. An organism that feeds by absorbing organic molecules from its surroundings and may cause infection by invading body tissue is called ______________________.

26. ______________________ is a minute microorganism characterized by a lack of independent metabolism and the ability to replicate only within living host cells; it also may cause infection by invading body tissue.

27. An abnormal hard spot(s) is called ______________________.

28. ______________________ is the swelling of tissue.

29. ______________________ is a herpes-type virus.

EXERCISE 33

Match the words in the first column with their correct definitions in the second column.

_____ 1. pressure ulcer
_____ 2. alopecia
_____ 3. cicatrix
_____ 4. fungus
_____ 5. nodule
_____ 6. bacteria
_____ 7. diaphoresis
_____ 8. cyst
_____ 9. ecchymosis
_____ 10. erythema
_____ 11. jaundice
_____ 12. edema
_____ 13. induration

a. loss of hair
b. small, flat, purple or blue discoloration caused by blood escaping into the skin or mucous membrane
c. yellow color to the skin
d. closed sac containing fluid
e. organism that feeds by absorbing organic molecules from its surroundings and may cause infection by invading body tissue
f. patches
g. profuse sweating
h. swelling of tissue
i. hard spot(s)
j. scar
k. redness
l. single-celled microorganisms that reproduce by cell division and may cause infection by invading body tissue
m. erosion of the skin caused by prolonged pressure
n. small knot

EXERCISE 34

Match the terms in the first column with their correct definitions in the second column.

______	1. keloid	a.	mole
______	2. leukoplakia	b.	severe itching
______	3. macule	c.	wart
______	4. nevus	d.	condition of white spots or patches on mucous membranes
______	5. pallor	e.	hemorrhages in the skin showing a purple-red color
______	6. papule	f.	skin elevation containing pus
______	7. petechiae	g.	overgrowth of scar tissue
______	8. pruritus	h.	small elevation of epidermis containing liquid
______	9. purpura	i.	individual urticaria lesion
______	10. pustule	j.	flat, colored spot on skin
______	11. ulcer	k.	small, solid skin elevation
______	12. verruca	l.	paleness
______	13. vesicle	m.	minute microorganism characterized by a lack of independent metabolism and the ability to replicate only within living host cells that may cause infection by invading body tissue
______	14. wheal	n.	pinpoint skin hemorrhages
______	15. virus	o.	erosion of the skin or mucous membrane
______	16. cytomegalovirus	p.	profuse sweating
		q.	herpes-type virus

EXERCISE 35

Spell each of the complementary terms not built from word parts on pp. 129-132 by having someone dictate them to you.

To hear and spell the terms, go to http://evolve.elsevier.com. Refer to p. 18 for your Evolve Access Information. Select Exercises & Review, Chapter 4, Chapter Exercises, Spelling.

☐ Place a check mark in the box if you have completed this exercise online.

1. ______________________	6. ______________________
2. ______________________	7. ______________________
3. ______________________	8. ______________________
4. ______________________	9. ______________________
5. ______________________	10. ______________________

11. ______________________
12. ______________________
13. ______________________
14. ______________________
15. ______________________
16. ______________________
17. ______________________
18. ______________________
19. ______________________
20. ______________________
21. ______________________
22. ______________________
23. ______________________
24. ______________________
25. ______________________
26. ______________________
27. ______________________
28. ______________________
29. ______________________

Abbreviations

BCC	basal cell carcinoma
bx	biopsy
CMV	cytomegalovirus
CA-MRSA	community-associated MRSA infection
decub	pressure ulcer
derm	dermatology
HA-MRSA	healthcare-associated MRSA infection
I&D	incision and drainage
ID	intradermal
MRSA	methicillin-resistant *Staphylococcus aureus*
SLE	systemic lupus erythematosus
SqCCA	squamous cell carcinoma
staph	staphylococcus
strep	streptococcus
subcut	subcutaneous
TD	transdermal

Refer to **Appendix C** for a complete list of abbreviations.

EXERCISE 36

Write the meaning for each of the abbreviations in the following sentences.

1. The most common form of skin cancer is **BCC** ______________ ______________ ______________.
2. It is rare to see cutaneous **CMV** ____________________ infections.
3. **SLE** ______________ ______________ ____________________ is a chronic relapsing disease, often with long periods of remission.
4. Long-term exposure to sunlight is by far the most frequent cause of **SqCCA** ______________ ______________ ______________.
5. The **bx** ______________ results were negative.
6. The medication was administered by **subcut** ____________________ injection.
7. **Staph** ______________ bacterium was cultured from the abscess.
8. The culture confirmed a **strep** ____________________ infection of the throat.
9. **I&D** ______________ ______________ ______________ is used to treat cutaneous abscesses, such as a furuncle.
10. Hormone replacement therapy is available in **TD** ____________________ administration.
11. The tuberculin test was administered by an **ID** ______________ injection.
12. The patient visited the **derm** ____________________ clinic for a psoriasis follow-up visit.
13. Débridement may be used to treat a **decub** ______________ ______________.
14. **MRSA** ______________ ______________ ______________ ______________ infections originating in a healthcare setting are called **HA-MRSA** ______________ ______________ ______________ ______________ ______________, whereas MRSA infections occurring in a person who has not recently been in a healthcare setting is called **CA-MRSA** ______________ ____________________________ ______________.

PRACTICAL APPLICATION

EXERCISE 37 *Interact with Medical Documents*

A. Below is an operative report. Complete the report by writing the medical terms in the blanks that correspond to the numbered definitions on the next page.

University Hospital and Medical Center

4700 North Main Street • Wellness, Arizona 54321 • (987) 555-3210

PATIENT NAME: Sandra Wharton **CASE NUMBER:** 76548-INT

DATE OF BIRTH: 10/03/19XX **DATE:** 07/27/20XX

OPERATIVE REPORT

CASE HISTORY: The patient is a 50-year-old white woman presenting to the 1. ________________ clinic for follow-up of a 2. ________________ located at the 3. ________________ aspect of her left eyebrow.

The patient's medical history is also significant for 4. ________________ ________________, primarily of the scalp and ears, as well as chronic 5. ________________, primarily of the forearms bilaterally.

INDICATIONS FOR PROCEDURE: Comparing today's exam with past medical records and photos from 10/20/20XX, the nevus shows changes that include hair loss, "crusty" surface, and some enlargement of the 6. ________________. The nevus has been present for approximately 3 years. Risks, benefits, indications, and expectations were discussed with the patient regarding biopsy, and she has agreed to proceed with 7. ________________.

PREOPERATIVE DIAGNOSIS: Dysplastic nevus, left eyebrow.

ANESTHESIA: Xylocaine 1% with epinephrine.

PROCEDURE: After written consent was obtained, the site was prepped with Betadine and draped in the usual sterile fashion. The skin was incised at the 8. ________________ pole of the lesion. The lesion was then excised, including a margin of clinically normal dermis. Specimen was submitted to 9. ________________. The superior pole was sutured. 10. ________________ was used to achieve hemostasis. Two A-T flaps were then constructed on superior aspect of upper left eyelid. Flaps and upper left eyelid undermined 2 to 3 mm. Flaps sutured with 6-0 Vicryl, followed by 6-0 nylon for closure. Pressure dressing was applied.

The patient tolerated the procedure well.

POSTOPERATIVE DIAGNOSIS: 11. ____________ revealed 12. ____________ ____________ ____________, nodular, transected at base.

____

William Hickman, MD

WH/mcm

1. study of skin
2. mole
3. pertaining to the middle
4. precancerous skin condition of horny tissue formation
5. noninfectious, inflammatory skin disease with redness, blisters, scabs, and itching
6. changes in tissue resulting from injury or disease
7. removal by cutting
8. pertaining to above
9. study of disease
10. destruction of tissue with a hot or cold instrument, electric current, or caustic substance
11. view of life
12. epithelial tumor arising from epidermis

B. Read the pathology report and answer the questions following it.

49785 LIGHT, Darla B.

File Patient Navigate Custom Fields Help

Patient Chart | Lab | Rad | Notes | Documents | Rx | Scheduling | Images | Billing

Name: **LIGHT, Darla B.** MR#: **49785** Sex: **F**
DOB: **6/15/19XX**

PATHOLOGY REPORT

DATE/TIME COLL: Jun 12 20XX 12:00 AM
DATE RECEIVED: Jun 12 20XX 8:00 PM
DATE REPORTED: Jun 22 20XX
REPORT STATUS: FINAL REPORT

HISTORY: Previous incidence of melanoma and basal cell carcinoma, no metastases

PRE-OP: Melanoma vs. compound nevi

PROCEDURE: Tissue biopsy

SPECIMEN: Skin biopsy, anterior, proximal right arm

GROSS DESCRIPTION: One container is received. Specimen in formalin labeled with the patient's name is a shave biopsy of gray-white hair bearing skin measuring 0.4 x 0.3 cm in surface dimension and averaging 0.1 cm in thickness. The epidermal surface contains a symmetric, smooth bordered, pigmented lesion measuring 0.3 cm in greatest diameter. The specimen is bisected and totally submitted.

MICROSCOPIC EXAMINATION: A microscopic examination has been performed.

DIAGNOSIS: Lesion, anterior, proximal right arm: benign compound nevus.

Electronically signed by: J. Alvarez, MD, Pathologist, 6/22/20XX 10:48 AM

Start | Log On/Off | Print | Edit

1. Identify singular and plural forms of medical terms used in the pathology report. Write "p" for plural and "s" for singular next to the terms. Refer to Table 2-2 on p. 37 for plural endings.
   a. melanoma ______
   b. melanomata ______
   c. nevi ______
   d. nevus ______
   e. metastasis ______
   f. metastases ______
   g. biopsy ______
   h. biopsies ______
2. The skin biopsy was obtained from:
   a. near the shoulder on the back of the right arm
   b. near the shoulder on the front of the right arm
   c. near the wrist on the back of the right arm
   d. near the wrist on the front of the right arm
3. Use your medical dictionary to find the meanings of the following terms used in the pathology report:
   a. compound ______________________
   b. pigmented ______________________
   c. bisected ______________________
   d. microscopic ______________________

EXERCISE 38 *Interpret Medical Terms*

To test your understanding of the terms introduced in this chapter, circle the words that correctly complete the sentences. The italicized words refer to the correct answer.

1. *Berry-shaped bacteria in grapelike clusters* are (**streptococci, staphylococci, pediculosis**).
2. The physician ordered lotions applied to the patient's *skin* to alleviate *dryness*, or (**pachyderma, dermatoconiosis, xeroderma**).
3. The injection given *within the skin* is called a(n) (**intradermal, epidermal, hypodermic**) injection.
4. The diagnosis of *onychomalacia* was given by the physician for (**ingrown nails, nail biting, softening of the nails**).
5. The *pinpoint hemorrhages*, or (**nevi, verrucae, petechiae**), were distributed over the patient's entire body.
6. The primary symptom of the disease was *profuse sweating*, or (**diaphoresis, ecchymosis, pruritus**).
7. The patient had an *abnormal condition of a fungus in the hair*; therefore the doctor recorded the diagnosis as (**onychocryptosis, trichomycosis, onychomycosis**).
8. The student nurse learned that the medical name for a *blister* was (**verruca, keloid, vesicle**).
9. The patient was to receive a *skin graft from her mother*, so the operation was listed as a (**dermatoplasty, dermatoautoplasty, dermatoheteroplasty**).
10. An *abnormal hard spot* is called (**edema, induration, virus**).
11. Another word for *jaundice* is (**erythroderma, leukoderma, xanthoderma**).
12. *Leiodermia* is a condition of (**striated, smooth, sweaty**) skin.
13. The *localized collection of pus* (**acne, abscess, cyst**) was incised and drained followed by débridement. A culture swab of the wound revealed methicillin-resistant *Staphylococcus aureus*.
14. *A technique of microscopically controlled serial excisions* (**cryosurgery, laser surgery, Mohs surgery**) was used to treat the patient's recurrent squamous cell carcinoma.
15. Antibiotics were not prescribed for the patient who presented with fever blisters, an infection caused by *a minute microorganism characterized by a lack of independent metabolism* (**bacteria, virus, fungus**).
16. *White skin (patches caused by depigmentation)* (**leiodermia, xeroderma, leukoderma**), *congenital, hereditary condition characterized by lack of pigment in skin, hair, and eyes* (**actinic keratosis, albinism, rosacea**), and *white patches on the skin caused by the destruction of melanocytes* (**vitiligo, Kaposi sarcoma, systemic lupus erythematosus**) are all forms of hypomelanosis, a condition characterized by a deficiency of melanin in the tissues.
17. *Small hemorrhages into the tissue, giving the skin a purple-red discoloration* (**pruritus, purpura, papule**) may be caused by blood disorders, vascular abnormalities, or trauma.

EXERCISE 39 *Read Medical Terms in Use*

Practice pronunciation of terms by reading aloud the following medical document. Use the pronunciation key following the medical term to assist you in saying the word.

To hear these terms, go to http://evolve.elsevier.com. Refer to p. 18 for your Evolve Access Information. Select Exercises & Review, Chapter 4, Chapter Exercises, Read Medical Terms in Use.

Emily visited the **dermatology** (*der*-ma-TOL-o-jē) clinic because of **pruritus** (prū-RĪ-tus) secondary to **dermatitis** (*der*-ma-TĪ-tis) involving her scalp, arms, and legs. A diagnosis of **psoriasis** (so-RĪ-a-sis) was made. **Eczema** (EK-ze-ma), **scabies** (SKĀ-bēz), and **tinea** (TIN-ē-a) were considered in the differential diagnosis. An emollient cream was prescribed. In addition the patient showed the **dermatologist** (der-ma-TOL-o-jist) the tender, discolored, thickened nail of her right great toe. Emily learned she had **onychomycosis** (*on*-i-kō-mī-KŌ-sis), for which she was given an additional prescription for an oral antifungal drug.

WEB LINK

For more information about diseases and disorders of the integumentary system and current treatments, visit the **American Academy of Dermatology** at ***www.aad.org.***

EXERCISE 40 *Comprehend Medical Terms In Use*

Test your comprehension of terms in the above medical document by circling the correct answer.

1. Emily sought medical attention because of:
   a. an eroded sore and inflammation of the skin
   b. severe itching and inflammation of the skin
   c. severe itching and thickness of the skin
   d. an eroded sore and thickening of the skin
2. T F An inflammatory disease of the skin involving sebaceous glands and hair follicles was considered in the differential diagnosis.
3. Emily was given an additional prescription for an abnormal condition of fungus in the:
   a. sudoriferous glands
   b. hair follicles
   c. sebaceous glands
   d. nails

CHAPTER REVIEW

ONLINE CHAPTER REVIEW

To access the Evolve website, go to http://evolve.elsevier.com. Refer to p. 18 for your Evolve Access Information. Select Exercises & Review, Chapter 4, then select Chapter Exercises, Practice Activities, Animations, or Games. Place a check mark in the box when you have completed an exercise or activity, watched an animation, or played a game. Have fun!

Chapter Exercises

Exercises in this section of your Evolve resources correlate to exercises in your textbook. You may have completed them as you worked through the chapter.

- ☐ Pronunciation
- ☐ Spelling
- ☐ Read Medical Terms in Use

Practice Activities

Practice in study mode, then test your learning in assessment mode. Keep track of your scores from assessment mode if you wish.

	SCORE
☐ Picture It	_______
☐ Define Word Parts	_______
☐ Build Medical Terms	_______
☐ Word Shop	_______
☐ Define Medical Terms	_______
☐ Use It	_______
☐ Hear It and Type It: Clinical Vignettes	_______

Animations

- ☐ Acne
- ☐ Pressure Ulcer

Games

- ☐ Name that Word Part
- ☐ Term Storm
- ☐ Term Explorer
- ☐ Termbusters
- ☐ Medical Millionaire
- ☐ Crossword puzzle

REVIEW OF WORD PARTS

Can you define and spell the following word parts?

Combining Forms

aut/o
bi/o
coni/o
crypt/o
cutane/o
derm/o
dermat/o
heter/o
hidr/o
kerat/o
myc/o
necr/o
onych/o
pachy/o
rhytid/o
seb/o
staphyl/o
strept/o
trich/o
ungu/o
xer/o

Prefixes

epi-
intra-
para-
per-
sub-
trans-

Suffixes

-a
-coccus (*pl.* -cocci)
-ectomy
-ia
-itis
-malacia
-opsy
-phagia
-plasty
-rrhea
-tome

REVIEW OF TERMS

Can you build, analyze, define, pronounce, and spell the following terms *built from word parts*?

Diseases and Disorders

dermatitis
dermatoconiosis
dermatofibroma
hidradenitis
leiodermia
leukoderma
onychocryptosis
onychomalacia
onychomycosis
onychophagia
pachyderma
paronychia
seborrhea
trichomycosis
xeroderma

Surgical

biopsy (bx)
dermatoautoplasty
dermatoheteroplasty
dermatome
dermatoplasty
onychectomy
rhytidectomy
rhytidoplasty

Complementary

dermatologist
dermatology (derm)
epidermal
erythroderma
hypodermic
intradermal (ID)
keratogenic
necrosis
percutaneous
staphylococcus (staph) (*pl.* staphylococci)
streptococcus (strep) (*pl.* streptococci)
subcutaneous (subcut)
transdermal (TD)
ungual
xanthoderma

Can you define, pronounce, and spell the following terms *not built from word parts?*

Diseases and Disorders

abrasion
abscess
acne
actinic keratosis
albinism
basal cell carcinoma (BCC)
candidiasis
carbuncle
cellulitis
contusion
eczema
fissure
furuncle
gangrene
herpes
impetigo
infection
Kaposi sarcoma
laceration
lesion
MRSA infection
pediculosis
psoriasis
rosacea
scabies
scleroderma
squamous cell carcinoma (SqCCA)
systemic lupus erythematosus (SLE)
tinea
urticaria
vitiligo

Surgical

cauterization
cryosurgery
débridement
dermabrasion
excision
incision
incision and drainage (I&D)
laser surgery
Mohs surgery
suturing

Complementary

alopecia
bacteria (*s.* bacterium)
cicatrix
cyst
cytomegalovirus (CMV)
diaphoresis
ecchymosis (*pl.* ecchymoses)
edema
erythema
fungus (*pl.* fungi)
induration
jaundice
keloid
leukoplakia
macule
nevus (*pl.* nevi)
nodule
pallor
papule
petechia (*pl.* petechiae)
pressure ulcer (decub)
pruritus
purpura
pustule
ulcer
verruca
vesicle
virus
wheal

ANSWERS

Exercise Figures

Exercise Figure

A. 1. horny tissue: kerat/o
2. hair: trich/o
3. skin: cutane/o, dermat/o, derm/o
4. sebum: seb/o
5. sweat: hidr/o

Exercise Figure

B. 1. nail: onych/o, ungu/o

Exercise Figure

C. 1. onych/o/myc/osis
2. par/onych/ia

Exercise Figure

D. 1. intra/derm/al
2. sub/cutane/ous, hypo/derm/ic
3. trans/derm/al

Exercise Figure

E. 1. staphyl/o/cocci
2. strept/o/cocci

Exercise 1

1. c
2. d
3. g
4. b
5. f
6. h
7. a

Exercise 2

1. sweat
2. skin
3. nail
4. hair
5. horny tissue, hard
6. skin
7. sebum (oil)
8. nail
9. skin

Exercise 3

1. trich/o
2. hidr/o
3. a. onych/o
   b. ungu/o
4. seb/o
5. a. derm/o
   b. dermat/o
   c. cutane/o
6. kerat/o

Exercise 4

1. death
2. grapelike clusters
3. hidden
4. thick
5. dust
6. fungus
7. life
8. other
9. twisted chains
10. dry
11. self
12. wrinkles

Exercise 5

1. myc/o
2. necr/o
3. heter/o
4. xer/o
5. pachy/o
6. strept/o
7. rhytid/o
8. staphyl/o
9. aut/o
10. crypt/o
11. coni/o
12. bi/o

Exercise 6

1. under, below
2. beside, beyond, around, abnormal
3. on, upon, over
4. within
5. through
6. through, across, beyond

Exercise 7

1. intra-
2. sub-
3. epi-
4. para-
5. per-
6. trans-

Exercise 8

1. c
2. e
3. a
4. j
5. i
6. h
7. d
8. b
9. f
10. k
11. l

Exercise 9

1. surgical repair
2. excision or surgical removal
3. softening
4. inflammation
5. instrument used to cut
6. eating, swallowing
7. flow, discharge
8. berry-shaped
9. view of, viewing
10. diseased or abnormal state, condition of
11. noun suffix, no meaning

Exercise 10

Pronunciation Exercise

Exercise 11

1. WR CV WR S
   dermat/o/coni/osis
   CF
   abnormal condition of the skin caused by dust
2. WR WR S
   hidr/aden/itis
   inflammation of the sweat glands
3. WR S
   dermat/itis
   inflammation of the skin
4. WR WR S
   pachy/derm/a
   thickening of the skin
5. WR CV S
   onych/o/malacia
   CF
   softening of the nails
6. WR CV WR S
   trich/o/myc/osis
   CF
   abnormal condition of a fungus in the hair
7. WR CV WR S
   dermat/o/fibr/oma
   CF
   fibrous tumor of the skin
8. P WR S
   par/onych/ia
   diseased state around the nail
9. WR CV WR S
   onych/o/crypt/osis
   CF
   abnormal condition of a hidden nail
10. WR CV S
    seb/o/rrhea
    CF
    discharge of sebum (excessive)
11. WR CV S
    onych/o/phagia
    CF
    eating the nails, nail biting
12. WR CV WR S
    xer/o/derm/a
    CF
    dry skin
13. WR CV WR S
    lei/o/derm/ia
    CF
    condition of smooth skin
14. WR CV WR S
    leuk/o/derm/a
    CF
    white skin

Exercise 12

1. pachy/derm/a
2. onych/o/myc/osis
3. seb/o/rrhea

4. dermat/itis
5. dermat/o/fibr/oma
6. onych/o/malacia
7. hidr/aden/itis
8. onych/o/crypt/osis
9. dermat/o/coni/osis
10. onych/o/phagia
11. par/onych/ia
12. xer/o/derm/a
13. lei/o/derm/ia
14. leuk/o/derm/a

Exercise 13
Spelling Exercise; see text pp. 105-106.

Exercise 14
Pronunciation Exercise

Exercise 15
1. systemic lupus erythematosus
2. abscess
3. fissure
4. abrasion
5. psoriasis
6. herpes
7. pediculosis
8. tinea
9. contusion
10. gangrene
11. lesion
12. Kaposi sarcoma
13. actinic keratosis
14. carbuncle
15. acne
16. laceration
17. furuncle
18. squamous cell
19. cellulitis
20. impetigo
21. eczema
22. scabies
23. urticaria
24. basal cell
25. scleroderma
26. candidiasis
27. infection
28. rosacea
29. albinism
30. MRSA infection
31. vitiligo

Exercise 16
1. f
2. j
3. g
4. l
5. n
6. c
7. i
8. k
9. e
10. b
11. h
12. a
13. d
14. m
15. p

Exercise 17
1. d
2. i
3. f
4. h
5. m
6. l
7. c
8. a
9. n
10. e
11. b
12. g
13. k
14. o
15. j
16. q

Exercise 18
Spelling Exercise; see text pp. 109-114.

Exercise 19
Pronunciation Exercise

Exercise 20
1. WR S
rhytid/ectomy
excision of wrinkles
2. WR S
bi/opsy
view of life (removal of living tissue)
3. WR CV WR CV S
dermat/o/aut/o/plasty
CF CF
surgical repair using one's own skin (for the skin graft)
4. WR S
onych/ectomy
excision of a nail
5. WR CV S
rhytid/o/plasty
CF
surgical repair of wrinkles
6. WR CV WR CV S
dermat/o/heter/o/plasty
CF CF
surgical repair using skin from others (for the skin graft)
7. WR S
derma/tome
instrument used to cut skin

Exercise 21
1. rhytid/ectomy
2. bi/opsy
3. dermat/o/heter/o/plasty
4. onych/ectomy
5. rhytid/o/plasty
6. dermat/o/plasty
7. derma/tome

Exercise 22
Spelling Exercise; see text p. 119.

Exercise 23
Pronunciation Exercise

Exercise 24
1. Mohs surgery
2. incision
3. cauterization
4. suturing
5. incision and drainage
6. débridement
7. excision
8. laser surgery
9. cryosurgery
10. dermabrasion

Exercise 25
1. i
2. h
3. g
4. d
5. a
6. e
7. b
8. f
9. j
10. c

Exercise 26
Spelling Exercise, see text p. 121.

Exercise 27
Pronunciation Exercise

Exercise 28
1. WR S
ungu/al
pertaining to the nail
2. P WR S
trans/derm/al
pertaining to through the skin
3. WR CV S
strept/o/coccus
CF
berry-shaped (bacterium) in twisted chains
4. P WR S
hypo/derm/ic
pertaining to under the skin
5. WR CV S
dermat/o/logy
CF
study of the skin
6. P WR S
sub/cutane/ous
pertaining to under the skin
7. WR CV S
staphyl/o/coccus
CF
berry-shaped (bacterium) in grapelike clusters
8. WR CV S
kerat/o/genic
CF
originating in horny tissue

9. WR CV S
dermat/o/logist
CF
physician who studies and treats skin (diseases)

10. WR S
necr/osis
abnormal condition of death (of cells and tissue)

11. P WR S
epi/derm/al
pertaining to upon the skin

12. WR CV WR S
xanth/o/derm/a
CF
yellow skin

13. WR CV WR S
erythr/o/derm/a
CF
red skin

14. P WR S
per/cutane/ous
pertaining to through the skin

Exercise 29

1. dermat/o/logy
2. necr/osis
3. ungu/al
4. staphyl/o/coccus
5. dermat/o/logist
6. intra/derm/al
7. epi/derm/al
8. sub/cutane/ous, hypo/derm/ic
9. strept/o/coccus
10. kerat/o/genic
11. erythr/o/derm/a
12. xanth/o/derm/a
13. per/cutane/ous, trans/derm/al

Exercise 30

Spelling Exercise; see text p. 124.

Exercise 31

Pronunciation Exercise

Exercise 32

1. cicatrix
2. diaphoresis
3. verruca
4. macule
5. jaundice
6. leukoplakia
7. petechia
8. ulcer
9. keloid
10. pallor
11. ecchymosis
12. pressure ulcer
13. nodule
14. cyst
15. pruritus
16. erythema
17. purpura
18. nevus
19. bacteria
20. alopecia
21. papule
22. wheal
23. pustule
24. vesicle
25. fungus
26. virus
27. induration
28. edema
29. cytomegalovirus

Exercise 33

1. m
2. a
3. j
4. e
5. n
6. l
7. g
8. d
9. b
10. k
11. c
12. h
13. i

Exercise 34

1. g
2. d
3. j
4. a
5. l
6. k
7. n
8. b
9. e
10. f
11. o
12. c
13. h
14. i
15. m
16. q

Exercise 35

Spelling Exercise; see text pp. 129-132.

Exercise 36

1. basal cell carcinoma
2. cytomegalovirus
3. systemic lupus erythematosus
4. squamous cell carcinoma
5. biopsy
6. subcutaneous
7. staphylococcus
8. streptococcus
9. incision and drainage
10. transdermal
11. intradermal
12. dermatology
13. pressure ulcer
14. methicillin-resistant *Staphylococcus aureus*, healthcare-associated methicillin-resistant *Staphylococcus aureus*, community-associated methicillin-resistant *Staphylococcus aureus*

Exercise 37

A. 1. dermatology
2. nevus
3. medial
4. actinic keratosis
5. eczema
6. lesion
7. excision
8. superior
9. pathology
10. cauterization
11. biopsy
12. basal cell carcinoma

B. 1. a. s
b. p
c. p
d. s
e. s
f. p
g. s
h. p
2. b
3. dictionary exercise

Exercise 38

1. staphylococci
2. xeroderma
3. intradermal
4. softening of the nails
5. petechiae
6. diaphoresis
7. trichomycosis
8. vesicle
9. dermatoheteroplasty
10. induration
11. xanthoderma
12. smooth
13. abscess
14. Mohs surgery
15. virus
16. leukoderma, albinism, vitiligo
17. purpura

Exercise 39

Reading Exercise

Exercise 40

1. b
2. *F*, acne is the condition described in the sentence.
3. d

NOTES

Chapter 5

Respiratory System

OUTLINE

OBJECTIVES

Upon completion of this chapter you will be able to:

1. Identify organs and structures of the respiratory system.
2. Define and spell word parts related to the respiratory system.
3. Define, pronounce, and spell disease and disorder terms related to the respiratory system.
4. Define, pronounce, and spell surgical terms related to the respiratory system.
5. Define, pronounce, and spell diagnostic terms related to the respiratory system.
6. Define, pronounce, and spell complementary terms related to the respiratory system.
7. Interpret the meaning of abbreviations related to the respiratory system.
8. Interpret, read, and comprehend medical language in simulated medical statements and documents.

ANATOMY

> **RESPIRATION**
> is also called **breathing,** or **ventilation.**

The respiratory system comprises the nose, pharynx, larynx, trachea, bronchi, and lungs. The upper respiratory tract includes the nose, pharynx, and larynx. The lower respiratory tract includes the trachea, bronchi, and lungs (Figure 5-1).

Function

The function of the respiratory system is the exchange of oxygen (O_2) and carbon dioxide (CO_2) between the atmosphere and body cells. This process is called **respiration** or **breathing**. During **external respiration**, air containing oxygen passes through the respiratory tract, beginning with the nose, pharynx, larynx, trachea, and, finally, bronchi to the lungs (inhalation). There, oxygen passes from the sacs in the lungs, called **alveoli**, to the blood in tiny blood vessels called **capillaries**. At the same time, carbon dioxide passes back from the capillaries to the alveoli and is expelled through the respiratory tract (exhalation) (Figure 5-2). During **internal respiration**, the body cells take on oxygen from the blood and simultaneously give back carbon dioxide, a waste produced when food and oxygen combine in cells. The carbon dioxide is transported by the blood back to the lungs for exhalation.

Organs of the Respiratory System

Term	Definition
nose	lined with mucous membrane and fine hairs; it acts as a filter to moisten and warm the entering air
nasal septum	partition separating the right and left nasal cavities
paranasal sinuses	air cavities within the cranial bones that open into the nasal cavities
pharynx	serves as a food and air passageway. Air enters from the nasal cavities and passes through the pharynx to the larynx. Food enters the pharynx from the mouth and passes into the esophagus; (also called the **throat**).
adenoids	lymphoid tissue located behind the nasal cavity
tonsils	lymphoid tissue located behind the mouth
larynx	location of the vocal cords. Air enters from the pharynx (also called the **voice box**).
epiglottis	flap of cartilage that automatically covers the opening of and keeps food from entering the larynx during swallowing
trachea	passageway for air to the bronchi; (also called the **windpipe**)
bronchus (*pl.* bronchi)	one of two branches from the trachea that conducts air into the lungs, where it divides and subdivides. The branchings resemble a tree; therefore, they are referred to as a **bronchial tree**.
bronchioles	smallest subdivision of the bronchial tree
alveolus (*pl.* alveoli)	air sacs at the end of the bronchioles. Oxygen and carbon dioxide are exchanged through the alveolar walls and the capillaries.
lungs	two spongelike organs in the thoracic cavity. The right lung consists of three lobes, and the left lung has two lobes.
pleura	double-folded serous membrane covering each lung and lining the thoracic cavity with a small space between, called the pleural cavity, which contains serous fluid

> **ADAM'S APPLE**
> is the largest ring of cartilage in the larynx and is also known as the ***thyroid cartilage.*** The name came from the belief that Adam, realizing he had sinned when he ate the forbidden fruit, was unable to swallow the apple lodged in his throat.

> **BRONCHI**
> originated from the Greek ***brecho,*** meaning ***to pour*** or ***wet.*** An ancient belief was that the esophagus carried solid food to the stomach and the bronchi carried liquids.

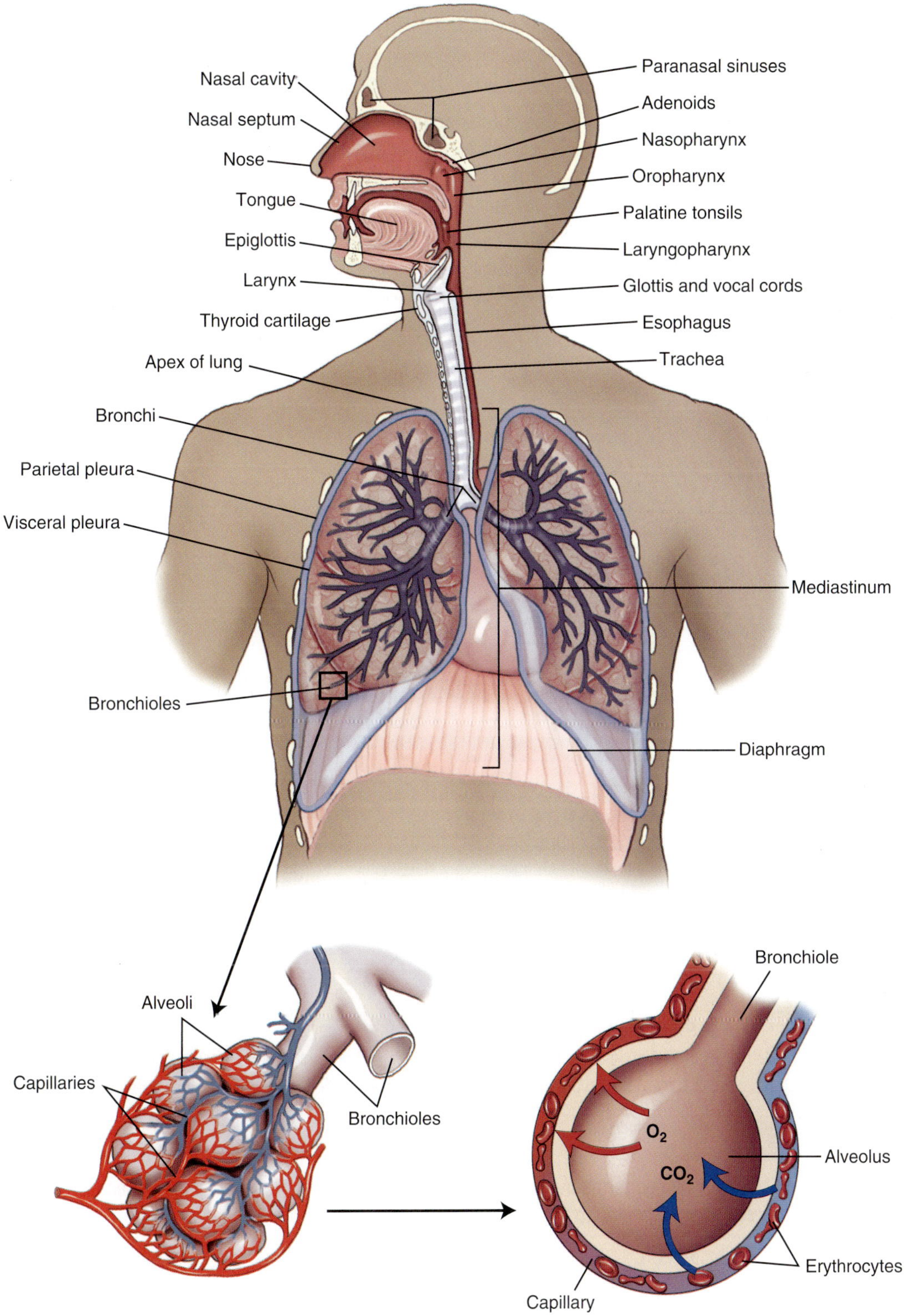

FIGURE 5-1
Organs of the respiratory system.

Organs of the Respiratory System—*cont'd*

Term	Definition
diaphragm	muscular partition that separates the thoracic cavity from the abdominal cavity. It aids in the breathing process by contracting and pulling air in, then relaxing and pushing air out.
mediastinum	space between the lungs. It contains the heart, esophagus, trachea, great blood vessels, and other structures.

MEDIASTINUM

literally means **to stand in the middle** because it is derived from the Latin **medius,** meaning **middle,** and **stare,** meaning **to stand.**

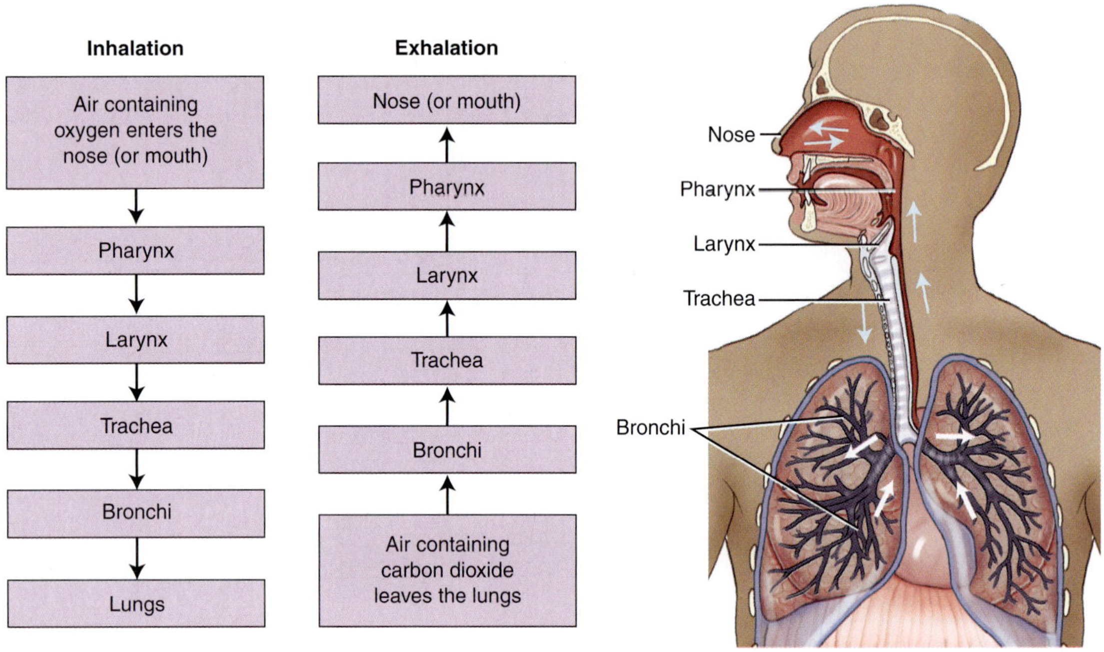

FIGURE 5-2
Flow of air.

A & P Booster
For students desiring more anatomy and physiology, go to http://evolve.elsevier.com. Refer to p. 18 for your Evolve Access Information. Select A & P Booster, Chapter 5.

EXERCISE 1

Match the anatomic terms in the first column with the correct definitions in the second column. *To check your answers, go to Answers, p. 211, at the back of this chapter.*

_____ 1. alveoli	a. tubes carrying air between the trachea and lungs
_____ 2. bronchi	b. passageway for air to the bronchi
_____ 3. larynx	c. located in the thoracic cavity
_____ 4. lungs	d. membrane covering the lung
_____ 5. pharynx	e. lymphoid tissue behind the nasal cavity
_____ 6. pleura	f. acts as food and air passageway
_____ 7. adenoids	g. location of the vocal cords
_____ 8. trachea	h. air sacs at the end of the bronchioles
	i. keeps food out of the trachea and larynx

EXERCISE 2

Fill in the blanks with the correct terms.

1. The partition that separates the right and left nasal cavities is called the _______________ _______________.
2. The _____________________ is a flap of cartilage that prevents food from entering the larynx.
3. The smallest subdivisions of the bronchial tree are the ____________________.
4. The _____________________ serves as a filter to moisten and warm air entering the body.
5. The thoracic cavity is separated from the abdominal cavity by the _____________________.
6. The space between the lungs is called the ____________________.
7. The lymphoid tissues located in the pharynx behind the mouth are called the _____________________.

WORD PARTS

Words parts you need to learn to complete this chapter are listed on the following pages. The exercises at the end of each list will help you learn their definitions and spelling.

Use the flashcards accompanying this text or electronic flashcards to assist you in memorizing the word parts for this chapter.

To use electronic flashcards, go to http://evolve.elsevier.com. Refer to p. 18 for your Evolve Access Information. Select Flashcards, Chapter 5.

Combining Forms of the Respiratory System

Combining Form	Definition
adenoid/o	adenoids
alveol/o	alveolus
bronchi/o, bronch/o	bronchus
diaphragmat/o, phren/o	diaphragm
epiglott/o	epiglottis
laryng/o	larynx
lob/o	lobe
nas/o, rhin/o	nose
pharyng/o	pharynx
pleur/o	pleura
pneum/o, pneumat/o, pneumon/o	lung, air
pulmon/o	lung
sept/o	septum (wall off, fence)
sinus/o	sinus
thorac/o	thorax (chest)
tonsill/o (NOTE: tonsil has one *l*, and the combining form has two *l*s.)	tonsil
trache/o	trachea

ADENOID

is derived from the Greek **aden**, meaning **gland**, and **eidos**, meaning **like**. The word was once used for the prostate gland. The first adenoid surgery was performed in 1868.

LOBE

literally means **the part that hangs down**, although it comes from the Greek **lobos**, meaning **capsule** or **pod**. Also applied to the lobe of an ear, liver, or brain.

Do not be concerned at this time about which word root to use for terms such as *lung* or *nose* that have more than one word root. As you continue to study and use medical terms you will become familiar with common usage of each word part.

EXERCISE FIGURE A

Fill in the blanks with combining forms in this diagram of the respiratory system. *To check your answers, go to p. 211.*

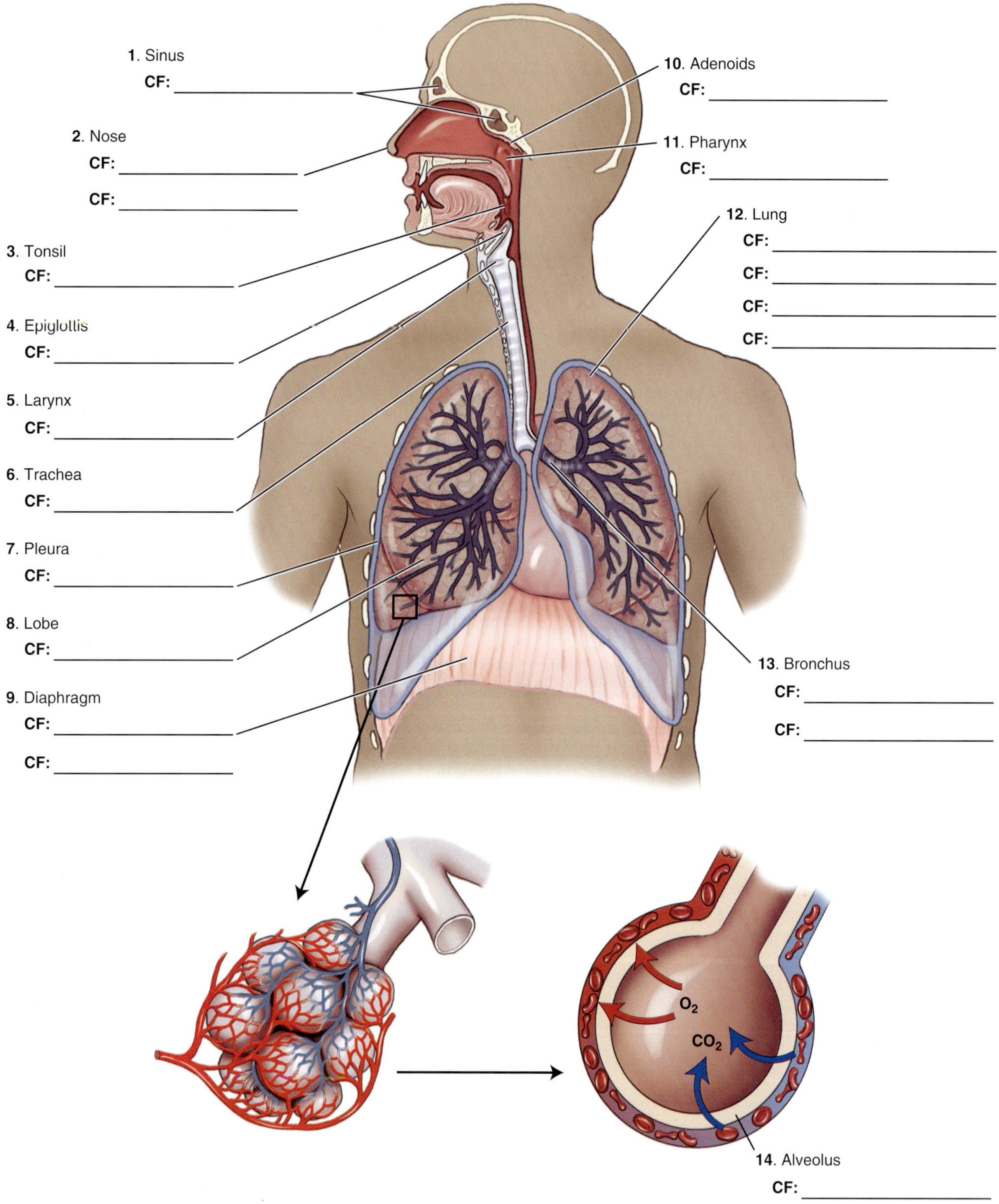

EXERCISE 3

Write the definitions of the following combining forms.

1. laryng/o ____________
2. bronchi/o, bronch/o ____________
3. pleur/o ____________
4. pneum/o ____________
5. tonsill/o ____________
6. pulmon/o ____________
7. diaphragmat/o ____________
8. trache/o ____________
9. alveol/o ____________
10. pneumon/o ____________
11. thorac/o ____________
12. adenoid/o ____________
13. pharyng/o ____________
14. rhin/o ____________
15. sinus/o ____________
16. lob/o ____________
17. epiglott/o ____________
18. pneumat/o ____________
19. nas/o ____________
20. sept/o ____________
21. phren/o ____________

EXERCISE 4

Write the combining form for each of the following terms.

1. nose a. ____________
   b. ____________
2. larynx ____________
3. lung, air a. ____________
   b. ____________
   c. ____________
4. lung ____________
5. tonsil ____________
6. trachea ____________
7. adenoids ____________
8. pleura ____________
9. diaphragm a. ____________
   b. ____________
10. sinus ____________
11. thorax ____________
12. alveolus ____________
13. pharynx ____________
14. bronchus a. ____________
    b. ____________
15. lobe ____________
16. epiglottis ____________
17. septum ____________

OXYGEN

was discovered in 1774 by Joseph Priestley. In 1775 Antoine-Laurent Lavoisier, a French chemist, noted that all the acids he knew contained oxygen. Because he thought it was an acid producer, he named it using the Greek ***oxys***, meaning ***sour***, and the suffix ***gen***, meaning ***to produce***.

Combining Forms Commonly Used with Respiratory System Terms

Combining Form	Definition
atel/o	imperfect, incomplete
capn/o	carbon dioxide
hem/o, hemat/o	blood
muc/o	mucus
orth/o	straight
ox/i, ox/o (NOTE: the combining vowels *o* and *i* are used with the word root *ox*.)	oxygen
phon/o	sound, voice
py/o	pus
somn/o	sleep
spir/o	breathe, breathing

EXERCISE 5

Write the definition of the following combining forms.

1. ox/o, ox/i ______________
2. spir/o ______________
3. muc/o ______________
4. atel/o ______________
5. orth/o ______________
6. py/o ______________
7. hem/o, hemat/o ______________
8. somn/o ______________
9. capn/o ______________
10. phon/o ______________

EXERCISE 6

Write the combining form for each of the following.

1. breathe, breathing ______________
2. oxygen a. ______________ b. ______________
3. imperfect, incomplete ______________
4. straight ______________
5. pus ______________
6. mucus ______________
7. blood a. ______________ b. ______________
8. sleep ______________
9. sound, voice ______________
10. carbon dioxide ______________

Prefixes

Prefix	Definition
a-, an- (NOTE: *an-* is used when the word root begins with a vowel.)	absence of, without
endo- (NOTE: the prefix *intra-*, introduced in Chapter 4, also means *within*.)	within
eu-	normal, good
pan-	all, total
poly-	many, much
tachy-	fast, rapid

EXERCISE 7

Write the definitions of the following prefixes.

1. endo- ____________________
2. a-, an- ____________________
3. pan- ____________________
4. eu- ____________________
5. poly- ____________________
6. tachy- ____________________

EXERCISE 8

Write the prefix for each of the following.

1. within ____________________
2. normal, good ____________________
3. without or absence of a. ____________________
   b. ____________________
4. all, total ____________________
5. many, much ____________________
6. fast, rapid ____________________

Suffixes

Suffix	Definition
-algia	pain
-ar, -ary, -eal	pertaining to
-cele	hernia or protrusion
-centesis	surgical puncture to aspirate fluid (with a sterile needle)
-ectasis	stretching out, dilatation, expansion
-emia	blood condition
-graphy	process of recording, radiographic imaging
-meter	instrument used to measure
-metry	measurement
-pexy	surgical fixation, suspension
-pnea	breathing
-rrhagia	rapid flow of blood
-scope	instrument used for visual examination
-scopic	pertaining to visual examination
-scopy	visual examination
-spasm	sudden, involuntary muscle contraction (spasmodic contraction)
-stenosis	constriction or narrowing
-stomy	creation of an artificial opening
-thorax	chest
-tomy	cut into or incision

Refer to **Appendix A** and **Appendix B** for alphabetical lists of word parts and their meanings.

EXERCISE 9

Match the suffixes in the first column with their correct definitions in the second column.

______	1. -algia	a. process of recording, radiographic imaging
______	2. -ar, -ary, -eal	b. stretching out, dilatation, expansion
______	3. -cele	c. surgical puncture to aspirate fluid
______	4. -centesis	d. measurement
______	5. -ectasis	e. pertaining to visual examination
______	6. -emia	f. pertaining to
______	7. -graphy	g. hernia or protrusion
______	8. -meter	h. instrument used to measure
______	9. -metry	i. rapid flow of blood
______	10. -scopic	j. blood condition
		k. pain

EXERCISE 10

Match the suffixes in the first column with their correct definitions in the second column.

______	1. -rrhagia	a. cut into or incision
______	2. -stomy	b. instrument used for visual examination
______	3. -tomy	c. rapid flow of blood
______	4. -pexy	d. constriction, narrowing
______	5. -scope	e. creation of an artificial opening
______	6. -scopy	f. sudden, involuntary muscle contraction
______	7. -spasm	g. chest
______	8. -stenosis	h. surgical fixation, suspension
______	9. -thorax	i. visual examination
______	10. -pnea	j. breathing

EXERCISE 11

Write the definitions of the following suffixes.

1. -thorax ______________________________
2. -ar, -ary, -eal ______________________________
3. -stenosis ______________________________
4. -cele ______________________________
5. -stomy ______________________________
6. -pexy ______________________________
7. -meter ______________________________
8. -spasm ______________________________
9. -algia ______________________________
10. -scopy ______________________________
11. -centesis ______________________________
12. -tomy ______________________________
13. -scope ______________________________
14. -rrhagia ______________________________
15. -ectasis ______________________________
16. -graphy ______________________________
17. -metry ______________________________
18. -emia ______________________________
19. -scopic ______________________________
20. -pnea ______________________________

ATELECTASIS

is derived from the Greek **ateles,** meaning **not perfect,** and **ektasis,** meaning **expansion**. It denotes an incomplete expansion of the lungs, especially at birth.

BRONCHOGENIC CARCINOMA/LUNG CANCER

Lung cancer, also referred to as *bronchogenic carcinoma*, is the most common cause of death due to cancer worldwide for both men and women. In 2010 there were nearly 225,520 cases of lung cancer and 157,300 deaths in the United States. About 6 out of 10 individuals die within a year of diagnosis; 87% of lung cancer is related to smoking. Categories of lung cancer, which are used to define treatment and determine diagnosis, are small cell and non–small cell.

Adenocarcinoma and **squamous cell carcinoma** are types of non–small cell lung cancer.

Symptoms include **cough, hemoptysis, dyspnea, hoarseness, fatigue,** and **weight loss**.

Thoracentesis, bronchoscopy, CT, and **PET scanning** are used for diagnosis. Treatment includes **surgery, chemotherapy**, and **radiation**.

MESOTHELIOMA

is a rare form of cancer most common in the pleura, the sac covering the lung, and lining the thoracic cavity, and is most often caused by inhalation exposure to asbestos.

Mesothelioma also occurs in the lining of the abdominal cavity and the lining around the heart as well.

MEDICAL TERMS

The terms you need to learn to complete this chapter are listed below and on the following pages. The exercises following each list will help you learn the definition and the spelling of each word.

Disease and Disorder Terms

Built from Word Parts

The following terms are built from word parts you have already learned and can be translated literally to find their meanings. Further explanation of terms beyond the definition of their word parts, if needed, is included in parentheses.

Term	Definition
adenoiditis (*ad*-e-noyd-Ī-tis)	inflammation of the adenoids
alveolitis (*al*-vē-o-LĪ-tis)	inflammation of the alveolus
atelectasis (*at*-e-LEK-ta-sis)	incomplete expansion (of the lung or portion of the lung) (Figure 5-3)
bronchiectasis (*bron*-kē-EK-ta-sis)	dilation of the bronchi (Exercise Figure B)
bronchitis (bron-KĪ-tis)	inflammation of the bronchi (see Figure 5-6)
bronchogenic carcinoma (bron-kō-JEN-ik) (*kar*-si-NŌ-ma)	cancerous tumor originating in a bronchus
bronchopneumonia (*bron*-kō-nū-MŌ-nē-a)	diseased state of the bronchi and lungs, (usually caused by infection)

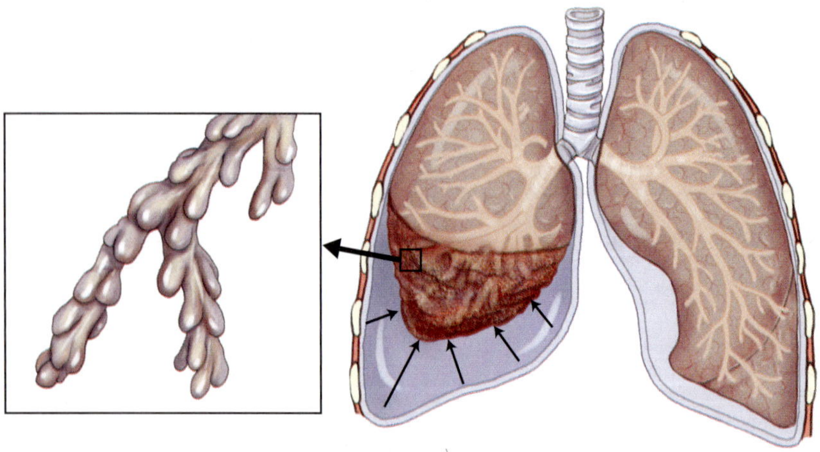

FIGURE 5-3
Atelectasis showing the collapsed alveoli.

EXERCISE FIGURE B

Fill in the blanks to label the diagram.

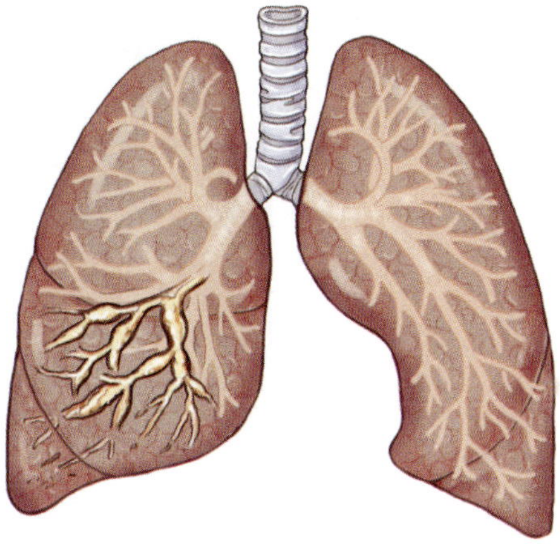

______ / ______
bronchus / dilation

Term	Definition
diaphragmatocele (*dī*-a-frag-MAT-ō-sēl)	hernia of the diaphragm
epiglottitis (*ep*-i-glo-TĪ-tis)	inflammation of the epiglottis
hemothorax (*hē*-mō-THOR-aks)	blood in the chest (pleural space) (Exercise Figure C)
laryngitis (*lar*-in-JĪ-tis)	inflammation of the larynx
laryngotracheobronchitis (LTB) (la-*ring*-gō-*trā*-kē-ō-bron-KĪ-tis)	inflammation of the larynx, trachea, and bronchi (the acute form is called **croup**)
lobar pneumonia (LŌ-bar) (nū-MŌ-nē-a)	pertaining to the lobe(s); diseased state of the lung (infection of one or more lobes of the lung)
nasopharyngitis (*nā*-zō-*far*-in-JĪ-tis)	inflammation of the nose and pharynx
pansinusitis (*pan*-sī-nu-SĪ-tis)	inflammation of all sinuses
pharyngitis (*far*-in-JĪ-tis)	inflammation of the pharynx
pleuritis (plū-RĪ-tis)	inflammation of the pleura (also called **pleurisy**) (Figure 5-4)
pneumatocele (nū-MAT-ō-sēl)	hernia of the lung (lung tissue protrudes through an opening in the chest)
pneumoconiosis (*nū*-mō-*kō*-nē-Ō-sis)	abnormal condition of dust in the lungs
pneumonia (nū-MŌ-nē-a)	diseased state of the lung (the infection and inflammation are caused by bacteria such as *Pneumococcus*, *Staphylococcus*, *Streptococcus*, and *Haemophilus*; viruses; and fungi) (Figure 5-5)

PNEUMOCONIOSIS

is the general name given for chronic inflammatory disease of the lung caused by excessive inhalation of mineral dust. When the disease is caused by a specific dust, it is named for the dust. For example, the disease caused by silica dust is called **silicosis**.

PNEUMOCYSTIS CARINII PNEUMONIA (PCP)

has officially been renamed ***Pneumocystis jiroveci*** pneumonia. Before the 1980s, PCP was rare. During the 1980s it became the most common opportunistic infection of patients with HIV or AIDS. Since the introduction of HAART (highly active antiretroviral therapy) for HIV infection, this infection is most commonly seen in newly diagnosed patients or those who do not follow the HAART regimen.

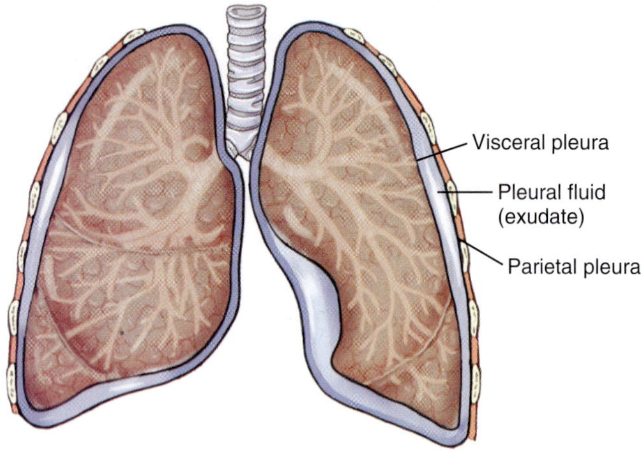

FIGURE 5-4
Pleuritis, also called pleurisy.

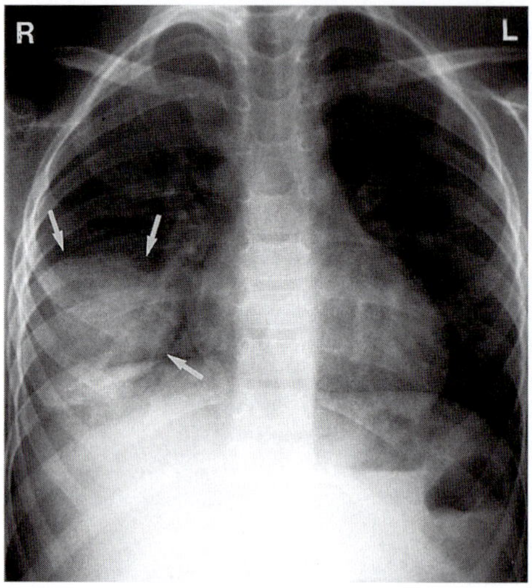

FIGURE 5-5
Chest radiograph revealing pneumonia of the right lung.

Disease and Disorder Terms—*cont'd*

Built from Word Parts

Term	Definition
pneumonitis (*nū*-mō-NĪ-tis)	inflammation of the lung
pneumothorax (*nū*-mō-THOR-aks)	air in the chest (pleural space), which causes collapse of the lung (often a result of an open chest wound) (Exercise Figure C)
pulmonary neoplasm (PUL-mō-*nar*-ē) (NĒ-ō-plazm)	pertaining to (in) the lung, new growth (tumor)
pyothorax (*pī*-ō-THOR-aks)	pus in the chest (pleural space) (also called **empyema**)
rhinitis (rī-NĪ-tis)	inflammation of the (mucous membranes) nose
rhinomycosis (*rī*-nō-mī-KŌ-sis)	abnormal condition of fungus in the nose
rhinorrhagia (*rī*-nō-RĀ-ja)	rapid flow of blood from the nose (also called **epistaxis**)
thoracalgia (*thor*-a-KAL-ja)	pain in the chest
tonsillitis (*ton*-sil-Ī-tis)	inflammation of the tonsils
tracheitis (*trā*-kē-Ī-tis)	inflammation of the trachea
tracheostenosis (*trā*-kē-ō-sten-Ō-sis)	narrowing of the trachea

CAM TERM

Traditional Chinese medicine (TCM) is an ancient healing system that uses herbal and nutritional therapy, acupuncture, massage, and therapeutic exercise to balance the Qi (vital energy) within the body to promote wellness and healing for body, mind, and spirit. Studies have demonstrated that a variety of TCM modalities can provide symptomatic relief and improvement in quality of life for patients with **asthma, allergic rhinitis, and other respiratory ailments.**

EPISTAXIS

and rhinorrhagia are both medical terms for **nosebleed**.

EXERCISE FIGURE C

Fill in the blanks to label the diagram.

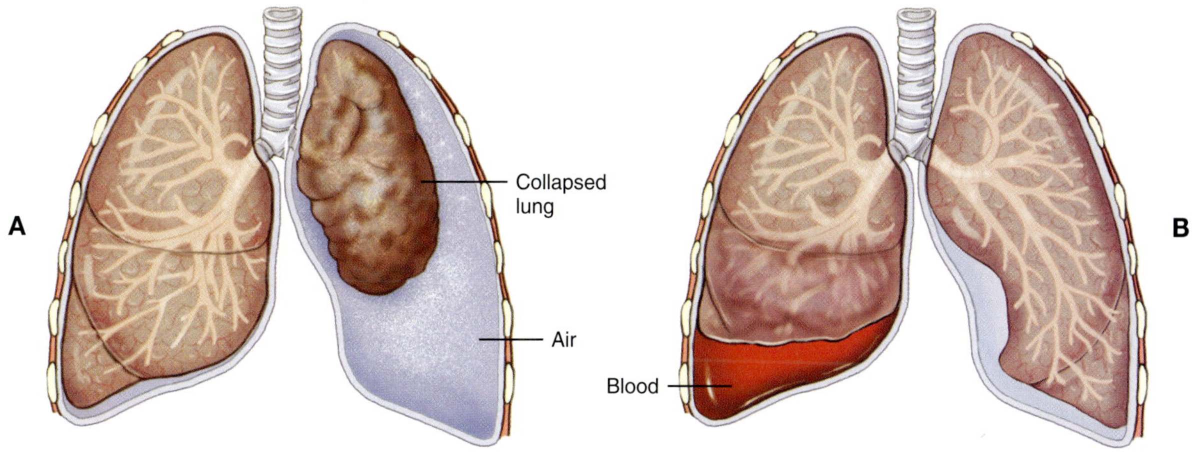

A. ______ / ______ / ______
air / CV / chest

B. ______ / ______ / ______
blood / CV / chest

EXERCISE 12

Practice saying aloud each of the disease and disorder terms built from word parts on pp. 160-162.

To hear the terms, go to http://evolve.elsevier.com. Refer to p. 18 for your Evolve Access Information. Select Exercises & Review, Chapter 5, Chapter Exercises, Pronunciation.

☐ Place a check mark in the box when you have completed this exercise.

EXERCISE 13

Analyze and define the following terms.

Example: diaphragmat / o / cele (WR / CV / S; CF) *hernia of the diaphragm*

1. pleuritis ______________________
2. nasopharyngitis ______________________
3. pneumothorax ______________________
4. pansinusitis ______________________
5. atelectasis ______________________
6. rhinomycosis ______________________
7. tracheostenosis ______________________
8. epiglottitis ______________________
9. thoracalgia ______________________
10. pulmonary neoplasm ______________________

11. bronchiectasis ______
12. tonsillitis ______
13. pneumoconiosis ______
14. bronchopneumonia ______
15. pneumonitis ______
16. laryngitis ______
17. pneumatocele ______
18. pyothorax ______
19. rhinorrhagia ______
20. bronchitis ______
21. pharyngitis ______
22. tracheitis ______
23. laryngotracheobronchitis ______
24. adenoiditis ______
25. hemothorax ______
26. lobar pneumonia ______
27. rhinitis ______
28. bronchogenic carcinoma ______
29. alveolitis ______
30. pneumonia ______

EXERCISE 14

Build disease and disorder terms for the following definitions with the word parts you have learned.

Example: inflammation of the tonsils tonsill / itis (WR / S)

1. pain in the chest ______ / ______ (WR / S)
2. abnormal condition of fungus (infection) in the nose ______ / ______ / ______ / ______ (WR / CV / WR / S)
3. hernia of the lung ______ / ______ / ______ (WR / CV / S)
4. pertaining to the lung; new growth (tumor) ______ / ______ (WR / S) ______ / ______ (P / S(WR))
5. inflammation of the larynx ______ / ______ (WR / S)

6. incomplete expansion (of the lung)
_____ / _____
WR / S

7. inflammation of the adenoids
_____ / _____
WR / S

8. inflammation of the larynx, trachea, and bronchi
_____ / _____ / _____ / _____ / _____ / _____
WR / CV / WR / CV / WR / S

9. dilation of the bronchi
_____ / _____
WR / S

10. inflammation of the pleura
_____ / _____
WR / S

11. abnormal condition of dust in the lung
_____ / _____ / _____ / _____
WR / CV / WR / S

12. inflammation of the lung
_____ / _____
WR / S

13. inflammation of all sinuses
_____ / _____ / _____
P / WR / S

14. narrowing of the trachea
_____ / _____ / _____
WR / CV / S

15. inflammation of the nose and pharynx
_____ / _____ / _____ / _____
WR / CV / WR / S

16. pus in the chest (pleural space)
_____ / _____ / _____
WR / CV / S

17. inflammation of the epiglottis
_____ / _____
WR / S

18. hernia of the diaphragm
_____ / _____ / _____
WR / CV / S

19. air in the chest (pleural space)
_____ / _____ / _____
WR / CV / S

20. diseased state of the bronchi and the lungs
_____ / _____ / _____ / _____
WR / CV / WR / S

21. rapid flow of blood from the nose
_____ / _____ / _____
WR / CV / S

22. inflammation of the pharynx
_____ / _____
WR / S

23. blood in the chest (pleural space) ______ / CV / ______
WR / CV / S

24. inflammation of the trachea ______ / ______
WR / S

25. inflammation of the bronchi ______ / ______
WR / S

26. pertaining to the lobe(s); diseased state of the lung(s) ______ / ______ ______ / ______
WR / S WR / S

27. inflammation of the (mucous membranes) nose ______ / ______
WR / S

28. cancerous tumor originating in a bronchus ______ / CV / ______
WR / CV / S

29. inflammation of the alveolus ______ / ______ ______ / ______
WR / S WR / S

30. diseased state of the lung ______ / ______
WR / S

EXERCISE 15

Spell each of the disease and disorder terms built from word parts on pp. 160-162 by having someone dictate them to you.

To hear and spell the terms, go to http://evolve.elsevier.com. Refer to p. 18 for your Evolve Access Information. Select Exercises & Review, Chapter 5, Chapter Exercises, Spelling.
☐ Place a check mark in the box if you have completed this exercise online.

1. ______
2. ______
3. ______
4. ______
5. ______
6. ______
7. ______
8. ______
9. ______
10. ______
11. ______
12. ______
13. ______
14. ______
15. ______
16. ______
17. ______
18. ______
19. ______
20. ______
21. ______
22. ______
23. ______
24. ______
25. ______
26. ______
27. ______
28. ______
29. ______
30. ______
31. ______

Disease and Disorder Terms

Not Built from Word Parts

In some of the following terms, you may recognize word parts; however, the terms cannot be translated literally to find their meanings.

Term	Definition
acute respiratory distress syndrome (ARDS) (a-KŪT) (RES-pi-ra-*tor*-ē) (di-STRES) (SIN-drōm)	respiratory failure as a result of disease or injury. Symptoms include dyspnea, tachypnea, and cyanosis (also called **adult respiratory distress syndrome**).
asthma (AZ-ma)	respiratory disease characterized by paroxysms of coughing, wheezing, and shortness of breath, which is caused by constriction of airways that is reversible between attacks
chronic obstructive pulmonary disease (COPD) (KRON-ik) (ob-STRUK-tiv) (PUL-mō-*nar*-ē) (di-ZĒZ)	a progressive lung disease that restricts air flow, which makes breathing difficult. Chronic bronchitis and emphysema are the two main components of COPD, but it may also be caused by chronic asthmatic bronchitis. Most COPD is a result of cigarette smoking.
coccidioidomycosis (kok-*sid*-ē-*oy*-dō-mī-KŌ-sis)	fungal disease affecting the lungs and sometimes other organs of the body (also called **valley fever** or **cocci**)
cor pulmonale (kōr) (*pul*-mō-NAL-ē)	serious cardiac disease associated with chronic lung disorders, such as emphysema
croup (krūp)	condition resulting from acute obstruction of the larynx, characterized by a barking cough, hoarseness, and stridor. It may be caused by viral or bacterial infection, allergy, or foreign body. Occurs mainly in children.
cystic fibrosis (CF) (SIS-tik) (fī-BRŌ-sis)	hereditary disorder of the exocrine glands characterized by excess mucus production in the respiratory tract, pancreatic deficiency, and other symptoms.
deviated septum (DĒ-vē-*āt*-ed) (SEP-tum)	one part of the nasal cavity is smaller because of malformation or injury of the nasal septum
emphysema (*em*-fi-SĒ-ma)	stretching of lung tissue caused by the alveoli becoming distended and losing elasticity (Figure 5-6)
epistaxis (*ep*-i-STAK-sis)	nosebleed (synonymous with **rhinorrhagia**)
influenza (*in*-flū-EN-za)	highly infectious respiratory disease caused by a virus (also called **flu**)
Legionnaire disease (lē-je-NĀR) (di-ZĒZ)	a lobar pneumonia caused by the bacterium *Legionella pneumophila*

ACUTE RESPIRATORY DISTRESS SYNDROME (ARDS)

is respiratory failure in an adult. In newborns the condition is referred to as **infant respiratory distress syndrome of newborn (IRDS)** or **hyaline membrane disease.**

ACUTE/CHRONIC

Acute, in reference to disease, means **sharp**, **sudden**, **short**, or **severe** type of disease. **Chronic**, in reference to disease, means a disease that continues for a long time.

REACTIVE AIRWAY DISEASE (RAD)

is a general term and not a specific diagnosis. It is used to describe a history of wheezing, coughing, and shortness of breath. In some people RAD may lead to **asthma**.

INFLUENZA PANDEMIC

is the sudden outbreak of a flu that becomes very widespread, affecting a region, a continent, or the world. Examples are H1N1 swine flu and H5N1 avian flu.

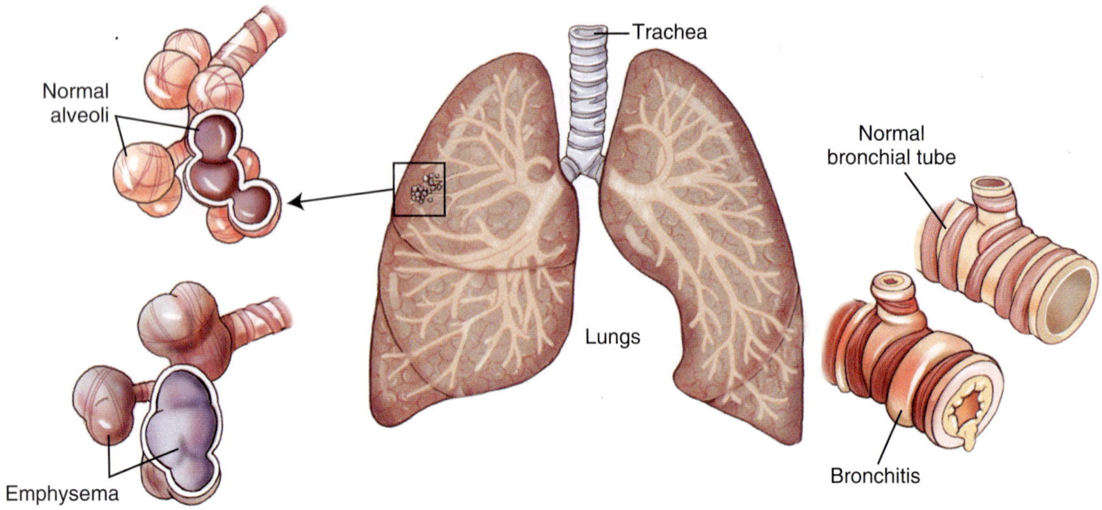

FIGURE 5-6
Emphysema and bronchitis.

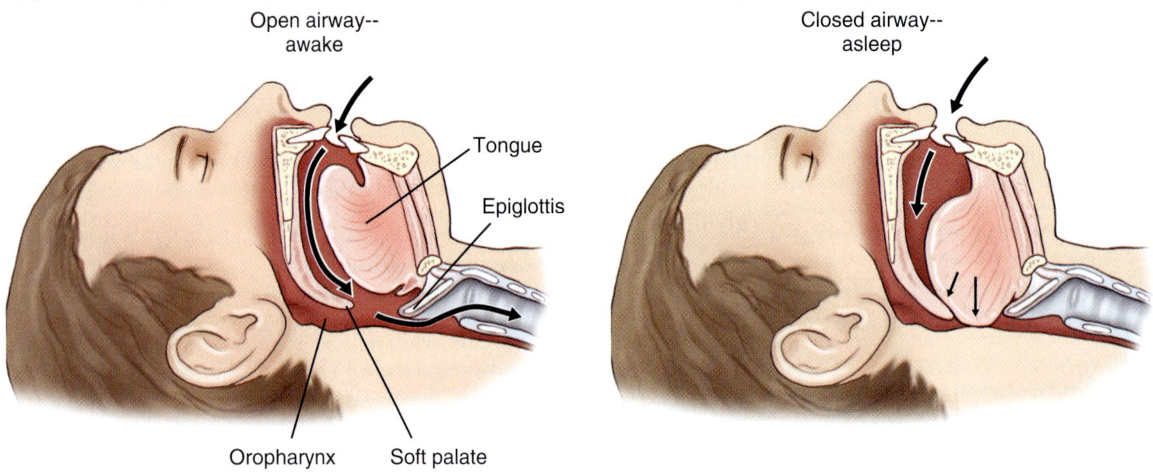

FIGURE 5-7
Obstructive sleep apnea (OSA). During sleep the absence of activity of the pharyngeal muscle structure allows the airway to close. OSA is associated with increased risk for elevated blood pressure, cardiovascular disease, diabetes, and stroke. Obesity is a major risk factor and weight loss can be an effective treatment. **Polysomnography** is used to diagnose OSA. Treatment includes the use of **CPAP (continuous positive airway pressure)** during sleep and **uvulopalatopharyngoplasty (UPPP),** a surgical procedure.

Disease and Disorder Terms—*cont'd*

Not Built from Word Parts

Term	Definition
obstructive sleep apnea (OSA) (ob-STRUK-tiv) (slēp) (AP-nē-a)	repetitive pharyngeal collapse during sleep, which leads to absence of breathing; can produce daytime drowsiness and elevated blood pressure (Figure 5-7)
pertussis (per-TUS-sis)	highly contagious bacterial infection of the respiratory tract characterized by an acute crowing inspiration, or whoop (also called **whooping cough**)

Term	Definition
pleural effusion (PLŪ-ral) (e-FŪ-zhun)	fluid in the pleural space caused by a disease process or trauma
pulmonary edema (PUL-mō-*nar*-ē) (e-DĒ-ma)	fluid accumulation in the alveoli and bronchioles
pulmonary embolism (PE) (***pl.*** **emboli)** (EM-bo-li) (PUL-mō-*nar*-ē) (EM-bo-lizm)	matter foreign to the circulation, carried to the pulmonary artery and its branches, where it blocks circulation to the lungs and can be fatal if of sufficient size or number. Blood clots broken loose from the deep veins of the lower extremities are the most common source of emboli.
tuberculosis (TB) (tū-*ber*-kū-LŌ-sis)	an infectious disease, caused by an acid-fast bacillus, most commonly spread by inhalation of small particles and usually affecting the lungs
upper respiratory infection (URI) (UP-er) (RES-pi-ra-*tor*-ē) (in-FEK-shun)	infection of the nasal cavity, pharynx, or larynx (commonly called a **cold**) (Figure 5-9)

TUBERCULOSIS (TB)

causes more deaths worldwide than any other infectious disease even though it is preventable and curable. The risk for active TB is higher in HIV-infected persons and drug users. The development of multidrug–resistant TB is becoming a problem in treatment of the disease.

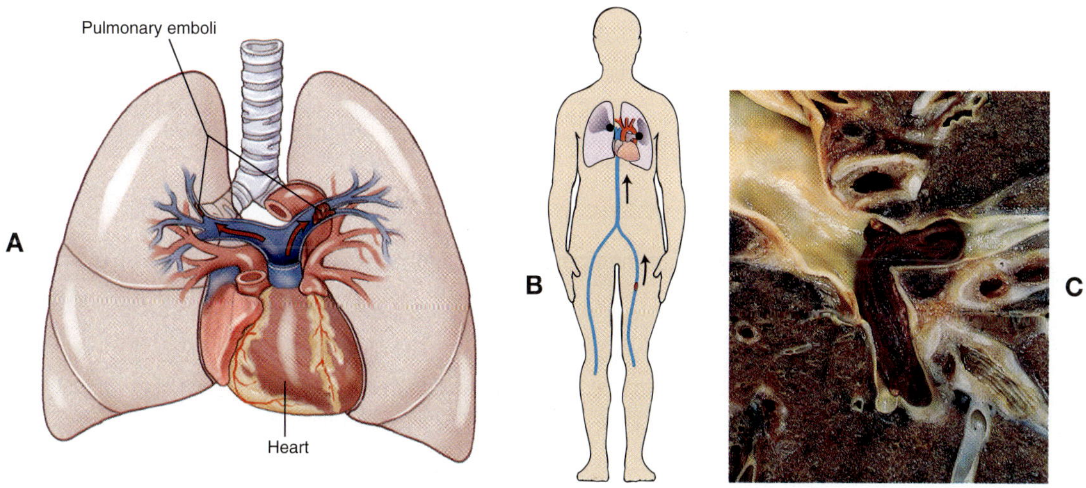

FIGURE 5-8

A, Bilateral pulmonary emboli. **B,** Pulmonary emboli usually originate in the deep veins of the lower extremities. **C,** Necropsy specimen of the lung showing a large embolus.

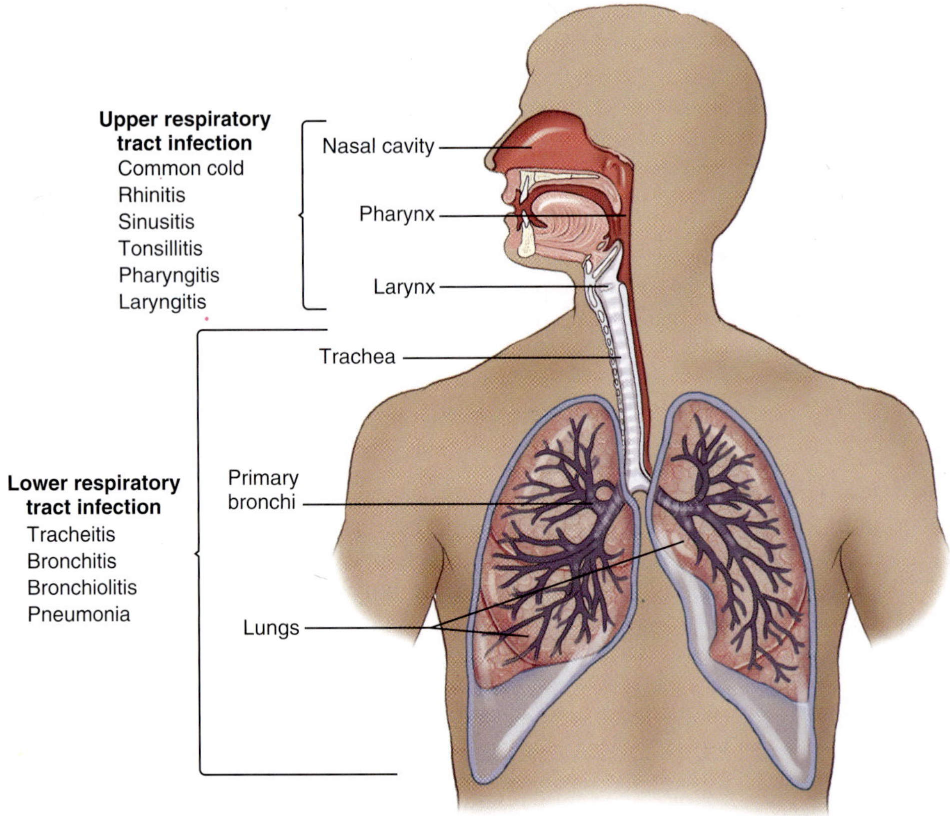

FIGURE 5-9
Upper and lower respiratory tract infections.

EXERCISE 16

Practice saying aloud each of the disease and disorder terms not built from word parts on pp. 167-169.

To hear the terms, go to http://evolve.elsevier.com. Refer to p. 18 for your Evolve Access Information. Select Exercises & Review, Chapter 5, Chapter Exercises, Pronunciation.

☐ Place a check mark in the box when you have completed this exercise.

EXERCISE 17

Fill in the blanks with the correct terms.

1. A disease characterized by lung tissue stretching that results from the alveoli losing elasticity and becoming distended is called ____________________.
2. ____________________ ____________________ is the name given to the fluid in the pleural space caused by a disease process or a trauma.

3. A cardiac condition that is associated with chronic lung disorders is called ____________ ____________.

4. A fungal disease affecting the lungs is called ____________.

5. ____________ ____________ is a hereditary disorder characterized by excess mucus production in the respiratory tract.

6. The medical name of the infectious respiratory disease commonly referred to as *flu* is ____________.

7. A progressive lung disease that restricts air flow ____________ ____________ ____________ ____________.

8. The medical name for the disease characterized by an acute crowing inspiration is ____________.

9. ____________ is a condition resulting from an acute obstruction of the larynx.

10. A chronic respiratory disease characterized by shortness of breath, wheezing, and paroxysmal coughing is called ____________.

11. A condition in which fluid accumulates in the alveoli and bronchioles is ____________ ____________.

12. A(n) ____________ ____________ ____________ generally refers to an infection involving the nasal cavity, pharynx, or larynx.

13. Foreign matter, such as a blood clot, carried to the pulmonary artery, where it blocks circulation to the lungs, is called a(n) ____________ ____________.

14. ____________ is another name for nosebleed.

15. A lobar pneumonia caused by the *Legionella pneumophila* bacterium is commonly called ____________ ____________.

16. ____________ ____________ is one part of the nasal cavity that is smaller than the other because of malformation or injury.

17. The diagnosis for repetitive pharyngeal collapse is ____________ ____________ ____________.

18. An infectious disease usually affecting the lungs and caused by inhaling infected small particles is ____________.

19. ____________ ____________ ____________ ____________ also called adult respiratory distress syndrome.

EXERCISE 18

Match the terms in the first column with the correct definitions in the second column.

_____ 1. asthma

_____ 2. chronic obstructive pulmonary disease

_____ 3. coccidioidomycosis

_____ 4. cor pulmonale

_____ 5. croup

_____ 6. cystic fibrosis

_____ 7. emphysema

_____ 8. epistaxis

_____ 9. influenza

_____ 10. Legionnaire disease

a. alveoli become distended and lose elasticity

b. caused by a virus (commonly called *flu*)

c. hereditary disorder characterized by excess mucus in the respiratory system

d. most often caused by cigarette smoking

e. nosebleed

f. cardiac disease associated with chronic lung disorders

g. condition resulting from acute obstruction of the larynx

h. also called *valley fever*

i. lobar pneumonia caused by the bacterium *Legionella pneumophila*

j. caused by restriction of airways that is reversible between attacks

EXERCISE 19

Match the terms in the first column with the correct definitions in the second column.

_____ 1. pertussis

_____ 2. pleural effusion

_____ 3. pulmonary edema

_____ 4. pulmonary embolism

_____ 5. upper respiratory infection

_____ 6. deviated septum

_____ 7. obstructive sleep apnea

_____ 8. tuberculosis

_____ 9. acute respiratory distress syndrome

a. respiratory failure as a result of disease or injury

b. fluid in the pleural space

c. fluid accumulation in alveoli and bronchioles

d. whooping cough

e. foreign material, carried to the pulmonary artery, where it blocks circulation to the lungs

f. commonly called a cold

g. unequal size of nasal cavities

h. repetitive pharyngeal collapse

i. an infectious disease usually affecting the lungs

EXERCISE 20

Spell each of the disease and disorder terms not built from word parts on pp. 167-169 by having someone dictate them to you.

To hear and spell the terms, go to http://evolve.elsevier.com. Refer to p. 18 for your Evolve Access Information. Select Exercises & Review, Chapter 5, Chapter Exercises, Spelling.
☐ Place a check mark in the box if you have completed this exercise online.

1. ______________________
2. ______________________
3. ______________________
4. ______________________
5. ______________________
6. ______________________
7. ______________________
8. ______________________
9. ______________________
10. ______________________
11. ______________________
12. ______________________
13. ______________________
14. ______________________
15. ______________________
16. ______________________
17. ______________________
18. ______________________
19. ______________________

Surgical Terms

Built from Word Parts

The following terms are built from word parts you have already learned and can be translated literally to find their meanings. Further explanation of terms beyond the definition of their word parts, if needed, is included in parentheses.

Term	Definition
adenoidectomy (*ad*-e-noyd-EK-to-mē)	excision of the adenoids (Exercise Figure D)
adenotome (AD-e-nō-*tōm*) (NOTE: the *oid* is missing from the word root *adenoid* in this term.)	surgical instrument used to cut the adenoids (Exercise Figure D)
bronchoplasty (BRON-kō-*plas*-tē)	surgical repair of a bronchus
laryngectomy (*lăr*-in-JEK-to-mē)	excision of the larynx
laryngoplasty (la-RING-gō-*plas*-tē)	surgical repair of the larynx

EXERCISE FIGURE D

Fill in the blanks to complete labeling of the diagram.

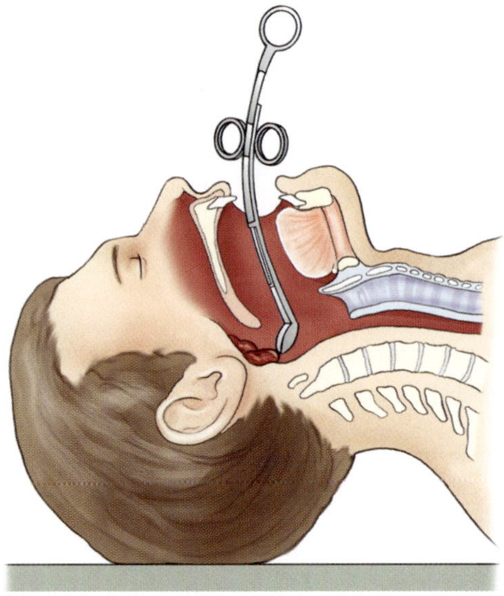

_______ / _______ performed using a(n) _______ / _______ / _______
adenoid / excision   adenoid / cv / surgical instrument used to cut

Surgical Terms—*cont'd*

Built from Word Parts

Term	Definition
laryngostomy (*lar*-in-GOS-to-mē)	creation of an artificial opening into the larynx
laryngotracheotomy (la-*ring*-gō-*trā*-kē-OT-o-mē)	incision of the larynx and trachea
lobectomy (lō-BEK-to-mē)	excision of a lobe (of the lung) (Figure 5-10)
pleuropexy (plū-rō-PEK-sē)	surgical fixation of the pleura
pneumobronchotomy (*nū*-mō-bron-KOT-o-mē)	incision of lung and bronchus
pneumonectomy (*nū*-mō-NEK-to-mē)	excision of a lung (see Figure 5-10)
rhinoplasty (RĪ-nō-*plas*-tē)	surgical repair of the nose
septoplasty (SEP-tō-*plas*-tē)	surgical repair of the (nasal) septum
septotomy (sep-TOT-o-mē)	incision into the (nasal) septum
sinusotomy (*sī*-nū-SOT-o-mē)	incision of a sinus

Term	Definition
thoracocentesis (*thor*-a-kō-sen-TĒ-sis)	surgical puncture to aspirate fluid from the chest cavity (also called **thoracentesis**) (Exercise Figure E)
thoracotomy (*thor*-a-KOT-o-mē)	incision into the chest cavity
tonsillectomy (*ton*-sil-EK-to-mē)	excision of the tonsils
tracheoplasty (TRĀ-kē-ō-*plas*-tē)	surgical repair of the trachea
tracheostomy (*trā*-kē-OS-to-mē)	creation of an artificial opening into the trachea (Figure 5-11)
tracheotomy (*trā*-kē-OT-o-mē)	incision of the trachea (Figure 5-11)

VIDEO-ASSISTED THORACIC SURGERY (VATS)

is the use of a thoracoscope and video equipment for an endoscopic approach to diagnose and treat thoracic conditions. It replaces the traditional thoracotomy, which required a large incision and greater recovery time.

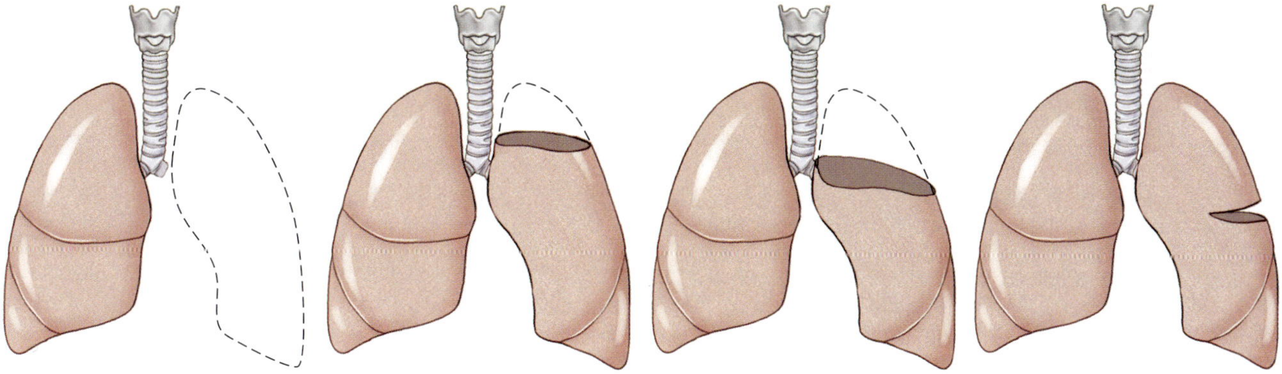

FIGURE 5-10
Types of lung resection. The diagram illustrates the amount of lung tissue removed with each type of surgery.

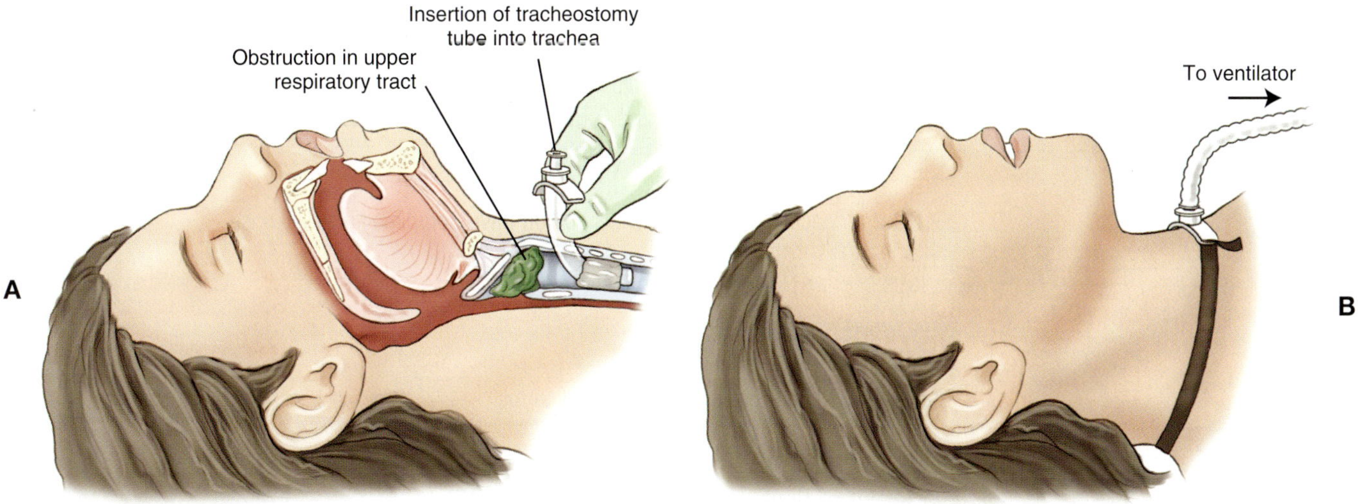

FIGURE 5-11
Tracheostomy. **A,** A tracheotomy is performed to establish an airway when normal breathing is obstructed. **B,** If the opening needs to be maintained, a tube is inserted, creating a tracheostomy. A tracheostomy may be temporary, as for prolonged mechanical ventilation to support breathing or it may be permanent, as in airway reconstruction after laryngeal cancer surgery.

EXERCISE FIGURE E

Fill in the blanks to complete labeling of the diagram.

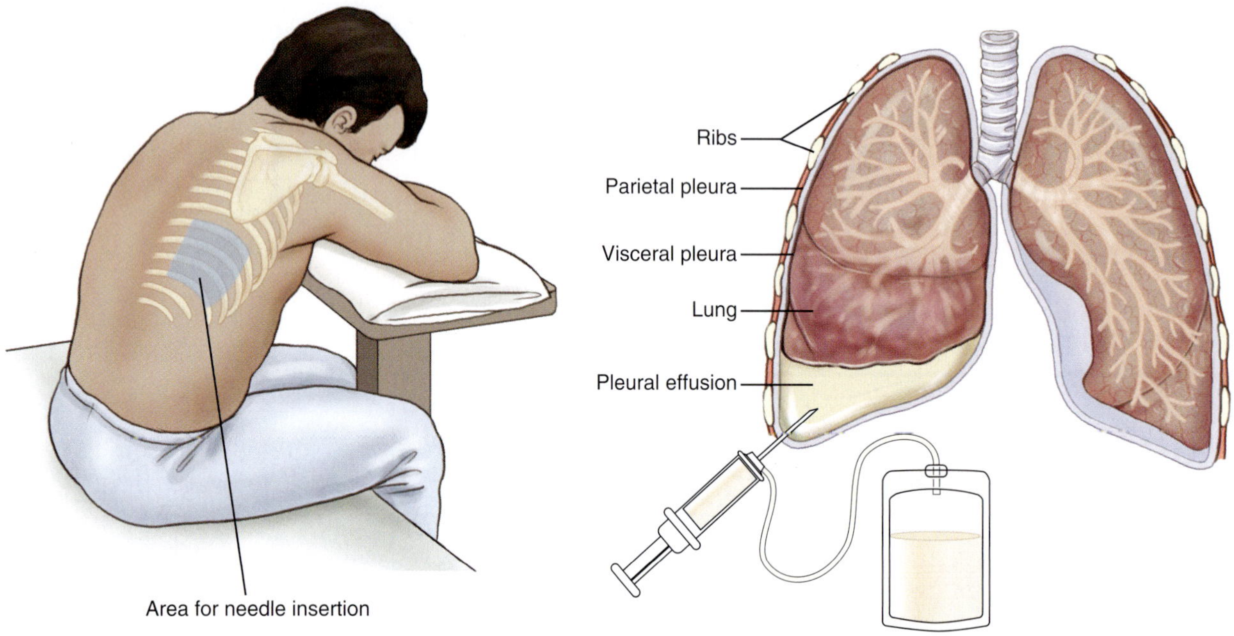

_____ / _____ / _____ is used for both diagnosis and treatment.
chest / cv / surgical puncture to remove fluid

EXERCISE 21

Practice saying aloud each of the surgical terms built from word parts on pp. 173-175.

To hear the terms, go to http://evolve.elsevier.com. Refer to p. 18 for your Evolve Access Information. Select Exercises & Review, Chapter 5, Chapter Exercises, Pronunciation.

☐ Place a check mark in the box when you have completed this exercise.

EXERCISE 22

Analyze and define the following surgical terms.

Example: pneumon/ectomy (WR / S) _excision of lung_

1. tracheotomy _____
2. laryngostomy _____
3. adenoidectomy _____

4. rhinoplasty ____________________
5. adenotome ____________________
6. tracheostomy ____________________
7. sinusotomy ____________________
8. laryngoplasty ____________________
9. pneumobronchotomy ____________________
10. bronchoplasty ____________________
11. lobectomy ____________________
12. laryngotracheotomy ____________________
13. tracheoplasty ____________________
14. thoracotomy ____________________
15. laryngectomy ____________________
16. thoracocentesis ____________________
17. tonsillectomy ____________________
18. pleuropexy ____________________
19. septoplasty ____________________
20. septotomy ____________________

EXERCISE 23

Build surgical terms for the following definitions by using the word parts you have learned.

Example: surgical fixation of the pleura pleur / o / pexy
WR / CV / S

1. surgical repair of the trachea ______ / ______ / ______
WR / CV / S

2. incision of larynx and trachea ______ / ______ / ______ / ______ / ______
WR / CV / WR / CV / S

3. surgical instrument used to cut the adenoids ______ / ______ / ______
WR / CV / S

4. incision into the chest cavity ______ / ______ / ______
WR / CV / S

5. creation of an artificial opening into the trachea ______ / ______ / ______
WR / CV / S

6. excision of the tonsils ______ / ______
   WR / S

7. incision of the trachea ______ / ___ / ______
   WR / CV / S

8. surgical repair of a bronchus ______ / ___ / ______
   WR / CV / S

9. excision of the larynx ______ / ______
   WR / S

10. surgical repair of the nose ______ / ___ / ______
   WR / CV / S

11. incision of a sinus ______ / ___ / ______
   WR / CV / S

12. surgical puncture to aspirate fluid from the chest cavity ______ / ___ / ______
   WR / CV / S

13. excision of the adenoids ______ / ______
   WR / S

14. surgical repair of the larynx ______ / ___ / ______
   WR / CV / S

15. excision of a lobe (of the lung) ______ / ______
   WR / S

16. incision of a lung and bronchus ______ / ___ / ______ / ___ / ______
   WR / CV / WR / CV / S

17. creation of an artificial opening into the larynx ______ / ___ / ______
   WR / CV / S

18. excision of a lung ______ / ______
   WR / S

19. incision into the septum ______ / ___ / ______
   WR / CV / S

20. surgical repair of the septum ______ / ___ / ______
   WR / CV / S

EXERCISE 24

Spell each of the surgical terms built from word parts on pp. 173-175 by having someone dictate them to you.

To hear and spell the terms, go to http://evolve.elsevier.com. Refer to p. 18 for your Evolve Access Information. Select Exercises & Review, Chapter 5, Chapter Exercises, Spelling.
☐ Place a check mark in the box if you have completed this exercise online.

1. ______________________
2. ______________________
3. ______________________
4. ______________________
5. ______________________
6. ______________________
7. ______________________
8. ______________________
9. ______________________
10. ______________________
11. ______________________
12. ______________________
13. ______________________
14. ______________________
15. ______________________
16. ______________________
17. ______________________
18. ______________________
19. ______________________
20. ______________________
21. ______________________

Diagnostic Terms

Built from Word Parts

The following terms are built from word parts you have already learned and can be translated literally to find their meanings. Further explanation of terms beyond the definition of their word parts, if needed, is included in parentheses.

Term	Definition
ENDOSCOPY	
bronchoscope (BRON-kō-skōp)	instrument used for visual examination of the bronchi (Table 5-1 and Exercise Figure F)
bronchoscopy (bron-KOS-ko-pē)	visual examination of the bronchi (Exercise Figure F)
endoscope (EN-dō-skōp)	instrument used for visual examination within (a hollow organ or body cavity). (Current trend is to use endoscopes for surgical procedures as well as for viewing.) (Table 5-1)
endoscopic (*en*-dō-SKOP-ik)	pertaining to visual examination within (a hollow organ or body cavity) (used to describe the practice of performing surgeries that use endoscopes)

EXERCISE FIGURE F

Fill in the blanks to complete labeling of the diagram.

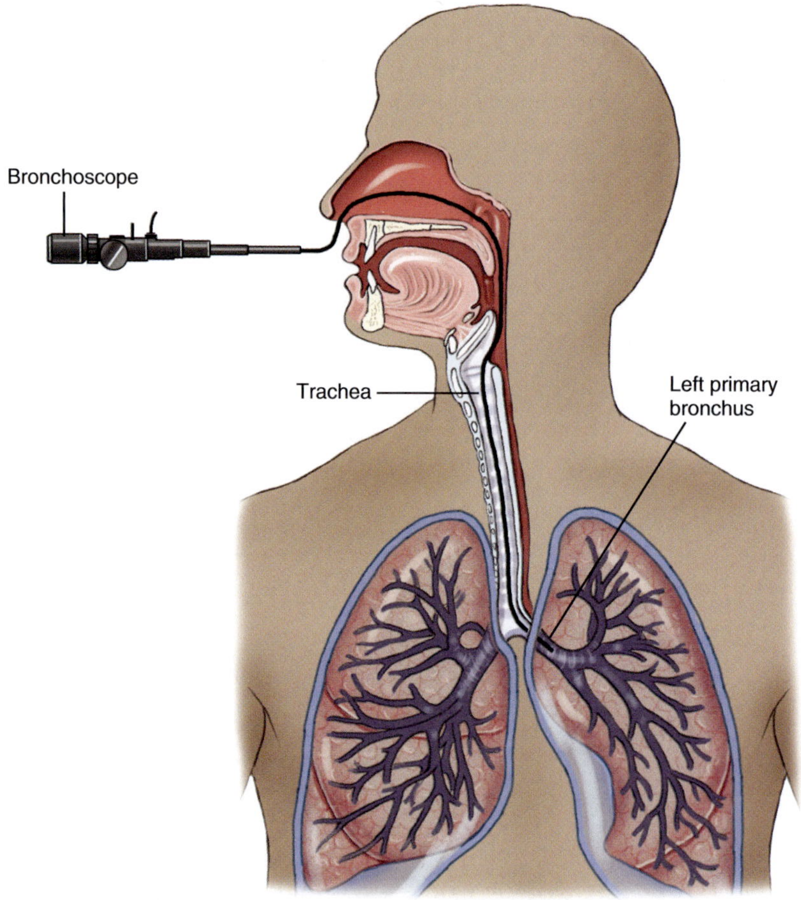

_______ / _______ / _______
bronchi / cv / visual examination

A bronchoscope is inserted through the nostril and passed through the throat, larynx, and trachea into the bronchus.

SCOPE

is taken from the Greek **skopein,** which means to **see** or to **view.** It also means **observing for a purpose.** To the ancient Greeks it meant "to look out for, to monitor, or to examine."

Today the following suffixes commonly are used:

- **-scope** describes the **instrument used to view or to examine,** such as in the term **endoscope** (means **instrument used for visual examination within** a hollow organ or body cavity).
- **-scopy** means **visual examination,** such as in the term **endoscopy (visual examination within** a hollow organ or body cavity).
- **-scopic** means **pertaining to visual examination,** such as in the term **endoscopic (pertaining to visual examination within** a hollow organ or body cavity).

Endoscopic surgery is used to describe modern surgery performed with the use of endoscopes. Most often the suffixes **-scope, -scopy,** and **-scopic** mean to **examine visually,** and that is the definition given in this text. However, the term **stethoscope** is an **instrument used for listening** to body sounds.

Diagnostic Terms—*cont'd*

Built from Word Parts

Term	Definition
endoscopy (en-DOS-ko-pē)	visual examination within (a hollow organ or body cavity) (Table 5-1)
laryngoscope (la-RING-go-skōp)	instrument used for visual examination of the larynx (Exercise Figure G)
laryngoscopy (*lar*-in-GOS-ko-pē)	visual examination of the larynx
thoracoscope (tho-RAK-ō-skōp)	instrument used for visual examination of the thorax (Table 5-1)
thoracoscopy (*thor*-a-KOS-ko-pē)	visual examination of the thorax (Table 5-1)

Term	Definition
PULMONARY FUNCTION	
capnometer (kap-NOM-e-ter)	instrument used to measure carbon dioxide (levels in expired gas) (Figure 5-12, *A*)
oximeter (ok-SIM-e-ter) (NOTE: the combining vowel is *i.*)	instrument used to measure oxygen (saturation in the blood) (Table 5-1)
spirometer (spī-ROM-e-ter)	instrument used to measure breathing (or lung volumes) (Figure 5-12, *B*)
spirometry (spī-ROM-e-trē)	a measurement of breathing (or lung volumes) (Figure 5-12, *B*)
SLEEP STUDIES	
polysomnography (PSG) (*pol*-ē-som-NOG-rah-fē)	process of recording many (tests) during sleep (performed to diagnose obstructive sleep apnea [see Figure 5-7]). Tests include **electrocardiography, electromyography, electroencephalography, air flow monitoring,** and **oximetry**.

A

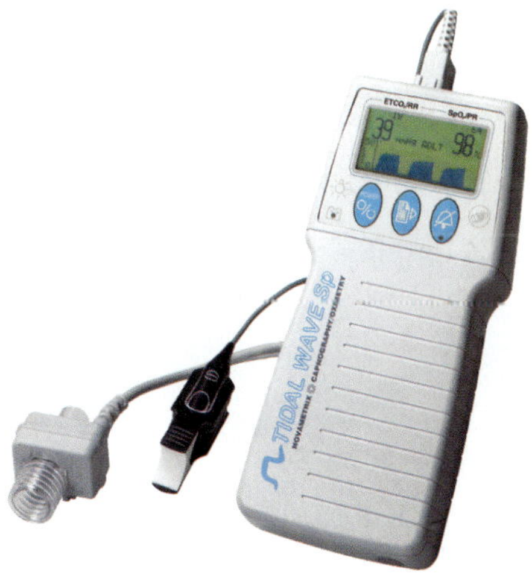

B

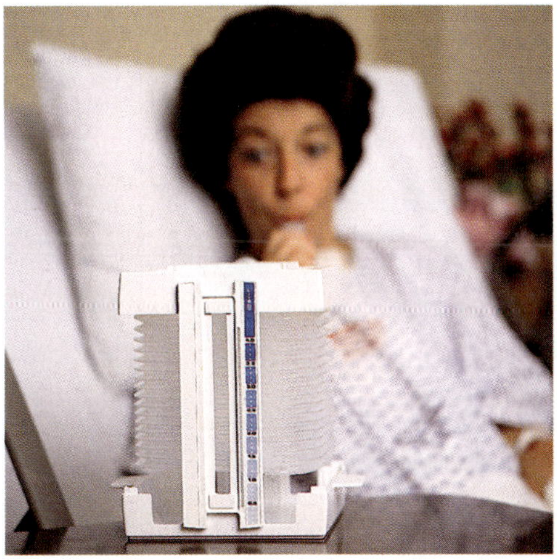

FIGURE 5-12
A, Capnometer; **B,** Spirometer.

TABLE 5-1

Types of Diagnostic Procedures

The following table illustrates the types of diagnostic procedures included in the **diagnostic term word lists** in this and subsequent chapters of this text.

Diagnostic Imaging

Diagnostic imaging is a generic term that covers radiology, ultrasonography, nuclear medicine, computed tomography, and magnetic resonance imaging.

Radiography produces images of internal organs by using ionizing radiation.

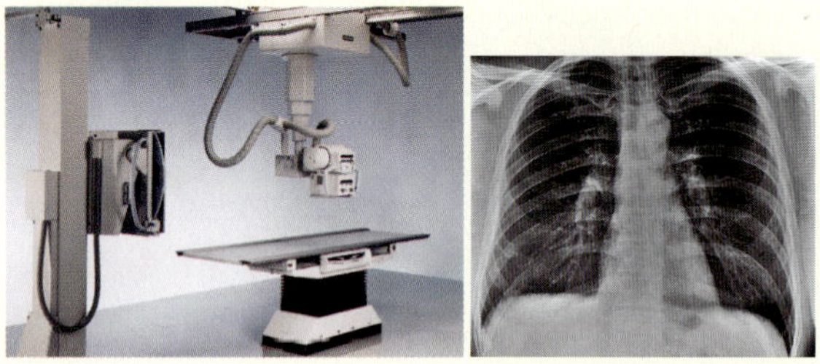

A B

A, Radiographic system with chest unit; **B,** chest radiograph.

Nuclear medicine produces scans by using radioactive material.

A

B

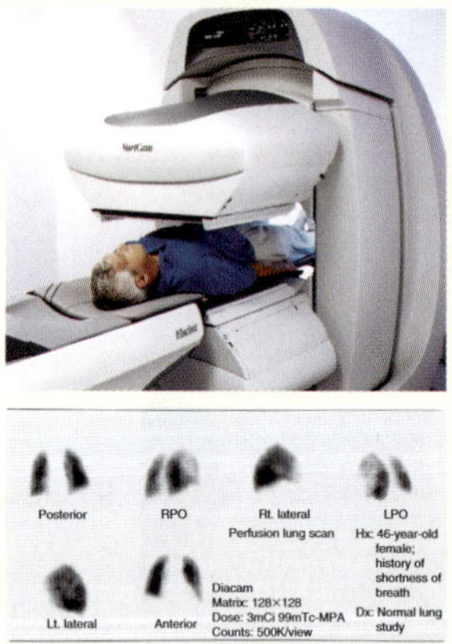

A, Nuclear medicine scanner; **B,** lung scan. Note: positron emission tomography (PET) is a nuclear medicine test.

Ultrasonography produces scans by using high-frequency sound waves.

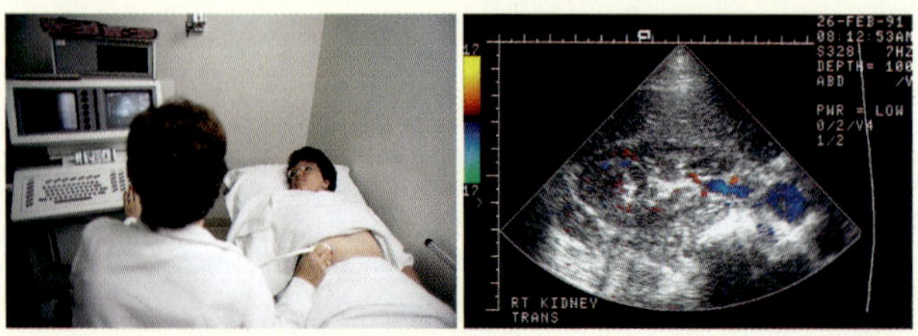

A B

A, Ultrasound scanner; **B,** ultrasound image of the kidney.

Computed tomography produces scans of computerized images of body organs in sectional slices.

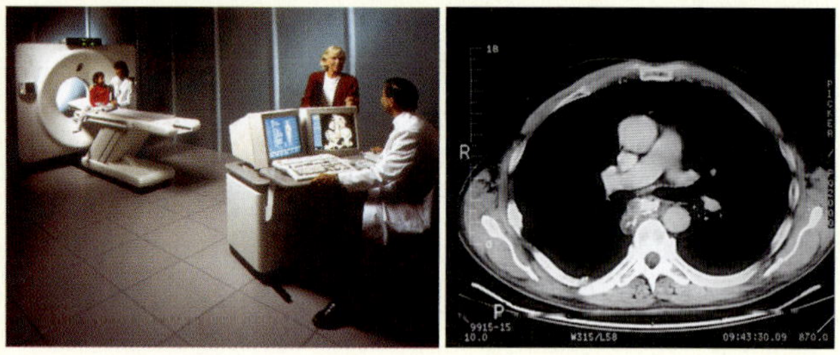

A B

A, Computed tomography scanner; **B,** scan of the chest with intravenous contrast media.

Magnetic resonance imaging produces scans that give information about the body's anatomy by placing the patient in a magnetic field.

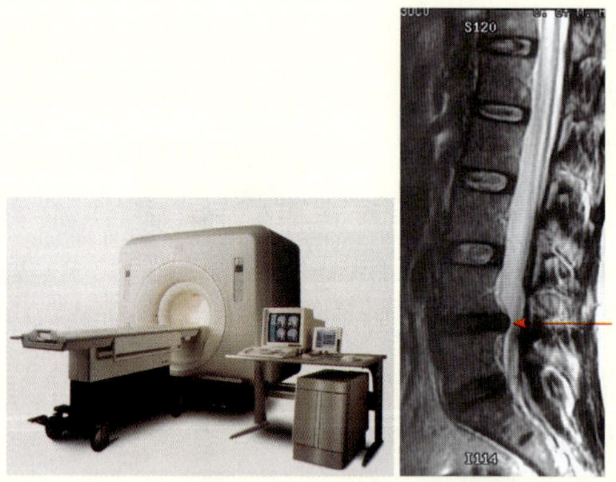

A B

A, Magnetic resonance scanner; **B,** sagittal scan of the lumbar spine with herniated disk (arrow).

TABLE 5-1

Types of Diagnostic Procedures—*cont'd*

Endoscopy

Endoscopy uses endoscopes, which are lighted, flexible instruments, to visually examine a hollow organ or body cavity, such as the bronchus.

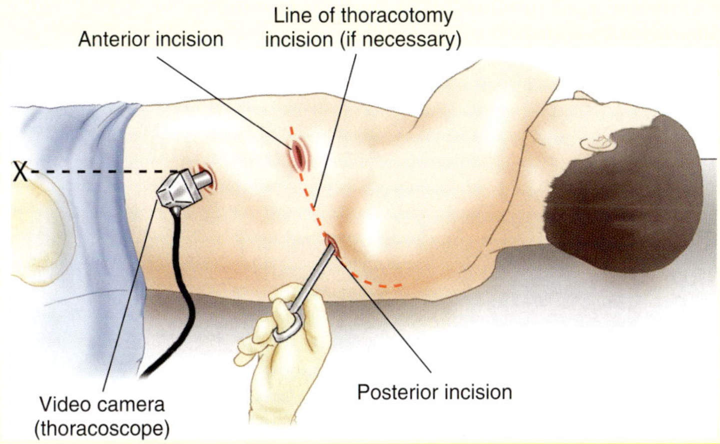

Laboratory

Laboratory procedures are performed on specimens such as blood, tissue, and urine.

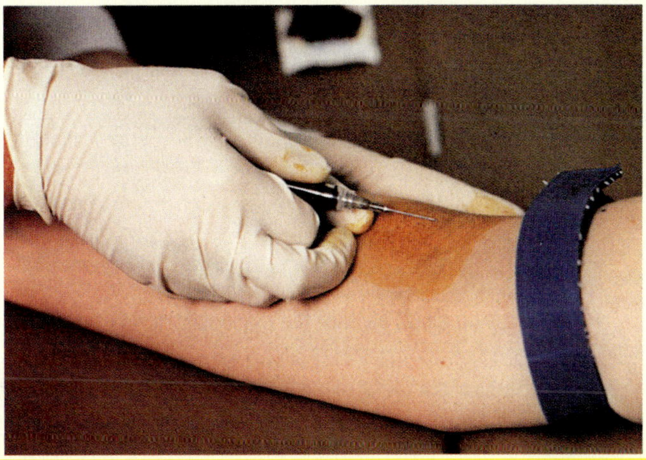

Pulmonary Function

Pulmonary function tests are performed in a variety of methods to determine lung function.

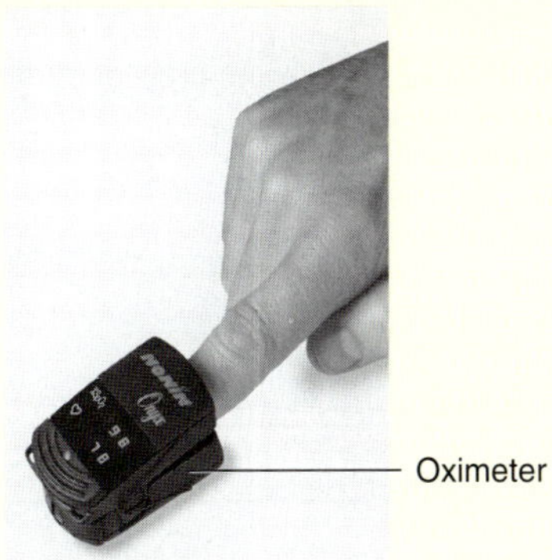

EXERCISE FIGURE G

Fill in the blanks to complete labeling of the diagram.

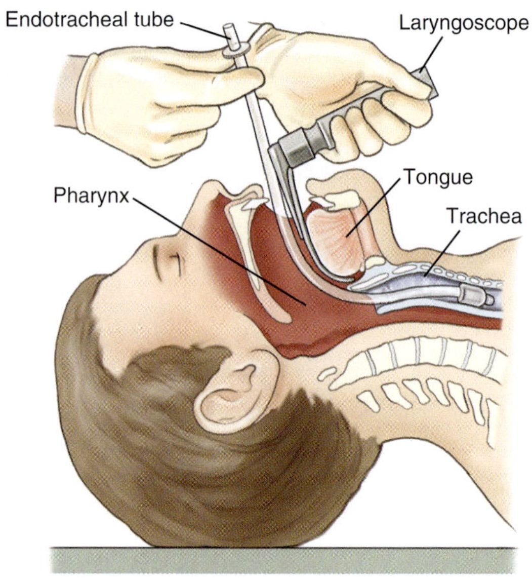

The physician is inserting a(an) ______ / ______ / ______ tube,
within / trachea / pertaining to

using a(an) ______ / ______ / ______ to
larynx / cv / instrument used for visual examination

guide the tube into place.

EXERCISE 25

Practice saying aloud each of the diagnostic terms built from word parts on pp. 179-181.

To hear the terms, go to http://evolve.elsevier.com. Refer to p. 18 for your Evolve Access Information. Select Exercises & Review, Chapter 5, Chapter Exercises, Pronunciation.

☐ Place a check mark in the box when you have completed this exercise.

EXERCISE 26

Analyze and define the following procedural terms.

Example: bronch / o / scopy (WR / CV / S; bronch/o = CF) — *visual examination of the bronchi*

1. spirometer ______
2. laryngoscope ______
3. capnometer ______
4. spirometry ______
5. oximeter ______
6. laryngoscopy ______

7. bronchoscope ______________________________
8. thoracoscope ______________________________
9. endoscope ______________________________
10. thoracoscopy ______________________________
11. endoscopic ______________________________
12. endoscopy ______________________________
13. polysomnography ______________________________

EXERCISE 27

Build diagnostic terms that correspond to the following definitions by using the word parts you have learned.

Example: instrument used to measure oxygen ox / i / meter
WR / CV / S

1. visual examination of the larynx ______ / ______ / ______
WR / CV / S

2. instrument used to measure breathing ______ / ______ / ______
WR / CV / S

3. instrument used to measure carbon dioxide ______ / ______ / ______
WR / CV / S

4. instrument used for visual examination of the larynx ______ / ______ / ______
WR / CV / S

5. visual examination of the bronchi ______ / ______ / ______
WR / CV / S

6. measurement of breathing ______ / ______ / ______
WR / CV / S

7. instrument used for visual examination of the bronchi ______ / ______ / ______
WR / CV / S

8. visual examination within (a hollow organ or body cavity) ______ / ______
P / S(WR)

9. instrument used for visual examination of the thorax ______ / ______ / ______
WR / CV / S

10. instrument used for visual examination (a hollow organ or body cavity) ______ / ______
P / S(WR)

11. visual examination within (of the thorax) ______ / ______ / ______
WR / CV / S

12. pertaining to visual examination within (a hollow organ or body cavity) ______ / ______
P / S(WR)

13. process of recording of many (tests) during sleep ______ / ______ / ______ / ______
P / WR / CV / S

EXERCISE 28

Spell each of the diagnostic terms built from word parts on pp. 179-181 by having someone dictate them to you.

To hear and spell the terms, go to http://evolve.elsevier.com. Refer to p. 18 for your Evolve Access Information. Select Exercises & Review, Chapter 5, Chapter Exercises, Spelling.
☐ Place a check mark in the box if you have completed this exercise online.

1. ______
2. ______
3. ______
4. ______
5. ______
6. ______
7. ______
8. ______
9. ______
10. ______
11. ______
12. ______
13. ______
14. ______

Diagnostic Terms

Not Built from Word Parts

In some of the following terms, you may recognize word parts; however, the terms cannot be translated literally to find their meanings.

Term	Definition
DIAGNOSTIC IMAGING	
chest computed tomography (CT) scan (chest) (kom-PŪ-ted) (tō-MOG-ra-fē) (skan)	computerized images of the chest created in sections sliced from front to back. Performed to diagnose tumors, abscesses, and pleural effusion. Computed tomography is used to visualize other body parts such as the abdomen and the brain (see Table 5-1).
chest radiograph (CXR) (chest) (RĀ-dē-ō-*graf*)	a radiographic image of the chest performed to evaluate the lungs and the heart (also called a **chest x-ray**) (see Table 5-1)
ventilation-perfusion scanning (VPS) (*ven*-ti-LĀ-shun) (per-FŪ-zhun)	a nuclear medicine procedure performed to diagnose a pulmonary embolism and other conditions (also called a **lung scan**) (see Table 5-1)
LABORATORY	
acid-fast bacilli (AFB) smear (AS-id-fast) (bah-SIL-ī) (smēr)	a test performed on sputum to determine the presence of acid-fast bacilli, which cause tuberculosis
PULMONARY FUNCTION	
arterial blood gases (ABGs) (ar-TĒ-rē-al) (blud) (GAS-es)	a test performed on arterial blood to determine levels of oxygen, carbon dioxide, and other gases present
peak flow meter (PFM) (pēk) (flō) (mē-ter)	a portable instrument used to measure how fast air can be pushed out of the lung; used to help monitor asthma and adjust medication accordingly (Figure 5-13)

HELICAL COMPUTED TOMOGRAPHY (CT) SCAN

of the chest, also called **spiral CT scan,** is an improvement over standard CT and is the preferred study to identify pulmonary embolism. Images are continually obtained as the patient passes through the gantry, which is part of the scanner. It produces a more concise and faster image, which can be performed with one breath hold.

X-RAY FILM AND RADIOGRAPH

are terms used interchangeably; however, they have different meanings. **X-ray film** is the material on which the image is exposed, whereas **radiograph** refers to the processed image. **Radiographic images**, referred to as **x-ray images** in former editions of this text, can be obtained as hard copy on x-ray film (radiograph) or as digital images stored electronically and viewed on a monitor.

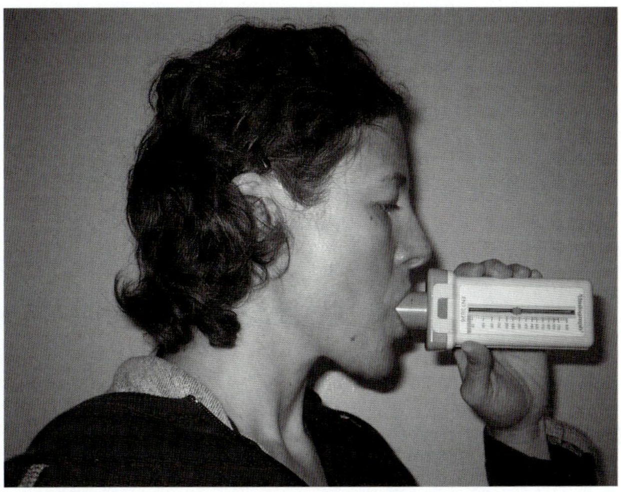

FIGURE 5-13
Peak flow meter.

Diagnostic Terms—*cont'd*

Not Built from Word Parts

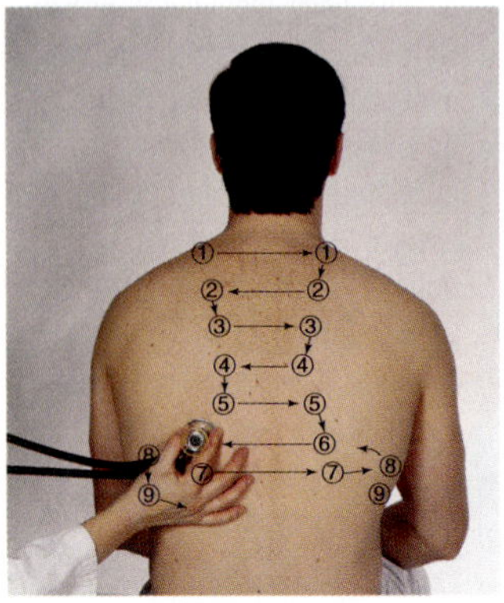

FIGURE 5-14
Auscultation.

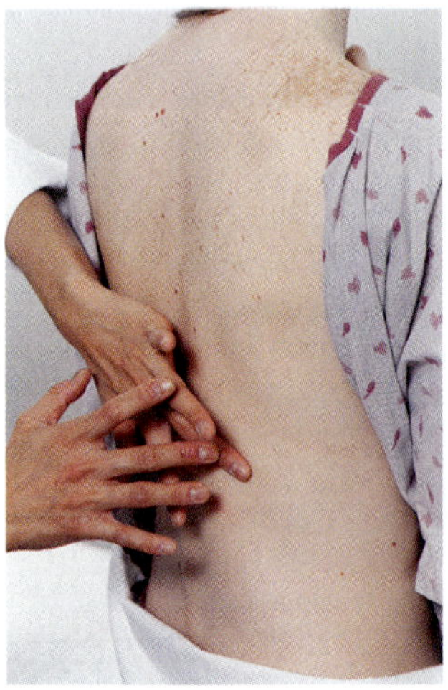

FIGURE 5-15
Percussion.

Term	Definition
PULMONARY FUNCTION—cont'd	
pulmonary function tests (PFTs) (PUL-mō-*nar*-ē) (FUNK-shun) (tests)	a group of tests performed to measure breathing and used to determine respiratory function; when abnormal, they are useful in distinguishing COPD from asthma
pulse oximetry (puls) (ok-SIM-e-trē)	a noninvasive method of measuring oxygen in the blood by using a device that attaches to the fingertip (see Table 5-1)
OTHER	
auscultation (*aws*-kul-TĀ-shun)	the act of listening for sounds within the body through a stethoscope. Used for assessing and/or diagnosing conditions of the lungs, pleura, heart and abdomen (Figure 5-14).
percussion (per-KUSH-un)	the act of tapping of a body surface with the fingers to determine the density of the part beneath by the sound obtained. A dull sound indicates the presence of fluid in a body space or cavity such as in the pleural space (Figure 5-15).
PPD (purified protein derivative) skin test	a test performed on individuals who have recently been exposed to tuberculosis. PPD of the tuberculin bacillus is injected intradermally. Positive tests indicate previous exposure, not necessarily active tuberculosis (also called **TB skin test**)
stethoscope (STETH-ō-skōp)	an instrument used to hear internal body sounds; used for performing auscultation and blood pressure measurement (Figure 5-16)

A

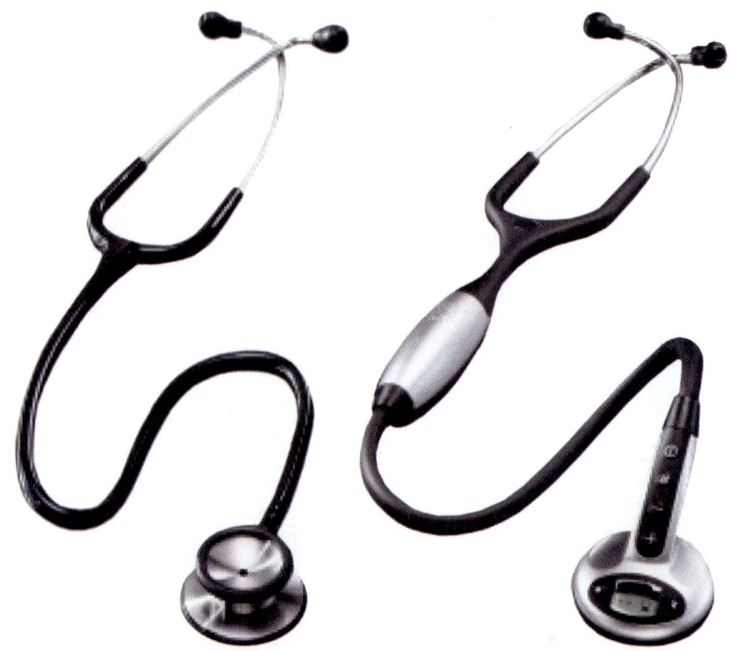

B

FIGURE 5-16
Stethoscope types. **A,** Acoustic. **B,** Electronic.

EXERCISE 29

Practice saying aloud each of the diagnostic terms not built from word parts on pp. 187-188.

To hear the terms, go to http://evolve.elsevier.com. Refer to p. 18 for your Evolve Access Information. Select Exercises & Review, Chapter 5, Chapter Exercises, Pronunciation.

☐ Place a check mark in the box when you have completed this exercise.

EXERCISE 30

Fill in the blanks with the correct terms.

1. ______________________ ______________ is a nuclear medicine procedure performed to diagnose pulmonary embolism and other conditions.
2. Computerized images of the chest, created in sections sliced from front to back, are called a(n) ______________ ______________ ______________ scan.
3. ______________ ______________ is performed to evaluate the lungs and the heart.
4. The test performed on arterial blood to determine levels of oxygen, carbon dioxide, and other gases present is called ______________ ______________ ______________.
5. A noninvasive test to measure oxygen in the blood is called ______________ ______________.
6. A test performed on sputum to diagnose tuberculosis is called ______________________ ______________ ______________.
7. __________ __________ __________ is the name of a group of tests performed on breathing to determine respiratory function or abnormalities.
8. ______________ ______________ ______________ is a test that, when positive, indicates an individual has been exposed to tuberculosis.
9. ______________ ______________ ______________ is used to measure how fast air can be pushed out of the lung.
10. The instrument used to hear internal body sounds is called a(n) ______________.
11. An act that involves tapping a body surface with the finger is called ______________.
12. The act of listening for sounds within the body through a stethoscope is called ______________.

EXERCISE 31

Match the terms in the first column with their correct definitions in the second column.

______	1. ventilation-perfusion scanning	a. computerized images of the chest
______	2. chest radiograph	b. a noninvasive method used to measure oxygen in the blood
______	3. chest CT scan	c. a blood test used to determine oxygen and other gases in the blood
______	4. acid-fast bacilli smear	d. a test for tuberculosis
______	5. pulse oximetry	e. chest x-ray
______	6. arterial blood gases	f. a nuclear medicine procedure used to diagnose pulmonary conditions
______	7. pulmonary function tests	g. injected intradermally
______	8. PPD skin test	h. tests performed on breathing
______	9. auscultation	i. an instrument to measure pulse waves
______	10. stethoscope	j. an instrument used for auscultation
______	11. peak flow meter	k. used to help monitor asthma
______	12. percussion	l. used for assessing and diagnosing conditions of the lung and pleura
		m. used to determine the presence of fluid in the pleural space

EXERCISE 32

Spell each of the diagnostic terms not built from word parts on pp. 187-188 by having someone dictate them to you.

To hear and spell the terms, go to http://evolve.elsevier.com. Refer to p. 18 for your Evolve Access Information. Select Exercises & Review, Chapter 5, Chapter Exercises, Spelling.
☐ Place a check mark in the box if you have completed this exercise online.

1. ______________________	7. ______________________
2. ______________________	8. ______________________
3. ______________________	9. ______________________
4. ______________________	10. ______________________
5. ______________________	11. ______________________
6. ______________________	12. ______________________

Complementary Terms

Built from Word Parts

The following terms are built from word parts you have already learned and can be translated literally to find their meanings. Further explanation of terms beyond the definition of their word parts, if needed, is included in parentheses.

Term	Definition
acapnia (a-CAP-nē-a)	condition of absence (less than normal level) of carbon dioxide (in the blood)
alveolar (al-VĒ-ō-lar)	pertaining to the alveolus
anoxia (a-NOK-sē-a)	condition of absence (deficiency) of oxygen
aphonia (ā-FŌ-nē-a)	condition of absence of voice
apnea (AP-nē-a)	absence of breathing
bronchoalveolar (*bron*-kō-al-VĒ-o-lar)	pertaining to the bronchi and alveoli
bronchospasm (BRON-kō-spaz-m)	spasmodic contraction in the bronchi
diaphragmatic (*dī*-a-frag-MAT-ik)	pertaining to the diaphragm (also called **phrenic**)
dysphonia (dis-FŌ-nē-a)	condition of difficult speaking (voice)
dyspnea (DISP-nē-a)	difficult breathing
endotracheal (*en*-dō-TRĀ-kē-al)	pertaining to within the trachea (see Exercise Figure G)
eupnea (ŪP-nē-a)	normal breathing
hypercapnia (*hī*-per-KAP-nē-a)	condition of excessive carbon dioxide (in the blood)
hyperpnea (*hī*-perp-NĒ-a)	excessive breathing
hypocapnia (*hī*-pō-KAP-nē-a)	condition of deficient carbon dioxide (in the blood)
hypopnea (hī-POP-nē-a)	deficient breathing
hypoxemia (*hī*-pok-SĒ-mē-a) (NOTE: the *o* from *hypo* has been dropped. The final vowel in a prefix may be dropped when the word to which it is added begins with a vowel.)	condition of deficient oxygen in the blood
hypoxia (hī-POK-sē-a) (NOTE: see note for hypoxemia.)	condition of deficient oxygen (to the tissues)

ANOXIA

literally means **without oxygen** or **absence of oxygen.** The term actually denotes an oxygen deficiency in the body tissues.

Complementary Terms—*cont'd*

Built from Word Parts

Term	Definition
intrapleural (*in*-tra-PLUR-al)	pertaining to within the pleura (space between the two pleural membranes)
laryngeal (lar-IN-jē-al)	pertaining to the larynx
laryngospasm (la-RING-gō-spaz-m)	spasmodic contraction of the larynx
mucoid (MŪ-koyd)	resembling mucus
mucous (MŪ-kus)	pertaining to mucus
nasopharyngeal (*nā*-zō-fa-RIN-jē-al)	pertaining to the nose and pharynx
orthopnea (or-THOP-nē-a)	able to breathe easier in a straight (upright) position
phrenalgia (fre-NAL-ja)	pain in the diaphragm (also called **diaphragmalgia**)
phrenospasm (FREN-ō-spaz-m)	spasm of the diaphragm
pulmonary (PUL-mō-*nar*-ē)	pertaining to the lungs
pulmonologist (*pul*-mon-OL-o-jist)	a physician who studies and treats diseases of the lung
pulmonology (*pul*-mon-OL-o-jē)	study of the lung (a branch of medicine dealing with diseases of the lung)
rhinorrhea (*rī*-nō-RĒ-a)	discharge from the nose (as in a cold)
tachypnea (tak-IP-nē-a)	rapid breathing
thoracic (thō-RAS-ik)	pertaining to the chest

MUCUS

is the noun that describes slimy fluid secreted by the mucous membrane. **Mucous** is the adjective that means pertaining to the mucous membrane. Pronunciation is the same for both terms.

EXERCISE 33

Practice saying aloud each of the complementary terms built from word parts on pp. 191-192.

To hear the terms, go to http://evolve.elsevier.com. Refer to p. 18 for your Evolve Access Information. Select Exercises & Review, Chapter 5, Chapter Exercises, Pronunciation.

☐ Place a check mark in the box when you have completed this exercise.

EXERCISE 34

Analyze and define the following complementary terms.

Example: hyper (P) / capn (WR) / ia (S) *condition of excessive carbon dioxide (in the blood)*

1. laryngeal ______
2. eupnea ______
3. mucoid ______
4. apnea ______
5. hypoxia ______
6. laryngospasm ______
7. endotracheal ______
8. anoxia ______
9. dysphonia ______
10. bronchoalveolar ______
11. dyspnea ______
12. hypocapnia ______
13. bronchospasm ______
14. orthopnea ______
15. hyperpnea ______
16. acapnia ______
17. hypopnea ______
18. hypoxemia ______
19. aphonia ______
20. rhinorrhea ______
21. thoracic ______
22. mucous ______
23. nasopharyngeal ______
24. diaphragmatic ______
25. intrapleural ______
26. pulmonary ______
27. phrenalgia ______
28. tachypnea ______
29. phrenospasm ______
30. pulmonologist ______
31. pulmonology ______
32. alveolar ______

EXERCISE 35

Build the complementary terms for the following definitions by using the word parts you have learned.

Example: pertaining to bronchi and alveoli bronch / o / alveol / ar
WR / CV / WR / S

1. condition of deficient oxygen ______ / ______ / ______
P / WR / S

2. resembling mucus ______ / ______
WR / S

3. able to breathe easier in a straight (upright) position ______ / ______ / ______
WR / CV / S

4. pertaining to within the trachea ______ / ______ / ______
P / WR / S

5. condition of absence of oxygen ______ / ______ / ______
P / WR / S

6. difficult breathing ______ / ______
P / S(WR)

7. pertaining to the larynx ______ / ______
WR / S

8. condition of excessive carbon dioxide (in the blood) ______ / ______ / ______
P / WR / S

9. normal breathing ______ / ______
P / S(WR)

10. condition of absence of voice ______ / ______ / ______
P / WR / S

11. spasmodic contraction of the larynx ______ / ______ / ______
WR / CV / S

12. condition of deficient carbon dioxide (in the blood) ______ / ______ / ______
P / WR / S

13. pertaining to the nose and pharynx ______ / ______ / ______ / ______
WR / CV / WR / S

14. pertaining to the diaphragm ______ / ______
WR / S

15. condition of absence of breathing ______ / ______
P / S(WR)

16. condition of deficient oxygen in the blood ______ / ______ / ______
P / WR / S

17. excessive breathing ______ / ______
P / S(WR)

18. spasmodic contraction in the bronchi ______ / ______ / ______
WR / CV / S

19. deficient breathing ______ / ______
P / S(WR)

20. condition of absence of carbon dioxide (in the blood) ______ / ______ / ______
P / WR / S

21. condition of difficulty in speaking (voice) ______ / ______ / ______
P / WR / S

22. discharge from the nose ______ / ______ / ______
WR / CV / S

23. pertaining to mucus ______ / ______
WR / S

24. pertaining to the chest ______ / ______
WR / S

25. pertaining to within the pleura ______ / ______ / ______
P / WR / S

26. pertaining to the lungs ______ / ______
WR / S

27. spasm of the diaphragm ______ / ______ / ______
WR / CV / S

28. rapid breathing ______ / ______
P / S(WR)

29. pain in the diaphragm ______ / ______
WR / S

30. pertaining to the alveolus ______ / ______
WR / S

31. study of the lung ______ / ______ / ______
WR / CV / S

32. a physician who studies and treats diseases of the lung ______ / ______ / ______
WR / CV / S

EXERCISE 36

Spell each of the complementary terms built from word parts on pp. 191-192 by having someone dictate them to you.

To hear and spell the terms, go to http://evolve.elsevier.com. Refer to p. 18 for your Evolve Access Information. Select Exercises & Review, Chapter 5, Chapter Exercises, Spelling.
☐ Place a check mark in the box if you have completed this exercise online.

1. ______________________
2. ______________________
3. ______________________
4. ______________________
5. ______________________
6. ______________________
7. ______________________
8. ______________________
9. ______________________
10. ______________________
11. ______________________
12. ______________________
13. ______________________
14. ______________________
15. ______________________
16. ______________________
17. ______________________
18. ______________________
19. ______________________
20. ______________________
21. ______________________
22. ______________________
23. ______________________
24. ______________________
25. ______________________
26. ______________________
27. ______________________
28. ______________________
29. ______________________
30. ______________________
31. ______________________
32. ______________________
33. ______________________

Complementary Terms

Not Built from Word Parts

In some of the following terms, you may recognize word parts; however, the terms cannot be translated literally to find their meanings.

Term	Definition
airway (AR-wā)	passageway by which air enters and leaves the lungs as well as a mechanical device used to keep the air passageway unobstructed
asphyxia (as-FIK-sē-a)	deprivation of oxygen for tissue use; suffocation
aspirate (AS-per-āt)	to withdraw fluid or suction fluid; also to draw foreign material into the respiratory tract
bronchoconstrictor (*bron*-kō-kon-STRIK-tor)	agent causing narrowing of the bronchi

Term	Definition
bronchodilator (*bron*-kō-dī-LĀ-tor)	agent causing the bronchi to widen
cough (kawf)	sudden, noisy expulsion of air from the lungs
hiccup (HIK-up)	sudden catching of breath with a spasmodic contraction of the diaphragm (also called **hiccough** and **singultus**)
hyperventilation (*hī*-per-*ven*-ti-LĀ-shun)	ventilation of the lungs beyond normal body needs
hypoventilation (*hī*-pō-*ven*-ti-LĀ-shun)	ventilation of the lungs that does not fulfill the body's gas exchange needs
mucopurulent (*mū*-kō-PŪR-ū-lent)	containing both mucus and pus
mucus (MŪ-kus)	slimy fluid secreted by the mucous membranes
nebulizer (NEB-ū-lī-zer)	device that creates a mist used to deliver medication for giving respiratory treatment (Figure 5-17)
nosocomial infection (nos-ō-KŌ-mē-al) (in-FEK-shun)	an infection acquired during hospitalization
paroxysm (PAR-ok-sizm)	periodic, sudden attack
patent (PĀ-tent)	open, the opposite of closed or compromised, thus allowing passage of air, as in patent trachea and bronchi (can be applied to any tubular passageway in the body, as in a patent artery, allowing passage of blood)
sputum (SPŪ-tum)	mucous secretion from the lungs, bronchi, and trachea expelled through the mouth
ventilator (VEN-ti-*lā*-tor)	mechanical device used to assist with or substitute for breathing (Figure 5-18)

SPUTUM

is derived from the Latin ***spuere***, meaning ***to spit***. In a 1693 dictionary it is defined as a "secretion thicker than ordinary spittle."

Refer to **Appendix D** for pharmacology terms related to the respiratory system.

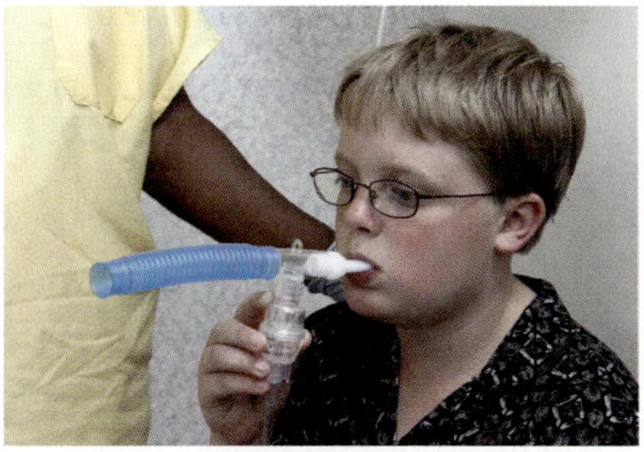

FIGURE 5-17
Nebulizer.

A

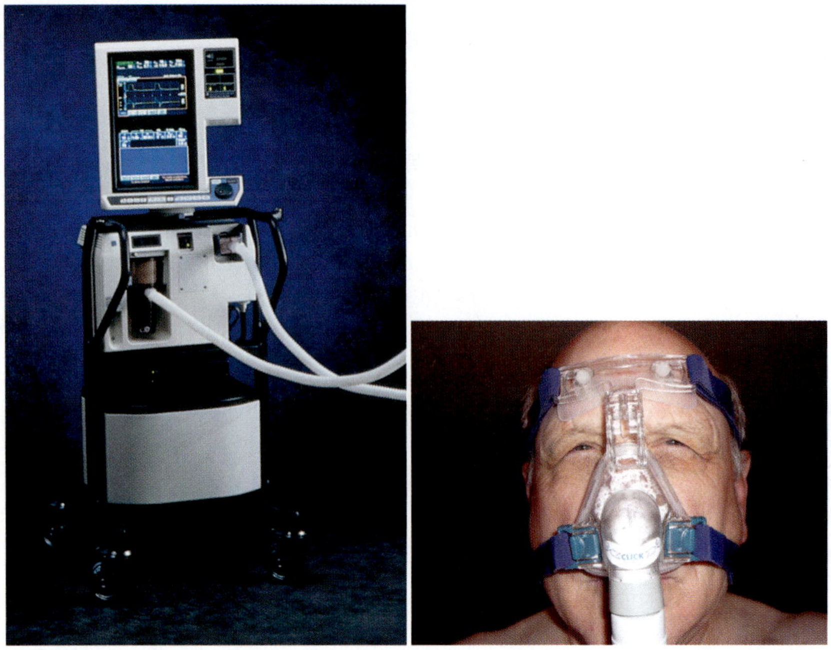

B

FIGURE 5-18

A, Invasive ventilator. Positive pressure ventilator is applied to the patient's airway through an endotracheal or tracheostomy tube and is used when spontaneous breathing is inadequate to sustain life. **B,** Noninvasive ventilator. CPAP (continuous positive airway pressure) is used for patients who can initiate their own breathing and is often used to treat obstructive sleep apnea.

EXERCISE 37

Practice saying aloud each of the complementary terms not built from word parts on pp. 196-197.

To hear the terms, go to http://evolve.elsevier.com. Refer to p. 18 for your Evolve Access Information. Select Exercises & Review, Chapter 5, Chapter Exercises, Pronunciation.

☐ Place a check mark in the box when you have completed this exercise.

EXERCISE 38

Fill in the blanks with the correct terms.

1. Another term for ventilation of the lungs beyond normal body needs is ____________________.
2. A device that creates a mist used to deliver medication for giving respiratory treatment is a(n) ____________________.
3. A(n) ____________________ is an agent that causes the air passages to widen.
4. A patient who has difficulty breathing can be attached to a mechanical breathing device called a(n) ____________________.
5. Another term for suffocation is ____________________.
6. Material made up of mucous secretions from the lungs, bronchi, and trachea is called ____________________.

7. To suction or withdraw fluid is to ________________.

8. A(n) ________________ is a mechanical device that keeps the air passageway unobstructed.

9. A sudden catching of breath with spasmodic contraction of the diaphragm is called a(n) ________________.

10. A sudden, noisy expulsion of air from the lung is a(n) ________________.

11. Material containing both mucus and pus is referred to as being ________________.

12. ________________ is the name given to ventilation of the lungs that does not fulfill the body's gas exchange needs.

13. An infection acquired during hospitalization is called ________________.

14. The term that applies to a periodic sudden attack is ________________.

15. An airway must be kept ________________ (open) for the patient to breathe.

16. An agent that causes bronchi to narrow is called a(n) ________________.

17. ________________ is the name given to the slimy fluid secreted by the mucous membranes.

EXERCISE 39

Match the terms in the first column with their correct definitions in the second column.

______ 1. airway	a. sudden, noisy expulsion of air from the lungs
______ 2. aspirate	b. mechanical device used to keep the air passageway unobstructed
______ 3. bronchoconstrictor	c. agent that narrows the bronchi
______ 4. bronchodilator	d. catching of breath with spasmodic contraction of diaphragm
______ 5. cough	e. mucus from throat and lungs
______ 6. hiccup	f. suffocation
______ 7. hyperventilation	g. ventilation of the lungs beyond normal body needs
______ 8. asphyxia	h. to draw foreign material into the respiratory tract
	i. agent that widens the bronchi

EXERCISE 40

Match the terms in the first column with their correct definitions in the second column.

_____ 1. hypoventilation
_____ 2. mucopurulent
_____ 3. mucus
_____ 4. nebulizer
_____ 5. nosocomial
_____ 6. patent
_____ 7. sputum
_____ 8. ventilator
_____ 9. paroxysm

a. open
b. mucous secretion from lungs, bronchi, and trachea, expelled through the mouth
c. respiratory treatment device that sends a mist
d. mechanical breathing device
e. ventilation of the lungs that does not fulfill the body's gas exchange needs
f. periodic, sudden attack
g. agent that widens air passages
h. containing both mucus and pus
i. slimy fluid secreted by mucous membranes
j. hospital-acquired infection

EXERCISE 41

Spell each of the complementary terms not built from word parts on pp. 196-197 by having someone dictate them to you.

To hear and spell the terms, go to http://evolve.elsevier.com. Refer to p. 18 for your Evolve Access Information. Select Exercises & Review, Chapter 5, Chapter Exercises, Spelling.
☐ Place a check mark in the box if you have completed this exercise online.

1. _____________________
2. _____________________
3. _____________________
4. _____________________
5. _____________________
6. _____________________
7. _____________________
8. _____________________
9. _____________________
10. _____________________
11. _____________________
12. _____________________
13. _____________________
14. _____________________
15. _____________________
16. _____________________
17. _____________________

Abbreviations

ABGs	arterial blood gases
AFB	acid-fast bacilli
ARDS	acute respiratory distress syndrome
CF	cystic fibrosis
CO_2	carbon dioxide
COPD	chronic obstructive pulmonary disease
CT	computed tomography
CXR	chest radiograph (chest x-ray)
flu	influenza
LLL	left lower lobe
LTB	laryngotracheobronchitis
LUL	left upper lobe
O_2	oxygen
OSA	obstructive sleep apnea
PE	pulmonary embolism
PFM	peak flow meter
PFTs	pulmonary function tests
PSG	polysomnography
RLL	right lower lobe
RML	right middle lobe
RUL	right upper lobe
SOB	shortness of breath
TB	tuberculosis
URI	upper respiratory infection
VPS	ventilation-perfusion scanning

Refer to **Appendix C** for a complete list of abbreviations.

EXERCISE 42

Write the meaning of the abbreviations in the following sentences.

1. A variety of tests are used to diagnose **COPD** ____________________

____________________ ____________________ ____________________,

including **PFTs** ____________________ ____________________

____________________, **CXR** ____________________

____________________, **ABGs** ____________________

____________________ ____________________, and chest **CT**

____________________ ____________________ scan. **SOB**

____________________ ____________________ ____________________ is

often a symptom of COPD ____________________ ____________________

____________________ ____________________.

2. **VPS** ______________________________ ______________ is very helpful in diagnosing **PE** ______________ ______________.
3. The lobes of the left lung are **LUL** ______________ ______________ ______________ and **LLL** ______________ ______________ ______________; the lobes of the right lung are **RUL** ______________ ______________ ______________, **RML** ______________ ______________ ______________, and **RLL** ______________ ______________ ______________.
4. **AFB** ______________________________ ______________ smear is used to support the diagnosis of **TB** ______________.
5. **PSG** ______________________________ is used to confirm the diagnosis of **OSA** ______________ ______________ ______________.
6. Respiration is the exchange of O_2 ______________ and CO_2 ______________ ______________ between the atmosphere and body cells.
7. Measurements obtained from using a **PFM** ______________ ______________ ______________ can be used to adjust medication for persons with asthma.

EXERCISE 43

Write the definition for the following abbreviations.

1. ARDS ______________ ______________ ______________ ______________
2. CF ______________ ______________
3. flu ______________
4. LTB ______________________________
5. URI ______________ ______________ ______________

Common Abbreviations Used in the Respiratory Care Department within a Healthcare Facility

BiPAP	bilevel positive airway pressure
CPT	chest physiotherapy
CPAP	continuous positive airway pressure
DPI	dry powder inhaler
HME	heat/moisture exchanger
IPPB	intermittent positive-pressure breathing
MDI	metered-dose inhaler
NPPV	noninvasive positive-pressure ventilator
PEP	positive expiratory pressure
SVN	small-volume nebulizer
VAP	ventilator-associated pneumonia

PRACTICAL APPLICATION

EXERCISE 44 *Interact with Medical Documents*

A. Complete the medical consultation report by writing the medical terms in the blanks. Use the list of definitions with the corresponding numbers following it.

University Hospital and Medical Center
4700 North Main Street • Wellness, Arizona 54321 • (987) 555-3210

PATIENT NAME: Victor Marquez
DATE OF BIRTH: 02/01/19XX
CASE NUMBER: 516987-RSP
DATE: 02/16/20XX

MEDICAL CONSULT REPORT

HISTORY: Victor Marquez is a 55-year-old Mexican-American man who came to the Emergency Department on 02/16/XX because of recent onset of 1. ___________ and 2. ___________. He has also had weight loss and has had the cough for the past 6 months. He denies hemoptysis, chest pain, fever, or night sweats. He has a history of smoking two packs of cigarettes a day for 40 years. It was decided that he should be admitted and scheduled for a 3. ___________ consultation.

PHYSICAL EXAMINATION: VITAL SIGNS: Blood pressure, 148/82 mm Hg. Temperature, 98.2. Pulse, 60. Respirations, 18. The chest is clear except for scattered rhonchi over left posterior lung. The heart is regular rhythm without murmur. He is in no acute distress. Pulses are full and equal throughout. There is mild clubbing of the fingers.

PULMONARY EXAM: 4. ___________ ___________ reveals a suspicious lesion in the left upper lobe of the lung with diffuse interstitial fibrotic lesions. Fiberoptic 5. ___________ shows edematous vocal cords with no obvious nodules. However, at the entry of the left bronchus, a lesion is observed that partially obstructs the opening. A biopsy and brush cytology of the specimen were obtained. 6. ___________ ___________ ___________ shows mild 7. ___________ .

IMPRESSION: It is my impression that the patient has 8. ___________ ___________.

DISPOSITION:
1. Obtain 9. ___________ ___________ ___________ to include lung volumes and diffusing capacity.
2. Obtain a CT scan of the chest and a 10. ___________ surgery consultation.

____

Miguel Valdez, MD

MV/mcm

1. sudden noisy expulsion of air from the lungs
2. difficult breathing
3. pertaining to the lungs
4. radiographic image used to evaluate the lungs and heart
5. visual examination of the bronchi
6. test performed on arterial blood to determine the presence of oxygen, carbon dioxide, and other gases
7. condition of deficient oxygen in the blood
8. cancerous tumor originating in the bronchus
9. a group of tests performed on breathing
10. pertaining to the chest

EXERCISE 44 *Interact with Medical Documents—cont'd*

B. Read the clinical case study and answer the questions following it.

Medical History: A 65-year-old man who has a history of nonproductive cough and shortness of breath of 3 weeks' duration was admitted to the hospital. He has smoked one pack of cigarettes daily for nearly 40 years.

Physical Examination: The patient is thin, has tachypnea, and is mildly cyanotic with a barrel chest. He uses accessory muscles of inspiration and pursed-lip breathing. Expiration is prolonged, breath sounds are diminished, and wheezing is present. Respiratory rate: 30 breaths/min, heart rate: 100 beats/min, blood pressure: 110/70, temperature: 38.2°C.

Diagnostic Studies: PA and lateral chest radiographs reveal pulmonary hyperinflation, a widened anteroposterior diameter, increased depth of the retrosternal air space, and a right lobe infiltrate consistent with pneumonia.

Arterial blood gases: PaO_2, 52 mm Hg; $PaCO_2$, 68 mm Hg; pH, 7.30

O_2 saturation measured by pulse oximetry at room air is 87%.

Diagnosis: Chronic obstructive pulmonary disease with respiratory insufficiency, pneumonia, hypoxia, hypercapnia, and respiratory acidosis.

1. Three tests used to determine the diagnosis are
   ____________ ____________;
   __________ __________ __________;
   ____________ ____________.
2. The patient was experiencing (excessive, deficient) carbon dioxide and (excessive, deficient) oxygen in the blood.
3. a. T F On physical examination the patient was experiencing rapid breathing.
   b. T F The patient was diagnosed as having COPD.
   c. T F A CXR was performed as one of the diagnostic studies.

EXERCISE 44 *Interact with Medical Documents—cont'd*

C. Below is a printed report of a CT scan of the chest. Refer to Table 5-1 for illustrations of a CT scanner and images.

Terms you have studied thus far are in bold. Note how they are used within a medical record.

NAME: Abigail Frank **MR #:** 7463802 **ACCESSION #:** 1503132
DATE OF EXAM: 11/16/20XX **PHYSICIAN:** Irene Buchanan, MD

CT CHEST W/CONTRAST AT 1117 HOURS

EXAM: **CT OF THE CHEST**

History: Cervical **cancer**

TECHNIQUE: Multiple contiguous axial images were obtained to the chest during the uneventful infusion of **intravenous** contrast.

FINDINGS: There has been interval decrease in size of **bilateral pulmonary metastases.** Again the largest is noted within the left lower **lobe** and measures 4.8 × 3.9 cm compared to 6.5 × 5.0 cm previously when measured at the same weight. Multiple smaller **lesions** within both **lungs** have decreased in size.

No significant **adenopathy** is identified. Postsurgical changes centrally within the right lower lobe are again noted with a surgical staple line in place.

There has been interval development of several patchy probably interstitial opacities within both lungs. Some are located adjacent to **metastases** that have decreased in size.

No new masses are noted. There is no pericardial or **pleural effusion.** The osseous structures remain within normal limits.

A left adrenal **nodule** remains essentially unchanged measuring approximately 2 cm in greatest dimension.

IMPRESSION: Interval decrease in size of **bilateral pulmonary metastases** as described following **chemotherapy** and **radiation therapy.**

Development of occasional patchy predominately interstitial opacities. Given the history of **chemotherapy** and **radiation therapy** this likely reflects a postradiation or post-therapeutic **pneumonitis** or hypersensitivity. Additional considerations are an infectious **pneumonitis** or hemorrhage. Continued follow-up is recommended. Stable small left adrenal **nodule.**

Transcribed By: MCM 11/16/20XX: 1641

Approved By: Radiologist: Brian Benson, DO

EXERCISE 45 *Interpret Medical Terms*

To test your understanding of the terms introduced in this chapter, circle the words that correctly complete the sentences. The italicized words refer to the correct answer.

1. The patient was admitted to the emergency department with a *severe nosebleed*, or (**rhinomycosis, epistaxis, nasopharyngitis**).
2. The accident caused damage to the *larynx*, necessitating a *surgical repair*, or a (**laryngectomy, laryngostomy, laryngoplasty**).
3. Mr. Prince was *able to breathe easier in an upright position*, so the nurse recorded that he had (**orthopnea, eupnea, dyspnea**).
4. The *test on arterial blood to determine oxygen and carbon dioxide levels* (**pulse oximetry, pulmonary function tests, arterial blood gases**) indicated that the patient was *deficient in oxygen*, or had (**dysphonia, hypoxia, hypocapnia**).
5. The physician informed the patient that a heart attack was not the cause of the *chest pain*, or (**thoracalgia, pneumothorax, thoracentesis**).
6. The patient reported dizziness brought on by *ventilation of the lungs beyond normal body needs*, or (**hyperventilation, hypoventilation, dysphonia**).
7. The physician wished the patient to have the medication given by *a device that delivers mist*, so he ordered that the treatment be given by (**airway, nebulizer, ventilator**).
8. The patient with *blood in the chest* was diagnosed as having a (**pneumothorax, pleuritis, hemothorax**).
9. After surgery, the patient had a *block in the circulation to the pulmonary artery* or (**pleural effusion, pulmonary edema, pulmonary embolism**).
10. The patient was diagnosed as having *a fungal disease affecting the lung*, or (**obstructive sleep apnea, tuberculosis, coccidioidomycosis**).
11. The physician ordered a *radiographic image of the chest* (**chest radiograph, chest CT scan, bronchoscopy**) because she suspected *an infection acquired during hospitalization*, or (**patent, nosocomial, paroxysm**) pneumonia.
12. The patient received an *intradermal injection* (**AFB, ABGs, PPD skin test**) *to determine if she had been exposed to TB.*
13. The patient was experiencing *rapid breathing* or (**phrenospasm, tachypnea, phrenalgia**).
14. To assess conditions of the lungs and pleura by listening, the nurse practicioner used a (**peak flow meter**, **stethoscope, chest radiograph**.)

EXERCISE 46 *Read Medical Terms in Use*

Practice pronouncing the terms by reading the following medical document. Use the pronunciation key following the medical terms to assist you in saying the word.

To hear these terms, go to http://evolve.elsevier.com. Refer to p. 18 for your Evolve Access Information. Select Chapter 5, Chapter Exercises, Read Medical Terms in Use.

A 24-year-old man visited the emergency department because of **dyspnea** (DISP-nē-a), **hyperpnea** (hī-perp-NĒ-a), **paroxysms** (PAR-ok-sizms) of **cough** (kawf), and the presence of thick, tenacious **mucus** (MŪ-kus). He had a history of **asthma** (AZ-ma) since the age of 12 years. A chest radiograph was negative for **pneumonia** (nū-MŌ-nē-a). **Arterial blood gases** (ar-TĒ-rē-al) (blud) (GAS-es) showed **hypoxemia** (hī-pok-SĒ-mē-a) but no **hypercapnia** (hī-per-KAP-nē–a). **Pulmonary function tests** (PUL-mō-ner-ē) (FUNK-shun) (tests) disclosed bronchoconstriction, which was corrected by a **bronchodilator** (*bron*-kō–dī-LĀ-tor). A **nebulizer** (NEB-ū-lī-zer) was prescribed for treatment. The asthma attack was probably precipitated by an episode of **bronchitis** (bron-KĪ-tis).

EXERCISE 47 *Comprehend Medical Terms in Use*

Test your comprehension of terms in the previous medical document by answering *T* for true and *F* for false.

_____ 1. The patient visited the emergency department because of many symptoms, one of which was sudden, periodic coughing.

_____ 2. Diagnostic procedures were performed to assist with the diagnosis. ABGs showed increased O_2 and decreased CO_2.

_____ 3. An agent that causes the bronchi to widen was used to treat the condition diagnosed with the PFTs.

_____ 4. The asthma attack was precipitated by narrowing of the bronchi.

WEB LINK

For additional information on diseases of the lung, visit the **American Lung Association** at ***www.lungusa.org***.

CHAPTER REVIEW

ONLINE CHAPTER REVIEW

To access the Evolve website, go to http://evolve.elsevier.com. Refer to p. 18 for your Evolve Access Information. Select Exercises & Review, Chapter 5, then select Chapter Exercises, Practice Activities, Animations, or Games. Place a check mark in the box when you have completed an exercise or activity, watched an animation, or played a game. Have fun!

Chapter Exercises

Exercises in this section of your Evolve resources correlate to exercises in your textbook. You may have completed them as you worked through the chapter.

- ☐ Pronunciation
- ☐ Spelling
- ☐ Read Medical Terms in Use

Practice Activities

Practice in study mode, then test your learning in assessment mode. Keep track of your scores from assessment mode if you wish.

	SCORE
☐ Picture It	_______
☐ Define Word Parts	_______
☐ Build Medical Terms	_______
☐ Word Shop	_______
☐ Define Medical Terms	_______
☐ Use It	_______
☐ Hear It and Type It: Clinical Vignettes	_______

Animations

- ☐ Atelectasis
- ☐ Asthma
- ☐ Pneumonia
- ☐ Pneumothorax
- ☐ Pulse oximeter
- ☐ Tuberculosis

Games

- ☐ Name that Word Part
- ☐ Term Storm
- ☐ Term Explorer
- ☐ Termbusters
- ☐ Medical Millionaire
- ☐ Crossword Puzzle

REVIEW OF WORD PARTS

Can you define and spell the following word parts?

Combining Forms

adenoid/o
alveol/o
atel/o
bronchi/o
bronch/o
capn/o
diaphragmat/o
epiglott/o
hem/o
hemat/o
laryng/o
lob/o
muc/o
nas/o
orth/o
ox/i
ox/o
pharyng/o
phon/o
phren/o
pleur/o
pneum/o
pneumat/o
pneumon/o
pulmon/o
py/o
rhin/o
sept/o
sinus/o
somn/o
spir/o
thorac/o
tonsill/o
trache/o

Prefixes

a-
an-
endo-
eu-
pan-
poly-
tachy-

Suffixes

-algia
-ar
-ary
-cele
-centesis
-eal
-ectasis
-emia
-graphy
-meter
-metry
-pexy
-pnea
-rrhagia
-scope
-scopic
-scopy
-spasm
-stenosis
-stomy
-thorax
-tomy

REVIEW OF TERMS

Can you define, pronounce, and spell the following terms *built from word parts?*

Diseases and Disorders

adenoiditis
alveolitis
atelectasis
bronchiectasis
bronchitis
bronchogenic carcinoma
bronchopneumonia
diaphragmatocele
epiglottitis
hemothorax
laryngitis
laryngotracheobronchitis (LTB)
lobar pneumonia
nasopharyngitis
pansinusitis
pharyngitis
pleuritis
pneumatocele
pneumoconiosis
pneumonia
pneumonitis
pneumothorax
pulmonary neoplasm
pyothorax
rhinitis
rhinomycosis
rhinorrhagia
thoracalgia
tonsillitis
tracheitis
tracheostenosis

Surgical

adenoidectomy
adenotome
bronchoplasty
laryngectomy
laryngoplasty
laryngostomy
laryngotracheotomy
lobectomy
pleuropexy
pneumobronchotomy
pneumonectomy
rhinoplasty
septoplasty
septotomy
sinusotomy
thoracocentesis
thoracotomy
tonsillectomy
tracheoplasty
tracheostomy
tracheotomy

Diagnostic

bronchoscope
bronchoscopy
capnometer
endoscope
endoscopic
endoscopy
laryngoscope
laryngoscopy
oximeter
polysomnography (PSG)
spirometer
spirometry
thoracoscope
thoracoscopy

Complementary

acapnia
alveolar
anoxia
aphonia
apnea
bronchoalveolar
bronchospasm
diaphragmatic
dysphonia
dyspnea
endotracheal
eupnea
hypercapnia
hyperpnea
hypocapnia
hypopnea
hypoxemia
hypoxia
intrapleural
laryngeal
laryngospasm
mucoid
mucous
nasopharyngeal
orthopnea
phrenalgia
phrenospasm
pulmonary
pulmonologist
pulmonology
rhinorrhea
tachypnea
thoracic

REVIEW OF TERMS—*cont'd*

Can you define, pronounce, and spell the following terms *not built from word parts?*

Diseases and Disorders	Diagnostic	Complementary
acute respiratory distress syndrome (ARDS)	acid-fast bacilli smear (AFB)	airway
asthma	arterial blood gases (ABGs)	asphyxia
chronic obstructive pulmonary disease (COPD)	auscultation	aspirate
coccidioidomycosis	chest computed tomography (CT) scan	bronchoconstrictor
cor pulmonale	chest radiograph (CXR)	bronchodilator
croup	peak flow meter (PFM)	cough
cystic fibrosis (CF)	percussion	hiccup
deviated septum	PPD skin test	hyperventilation
emphysema	pulmonary function tests (PFTs)	hypoventilation
epistaxis	pulse oximetry	mucopurulent
influenza (flu)	stethoscope	mucus
Legionnaire disease	ventilation-perfusion scanning (VPS)	nebulizer
obstructive sleep apnea (OSA)		nosocomial infection
pertussis		paroxysm
pleural effusion		patent
pulmonary edema		sputum
pulmonary embolism (PE)		ventilator
tuberculosis (TB)		
upper respiratory infection (URI)		

ANSWERS

Exercise Figures

Exercise Figure

A. 1. sinus: sinus/o
2. nose: nas/o, rhin/o
3. tonsil: tonsill/o
4. epiglottis: epiglott/o
5. larynx: laryng/o
6. trachea: trache/o
7. pleura: pleur/o
8. lobe: lob/o
9. diaphragm: diaphragmat/o, phren/o
10. adenoids: adenoid/o
11. pharynx: pharyng/o
12. lung: pneum/o, pneumat/o, pneumon/o, pulmon/o
13. bronchus: bronch/o, bronchi/o
14. alveolus: alveol/o

Exercise Figure

B. bronchi/ectasis

Exercise Figure

C. A. pneum/o/thorax
B. hem/o/thorax

Exercise Figure

D. adenoid/ectomy, aden/o/tome

Exercise Figure

E. thorac/o/centesis

Exercise Figure

F. bronch/o/scopy

Exercise Figure

G. endo/trache/al, laryng/o/scope

Exercise 1

1. h
2. a
3. g
4. c
5. f
6. d
7. e
8. b

Exercise 2

1. nasal septum
2. epiglottis
3. bronchioles
4. nose
5. diaphragm
6. mediastinum
7. tonsils

Exercise 3

1. larynx
2. bronchus
3. pleura
4. lung, air
5. tonsil
6. lung
7. diaphragm
8. trachea
9. alveolus
10. lung, air
11. thorax (chest)
12. adenoids
13. pharynx
14. nose
15. sinus
16. lobe
17. epiglottis
18. lung, air
19. nose
20. septum
21. diaphragm

Exercise 4

1. a. nas/o
   b. rhin/o
2. laryng/o
3. a. pneum/o
   b. pneumat/o
   c. pneumon/o
4. pulmon/o
5. tonsill/o
6. trache/o
7. adenoid/o
8. pleur/o
9. a. diaphragmat/o
   b. phren/o
10. sinus/o
11. thorac/o
12. alveol/o
13. pharyng/o
14. a. bronchi/o
    b. bronch/o
15. lob/o
16. epiglott/o
17. sept/o

Exercise 5

1. oxygen
2. breathe, breathing
3. mucus
4. imperfect, incomplete
5. straight
6. pus
7. blood
8. sleep
9. carbon dioxide
10. sound, voice

Exercise 6

1. spir/o
2. a. ox/o
   b. ox/i
3. atel/o
4. orth/o
5. py/o
6. muc/o
7. a. hem/o
   b. hemat/o
8. somn/o
9. phon/o
10. capn/o

Exercise 7

1. within
2. without, absence of
3. all, total
4. normal, good
5. many, much
6. fast, rapid

Exercise 8

1. endo-
2. eu-
3. a. a-
   b. an-
4. pan-
5. poly-
6. tachy-

Exercise 9

1. k
2. f
3. g
4. c
5. b
6. j
7. a
8. h
9. d
10. e

Exercise 10

1. c
2. e
3. a
4. h
5. b
6. i
7. f
8. d
9. g
10. j

Exercise 11

1. chest
2. pertaining to
3. constriction, narrowing
4. hernia, protrusion
5. creation of an artificial opening
6. surgical fixation or suspension
7. instrument used to measure
8. sudden, involuntary muscle contraction
9. pain
10. visual examination
11. surgical puncture to aspirate fluid
12. cut into, incision
13. instrument used for visual examination
14. rapid flow of blood
15. stretching out, dilatation, expansion
16. process of recording, radiographic imaging
17. measurement
18. blood condition
19. pertaining to visual examination
20. breathing

Exercise 12

Pronunciation Exercise

Exercise 13

1. WR S
pleur/itis
inflammation of the pleura

2. WR CV WR S
nas/o/pharyng/itis
CF
inflammation of the nose and pharynx

3. WR CV S
pneum/o/thorax
CF
air in the chest

4. P WR S
pan/sinus/itis
inflammation of all sinuses

5. WR S
atel/ectasis
incomplete expansion (or collapsed lung)

6. WR CV WR S
rhin/o/myc/osis
CF
abnormal condition of fungus in the nose

7. WR CV S
trache/o/stenosis
CF
narrowing of the trachea

8. WR S
epiglott/itis
inflammation of the epiglottis

9. WR S
thorac/algia
pain in the chest

10. WR S P S(WR)
pulmon/ary neo/plasm
pertaining to (in) the lung new growth (tumor)

11. WR S
bronchi/ectasis
dilation of the bronchi

12. WR S
tonsill/itis
inflammation of the tonsils

13. WR CV WR S
pneum/o/coni/osis
CF
abnormal condition of dust in the lungs

14. WR CV WR S
bronch/o/pneumon/ia
CF
diseased state of bronchi and lungs

15. WR S
pneumon/itis
inflammation of the lung

16. WR S
laryng/itis
inflammation of the larynx

17. WR CV S
pneumat/o/cele
CF
hernia of the lung

18. WR CV S
py/o/thorax
CF
pus in the chest (pleural space)

19. WR CV S
rhin/o/rrhagia
CF
rapid flow of blood from the nose

20. WR S
bronch/itis
inflammation of the bronchi

21. WR S
pharyng/itis
inflammation of the pharynx

22. WR S
trache/itis
inflammation of the trachea

23. WR CV WR CV WR S
laryng/o/trache/o/bronch/itis
CF CF
inflammation of the larynx, trachea, and bronchi

24. WR S
adenoid/itis
inflammation of the adenoids

25. WR CV S
hem/o/thorax
CF
blood in the chest (pleural space)

26. WR S WR S
lob/ar pneumon/ia
pertaining to the lobe, diseased state of a lung

27. WR S
rhin/itis
inflammation of the nose

28. WR CV S WR S
bronch/o/genic carcin/oma
CF
cancerous tumor originating in a bronchus

29. WR S
alveol/itis
inflammation of the alveolus

30. WR S
pneumon/ia
diseased state of the lung

Exercise 14

1. thorac/algia
2. rhin/o/myc/osis
3. pneumat/o/cele
4. pulmon/ary neo/plasm
5. laryng/itis
6. atel/ectasis
7. adenoid/itis
8. laryng/o/trache/o/bronch/itis
9. bronchi/ectasis
10. pleur/itis
11. pneum/o/coni/osis
12. pneumon/itis
13. pan/sinus/itis
14. trache/o/stenosis
15. nas/o/pharyng/itis
16. py/o/thorax
17. epiglott/itis
18. diaphragmat/o/cele
19. pneum/o/thorax
20. bronch/o/pneumon/ia
21. rhin/o/rrhagia
22. pharyng/itis
23. hem/o/thorax
24. trache/itis
25. bronch/itis
26. lob/ar pneumon/ia
27. rhin/itis
28. bronch/o/genic carcin/oma
29. alveol/itis
30. pneumon/ia

Exercise 15

Spelling Exercise; see text pp. 160-162.

Exercise 16

Pronunciation Exercise

Exercise 17

1. emphysema
2. pleural effusion
3. cor pulmonale
4. coccidioidomycosis
5. cystic fibrosis
6. influenza
7. chronic obstructive pulmonary disease
8. pertussis
9. croup
10. asthma
11. pulmonary edema
12. upper respiratory infection
13. pulmonary embolism
14. epistaxis
15. Legionnaire disease
16. deviated septum
17. obstructive sleep apnea
18. tuberculosis
19. acute respiratory distress syndrome

Exercise 18

1. j
2. d
3. h
4. f
5. g
6. c
7. a
8. e
9. b
10. i

Exercise 19

1. d
2. b
3. c
4. e
5. f
6. g
7. h
8. i
9. a

Exercise 20

Spelling Exercise; see text pp. 167-169.

Exercise 21

Pronunciation Exercise

Exercise 22

1. WR CV S
   trache/o/tomy
   CF
   incision of the trachea
2. WR CV S
   laryng/o/stomy
   CF
   creation of an artificial opening into the larynx
3. WR S
   adenoid/ectomy
   excision of the adenoids
4. WR CV S
   rhin/o/plasty
   CF
   surgical repair of the nose
5. WR CV S
   aden/o/tome
   CF
   surgical instrument used to cut the adenoids
6. WR CV S
   trache/o/stomy
   CF
   creation of an artificial opening into the trachea
7. WR CV S
   sinus/o/tomy
   CF
   incision of a sinus
8. WR CV S
   laryng/o/plasty
   CF
   surgical repair of the larynx
9. WR CV WR CV S
   pneum/o/bronch/o/tomy
   CF CF
   incision of lung and bronchus
10. WR CV S
    bronch/o/plasty
    CF
    surgical repair of a bronchus
11. WR S
    lob/ectomy
    excision of a lobe (of the lung)
12. WR CV WR CV S
    laryng/o/trache/o/tomy
    CF CF
    incision of larynx and trachea
13. WR CV S
    trache/o/plasty
    CF
    surgical repair of the trachea
14. WR CV S
    thorac/o/tomy
    CF
    incision into the chest cavity
15. WR S
    laryng/ectomy
    excision of the larynx
16. WR CV S
    thorac/o/centesis
    CF
    surgical puncture to aspirate fluid from the chest cavity
17. WR S
    tonsill/ectomy
    excision of the tonsils
18. WR CV S
    pleur/o/pexy
    CF
    surgical fixation of the pleura
19. WR CV S
    sept/o/plasty
    CF
    surgical repair of the septum
20. WR CV S
    sept/o/tomy
    CF
    incision into the septum

Exercise 23

1. trache/o/plasty
2. laryng/o/trache/o/tomy
3. aden/o/tome
4. thorac/o/tomy
5. trache/o/stomy
6. tonsill/ectomy
7. trache/o/tomy
8. bronch/o/plasty
9. laryng/ectomy
10. rhin/o/plasty
11. sinus/o/tomy
12. thorac/o/centesis
13. adenoid/ectomy
14. laryng/o/plasty
15. lob/ectomy
16. pneum/o/bronch/o/tomy
17. laryng/o/stomy
18. pneumon/ectomy
19. sept/o/tomy
20. sept/o/plasty

Exercise 24

Spelling Exercise; see text pp. 173-175.

Exercise 25

Pronunciation Exercise

Exercise 26

1. WR CV S
   spir/o/meter
   CF
   instrument used to measure breathing
2. WR CV S
   laryng/o/scope
   CF
   instrument used for visual examination of the larynx
3. WR CV S
   capn/o/meter
   CF
   instrument used to measure carbon dioxide

4. WR CV S
spir/o/metry
CF
measurement of breathing
5. WR CV S
ox/i/meter
CF
instrument used to measure oxygen
6. WR CV S
laryng/o/scopy
CF
visual examination of the larynx
7. WR CV S
bronch/o/scope
CF
instrument used for visual examination of the bronchi
8. WR CV S
thorac/o/scope
CF
instrument used for visual examination of the thorax
9. P S(WR)
endo/scope
instrument used for visual examination within (a hollow organ or body cavity)
10. WR CV S
thorac/o/scopy
CF
visual examination of the thorax
11. P S(WR)
endo/scopic
pertaining to visual examination within (a hollow organ or body cavity)
12. P S(WR)
endo/scopy
visual examination within (a hollow organ or body cavity)
13. P WR CV S
poly/somn/o/graphy
CF
process of recording many (tests) during sleep

Exercise 27

1. laryng/o/scopy
2. spir/o/meter
3. capn/o/meter
4. laryng/o/scope
5. bronch/o/scopy
6. spir/o/metry
7. bronch/o/scope
8. endo/scopy
9. thorac/o/scope
10. endo/scope
11. thorac/o/scopy
12. endo/scopic
13. poly/somn/o/graphy

Exercise 28

Spelling Exercise; see text pp. 179-181.

Exercise 29

Pronunciation Exercise

Exercise 30

1. ventilation-perfusion scanning
2. chest computed tomography
3. chest radiograph
4. arterial blood gases
5. pulse oximetry
6. acid-fast bacilli smear
7. pulmonary function tests
8. PPD skin test
9. peak flow meter
10. stethoscope
11. percussion
12. auscultation

Exercise 31

1. f
2. e
3. a
4. d
5. b
6. c
7. h
8. g
9. l
10. j
11. k
12. m

Exercise 32

Spelling Exercise; see text pp. 187-188.

Exercise 33

Pronunciation Exercise

Exercise 34

1. WR S
laryng/eal
pertaining to the larynx
2. P S(WR)
eu/pnea
normal breathing
3. WR S
muc/oid
resembling mucus
4. P S(WR)
a/pnea
absence of breathing
5. P WR S
hyp/ox/ia
condition of deficient oxygen (to tissues)
6. WR CV S
laryng/o/spasm
CF
spasmodic contraction of the larynx
7. P WR S
endo/trache/al
pertaining to within the trachea
8. P WR S
an/ox/ia
condition of absence of oxygen
9. P WR S
dys/phon/ia
condition of difficulty in speaking (voice)
10. WR CV WR S
bronch/o/alveol/ar
CF
pertaining to the bronchi and alveoli
11. P S(WR)
dys/pnea
difficult breathing
12. P WR S
hypo/capn/ia
condition of deficient in carbon dioxide (in the blood)
13. WR CV S
bronch/o/spasm
CF
spasmodic contraction in the bronchus
14. WR CV S
orth/o/pnea
CF
able to breathe easier in a straight (upright) position
15. P S(WR)
hyper/pnea
excessive breathing
16. P WR S
a/capn/ia
condition of absence of carbon dioxide (in the blood)
17. P S(WR)
hypo/pnea
deficient breathing
18. P WR S
hyp/ox/emia
condition of deficient oxygen in the blood
19. P WR S
a/phon/ia
condition of absence of voice
20. WR CV S
rhin/o/rrhea
CF
discharge from the nose
21. WR S
thorac/ic
pertaining to the chest
22. WR S
muc/ous
pertaining to mucus
23. WR CV WR S
nas/o/pharyng/eal
CF
pertaining to the nose and pharynx
24. WR S
diaphragmat/ic
pertaining to the diaphragm

25. P WR S
intra/pleur/al
pertaining to within the pleura
26. WR S
pulmon/ary
pertaining to the lungs
27. WR S
phren/algia
pain in the diaphragm
28. P S(WR)
tachy/pnea
rapid breathing
29. WR CV S
phren/o/spasm
spasm of the diaphragm
30. WR CV S
pulmon/o/logist
CF
a physician who studies and treats diseases of the lung
31. WR CV S
pulmon/o/logy
CF
study of the lung
32. WR S
alveol/ar
pertaining to the alveolus

Exercise 35
1. hyp/ox/ia
2. muc/oid
3. orth/o/pnea
4. endo/trache/al
5. an/ox/ia
6. dys/pnea
7. laryng/eal
8. hyper/capn/ia
9. eu/pnea
10. a/phon/ia
11. laryng/o/spasm
12. hypo/capn/ia
13. nas/o/pharyng/eal
14. diaphragmat/ic
15. a/pnea
16. hyp/ox/emia
17. hyper/pnea
18. bronch/o/spasm
19. hypo/pnea
20. a/capn/ia
21. dys/phon/ia
22. rhin/o/rrhea
23. muc/ous
24. thorac/ic
25. intra/pleur/al
26. pulmon/ary
27. phren/o/spasm
28. tachy/pnea
29. phren/algia
30. alveol/ar
31. pulmon/o/logy
32. pulmon/o/logist

Exercise 36
Spelling Exercise; see text pp. 191-192.

Exercise 37
Pronunciation Exercise

Exercise 38
1. hyperventilation
2. nebulizer
3. bronchodilator
4. ventilator
5. asphyxia
6. sputum
7. aspirate
8. airway
9. hiccup (hiccough)
10. cough
11. mucopurulent
12. hypoventilation
13. nosocomial
14. paroxysm
15. patent
16. bronchoconstrictor
17. mucus

Exercise 39
1. b
2. h
3. c
4. i
5. a
6. d
7. g
8. f

Exercise 40
1. e
2. h
3. i
4. c
5. j
6. a
7. b
8. d
9. f

Exercise 41
Spelling Exercise; see text pp. 196-197.

Exercise 42
1. chronic obstructive pulmonary disease; pulmonary function tests, chest radiograph, arterial blood gases, computed tomography, shortness of breath, chronic obstructive pulmonary disease
2. ventilation-perfusion scanning; pulmonary embolism
3. left upper lobe; left lower lobe; right upper lobe, right middle lobe, right lower lobe
4. acid-fast bacilli; tuberculosis
5. polysomnography; obstructive sleep apnea
6. oxygen; carbon dioxide
7. peak flow meter

Exercise 43
1. acute respiratory distress syndrome
2. cystic fibrosis
3. influenza
4. laryngotracheobronchitis
5. upper respiratory infection

Exercise 44
A. 1. cough
2. dyspnea
3. pulmonary
4. chest radiograph
5. bronchoscopy
6. arterial blood gases
7. hypoxemia
8. bronchogenic carcinoma
9. pulmonary function tests
10. thoracic

B. 1. chest radiograph, arterial blood gases, pulse oximetry
2. excessive, deficient
3. a. T
b. T
c. T

Exercise 45
1. epistaxis
2. laryngoplasty
3. orthopnea
4. arterial blood gases, hypoxia
5. thoracalgia
6. hyperventilation
7. nebulizer
8. hemothorax
9. pulmonary embolism
10. coccidioidomycosis
11. chest radiograph, nosocomial
12. PPD skin test
13. tachypnea
14. stethoscope

Exercise 46
Reading Exercise

Exercise 47
1. *T*
2. *F*, "hypoxemia" means deficient oxygen in the blood; "hypercapnia" means excessive carbon dioxide in the blood.
3. *T*
4. *F*, "bronchitis" means inflammation of the bronchi

Chapter 6

Urinary System

OUTLINE

OBJECTIVES

Upon completion of this chapter you will be able to:

1. Identify organs and structures of the urinary system.
2. Define and spell word parts related to the urinary system.
3. Define, pronounce, and spell disease and disorder terms related to the urinary system.
4. Define, pronounce, and spell surgical terms related to the urinary system.
5. Define, pronounce, and spell diagnostic terms related to the urinary system.
6. Define, pronounce, and spell complementary terms related to the urinary system.
7. Interpret the meaning of abbreviations related to the urinary system.
8. Interpret, read, and comprehend medical language in simulated medical statements and documents.

ANATOMY

Organs of the urinary system are the kidneys, ureters, bladder, and urethra (Figures 6-1, 6-2, and 6-3).

Function

The urinary system removes waste material from the body, regulates fluid volume, and maintains electrolyte concentration in the body fluid. The kidneys secrete urine formed from water and waste materials such as urea, potassium chloride, sodium chloride, phosphates, and other elements. Urine is collected in the renal pelvis of the kidney and is transported through the ureters into the bladder, where it is stored until it can be eliminated. Urine passes from the bladder through the urethra and urinary meatus to the outside of the body (Figure 6-4).

Organs of the Urinary System

Term	Definition
kidneys	two bean-shaped organs located on each side of the vertebral column on the posterior wall of the abdominal cavity behind the parietal peritoneum. Their function is to remove waste products from the blood and to aid in maintaining water and electrolyte balances.
nephron	urine-producing microscopic structure. Approximately 1 million nephrons are located in each kidney.
glomerulus (*pl.* glomeruli)	cluster of capillaries at the entrance of the nephron. The process of filtering the blood, thereby forming urine, begins here.
renal pelvis	funnel-shaped reservoir that collects the urine and passes it to the ureter
hilum	indentation on the medial side of the kidney where the ureter leaves the kidney
ureters	two slender tubes, approximately 10 to 13 inches (26 to 33 cm) long, that receive the urine from the kidneys and carry it to the posterior portion of the bladder
urinary bladder	muscular, hollow organ that temporarily holds the urine. As it fills, the thick, muscular wall becomes thinner, and the organ increases in size.
urethra	lowest part of the urinary tract, through which the urine passes from the urinary bladder to the outside of the body. This narrow tube varies in length by sex. It is approximately 1.5 inches (3.8 cm) long in the female and approximately 8 inches (20 cm) in the male, in whom it is also part of the reproductive system. It carries seminal fluid (semen) at the time of ejaculation.
urinary meatus	opening through which the urine passes to the outside

BLADDER

is a derivative of the Anglo-Saxon **blaeddre,** meaning a **blister** or **windbag.**

A & P Booster

For students desiring more anatomy and physiology, go to http://evolve.elsevier.com. Refer to p. 18 for your Evolve Access Information. Select A & P Booster, Chapter 6.

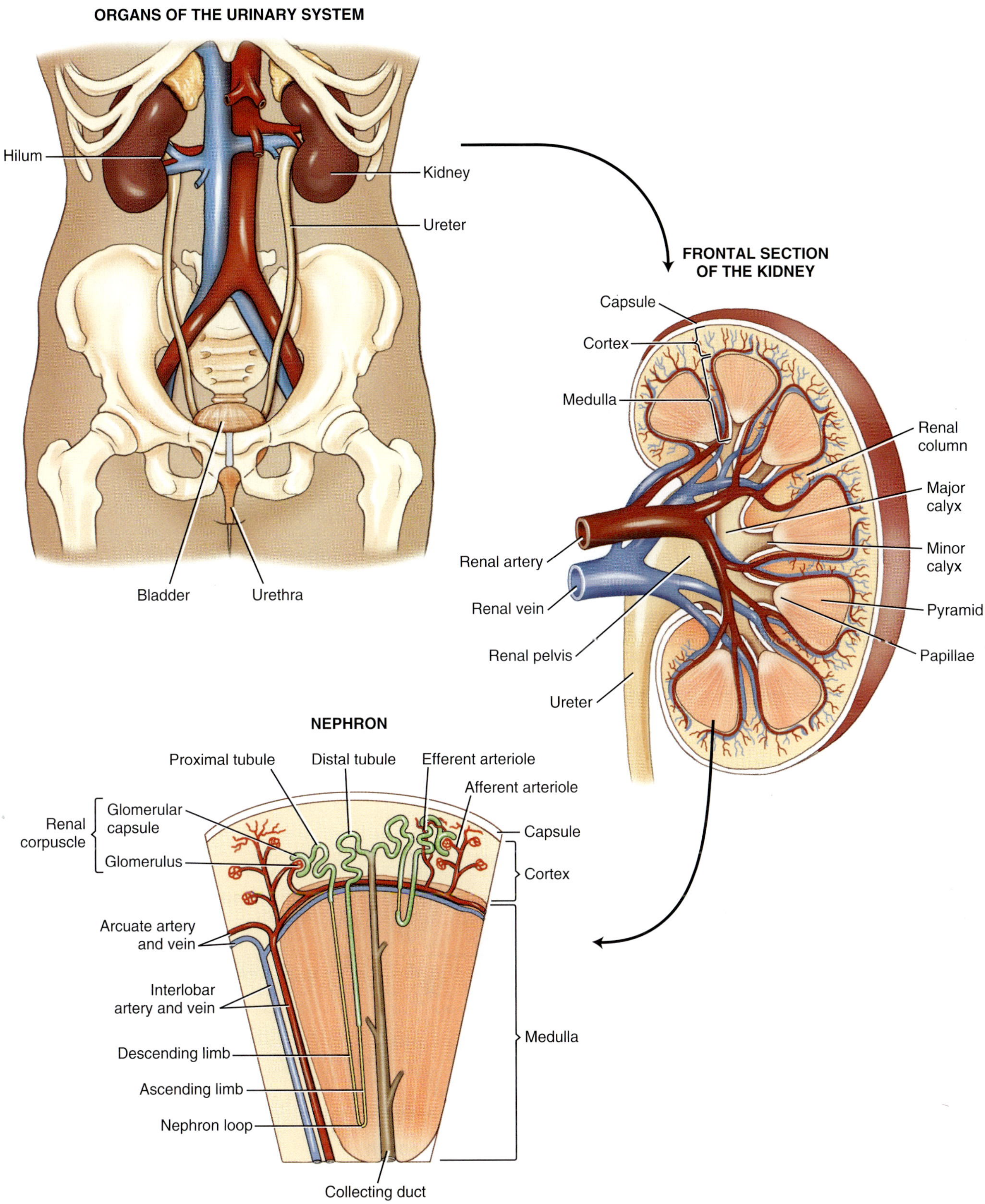

FIGURE 6-1
The urinary system.

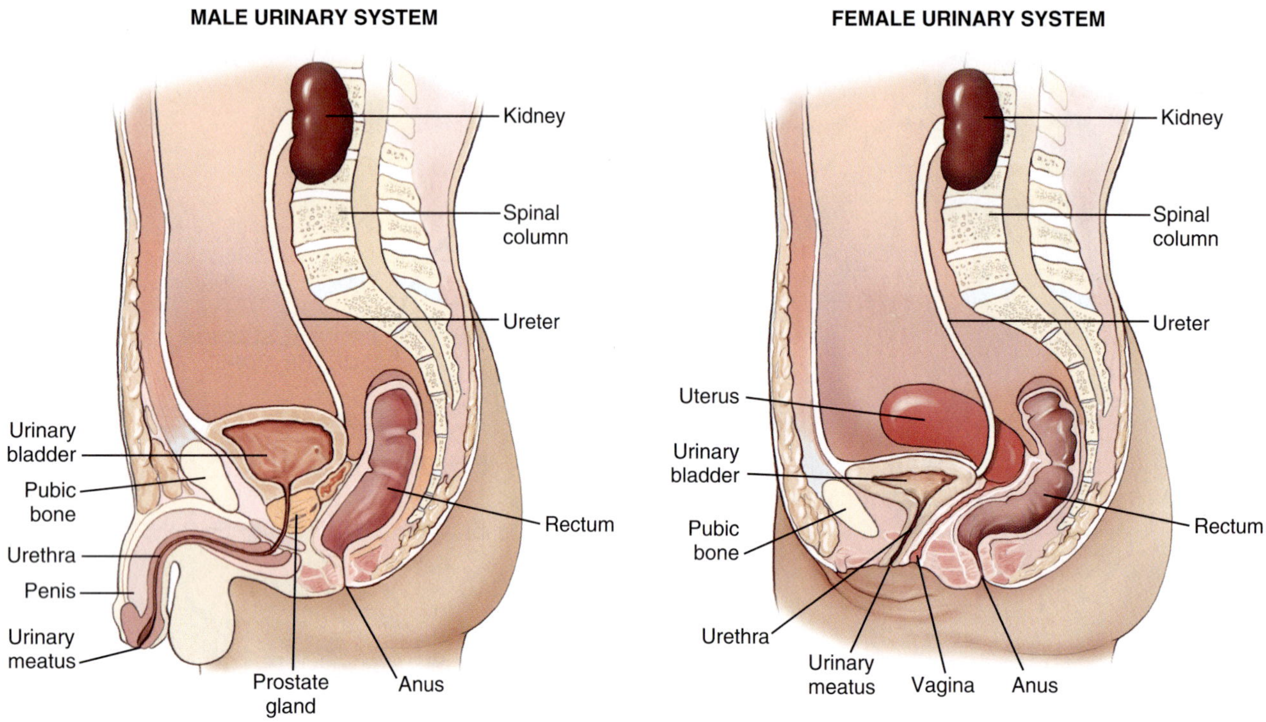

FIGURE 6-2
Male and female urinary systems, sagittal view. The male urethra is approximately 8 inches (20 cm) in length compared with the female urethra, which is approximately 1.5 inches (3.8 cm) in length.

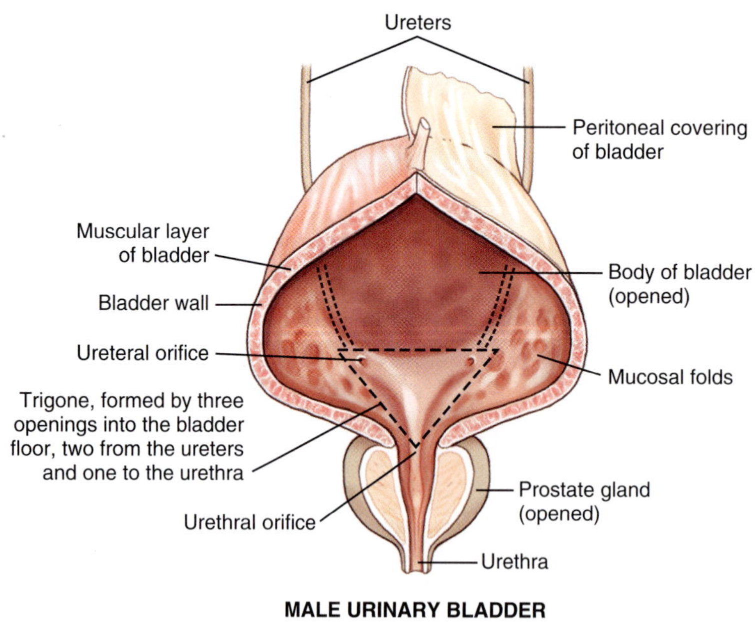

FIGURE 6-3
Male urinary bladder.

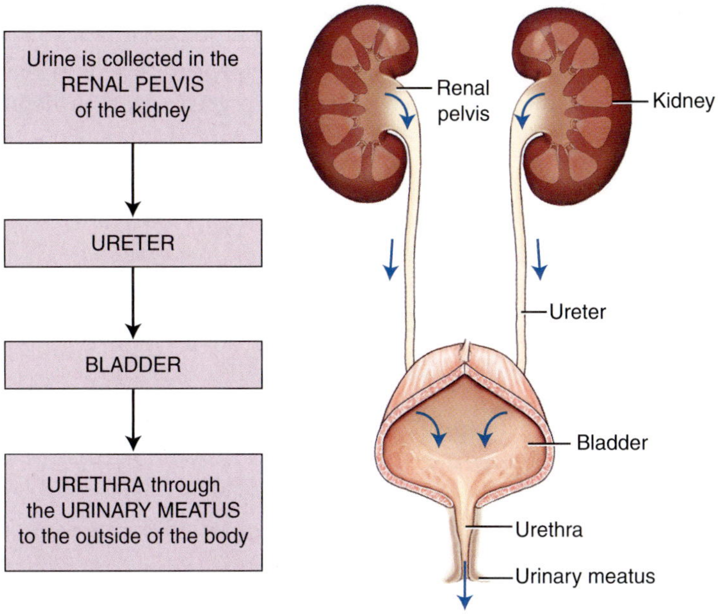

FIGURE 6-4
Flow of urine.

EXERCISE 1

Match the anatomic terms in the first column with the correct definitions in the second column. *To check your answers to the exercises in this chapter, go to Answers, p. 263, at the end of the chapter.*

_____ 1. kidney(s)
_____ 2. glomerulus
_____ 3. nephron
_____ 4. ureters
_____ 5. urinary bladder
_____ 6. urinary meatus
_____ 7. urethra

a. stores urine
b. outside opening through which the urine passes
c. carry urine from the kidneys to the urinary bladder
d. cluster of capillaries in the kidney where the urine begins to form
e. carries urine from the bladder to the urinary meatus
f. kidney's urine-producing unit
g. organs that remove waste products from the blood

GLOMERULUS

is derived from the Latin **glomus,** which means **ball of thread.** It was thought that the rounded cluster of capillary loops at the nephron's entrance resembled thread in a ball.

MEATUS

is derived from the Latin **meare,** meaning **to pass** or **to go.** Other anatomic passages share the same name, such as the auditory meatus.

PYELOS

is the Greek word for **tub-shaped vessel,** which describes the kidney's shape.

WORD PARTS

Word parts you need to know to complete this chapter are listed on the following pages. The exercises at the end of each list will help you learn their definitions and spellings.

Use the flashcards accompanying this text or electronic flashcards to assist you in memorizing the word parts for this chapter.

To use electronic flashcards, go to http://evolve.elsevier.com. Refer to p. 18 for your Evolve Access Information. Select Flashcards, Chapter 6.

Combining Forms of the Urinary System

Combining Form	Definition
cyst/o, vesic/o (NOTE: these refer to the *urinary bladder* unless otherwise identified.)	bladder, sac
glomerul/o	glomerulus
meat/o	meatus (opening)
nephr/o, ren/o	kidney
pyel/o	renal pelvis
ureter/o	ureter
urethr/o	urethra

EXERCISE FIGURE A

Fill in the blanks with combining forms for this diagram of the urinary system. *To check your answers, go to p. 263.*

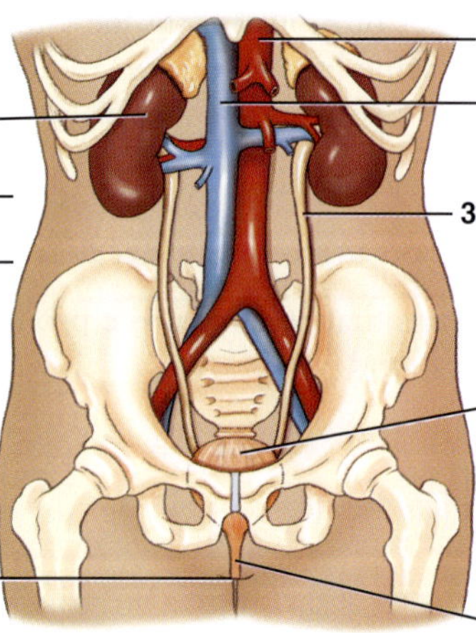

EXERCISE FIGURE B

Fill in the blanks with combining forms to label this diagram of the internal kidney structure.

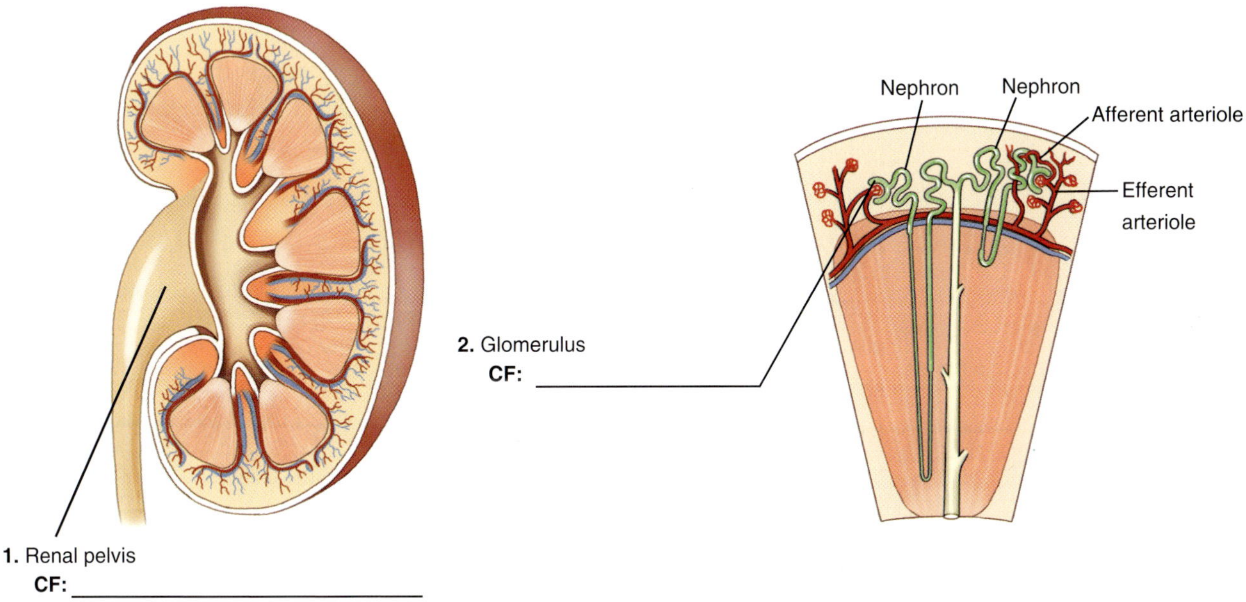

EXERCISE 2

Write the definitions of the following combining forms.

1. glomerul/o ____________
2. vesic/o ____________
3. nephr/o ____________
4. pyel/o ____________
5. ureter/o ____________
6. cyst/o ____________
7. urethr/o ____________
8. ren/o ____________
9. meat/o ____________

EXERCISE 3

Write the combining form for each of the following terms.

1. kidney a. ____________ b. ____________
2. bladder, sac a. ____________ b. ____________
3. ureter ____________
4. renal pelvis ____________
5. glomerulus ____________
6. urethra ____________
7. meatus ____________

Combining Forms Commonly Used with Urinary System Terms

Combining Form	Definition
albumin/o	albumin
azot/o	urea, nitrogen
blast/o	developing cell, germ cell
glyc/o, glycos/o	sugar
hydr/o	water
lith/o	stone, calculus
noct/i (NOTE: the combining vowel is i.)	night
olig/o	scanty, few
son/o	sound
tom/o	cut, section
urin/o, ur/o	urine, urinary tract

EXERCISE 4

Write the definitions of the following combining forms.

1. hydr/o ____________
2. azot/o ____________
3. noct/i ____________
4. lith/o ____________
5. tom/o ____________
6. albumin/o ____________
7. urin/o ____________
8. son/o ____________
9. glyc/o ____________
10. blast/o ____________
11. olig/o ____________
12. ur/o ____________
13. glycos/o ____________

EXERCISE 5

Write the combining form for each of the following.

1. sugar a. ____________ b. ____________
2. sound ____________
3. urine, urinary tract a. ____________ b. ____________
4. water ____________
5. developing cell, germ cell ____________
6. cut, section ____________
7. albumin ____________
8. night ____________
9. urea, nitrogen ____________
10. stone, calculus ____________
11. scanty, few ____________

Suffixes

Suffix	Definition
-gram	record, radiographic image
-iasis, -esis	condition
-lysis	loosening, dissolution, separating
-megaly	enlargement
-ptosis	drooping, sagging, prolapse
-rrhaphy	suturing, repairing
-tripsy	surgical crushing
-trophy	nourishment, development
-uria	urine, urination

Refer to **Appendix A** and **Appendix B** for alphabetized lists of word parts and their meanings.

EXERCISE 6

Match the suffixes in the first column with their correct definitions in the second column.

______ 1.	-iasis, -esis	a. nourishment, development
______ 2.	-lysis	b. urine, urination
______ 3.	-megaly	c. condition
______ 4.	-rrhaphy	d. enlargement
______ 5.	-ptosis	e. surgical crushing
______ 6.	-tripsy	f. suturing, repairing
______ 7.	-trophy	g. drooping, sagging, prolapse
______ 8.	-uria	h. record, radiographic image
______ 9.	-gram	i. loosening, dissolution, separating

EXERCISE 7

Write the definitions of the following suffixes.

1. -rrhaphy ____________________
2. -lysis ____________________
3. -iasis, -esis ____________________
4. -trophy ____________________
5. -uria ____________________
6. -megaly ____________________
7. -ptosis ____________________
8. -tripsy ____________________
9. -gram ____________________

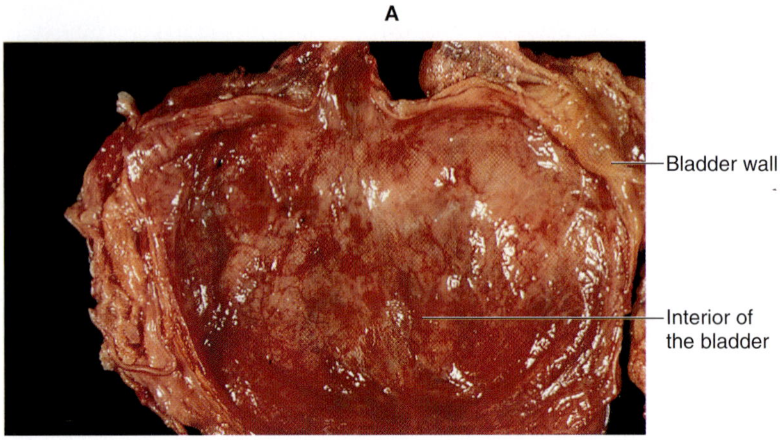

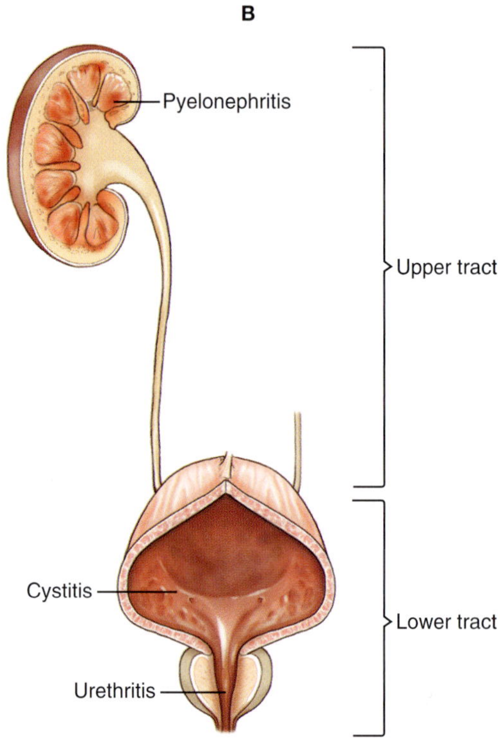

FIGURE 6-5
Urinary tract infection. **A,** Acute cystitis. The swollen and red mucosa demonstrates inflammation. Cystitis is more common in women because the urethra is short, allowing easy access of bacteria to the urinary bladder. **B,** Upper and lower urinary tract infections. If cystitis is not treated promptly, the infection can spread to the kidneys, causing pyelonephritis.

UREMIA, ALSO CALLED AZOTEMIA

translated literally is **urine in the blood;** however, the term means **urea** and other waste products **in the blood.**

The term was first used by Pierre Piorry, a French physician (1794-1879). He also created the medical terms *toxin*, *toxemia*, and *septicemia*.

EXERCISE FIGURE C

Fill in the blanks to label the diagram.

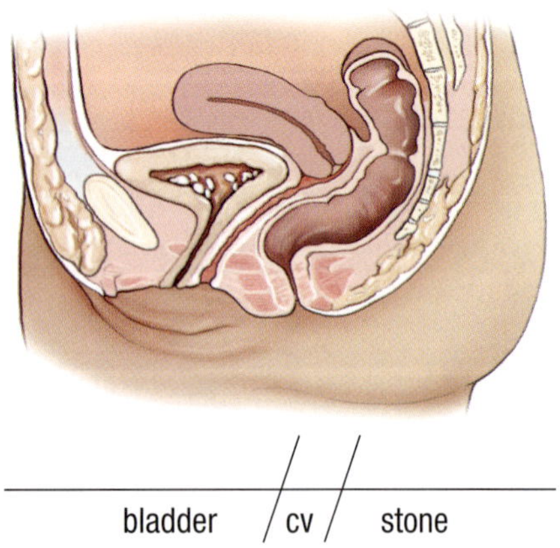

MEDICAL TERMS

The terms you need to learn to complete this chapter are listed next. The exercises following each list will help you learn the definition and the spelling of each word.

Disease and Disorder Terms

Built from Word Parts

The following terms are built from word parts you have already learned and can be translated literally to find their meanings. Further explanation of terms beyond the definition of their word parts, if needed, is included in parentheses.

Term	Definition
azotemia (*az*-ō-TĒ-mē-a)	condition of urea in the blood (a toxic condition resulting from disease of the kidney in which waste products are in the blood that are normally excreted by the kidney); (also called **uremia.**)
cystitis (sis-TĪ-tis)	inflammation of the bladder (Figure 6-5)
cystocele (SIS-tō-sēl)	protrusion of the bladder
cystolith (SIS-tō-lith)	stone in the bladder (Exercise Figure C)
glomerulonephritis (glō-*mer*-ū-lō-ne-FRĪ-tis)	inflammation of the glomeruli of the kidney

Term	Definition
hydronephrosis (*hī*-drō-ne-FRŌ-sis)	abnormal condition of water in the kidney (distention of the renal pelvis with urine because of an obstruction)
nephritis (ne-FRĪ-tis)	inflammation of a kidney
nephroblastoma (*nef*-rō-blas-TŌ-ma)	kidney tumor containing developing cells (malignant tumor) (also called **Wilms' tumor**)
nephrohypertrophy (*nef*-rō-hī-PER-tro-fē) (NOTE: the prefix *hyper-* appears in the middle of this term.)	excessive development (increase in size) of the kidney
nephrolithiasis (*nef*-rō-lith-Ī-a-sis)	condition of stone(s) in the kidney
nephroma (nef-RŌ-ma)	tumor of the kidney
nephromegaly (*nef*-rō-MEG-a-lē)	enlargement of a kidney
nephroptosis (*nef*-rop-TŌ-sis)	drooping kidney
pyelitis (*pī*-e-LĪ-tis)	inflammation of the renal pelvis
pyelonephritis (*pī*-e-lō-ne-FRĪ-tis)	inflammation of the renal pelvis and the kidney (Figures 6-5, *B*, and 6-6)
ureteritis (ū-*rē*-ter-Ī-tis)	inflammation of a ureter
ureterocele (ū-RĒ-ter-ō-*sēl*)	protrusion of a ureter (distally into the bladder)
ureterolithiasis (ū-*rē*-ter-ō-lith-Ī-a-sis)	condition of stones in the ureters
ureterostenosis (ū-*rē*-ter-ō-sten-Ō-sis)	narrowing of the ureter
urethrocystitis (ū-*rē*-thrō-sis-TĪ-tis)	inflammation of the urethra and the bladder

NEPHROPTOSIS

is also known as a **floating kidney** and occurs when the kidney is no longer held in place and drops out of its normal position. The kidney is normally held in position by connective and adipose tissue, so it is prone to injury and also may cause the ureter to twist. Truck drivers and horseback riders are prone to this condition.

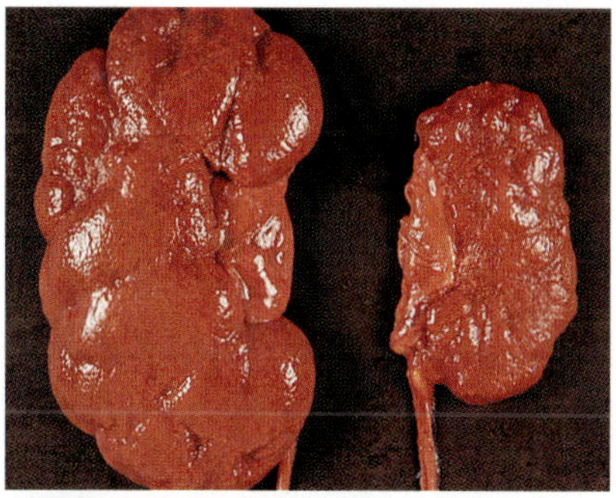

FIGURE 6-6
Kidney on left of illustration, chronic pyelonephritis. *Kidney on right of illustration,* normal size with some scarring.

EXERCISE 8

Practice saying aloud each of the disease and disorder terms built from word parts on pp. 226-227.

To hear the terms, go to http://evolve.elsevier.com. Refer to p. 18 for your Evolve Access Information. Select Chapter 6, Chapter Exercises, Pronunciation.

☐ Place a check mark in the box when you have completed this exercise.

EXERCISE 9

Analyze and define the following terms.

Example: glomerul (WR) / o (CV) / nephr (WR) / itis (S) — glomerul/o = CF — inflammation of the glomeruli of the kidney

1. nephroma ________________
2. cystolith ________________
3. nephrolithiasis ________________
4. azotemia ________________
5. nephroptosis ________________
6. cystocele ________________
7. nephrohypertrophy ________________
8. cystitis ________________
9. pyelitis ________________
10. ureterocele ________________
11. hydronephrosis ________________
12. nephromegaly ________________
13. ureterolithiasis ________________
14. pyelonephritis ________________
15. ureteritis ________________
16. nephritis ________________
17. urethrocystitis ________________
18. ureterostenosis ________________
19. nephroblastoma ________________

EXERCISE 10

Build disease and disorder terms for the following definitions with the word parts you have learned.

Example: inflammation of the ureter ureter / itis
WR / S

1. enlargement of the kidney ______ / ______ / ______
WR / CV / S

2. inflammation of the bladder ______ / ______
WR / S

3. excessive development of the kidney ______ / ______ / ______ / ______
WR / CV / P / S

4. inflammation of the urethra and bladder ______ / ______ / ______ / ______
WR / CV / WR / S

5. protrusion of the bladder ______ / ______ / ______
WR / CV / S

6. abnormal condition of water in the kidney ______ / ______ / ______ / ______
WR / CV / WR / S

7. stone in the bladder ______ / ______ / ______
WR / CV / WR

8. inflammation of the glomeruli of the kidney ______ / ______ / ______ / ______
WR / CV / WR / S

9. tumor of the kidney ______ / ______
WR / S

10. a drooping kidney ______ / ______ / ______
WR / CV / S

11. inflammation of a kidney ______ / ______
WR / S

12. condition of stones in the kidney ______ / ______ / ______ / ______
WR / CV / WR / S

13. protrusion of a ureter ______ / ______ / ______
WR / CV / S

14. inflammation of the renal pelvis ______ / ______
WR / S

15. condition of urea in the blood ______ / ______
WR / S

16. narrowing of the ureter ______ / ______ / ______
WR / CV / S

17. inflammation of the renal pelvis and the kidney

_____ / _____ / _____ / _____
WR / CV / WR / S

18. condition of stones in the ureters

_____ / _____ / _____ / _____
WR / CV / WR / S

19. kidney tumor containing developing cells

_____ / _____ / _____ / _____
WR / CV / WR / S

EXERCISE 11

Spell each of the disease and disorder terms built from word parts on pp. 226-227 by having someone dictate them to you.

To hear and spell the terms, go to http://evolve.elsevier.com. Refer to p. 18 for your Evolve Access Information. Select Exercises & Review, Chapter 6, Chapter Exercises, Spelling.

☐ Place a check mark in the box if you have completed this exercise online.

1. ____________ 11. ____________
2. ____________ 12. ____________
3. ____________ 13. ____________
4. ____________ 14. ____________
5. ____________ 15. ____________
6. ____________ 16. ____________
7. ____________ 17. ____________
8. ____________ 18. ____________
9. ____________ 19. ____________
10. ____________ 20. ____________

Disease and Disorder Terms

Not Built from Word Parts

In some of the following terms, you may recognize word parts you have already learned; however, the full meaning of the terms cannot be discerned by the definition of their word parts.

Term	Definition
epispadias (*ep*-i-SPĀ-dē-as)	congenital defect in which the urinary meatus is located on the upper surface of the penis
hypospadias (*hī*-pō-SPĀ-dē-as)	congenital defect in which the urinary meatus is located on the underside of the penis; a similar defect can occur in the female (Figure 6-7)

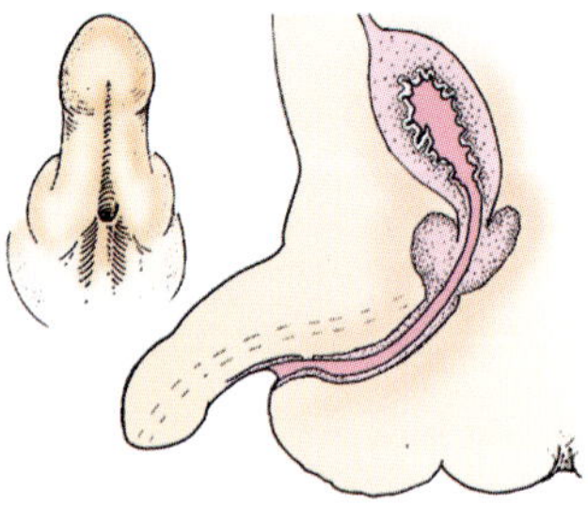

FIGURE 6-7
Hypospadias.

Term	Definition
polycystic kidney disease (*pol*-ē-SIS-tik) (KID-nē) (di-ZĒZ)	condition in which the kidney contains many cysts and is enlarged (Figure 6-8)
renal calculus (pl. calculi) (RĒ-nal) (KAL-kū-lus) (KAL-kū-lī)	stone in the kidney
renal failure (RĒ-nal) (FĀL-ūr)	loss of kidney function resulting in its inability to remove waste products from the body and maintain electrolyte balance
renal hypertension (RĒ-nal) (*hī*-per-TEN-shun)	elevated blood pressure resulting from kidney disease
urinary retention (Ū-rin-*ār*-ē) (rē-TEN-shun)	abnormal accumulation of urine in the bladder because of an inability to urinate
urinary suppression (Ū-rin-*ār*-ē) (sū-PRESH-un)	sudden stoppage of urine formation
urinary tract infection (UTI) (Ū-rin-*ār*-ē) (trakt) (in-FEK-shun)	infection of one or more organs of the urinary tract (see Figure 6-5)

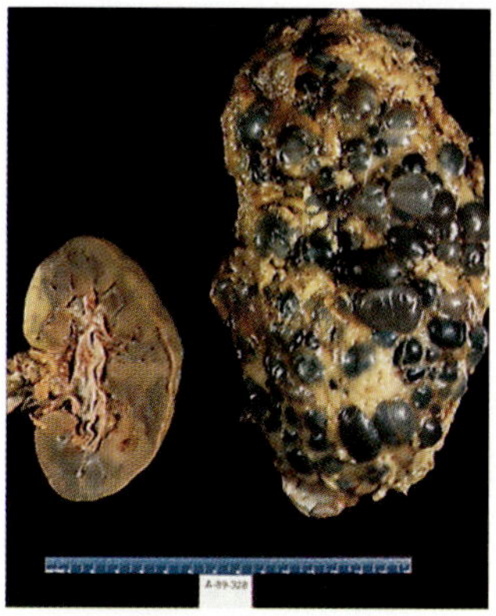

FIGURE 6-8
Polycystic kidney disease.

RENAL FAILURE

Acute renal failure (ARF) is a sudden and severe reduction in renal function resulting in a collection of metabolic waste in the body. ARF may be caused by excessive bleeding, trauma, or severe infection. Prompt treatment can reverse the condition and recovery can occur.

Chronic renal failure (CRF), unlike ARF, is a progresive, irreversible, loss of renal function, and the onset of uremia. Hypertension, diabetes mellitus, and glomerulonephritis may cause CRF. Dialysis and kidney transplant are used in treating this disease.

End-stage renal disease (ESRD) is what chronic renal failure is called when kidney function is too poor to sustain life.

EXERCISE 12

Practice saying aloud each of the disease and disorder terms not built from word parts on pp. 230-231.

To hear the terms, go to http://evolve.elsevier.com. Refer to p. 18 for your Evolve Access Information. Select Exercises & Review, Chapter 6, Chapter Exercises, Pronunciation.

☐ Place a check mark in the box when you have completed this exercise.

EXERCISE 13

Fill in the blanks with the correct terms.

1. Stone in the kidney is also called ________________ ________________.
2. The inability to urinate, which results in an abnormal amount of urine in the bladder, is known as ________________ ________________.
3. The name given to a condition in which a kidney is enlarged and contains many cysts is ________________ ________________ ________________.
4. The condition in which the urinary meatus is located on the underside of the penis is called ________________.
5. Elevated blood pressure resulting from kidney disease is ________________ ________________.

CAM TERM

Biologically based therapies, one of NCCAM's five major classifications of CAM, are therapies that use substances found in nature such as herbs, foods, minerals, and vitamins. Standardized extracts of cranberries have repeatedly been found to be effective in reducing the number of recurrent **urinary tract infections** in women.

6. Sudden stoppage of urine formation is referred to as ________________ ________________.
7. ________________ is a condition in which the urinary meatus is located on the upper surface of the penis.
8. Infection of one or more organs of the urinary system is called ________________ ________________ ________________.
9. Loss of kidney function is called ________________ ________________.

EXERCISE 14

Match the terms in the first column with the correct definitions in the second column.

_____ 1.	epispadias	a.	enlarged kidney with many cysts
_____ 2.	hypospadias	b.	sudden stoppage of urine formation
_____ 3.	renal calculus	c.	urinary meatus on the upper surface of the penis
_____ 4.	renal hypertension	d.	kidney stone
_____ 5.	polycystic kidney disease	e.	inability to urinate
_____ 6.	urinary retention	f.	urinary meatus on the underside of the penis
_____ 7.	urinary suppression	g.	infection of one or more organs of the urinary system
_____ 8.	urinary tract infection	h.	characterized by elevated blood pressure
_____ 9.	renal failure	i.	inability to remove waste products from the body and maintain electrolyte balance
		j.	excessive amount of urine

EXERCISE 15

Spell each of the disease and disorder terms not built from word parts on pp. 226-227 by having someone dictate them to you.

To hear and spell the terms, go to http://evolve.elsevier.com. Refer to p. 18 for your Evolve Access Information. Select Exercises & Review, Chapter 6, Chapter Exercises, Spelling.
☐ Place a check mark in the box if you have completed this exercise online.

1. ________________________
2. ________________________
3. ________________________
4. ________________________
5. ________________________
6. ________________________
7. ________________________
8. ________________________
9. ________________________

Surgical Terms

Built from Word Parts

The following terms are built from word parts you have already learned and can be translated literally to find their meanings. Further explanation of terms beyond the definition of their word parts, if needed, is included in parentheses.

Term	Definition
cystectomy (sis-TEK-to-mē)	excision of the bladder
cystolithotomy (*sis*-tō-li-THOT-o-mē)	incision of the bladder to remove a stone
cystorrhaphy (sist-OR-a-fē)	suturing the bladder
cystostomy (sis-TOS-to-mē)	creating an artificial opening into the bladder (Exercise Figure D)
cystotomy, vesicotomy (sis-TOT-o-mē) (*ves*-i-KOT-o-mē)	incision of the bladder
lithotripsy (LITH-ō-trip-sē)	surgical crushing of a stone (Exercise Figure E)
meatotomy (*mē*-a-TOT-o-mē)	incision of the meatus (to enlarge it)
nephrectomy (ne-FREK-to-mē)	excision of a kidney
nephrolithotomy (*nef*-rō-li-THOT-o-mē)	incision of the kidney to remove a stone (Figure 6-9)
nephrolithotripsy (*nef*-rō-LITH-o-trip-sē)	surgical crushing of a stone in the kidney (Figure 6-9)
nephrolysis (ne-FROL-i-sis)	separating the kidney (from other body structures)
nephropexy (NEF-rō-*peks*-ē)	surgical fixation of the kidney
nephrostomy (nef-ROS-to-mē)	creation of an artificial opening into the kidney (Exercise Figure F)
pyelolithotomy (*pī*-el-ō-lith-OT-o-mē)	incision of the renal pelvis to remove a stone (Exercise Figure G)
pyeloplasty (PĪ-el-ō-*plas*-tē)	surgical repair of the renal pelvis
ureterectomy (ū-*rē*-ter-EK-to-mē)	excision of a ureter
ureterostomy (ū-*rē*-ter-OS-to-mē)	creation of an artificial opening into the ureter
urethroplasty (ū-RĒ-thrō-*plas*-tē)	surgical repair of the urethra
vesicourethral suspension (*ves*-i-kō-ū-RĒ-thral) (*sus*-PEN-shun)	suspension pertaining to the bladder and urethra

EXERCISE FIGURE D

Fill in the blanks to label the diagram.

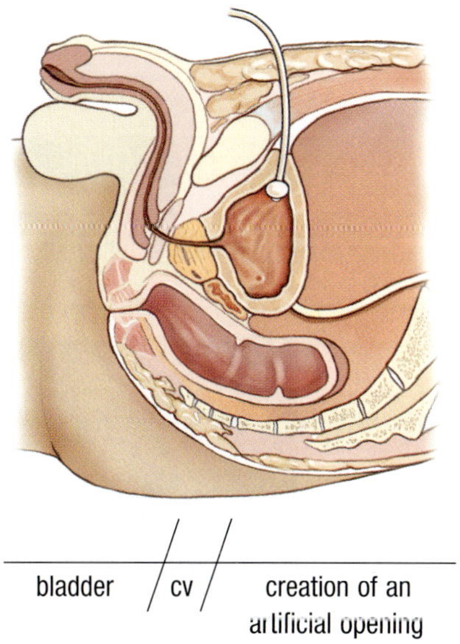

STRESS INCONTINENCE

is the involuntary intermittent leakage of urine as a result of pressure, from a cough or a sneeze, on the weakened area around the urethra and bladder. The Marshall-Marchetti Krantz technique, or **vesicourethral suspension** with a midurethral sling is a suspension surgery performed on patients with stress incontinence.

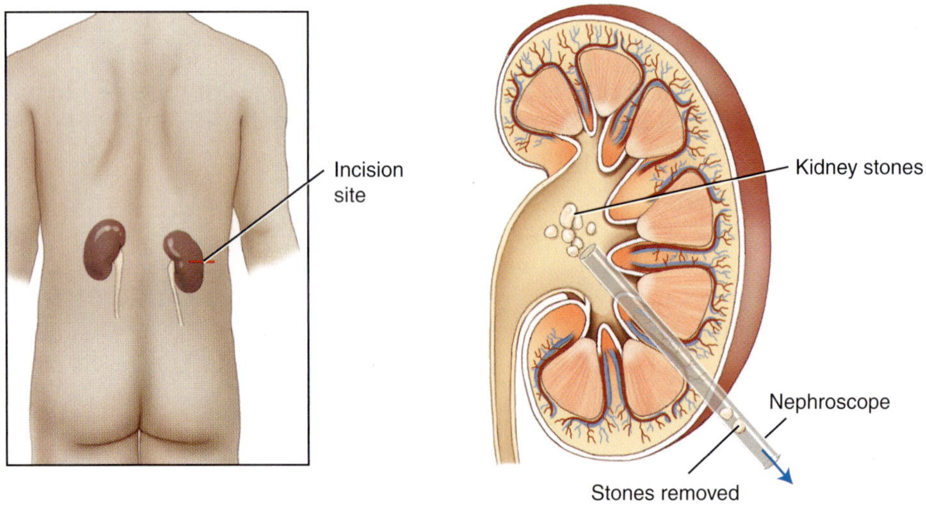

FIGURE 6-9
Percutaneous nephrolithotomy or percutaneous lithotripsy uses a small incision in the back to remove medium or larger-size kidney stones. A nephroscope is passed into the kidney through the incision. In a **nephrolithotomy**, the surgeon removes the stone through the nephroscope. In a **nephrolithotripsy**, the stone is broken into fragments by a lithotripter and then removed through the nephroscope.

EXERCISE FIGURE E

Fill in the blanks to complete the labeling of the diagram.

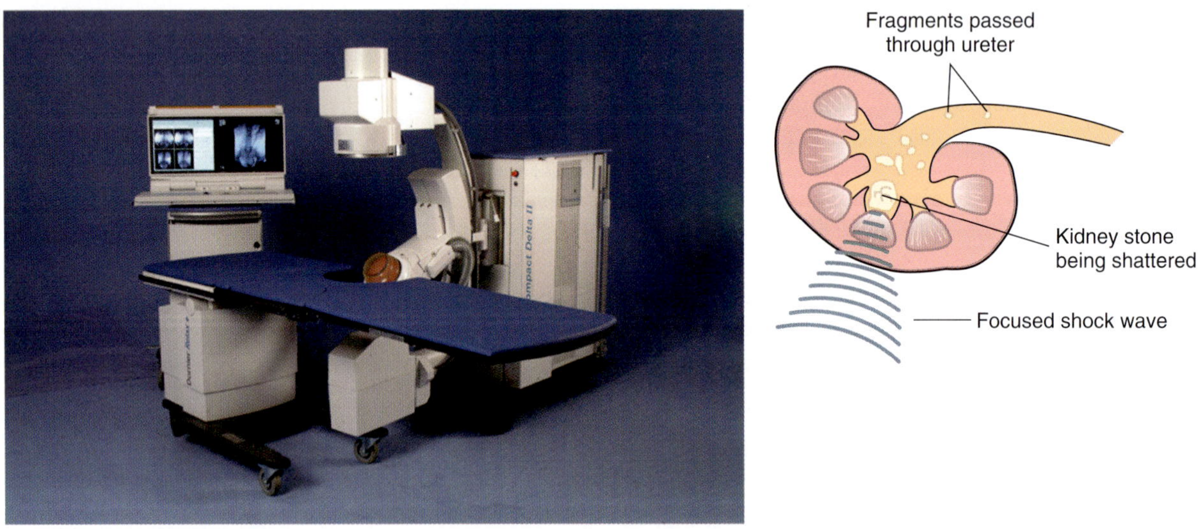

Extracorporeal shock wave ______ / ______ / ______
stone / cv / surgical crushing

ESWL breaks down the kidney stone into fragments by shock waves from outside the body. The broken fragments are eliminated from the body with the passing of urine.

EXERCISE FIGURE F

Fill in the blanks to label the diagram.

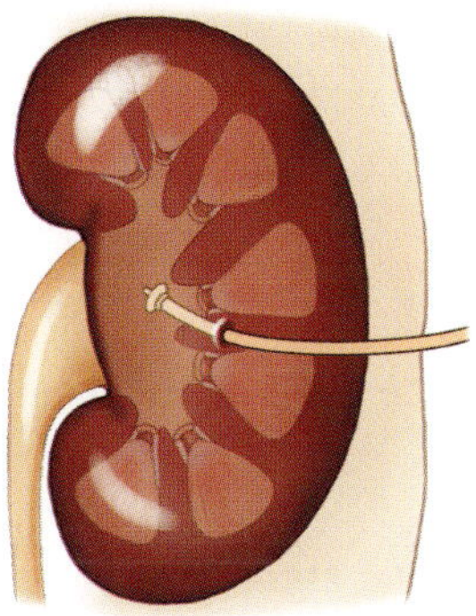

Percutaneous ________ / ________ / ________
kidney / cv / creation of an artificial opening

EXERCISE FIGURE G

Fill in the blanks to label the diagram.

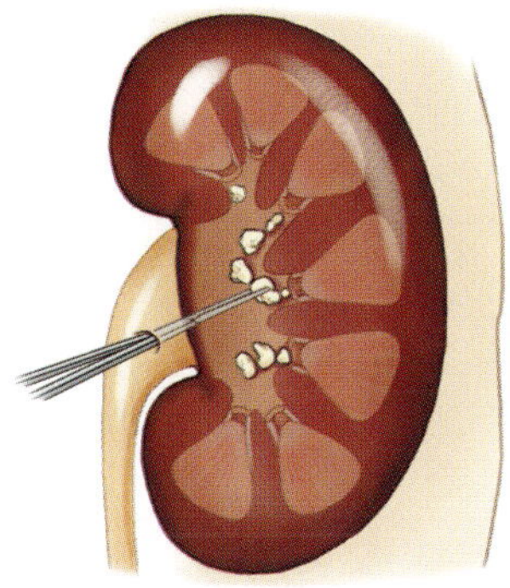

________ / ________ / ________ / ________ / ________
renal pelvis / cv / stone / cv / incision

EXERCISE 16

Practice saying aloud each of the surgical terms built from word parts on p. 223.

To hear the terms, go to http://evolve.elsevier.com. Refer to p. 18 for your Evolve Access Information. Select Exercises & Review, Chapter 6, Chapter Exercises, Pronunciation.

☐ Place a check mark in the box when you have completed this exercise.

EXERCISE 17

Analyze and define the following surgical terms.

1. vesicotomy ________
2. cystotomy ________
3. nephrostomy ________
4. nephrolysis ________
5. cystectomy ________
6. pyelolithotomy ________
7. nephropexy ________
8. cystolithotomy ________
9. nephrectomy ________
10. ureterectomy ________
11. cystostomy ________
12. pyeloplasty ________
13. cystorrhaphy ________

14. meatotomy ____________________
15. lithotripsy ____________________
16. urethroplasty ____________________
17. vesicourethral (suspension) ____________________
18. nephrolithotomy ____________________
19. ureterostomy ____________________
20. nephrolithotripsy ____________________

EXERCISE 18

Build surgical terms for the following definitions by using the word parts you have learned.

1. creation of an artificial opening into the ureter ______ WR / CV / S
2. excision of a kidney ______ WR / S
3. incision of the kidney to remove a stone ______ WR / CV / WR / CV / S
4. suturing of the bladder ______ WR / CV / S
5. separating the kidney (from other structures) ______ WR / CV / S
6. creation of an artificial opening into the kidney ______ WR / CV / S
7. surgical repair of the urethra ______ WR / CV / S
8. excision of the bladder ______ WR / S
9. incision of the meatus ______ WR / CV / S
10. incision of the bladder a. ______ WR / CV / S
    b. ______ WR / CV / S
11. surgical repair of the renal pelvis ______ WR / CV / S

12. excision of the ureter ______ / ______
WR / S

13. surgical fixation of the kidney ______ /CV/ ______
WR /CV/ S

14. incision into the bladder to remove a stone ______ /CV/ ______ /CV/ ______
WR /CV/ WR /CV/ S

15. surgical crushing of a stone ______ /CV/ ______
WR /CV/ S

16. pertaining to the bladder and urethra ______ /CV/ ______ / ______
WR (suspension) /CV/ WR / S

17. creation of an artificial opening into the bladder ______ /CV/ ______
WR /CV/ S

18. incision through the kidney into the renal pelvis to remove a stone ______ /CV/ ______ /CV/ ______
WR /CV/ WR /CV/ WR

19. surgical crushing of a stone in the kidney ______ /CV/ ______ /CV/ ______
WR /CV/ WR /CV/ S

EXERCISE 19

Spell each of the surgical terms built from word parts on p. 223 by having someone dictate them to you.

To hear and spell the terms, go to http://evolve.elsevier.com. Refer to p. 18 for your Evolve Access Information. Select Exercises & Review, Chapter 6, Chapter Exercises, Spelling.

☐ Place a check mark in the box if you have completed this exercise online.

1.	______	11.	______
2.	______	12.	______
3.	______	13.	______
4.	______	14.	______
5.	______	15.	______
6.	______	16.	______
7.	______	17.	______
8.	______	18.	______
9.	______	19.	______
10.	______	20.	______

Surgical Terms

Not Built from Word Parts

In some of the following terms, you may recognize word parts you have already learned; however, the full meaning of the terms cannot be discerned by the definition of their word parts.

Term	Definition
extracorporeal shock wave lithotripsy (ESWL) (*eks*-tra-kor-POR-ē-al) (LITH-ō-*trip*-sē)	a noninvasive treatment for removal of kidney stone(s) or ureteral stone(s). By using ultrasound and fluoroscopic imaging, the stone is positioned at a focal point. Repeated firing of shock waves renders the stone into fragments that pass from the body in the urine (also called **shock wave lithotripsy [SWL]**) (see Exercise Figure E).
fulguration (*ful*-gū-RĀ-shun)	destruction of living tissue with an electric spark (a method commonly used to destroy bladder growths) (Figure 6-10)
renal transplant (RĒ-nal) (TRANS-plant)	surgical implantation of a donor kidney to replace a nonfunctioning kidney (Figure 6-11)

EXTRACORPOREAL

means occurring **outside the body.**

RENAL REPLACEMENT THERAPIES

- Hemodialysis
- Peritoneal dialysis
- Kidney transplant

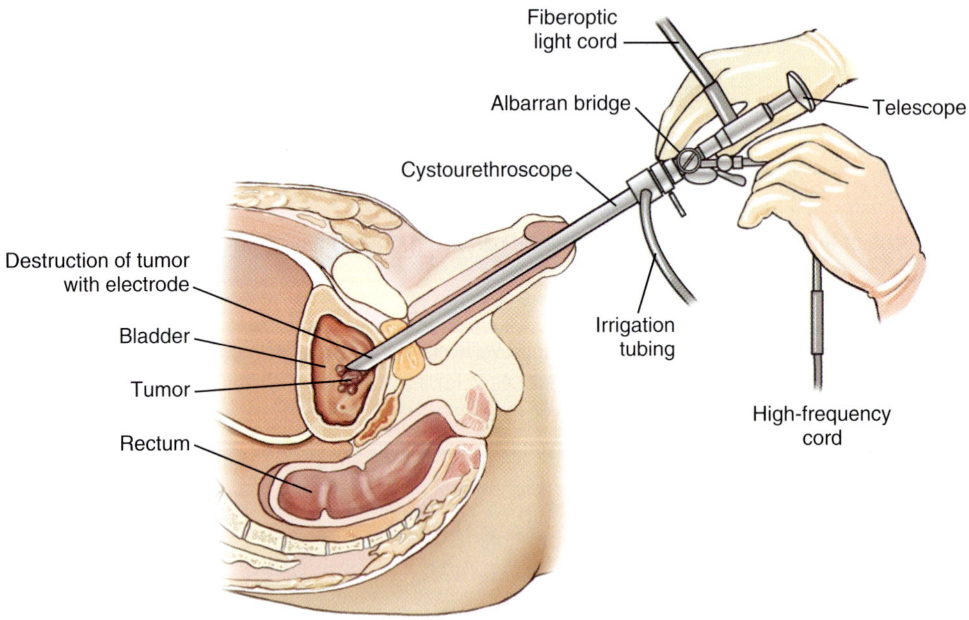

FIGURE 6-10
Bladder fulguration.

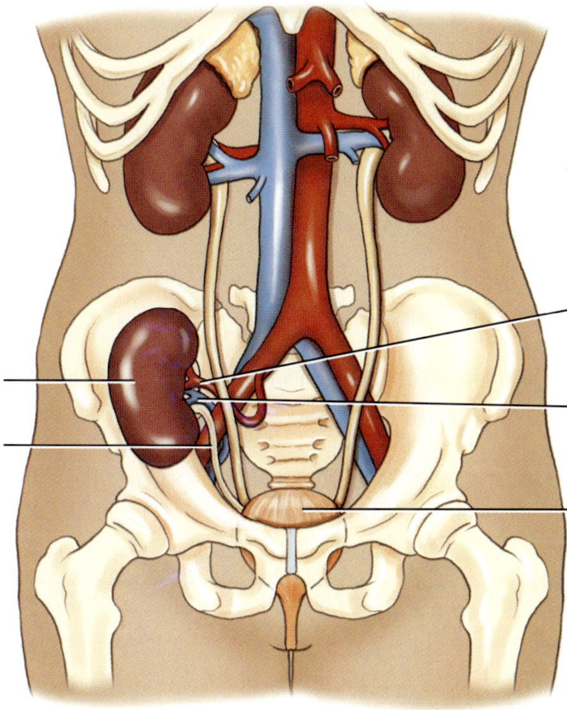

FIGURE 6-11
Renal transplant showing donor kidney and blood vessels in place. Recipient's kidney is not always removed unless it is infected or is a cause of hypertension

EXERCISE 20

Practice saying aloud each of the surgical terms not built from word parts on p. 238.

To hear the terms, go to http://evolve.elsevier.com. Refer to p. 18 for your Evolve Access Information. Select Exercises & Review, Chapter 6, Chapter Exercises, Pronunciation.

☐ Place a check mark in the box when you have completed this exercise.

EXERCISE 21

1. The surgical implantation of a donor kidney to replace a nonfunctioning kidney is called ______________ ______________.
2. The destruction of living tissue with an electric spark is ______________.
3. ______________ ______________ ______________ ______________ is a noninvasive treatment for removal of kidney or ureteral stones.

EXERCISE 22

Match the terms in the first column with their correct definitions in the second column.

_____ 1.	fulguration	a. used to replace a nonfunctioning kidney
_____ 2.	renal transplant	b. used to destroy bladder growths
_____ 3.	ESWL	c. also called shock wave lithotripsy

EXERCISE 23

Spell each of the surgical terms not built from word parts on p. 238 by having someone dictate them to you.

To hear and spell the terms, go to http://evolve.elsevier.com. Refer to p. 18 for your Evolve Access Information. Select Exercises & Review, Chapter 6, Chapter Exercises, Spelling.
☐ Place a check mark in the box if you have completed this exercise online.

1. ______________________________
2. ______________________________
3. ______________________________

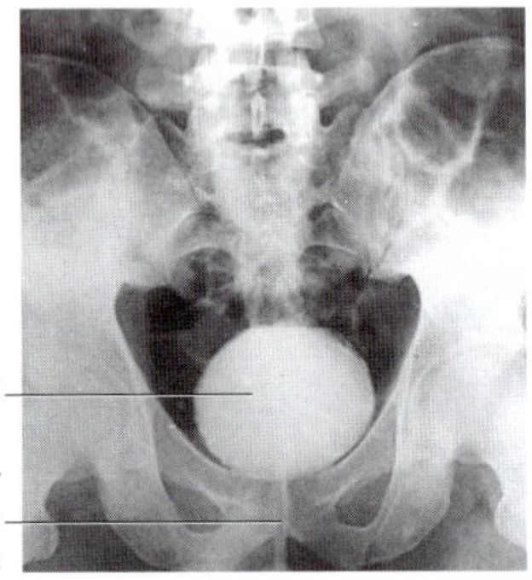

FIGURE 6-12
Cystogram.

SPIRAL/HELICAL CT

scans are replacing **intravenous urograms** to detect **urinary tract stones** and **perirenal infections**. Intravenous contrast media is not required.

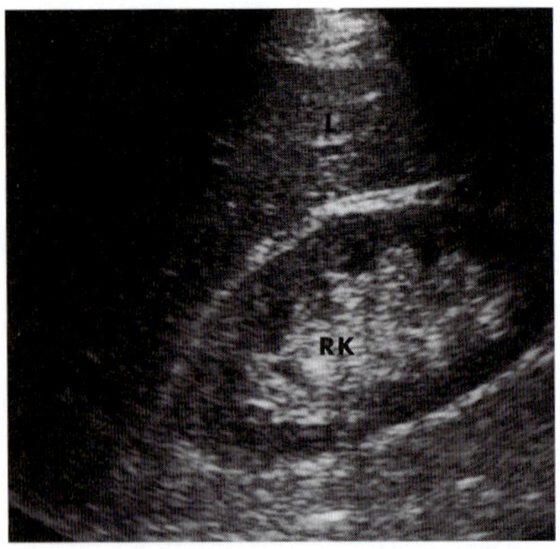

FIGURE 6-13
Nephrosonogram (ultrasound) of the right kidney, sagittal view.

Diagnostic Terms

Built from Word Parts

The following terms are built from word parts you have already learned and can be translated literally to find their meanings. Further explanation of terms beyond the definition of their word parts, if needed, is included in parentheses.

Review Table 5-1, Types of Diagnostic Procedures, p. 182 before proceeding.

Term	Definition
DIAGNOSTIC IMAGING	
cystogram (SIS-tō-gram)	radiographic image of the bladder (Figure 6-12)
cystography (sis-TOG-ra-fē)	radiographic imaging of the bladder
intravenous urogram (IVU) (*in*-tra-VĒ-nus) (Ū-rō-gram)	radiographic image of the urinary tract (with contrast medium injected intravenously) (also called **intravenous pyelogram [IVP]**)
nephrogram (NEF-rō-gram)	radiographic image of the kidney
nephrography (ne-FROG-ra-fē)	radiographic imaging of the kidney (also called **renogram**)
nephrosonography (*nef*-rō-so-NOG-ra-fē)	process of recording the kidney using sound (an ultrasound test) (Figure 6-13)

Term	Definition
nephrotomogram (*nef*-rō-TŌ-mō-gram)	sectional radiographic image of the kidney (Figure 6-14)
renogram (RĒ-nō-gram)	(graphic) record of the kidney (a nuclear medicine test produced by radioactivity after injecting a radiopharmaceutical, or radioactive material, into the blood) (also called **renal scan** or **nephrogram**)
retrograde urogram (RET-rō-grād) (Ū-ro-gram)	radiographic image of the urinary tract (retrograde means to move in a direction opposite from normal; contrast medium is instilled through urethral catheters by a cystoscope) (Exercise Figure H)
voiding cystourethrography (VCUG) (VOID-ing) (*sis*-tō-*ū*-rē-THROG-ro-fe)	radiographic imaging of the bladder and the urethra (Figure 6-15). (Radiopaque dye is instilled in the bladder. Radiographic images called voiding cystourethrograms are taken of the bladder and during urination of the dye.)
ENDOSCOPY	
cystoscope (SIS-tō-skōp)	instrument used for visual examination of the bladder
cystoscopy (sis-TOS-ko-pē)	visual examination of the bladder (Figure 6-16)
nephroscopy (ne-FROS-ko-pē)	visual examination of the kidney (Figure 6-17)
ureteroscopy (ū-*rē*-ter-OS-ko-pē)	visual examination of the ureter
urethroscope (*ū*-RĒ-thrō-skōp)	instrument used for visual examination of the urethra

Ultrasonography (US), computed tomography (CT), and **magnetic resonance imaging (MRI)** can be used in evaluating structure and function of the urinary system organs. See Table 5-1, p. 182.

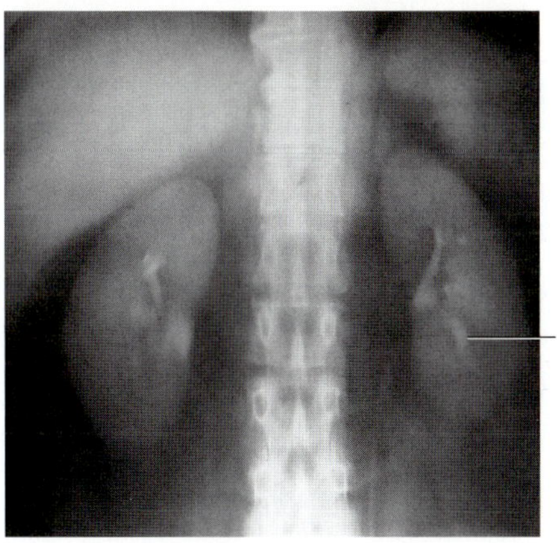

FIGURE 6-14
Nephrotomogram.

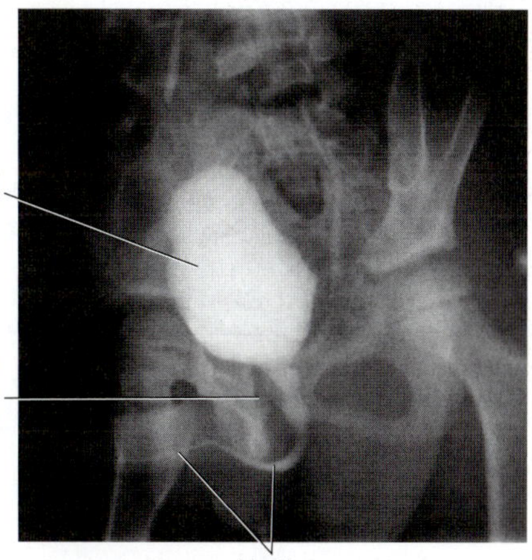

FIGURE 6-15
Voiding cystourethrogram, male.

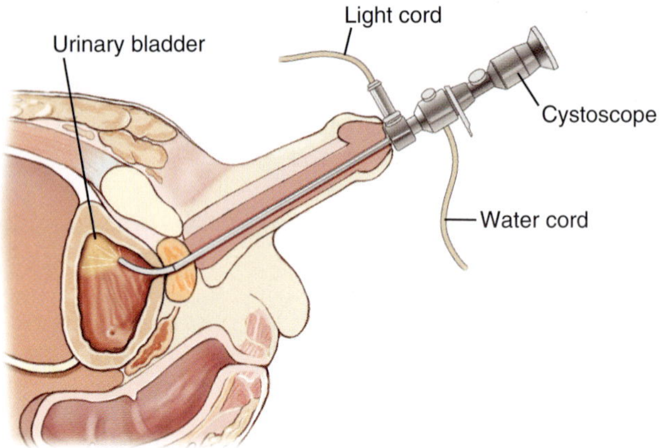

FIGURE 6-16
Cystoscopy.

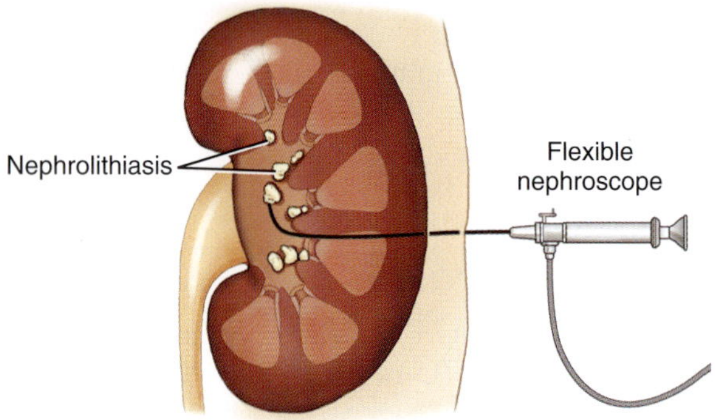

FIGURE 6-17
Nephroscopy.

EXERCISE FIGURE H

Fill in the blanks to label the diagram.

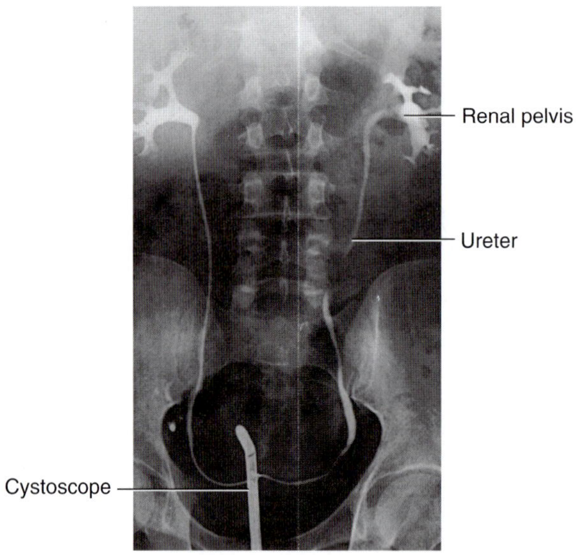

Retrograde ____________ / ____ / ____________.
urinary tract / cv / radiographic image.

A urethral catheter is passed by use of a cystoscope, and contrast material is injected to show urinary system structures.

EXERCISE 24

Practice saying aloud each of the diagnostic terms built from word parts on pp. 240-241.

To hear the terms, go to http://evolve.elsevier.com. Refer to p. 18 for your Evolve Access Information. Select Exercises & Review, Chapter 6, Chapter Exercises, Pronunciation.

☐ Place a check mark in the box when you have completed this exercise.

EXERCISE 25

Analyze and define the following diagnostic terms.

1. (voiding) cystourethrography ______________________
2. cystography ______________________
3. urethroscope ______________________
4. nephrosonography ______________________
5. cystoscope ______________________
6. nephrotomogram ______________________
7. cystogram ______________________
8. nephrogram ______________________
9. cystoscopy ______________________
10. nephrography ______________________
11. (intravenous) urogram ______________________
12. (retrograde) urogram ______________________
13. renogram ______________________
14. nephroscopy ______________________
15. ureteroscopy ______________________

EXERCISE 26

Build diagnostic terms that correspond to the following definitions by using the word parts you have learned.

1. visual examination of the bladder ______ / ______ / ______
   WR / CV / S
2. sectional radiographic image of the kidney ______ / ______ / ______ / ______ / ______
   WR / CV / WR / CV / S
3. radiographic image of the urinary tract (with contrast medium injected intravenously)
   intravenous ______ / ______ / ______
   WR / CV / S
4. instrument used for visual examination of the urethra ______ / ______ / ______
   WR / CV / S
5. process of radiographic recording the kidney using sound ______ / ______ / ______ / ______ / ______
   WR / CV / WR / CV / S
6. radiographic image of the bladder ______ / ______ / ______
   WR / CV / S
7. instrument used for visual examination of the bladder ______ / ______ / ______
   WR / CV / S
8. radiographic imaging of the bladder and the urethra
   voiding ______ / ______ / ______ / ______ / ______
   WR / CV / WR / CV / S
9. radiographic imaging of the bladder ______ / ______ / ______
   WR / CV / S
10. radiographic image of the kidney ______ / ______ / ______
    WR / CV / S
11. (graphic) record of the kidney (produced by radioactivity after injecting a radiopharmaceutical material into the blood) ______ / ______ / ______
    WR / CV / S

12. radiographic imaging of the kidney

_______ / _______ / _______
WR / CV / S

13. radiographic image of the urinary tract (with contrast medium instilled through the urethral catheters in a direction opposite from normal)

retrograde _______ / _______ / _______
WR / CV / S

14. visual examination of the kidney

_______ / _______ / _______
WR / CV / S

15. visual examination of the ureter

_______ / _______ / _______
WR / CV / S

EXERCISE 27

Spell each of the diagnostic terms built from word parts on pp. 240-241 by having someone dictate them to you.

To hear and spell the terms, go to http://evolve.elsevier.com. Refer to p. 18 for your Evolve Access Information. Select Exercises & Review, Chapter 6, Chapter Exercises, Spelling.

☐ Place a check mark in the box if you have completed this exercise online.

1. _______________
2. _______________
3. _______________
4. _______________
5. _______________
6. _______________
7. _______________
8. _______________
9. _______________
10. _______________
11. _______________
12. _______________
13. _______________
14. _______________
15. _______________

Diagnostic Terms

Not Built from Word Parts

In some of the following terms, you may recognize word parts you have already learned; however, the full meaning of the terms cannot be discerned by the definition of their word parts.

Term	Definition
DIAGNOSTIC IMAGING	
KŪB (kidney, ureter, and bladder) (NOTE: KUB is pronounced K-Ū-B, and not cub.)	a simple radiographic image of the abdomen. It is often used to view the kidneys, ureters, and bladder to determine size, shape, and location. Also used to identify calculi in the kidney, ureters, or bladder, or to diagnose intestinal obstruction; (also called **flat plate of the abdomen**)
LABORATORY	
blood urea nitrogen (BUN) (ū-RĒ-a) (NĪ-trō-jen)	a blood test that measures the amount of urea in the blood; used to determine kidney function. An increased BUN indicates renal dysfunction.
creatinine (crē-AT-i-nin)	a blood test that measures the amount of creatinine in the blood. An elevated amount may indicate impaired kidney function.
specific gravity (SG) (spe-SIF-ik) (GRAV-i-tē)	a test performed on a urine specimen to measure the concentrating or diluting ability of the kidneys
urinalysis (UA) (*ū*-rin-AL-is-is)	multiple routine tests performed on a urine specimen

BUN

The abbreviation BUN for blood urea nitrogen is commonly used in the healthcare setting. It is pronounced B-Ū-N and not bun.

EXERCISE 28

Practice saying aloud each of the diagnostic terms not built from word parts on p. 246.

To hear terms, go to http://evolve.elsevier.com. Refer to p. 18 for your Evolve Access Information. Select Exercises & Review, Chapter 6, Chapter Exercises, Pronunciation.

☐ Place a check mark in the box when you have completed this exercise.

EXERCISE 29

Fill in the blanks with the correct terms.

1. The radiographic image of the abdomen used to view the kidneys, ureters, and bladder to determine size, shape, and location is called ________________.
2. A test performed on a urine specimen to measure concentrating and diluting ability of the kidneys is called ________________ ________________.
3. ________________ ________________ ________________ measures the amount of urea in the blood.
4. Multiple routine tests performed on a urine specimen are referred to as a(n) ________________________.
5. ________________________ is a blood test that measures the amount of creatinine in the blood.

EXERCISE 30

Match the terms in the first column with their correct definitions in the second column.

_____ 1. specific gravity
_____ 2. blood urea nitrogen
_____ 3. urinalysis
_____ 4. KUB
_____ 5. creatinine

a. a radiographic image of the kidneys, ureters, and bladder
b. a blood test that measures the amount of urea in the blood
c. a urine test to measure concentrating or diluting abilities of the kidneys
d. multiple routine tests performed on a urine sample
e. a radiographic image of the kidneys, urethra, and bladder
f. a test on blood that if elevated may indicate impaired kidney function

EXERCISE 31

Spell each of the diagnostic terms not built from word parts on p. 246 by having someone dictate them to you.

To hear and spell the terms, go to http://evolve.elsevier.com. Refer to p. 18 for your Evolve Access Information. Select Exercises & Review, Chapter 6, Chapter Exercises, Spelling.
☐ Place a check mark in the box if you have completed this exercise online.

1. ________________________
2. ________________________
3. ________________________
4. ________________________
5. ________________________

Complementary Terms

Built from Word Parts

The following terms are built from word parts you have already learned and can be translated literally to find their meanings. Further explanation of terms beyond the definition of their word parts, if needed, is included in parentheses.

Term	Definition
albuminuria (*al*-bū-min-Ū-rē-a)	albumin in the urine (albumin is an important protein in the blood, but when found in the urine, it indicates a kidney problem)
anuria (an-Ū-rē-a)	absence of urine (failure of the kidney to produce urine)
diuresis (*dī*-ū-RĒ-sis) (NOTE: the *a* is dropped from dia- because uresis begins with a vowel.)	condition of urine passing through (increased amount of urine)
dysuria (dis-Ū-rē-a)	difficult or painful urination
glycosuria (*glī*-kō-SŪ-rē-a)	sugar (glucose) in the urine
hematuria (*hēm*-a-TŪ-rē-a)	blood in the urine
meatal (mē-Ā-tal)	pertaining to the meatus
nephrologist (ne-FROL-o-jist)	a physician who studies and treats diseases of the kidney
nephrology (ne-FROL-o-jē)	study of the kidney (a branch of medicine dealing with diseases of the kidney)
nocturia (nok-TŪ-rē-a)	night urination
oliguria (*ol*-i-GŪ-rē-a)	scanty urine (amount)
polyuria (*pol*-ē-Ū-rē-a)	much (excessive) urine
pyuria (pī-Ū-rē-a)	pus in the urine
urinary (Ū-rin-*ār*-ē)	pertaining to urine
urologist (ū-ROL-o-jist)	a physician who studies and treats diseases of the urinary tract
urology (ū-ROL-o-jē)	study of the urinary tract (a branch of medicine dealing with diseases of the male and female urinary systems and the male reproductive system)

UROLOGIST/ NEPHROLOGIST

A **urologist** treats diseases of the male and female urinary system and the male reproductive system both medically and surgically. A **nephrologist** treats kidney diseases and prescribes dialysis therapy.

EXERCISE 32

Practice saying aloud each of the complementary terms built from word parts on p. 248.

To hear the terms, go to http://evolve.elsevier.com. Refer to p. 18 for your Evolve Access Information. Select Exercises & Review, Chapter 6, Chapter Exercises, Pronunciation.

☐ Place a check mark in the box when you have completed this exercise.

EXERCISE 33

Analyze and define the following complementary terms.

1. nocturia ______________________________
2. urologist ______________________________
3. oliguria ______________________________
4. nephrologist ______________________________
5. hematuria ______________________________
6. urology ______________________________
7. polyuria ______________________________
8. albuminuria ______________________________
9. anuria ______________________________
10. diuresis ______________________________
11. pyuria ______________________________
12. urinary ______________________________
13. glycosuria ______________________________
14. dysuria ______________________________
15. nephrology ______________________________
16. nephrologist ______________________________

EXERCISE 34

Build the complementary terms for the following definitions by using the word parts you have learned.

1. night urination ______ / ______ (WR / S)
2. scanty urine ______ / ______ (WR / S)
3. pus in the urine ______ / ______ (WR / S)
4. physician who studies and treats the urinary tract ______ / ______ / ______ (WR / CV / S)
5. much (excessive) urine ______ / ______ (P / S(WR))
6. physician who studies and treats diseases of the kidney ______ / ______ / ______ (WR / CV / S)
7. pertaining to urine ______ / ______ (WR / S)
8. blood in the urine ______ / ______ (WR / S(WR))
9. study of the urinary tract ______ / ______ / ______ (WR / CV / S)
10. condition of urine passing through (increased amount of urine) ______ / ______ / ______ (P / WR / S)
11. absence of urine ______ / ______ (P / S(WR))
12. sugar in the urine ______ / ______ (WR / S(WR))
13. difficult or painful urination ______ / ______ (P / S(WR))
14. albumin in the urine ______ / ______ (WR / S(WR))
15. pertaining to the meatus ______ / ______ (WR / S)
16. study of the kidney ______ / ______ / ______ (WR / CV / S)

EXERCISE 35

Spell each of the complementary terms built from word parts on p. 248 by having someone dictate them to you.

To hear and spell the terms, go to http://evolve.elsevier.com. Refer to p. 18 for your Evolve Access Information. Select Exercises & Review, Chapter 6, Chapter Exercises, Spelling.
☐ Place a check mark in the box if you have completed this exercise online.

1. ______________________
2. ______________________
3. ______________________
4. ______________________
5. ______________________
6. ______________________
7. ______________________
8. ______________________
9. ______________________
10. ______________________
11. ______________________
12. ______________________
13. ______________________
14. ______________________
15. ______________________
16. ______________________

CATHETER

is derived from the Greek **katheter,** meaning a **thing let down.** A catheter lets down the urine from the bladder.

ENURESIS

Nocturnal enuresis, or bed-wetting, has been described in early literature and continues to be a problem affecting 15% to 20% of school-aged children. There is no one cause for bed wetting. **Diurnal eneuresis** is daytime wetting, which may be caused by a small bladder. Various treatments are used to treat diurnal eneuresis. Children generally outgrow daytime wetting.

Complementary Terms

Not Built from Word Parts

In some of the following terms, you may recognize word parts you have already learned; however, the full meaning of the terms cannot be discerned by the definition of their word parts.

Term	Definition
catheter (cath) (KATH-e-ter)	flexible, tubelike device, such as a urinary catheter, for withdrawing or instilling fluids
distended (dis-TEN-ded)	stretched out (a bladder is distended when filled with urine)
enuresis (*en*-ū-RĒ-sis)	involuntary urination
hemodialysis (HD) (*hē*-mō-dī-AL-i-sis)	procedure for removing impurities from the blood because of an inability of the kidneys to do so (Figure 6-18)
incontinence (in-KON-ti-nens)	inability to control bladder and/or bowels
micturate (MIK-tū-rāt)	to urinate or void

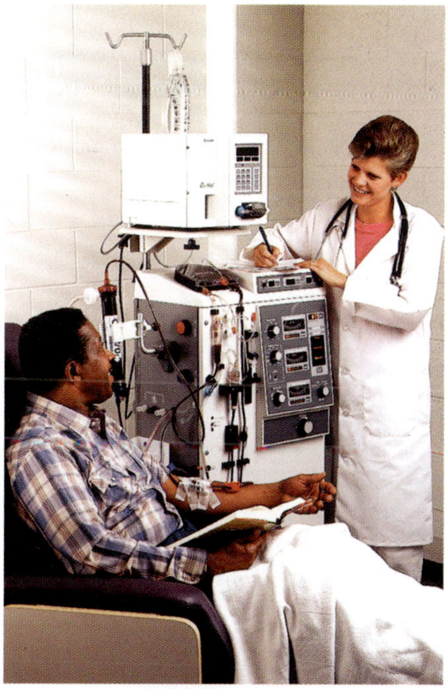

FIGURE 6-18
Hemodialysis.

MICTURATE

is derived from the Latin **mictus,** meaning **a making of water.** The noun form of micturate is **micturition.** Note the spelling of each. **Micturition** is often misspelled as **micturation.**

Complementary Terms—*cont'd*

Not Built from Word Parts

Term	Definition
peritoneal dialysis (*păr*-i-tō-NĒ-al) (dī-AL-i-sis)	procedure for removing toxic wastes when the kidney is unable to do so; the peritoneal cavity is used as the receptacle for the fluid used in the dialysis (Figure 6-19)
stricture (STRIK-chūr)	abnormal narrowing, such as a urethral stricture
urinal (Ū-rin-al)	receptacle for urine
urinary catheterization (Ū-rin-*ār*-ē) (*kath*-e-*ter*-i-ZĀ-shun)	passage of a catheter into the urinary bladder to withdraw urine (Exercise Figure I)
urodynamics (*ū*-rō-dī-NAM-iks)	pertaining to the force and flow of urine within the urinary tract
void (voyd)	to empty or evacuate waste material, especially urine

URODYNAMIC STUDIES

examines the process of voiding and tests bladder tone, capacity, and pressure along with urine flow and perineal muscle function. **Prostatic cancer,** prostatic hypertrophy, and urethral stricture will diminish urine flow rate.

EXERCISE FIGURE I

Fill in the blanks to complete labeling of the diagram.

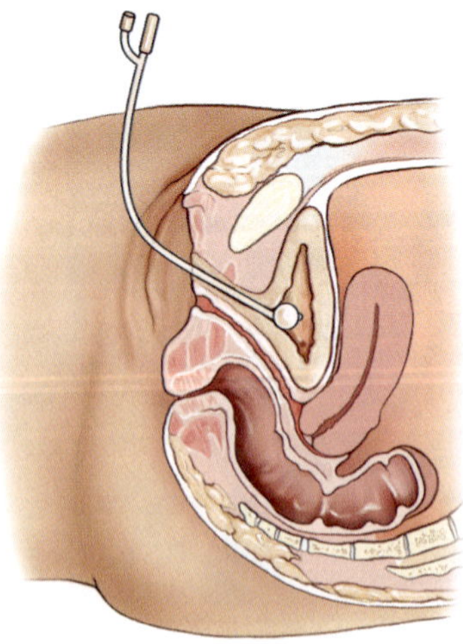

_____ / _____
urine / pertaining to
catheterization. A catheter has been inserted through the urethra and urine has been drained. The balloon on the end of the catheter has been inflated to hold the catheter in the bladder for a period of time. This type of catheter is called a **retention catheter**; commonly referred to as a **Foley catheter.**

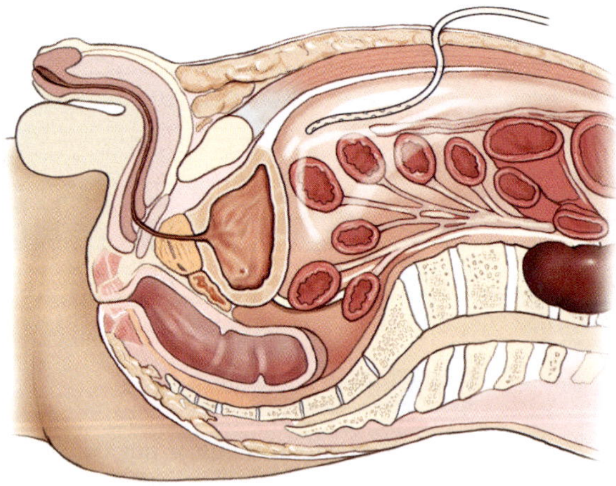

FIGURE 6-19
Peritoneal dialysis. A sterile dialyzing fluid is instilled into the peritoneal cavity by gravity and dwells there for a period of time ordered by the physician. The fluid, containing the nitrogenous wastes and excess water that a healthy kidney normally removes, is drained from the cavity.

EXERCISE 36

Practice saying aloud each of the complementary terms not built from word parts on pp. 251-252.

To hear the terms, go to http://evolve.elsevier.com. Refer to p. 18 for your Evolve Access Information. Select Exercises & Review, Chapter 6, Chapter Exercises, Pronunciation.

☐ Place a check mark in the box when you have completed this exercise.

EXERCISE 37

Fill in the blanks with the correct terms.

1. A receptacle for urine is a(n) ________________________.
2. The procedure for removing impurities from the blood because of the inability of the kidneys to do so is called ________________________.
3. A ________________________ bladder is stretched out.
4. A flexible, tubelike device for withdrawing or instilling fluids is a(n) ________________________.
5. The inability to control the bladder and/or bowels is called ________________________.
6. The passage of a catheter into the urinary bladder to withdraw urine is a(n) ________________________ ________________________.
7. To remove toxic wastes caused by kidney insufficiency by placing dialyzing fluid in the peritoneal cavity is called ________________________ ________________________.
8. To void is to ________________________ ________________________ ________________________.
9. An abnormal narrowing is a(n) ________________________.
10. Involuntary urination is called ________________________.
11. ________________________ is another word for void, or urinate.
12. ________________________ is the name given to the force and flow of urine.

EXERCISE 38

Match the terms in the first column with their correct definitions in the second column.

_____ 1. catheter
_____ 2. urinary catheterization
_____ 3. distended
_____ 4. void
_____ 5. hemodialysis
_____ 6. incontinence

a. to evacuate or empty waste material, especially urine
b. overdevelopment of the kidney
c. inability to control the bladder and/or bowels
d. process for removing impurities from the blood when the kidneys are unable to do so
e. flexible, tubelike device for withdrawing or instilling fluids
f. stretched out
g. passage of a tubelike device into the urinary bladder to remove urine

EXERCISE 39

Match the terms in the first column with their correct definitions in the second column.

_____ 1. micturate, or urinate
_____ 2. peritoneal dialysis
_____ 3. stricture
_____ 4. urinal
_____ 5. enuresis
_____ 6. urodynamics

a. to void liquid waste
b. receptacle for urine
c. force and flow of urine within the urinary tract
d. absence of urine
e. use of peritoneal cavity to hold dialyzing fluid in the removal of toxic wastes
f. involuntary urination
g. narrowing

EXERCISE 40

Spell each of the complementary terms not built from word parts on pp. 251-252 by having someone dictate them to you.

To hear and spell the terms, go to http://evolve.elsevier.com. Refer to p. 18 for your Evolve Access Information. Select Exercises & Review, Chapter 6, Chapter Exercises, Spelling.
☐ Place a check mark in the box if you have completed this exercise online.

1. ____________	7. ____________
2. ____________	8. ____________
3. ____________	9. ____________
4. ____________	10. ____________
5. ____________	11. ____________
6. ____________	12. ____________

Refer to **Appendix D** for pharmacology terms related to the urinary system.

Abbreviations

ARF	acute renal failure
BUN	blood urea nitrogen
cath	catheterization, catheter
CRF	chronic renal failure
ESRD	end-stage renal disease
ESWL	extracorporeal shock wave lithotripsy
HD	hemodialysis
IVP	intravenous pyelogram
IVU	intravenous urogram
OAB	overactive bladder
SG	specific gravity
UA	urinalysis
UTI	urinary tract infection
VCUG	voiding cystourethrogram

Refer to **Appendix C** for a complete list of abbreviations.

EXERCISE 41

1. When imaging is used to diagnose obstructive uropathy, a KUB is usually performed first. An **IVU** _______________ _______________, also called **IVP** _______________ _______________, is usually best for confirming or excluding obstruction and determining its level and cause. For further examination a **VCUG** _______________ ____________________________ may be performed to evaluate the posterior urethra and check for vesicoureteral reflux.
2. **SG** _______________ _______________ is one of many tests performed on the urine specimen during a **UA** _______________. It measures the concentration of particles, including water and electrolytes in the urine.
3. **BUN** _______________ _______________ _______________ is a laboratory test done on a blood sample to determine kidney function.
4. The number, size, and type of stones are important in determining if **ESWL** _______________ _______________ _______________ _______________ is the best method for treating renal calculi.
5. Bladder **cath** _______________ carries the risk of **UTI** _______________ _______________ _______________; therefore it is sometimes preferable to use other methods for obtaining urine specimens and managing incontinence.
6. Peritoneal dialysis, **HD** _______________, and renal transplant are known as renal replacement therapies.
7. **ARF** _______________ _______________ _______________ is sudden and full recovery can occur with prompt treatment. **CRF** _______________ _______________ _______________ is irreversible and progressive. **ESRD** _______________ _______________ _______________ _______________ is when kidney function will not sustain life. A kidney transplant or renal dialysis may be used as treatment.
8. Urge incontinence is another name for **OAB** _______________ _______________ and involves a sudden, strong need to urinate. As the bladder contracts, leakage of urine occurs.

PRACTICAL APPLICATION

EXERCISE 42 *Interact with Medical Documents*

A. Complete the discharge summary report by writing the medical terms in the blanks. Use the list of definitions with the corresponding numbers.

University Hospital and Medical Center
4700 North Main Street • Wellness, Arizona 54321 • (987) 555-3210

PATIENT NAME: Bruno Oliver
DATE OF BIRTH: 07/30/19XX

CASE NUMBER: 83658-URI
DATE OF ADMISSION: 09/20/20XX
DATE OF DISCHARGE: 09/27/20XX

DISCHARGE SUMMARY

Bruno Oliver is a 32-year-old white man, appearing his stated age, who was admitted to the hospital after presenting himself to the emergency department on 09/20XX in acute distress. He complained of intermittent pain in the right posterior lumbar area, radiating to the right flank. He has a family history of 1. ____________________ and has been treated for this condition two other times in the past 10 years.

This patient was admitted to the 2. ____________________ Unit and was administered intravenous morphine sulfate for pain control. VITAL SIGNS: Low-grade temperature of 99.4. Initial blood pressure was 146/92 mm Hg.

The white blood count, hemoglobin, and hematocrit were normal. The urinalysis showed microscopic 3. ____________________ .

A 4. __________ revealed 5. ____________________ in the region of the right renal pelvis. A 6. ____________________ with a right retrograde 7. __________ confirmed the presence of the three stones in the right kidney. Minimal ureteral obstruction was present.

A percutaneous 8. ____________________________________ was completed with no complications. A ureteral stent was inserted as was an indwelling Foley 9. __________ . Drainage from the right kidney was pale yellow in 48 hours. The Foley catheter was removed 3 days postoperatively.

At discharge, the patient is voiding without difficulty. The stones were sent to the laboratory for analysis. The report indicated that they were calcium oxalate.

The patient is to follow up with his urologist in a week to have his ureteral stent removed.

____
Betsy Begay, MD

BB/mcm

1. condition of stones in the kidney
2. study of the urinary tract
3. blood in the urine
4. radiographic image of the abdomen
5. stones
6. visual examination of the bladder
7. radiographic image of the urinary tract
8. incision into the kidney to remove a stone
9. flexible, tubelike device

EXERCISE 42 *Interact with Medical Documents—cont'd*

B. Read the operative report and answer the questions following it.

OPERATIVE REPORT

Patient Name: John Allen
Date of Operation: May 21, 20XX
Preoperative Diagnosis: Urinary tract obstruction
Postoperative Diagnosis: Ureterolithiasis

Surgery Performed: Ureteroscopy with calculus extraction

Indications: The patient, a 31-year-old previously healthy man, presented with complaints of flank pain, oliguria, nausea, and chills. The patient denied gross hematuria. A spiral CT scan revealed presence of a ureteral stone.

Procedure: The patient was placed in the dorsal lithotomy position. The area was draped and prepared in the standard manner. Thirty mL of topical anesthesia (1% Lidocaine) was administered, and a penile clamp was applied to ensure retention. The ureteroscope was inserted, with access to the middle third of the ureter gained by passing a guidewire under fluoroscopic control. The guidewire was advanced beyond the stone, and the calculus was delivered through the ureter, engaged in a retrieval basket, and removed. The patient tolerated the procedure well and left the operating room in good condition.

Melvin Peterson, MD, Urologist

1. The patient presented with a complaint of
   a. difficult or painful urination.
   b. excessive urine.
   c. scanty urine.
   d. pus in the urine.

2. The presence of a ureteral stone was revealed by
   a. radiographic imaging.
   b. magnetic resonance imaging.
   c. ultrasound.
   d. computed tomography.

3. T F More than one stone was removed from the ureter.

4. Ureteroscope and ureteral are terms not included in the chapter. Using your knowledge of the meaning of word parts, define these terms.

   a. ureteral ____________________

   b. ureteroscope ____________________

EXERCISE 43 *Interpret Medical Terms*

To test your understanding of the terms introduced in this chapter, circle the words that correctly complete the sentences. The italicized words refer to the correct answer.

1. The patient was diagnosed with a *drooping kidney*, or (**nephromegaly, nephrohypertrophy, nephroptosis**).
2. The patient's radiographic image showed *stones in the ureter*, or a condition known as (**ureterocele, ureterolithiasis, ureterostenosis**).
3. The patient was scheduled for a right ureteral pelvic junction *ESWL*, a surgical treatment, to (**separate tissue, create an artificial opening, remove a stone**).

4. The physician first suspected diabetes when told of the *excessive amounts of urine* voided, or (**oliguria, polyuria, dysuria**).
5. The physician told the patient with the drooping kidney that it was necessary to *secure the kidney in place* by performing a (**nephropexy, nephrolysis, nephrotripsy**).
6. The patient had a *sudden stoppage of urine formation*, or (**urinary suppression, urinary retention, azoturia**).
7. The patient was scheduled for a *radiographic image of the urinary bladder*, or a (**cystoscopy, cystogram, cystography**).
8. The patient's mother informed the doctor of her son's *involuntary urination*, or (**diuresis, dysuria, enuresis**).
9. The patient was admitted to the hospital for *kidney and ureteral infection*, or (**polycystic kidney disease, urinary retention, urinary tract infection**).
10. *UA* is the abbreviation for (**urine, urinary, urinalysis**).
11. Percutaneous *nephrolithotripsy* is a (**surgical procedure**, **disease**, **diagnostic procedure**).

EXERCISE 44 *Read Medical Terms in Use*

Practice pronunciation of the terms by reading the following medical document. Use the pronunciation key following the medical terms to assist you in saying the word.

To hear these terms, go to http://evolve.elsevier.com. Refer to p. 18 for your Evolve Access Information. Select Exercises & Review, Chapter 6, Chapter Exercises, Read Medical Terms in Use.

A 76-year-old woman consulted with her primary care physician because of **hematuria** (*hēm*-a-TŪ-rē-a) and **dysuria** (dis-Ū-rē-a). She was referred to a **urologist** (ū-ROL-o-jist). **Urinalysis** (ū-rin-AL-is-is) disclosed 1+ albumin and mild **pyuria** (pī-Ū-rē-a) in addition to the hematuria. A spiral CT scan was obtained. Mild **nephrolithiasis** (*nef*-rō-lith-Ī-a-sis) was observed but no **hydronephrosis** (*hī*-drō-ne-FRŌ-sis). Finally a **cystoscopy** (sis-TOS-ko-pē) was performed, which showed mild **cystitis** (sis-TĪ-tis). A **urinary tract infection** (Ū-rin-*ār*-ē) (trakt) (in-FEK-shun) was diagnosed and the patient responded favorably to antibiotics. The urologist did not advise **lithotripsy** (LITH-ō-trip-sē) for the **renal calculi** (RĒ-nal) (KAL-kū-lī).

EXERCISE 45 *Comprehend Medical Terms in Use*

Test your comprehension of terms in the previous medical document by circling the correct answer.

1. Symptoms that prompted the patient to seek treatment from the urologist were:
   a. scanty urine and painful urination
   b. painful urination and bloody urine
   c. pus and blood in the urine
   d. sugar and blood in the urine
2. Which of the following was rejected as treatment for kidney stones?
   a. urinalysis
   b. intravenous urogram
   c. cystoscopy
   d. lithotripsy
3. The CT image revealed which of the following was not present in the kidney?
   a. water
   b. blood
   c. stones
   d. tumor

CHAPTER REVIEW

ONLINE CHAPTER REVIEW

To access the Evolve website, go to http://evolve.elsevier.com. Refer to p. 18 for your Evolve Access Information. Select Exercises & Review, Chapter 3, then select Chapter Exercises, Practice Activities, Animations, or Games. Place a check mark in the box when you have completed an exercise or activity, watched an animation, or played a game. Have fun!

Chapter Exercises

Exercises in this section of your Evolve resources correlate to exercises in your textbook. You may have completed them as you worked through the chapter.

- ☐ Pronunciation
- ☐ Spelling
- ☐ Read Medical Terms in Use

Practice Activities

Practice in study mode, then test your learning in assessment mode. Keep track of your scores from assessment mode if you wish.

	SCORE
☐ Picture It	_____
☐ Define Word Parts	_____
☐ Build Medical Terms	_____
☐ Word Shop	_____
☐ Define Medical Terms	_____
☐ Use It	_____
☐ Hear It and Type It: Clinical Vignettes	_____

Animations

- ☐ Bladder infection
- ☐ Cystourethrogram
- ☐ Nephrostomy

Games

- ☐ Name that Word Part
- ☐ Term Storm
- ☐ Term Explorer
- ☐ Termbusters
- ☐ Medical Millionaire
- ☐ Crossword Puzzle

REVIEW OF WORD PARTS

Can you define and spell the following word parts?

Combining Forms

albumin/o
azot/o
blast/o
cyst/o
glomerul/o
glyc/o
glycos/o
hydr/o
lith/o
meat/o
nephr/o
noct/i
olig/o
pyel/o
ren/o
son/o
tom/o
ureter/o
urethr/o
ur/o
urin/o
vesic/o

Suffixes

-esis
-gram
-iasis
-lysis
-megaly
-ptosis
-rrhaphy
-tripsy
-trophy
-uria

REVIEW OF TERMS

Can you define, pronounce, and spell the following terms *built from word parts*?

Diseases and Disorders

azotemia
cystitis
cystocele
cystolith
glomerulonephritis
hydronephrosis
nephritis
nephroblastoma
nephrohypertrophy
nephrolithiasis
nephroma
nephroptosis
pyelitis
pyelonephritis
ureteritis
ureterocele
ureterolithiasis
ureterostenosis
urethrocystitis

Surgical

cystectomy
cystolithotomy
cystorrhaphy
cystostomy
cystotomy
lithotripsy
meatotomy
nephrectomy
nephrolithotomy
nephrolithotripsy
nephrolysis
nephropexy
nephrostomy
pyelolithotomy
pyeloplasty
ureterectomy
ureterostomy
urethroplasty
vesicourethral suspension
vesicotomy

Diagnostic

cystogram
cystography
cystoscope
cystoscopy
intravenous urogram (IVU)
nephrogram
nephrography
nephroscopy
nephrosonography
nephrotomogram
renogram
retrograde urogram
ureteroscopy
urethroscope
voiding cystourethrography (VCUG)

Complementary

albuminuria
anuria
diuresis
dysuria
glycosuria
hematuria
meatal
nephrologist
nephrology
nocturia
oliguria
polyuria
pyuria
urinary
urologist
urology

Can you define, pronounce, and spell the following terms *not built from word parts*?

Diseases and Disorders	Surgical	Diagnostic	Complementary
epispadias	extracorporeal shock wave lithotripsy (ESWL)	blood urea nitrogen (BUN)	catheter (cath)
hypospadias	fulguration	creatinine	distended
polycystic kidney disease	renal transplant	KUB	enuresis
renal calculus (*pl.* calculi)		specific gravity (SG)	hemodialysis (HD)
renal failure		urinalysis (UA)	incontinence
renal hypertension			micturate
urinary retention			peritoneal dialysis
urinary suppression			stricture
urinary tract infection (UTI)			urinal
			urinary catheterization
			urodynamics
			void

ANSWERS

Exercise Figures

Exercise Figure

A. 1. kidney: nephr/o, ren/o
   2. meatus: meat/o
   3. ureter: ureter/o
   4. bladder: cyst/o, vesic/o
   5. urethra: urethr/o

Exercise Figure

B. 1. renal pelvis: pyel/o
   2. glomerulus: glomerul/o

Exercise Figure

C. cyst/o/lith

Exercise Figure

D. cyst/o/stomy

Exercise Figure

E. lith/o/tripsy

Exercise Figure

F. nephr/o/stomy

Exercise Figure

G. pyel/o/lith/o/tomy

Exercise Figure

H. ur/o/gram

Exercise Figure

I. urin/ary

Exercise 1

1. g
2. d
3. f
4. c
5. a
6. b
7. e

Exercise 2

1. glomerulus
2. bladder, sac
3. kidney
4. renal pelvis
5. ureter
6. bladder, sac
7. urethra
8. kidney
9. meatus

Exercise 3

1. a. nephr/o
   b. ren/o
2. a. cyst/o
   b. vesic/o
3. ureter/o
4. pyel/o
5. glomerul/o
6. urethr/o
7. meat/o

Exercise 4

1. water
2. urea, nitrogen
3. night
4. stone, calculus
5. cut, section
6. albumin
7. urine, urinary tract
8. sound
9. sugar
10. developing cell, germ cell
11. scanty, few
12. urine, urinary tract
13. sugar

Exercise 5

1. a. glyc/o
   b. glycos/o
2. son/o
3. a. urin/o
   b. ur/o
4. hydr/o
5. blast/o
6. tom/o
7. albumin/o
8. noct/i
9. azot/o
10. lith/o
11. olig/o

Exercise 6

1. c
2. i
3. d
4. f
5. g
6. e
7. a
8. b
9. h

Exercise 7

1. suturing, repairing
2. loosening, dissolution, separating
3. condition
4. nourishment, development
5. urine, urination
6. enlargement
7. drooping, sagging, prolapse
8. surgical crushing
9. record, radiographic image

Exercise 8

Pronunciation Exercise

Exercise 9

1. WR S
   nephr/oma
   tumor of the kidney
2. WR CV WR
   cyst/o/lith
   CF
   stone in the bladder
3. WR CV WR S
   nephr/o/lith/iasis
   CF
   condition of stone(s) in the kidney
4. WR S
   azot/emia
   condition of urea in the blood
5. WR CV S
   nephr/o/ptosis
   CF
   drooping kidney
6. WR CV S
   cyst/o/cele
   CF
   protrusion of the bladder
7. WR CV P S
   nephr/o/hyper/trophy
   CF
   excessive development of the kidney
8. WR S
   cyst/itis
   inflammation of the bladder
9. WR S
   pyel/itis
   inflammation of the renal pelvis
10. WR CV S
    ureter/o/cele
    CF
    protrusion of a ureter
11. WR CV WR S
    hydr/o/nephr/osis
    CF
    abnormal condition of water in the kidney
12. WR CV S
    nephr/o/megaly
    CF
    enlargement of a kidney
13. WR CV WR S
    ureter/o/lith/iasis
    CF
    condition of stones(s) in the ureters
14. WR CV WR S
    pyel/o/nephr/itis
    CF
    inflammation of the renal pelvis and the kidney
15. WR S
    ureter/itis
    inflammation of a ureter

16. WR S
nephr/itis
inflammation of a kidney

17. WR CV WR S
urethr/o/cyst/itis
CF
inflammation of the urethra and bladder

18. WR CV S
ureter/o/stenosis
CF
narrowing of the ureter

19. WR CV WR S
nephr/o/blast/oma
CF
kidney tumor containing developing cells

Exercise 10

1. nephr/o/megaly
2. cyst/itis
3. nephr/o/hyper/trophy
4. urethr/o/cyst/itis
5. cyst/o/cele
6. hydr/o/nephr/osis
7. cyst/o/lith
8. glomerul/o/nephr/itis
9. nephr/oma
10. nephr/o/ptosis
11. nephr/itis
12. nephr/o/lith/iasis
13. ureter/o/cele
14. pyel/itis
15. azot/emia
16. ureter/o/stenosis
17. pyel/o/nephr/itis
18. ureter/o/lith/iasis
19. nephr/o/blast/oma

Exercise 11

Spelling Exercise, see text p. 230.

Exercise 12

Pronunciation Exercise

Exercise 13

1. renal calculus
2. urinary retention
3. polycystic kidney disease
4. hypospadias
5. renal hypertension
6. urinary suppression
7. epispadias
8. urinary tract infection
9. renal failure

Exercise 14

1. c
2. f
3. d
4. h
5. a
6. e
7. b
8. g
9. i

Exercise 15

Spelling Exercise; see text p. 232.

Exercise 16

Pronunciation Exercise

Exercise 17

1. WR CV S
vesic/o/tomy
CF
incison of the bladder

2. WR CV S
cyst/o/tomy
CF
incison of the bladder

3. WR CV S
nephr/o/stomy
CF
creation of an artificial opening into the kidney

4. WR CV S
nephr/o/lysis
CF
separating the kidney

5. WR S
cyst/ectomy
excision of the bladder

6. WR CV WR CV S
pyel/o/lith/o/tomy
CF CF
incision of the renal pelvis to remove a stone

7. WR CV S
nephr/o/pexy
CF
surgical fixation of the kidney

8. WR CV WR CV S
cyst/o/lith/o/tomy
CF CF
incision of the bladder to remove a stone

9. WR S
nephr/ectomy
excision of a kidney

10. WR S
ureter/ectomy
excision of a ureter

11. WR CV S
cyst/o/stomy
CF
creation of an artificial opening into the bladder

12. WR CV S
pyel/o/plasty
CF
surgical repair of the renal pelvis

13. WR CV S
cyst/o/rrhaphy
CF
suturing of the bladder

14. WR CV S
meat/o/tomy
CF
incision of the meatus

15. WR CV S
lith/o/tripsy
CF
surgical crushing of a stone

16. WR CV S
urethr/o/plasty
CF
surgical repair of the urethra

17. WR CV WR S
vesic/o/urethr/al (suspension)
CF
suspension pertaining to the bladder and urethra

18. WR CV WR CV S
nephr/o/lith/o/tomy
CF CF CF
incision of the kidney to remove a stone

19. WR CV S
ureter/o/stomy
CF
creation of an artificial opening into the ureter

20. nephr/o/lith/o/tripsy
surgical crushing of stone in the kidney

Exercise 18

1. ureter/o/stomy
2. nephr/ectomy
3. nephr/o/lith/o/tomy
4. cyst/o/rrhaphy
5. nephr/o/lysis
6. nephr/o/stomy
7. urethr/o/plasty
8. cyst/ectomy
9. meat/o/tomy
10. a. cyst/o/tomy
    b. vesic/o/tomy
11. pyel/o/plasty
12. ureter/ectomy
13. nephr/o/pexy
14. cyst/o/lith/o/tomy
15. lith/o/tripsy
16. vesic/o/urethr/al (suspension)
17. cyst/o/stomy
18. pyel/o/lith/o/tomy
19. nephr/o/lith/o/tripsy

Exercise 19
Spelling Exercise; see text p. 237.

Exercise 20
Pronunciation Exercise

Exercise 21
1. renal transplant
2. fulguration
3. extracorporeal shock wave lithotripsy

Exercise 22
1. b 2. a 3. c

Exercise 23
Spelling Exercise; see text p. 240.

Exercise 24
Pronunciation Exercise

Exercise 25
1. WR CV WR CV S
(voiding) cyst/o/urethr/o/graphy
CF CF
radiographic imaging of the bladder and the urethra
2. WR CV S
cyst/o/graphy
CF
radiographic imaging of the bladder
3. WR CV S
urethr/o/scope
CF
instrument used for visual examination of the urethra
4. WR CV WR CV S
nephr/o/son/o/graphy
CF CF
process of recording the kidney with sound
5. WR CV S
cyst/o/scope
CF
instrument used for visual examination of the bladder
6. WR CV WR CV S
nephr/o/tom/o/gram
CF CF
sectional radiographic image of the kidney
7. WR CV S
cyst/o/gram
CF
radiographic image of the bladder
8. WR CV S
nephr/o/gram
CF
radiographic image of the kidney
9. WR CV S
cyst/o/scopy
CF
visual examination of the bladder
10. WR CV S
nephr/o/graphy
CF
radiographic imaging of the kidney
11. WR CV S
(intravenous) ur/o/gram
CF
radiographic image of the urinary tract (with contrast medium injected intravenously)
12. WR CV S
(retrograde) ur/o/gram
CF
radiographic image of the urinary tract
13. WR CV S
ren/o/gram
CF
(graphic) record of the kidney
14. WR CV S
nephr/o/scopy
CF
visual examination of the kidney
15. WR CV S
ureter/o/scopy
CF
visual examination of the ureter

Exercise 26
1. cyst/o/scopy
2. nephr/o/tom/o/gram
3. intravenous ur/o/gram
4. urethr/o/scope
5. nephr/o/son/o/graphy
6. cyst/o/gram
7. cyst/o/scope
8. (voiding) cyst/o/urethr/o/graphy
9. cyst/o/graphy
10. nephr/o/gram
11. ren/o/gram
12. nephr/o/graphy
13. (retrograde) ur/o/gram
14. nephr/o/scopy
15. ureter/o/scopy

Exercise 27
Spelling Exercise; see text p. 245.

Exercise 28
Pronunciation Exercise

Exercise 29
1. KUB
2. specific gravity
3. blood urea nitrogen
4. urinalysis
5. creatinine

Exercise 30
1. c.
2. b
3. d
4. a
5. f

Exercise 31
Spelling Exercise; see text p. 247.

Exercise 32
Pronunciation Exercise

Exercise 33
1. WR S
noct/uria
night urination
2. WRCV S
ur/o/logist
CF
physician who studies and treats (diseases of) the urinary tract
3. WR S
olig/uria
scanty urine
4. WR CV S
nephr/o/logist
CF
physician who studies and treats diseases of the kidney
5. WR S
hemat/uria
blood in the urine
6. WR CV S
ur/o/logy
CF
study of the urinary tract
7. P S(WR)
poly/uria
much (excessive) urine
8. WR S
albumin/uria
albumin in the urine
9. P S(WR)
an/uria
absence of urine
10. P WR S
di/ur/esis
condition of urine passing through (increased excretion of urine)
11. WR S
py/uria
pus in the urine

12. WR S
    urin/ary
    pertaining to urine
13. WR S
    glycos/uria
    sugar in the urine
14. P S(WR)
    dys/uria
    difficult or painful urination
15. WR CV S
    nephr/o/logy
    CF
    study of the kidney
16. WR CV S
    nephr/o/logist
    CF
    physician who studies and treats diseases of the kidney

Exercise 34
1. noct/uria
2. olig/uria
3. py/uria
4. ur/o/logist
5. poly/uria
6. nephr/o/logist
7. urin/ary
8. hemat/uria
9. ur/o/logy
10. di/ur/esis
11. an/uria
12. glycos/uria
13. dys/uria
14. albumin/uria
15. meat/al
16. nephr/o/logy

Exercise 35
Spelling Exercise; see text p. 251.

Exercise 36
Pronunciation Exercise

Exercise 37
1. urinal
2. hemodialysis
3. distended
4. catheter
5. incontinence
6. urinary catheterization
7. peritoneal dialysis
8. evacuate waste material
9. stricture
10. enuresis
11. micturate
12. urodynamics

Exercise 38
1. e
2. g
3. f
4. a
5. d
6. c

Exercise 39
1. a
2. e
3. g
4. b
5. f
6. c

Exercise 40
Spelling Exercise; see text p. 255.

Exercise 41
1. intravenous urogram; intravenous pyelogram; voiding cystourethrogram
2. specific gravity; urinalysis
3. blood urea nitrogen
4. extracorporeal shock wave lithotripsy
5. catheterization; urinary tract infection
6. hemodialysis
7. acute renal failure, chronic renal failure, end stage renal disease.
8. overactive bladder

Exercise 42
A. 1. nephrolithiasis
2. urology
3. hematuria
4. KUB
5. calculi
6. cystoscopy
7. urogram
8. nephrolithotomy
9. catheter

B. 1. c
2. d
3. *F,* calculus is singular for stone
4. a. pertaining to the ureter
   b. instrument used for visual examination of the ureter

Exercise 43
1. nephroptosis
2. ureterolithiasis
3. remove a stone
4. polyuria
5. nephropexy
6. urinary suppression
7. cystogram
8. enuresis
9. urinary tract infection
10. urinalysis
11. surgical procedure

Exercise 44
Reading Exercise

Exercise 45
1. b.
2. d
3. a

NOTES

Chapter 7

Male Reproductive System

OUTLINE

OBJECTIVES

Upon completion of this chapter you will be able to:

1. Identify organs and structures of the male reproductive system.
2. Define and spell word parts related to the male reproductive system.
3. Define, pronounce, and spell disease and disorder terms related to the male reproductive system.
4. Define, pronounce, and spell surgical terms related to the male reproductive system.
5. Define, pronounce, and spell diagnostic terms related to the male reproductive system.
6. Define, pronounce, and spell complementary terms related to the male reproductive system.
7. Interpret the meaning of abbreviations related to the male reproductive system.
8. Interpret, read, and comprehend medical language in simulated medical statements and documents.

ANATOMY

The organs of the male reproductive system are the genitalia, visible on the outside of the body, and include the testes, scrotum and penis, vas deferens, seminal vesicles, and prostate gland. The urethra and penis are shared with the urinary system.

Function

The function of the male reproductive system is to produce, sustain, and transport sperm, the male reproductive cell, and to secrete the hormone testosterone (Figures 7-1 and 7-2).

Organs of the Male Reproductive System

Term	Definition
testis, or testicle (*pl.* testes, or testicles)	primary male sex organs, paired, oval-shaped, and enclosed in a sac called the **scrotum**. The testes produce spermatozoa (sperm cells) and the hormone testosterone.
sperm (spermatozoon, *pl.* spermatozoa)	the microscopic male germ cell, which, when united with the ovum, produces a zygote (fertilized egg) that with subsequent development becomes an embryo (Figures 7-2 and 7-3)
testosterone	the principal male sex hormone. Its chief function is to stimulate the development of the male reproductive organs and secondary sex characteristics such as facial hair.
seminiferous tubules	approximately 900 coiled tubes within the testes in which spermatogenesis occurs
epididymis	coiled duct atop each of the testes that provides for storage, transit, and maturation of spermatozoa; continuous with the vas deferens
vas deferens, ductus deferens, or seminal duct	duct carrying the sperm from the epididymis to the urethra. The **spermatic cord** encloses each vas deferens with nerves, lymphatics, arteries, and veins. The urethra also connects with the urinary bladder and carries urine outside the body. A circular muscle constricts during intercourse to prevent urination.
seminal vesicles	two main glands located at the base of the bladder that open into the vas deferens. The glands secrete a thick fluid, which forms part of the semen.
prostate gland	encircles the upper end of the urethra. The prostate gland secretes a fluid that aids in the movement of the sperm and ejaculation.
scrotum	sac suspended on both sides of and just behind the penis. The testes are enclosed in the scrotum.

PROSTATE

is derived from the Greek **pro**, meaning **before**, and **statis**, meaning **standing** or **sitting**. Anatomically it is the gland standing before the bladder.

Term	Definition
penis	male organ of urination and copulation (sexual intercourse)
glans penis	enlarged tip on the end of the penis
prepuce	fold of skin covering the glans penis in uncircumcised males (foreskin of the penis)
semen	composed of sperm, seminal fluids, and other secretions
genitalia (genitals)	reproductive organs (male or female)

A & P Booster
For students desiring more anatomy and physiology, go to http://evolve.elsevier.com. Refer to p. 18 for your Evolve Access Information. Select A & P Booster, Chapter 7.

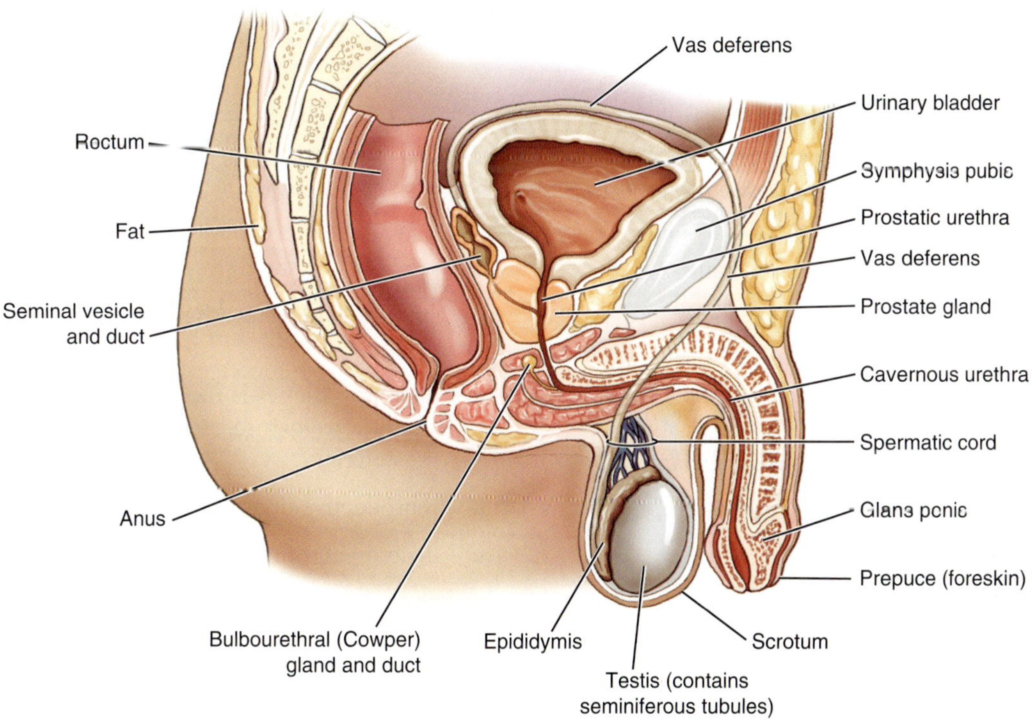

FIGURE 7-1
Male reproductive organs and associated structures.

Sperm formed in the SEMINIFEROUS TUBULES in the testes

↓

EPIDIDYMIS

↓

VAS DEFERENS through the SEMINAL VESICLE and duct

↓

URETHRA through the PROSTATE GLAND through the penis to the outside of the body

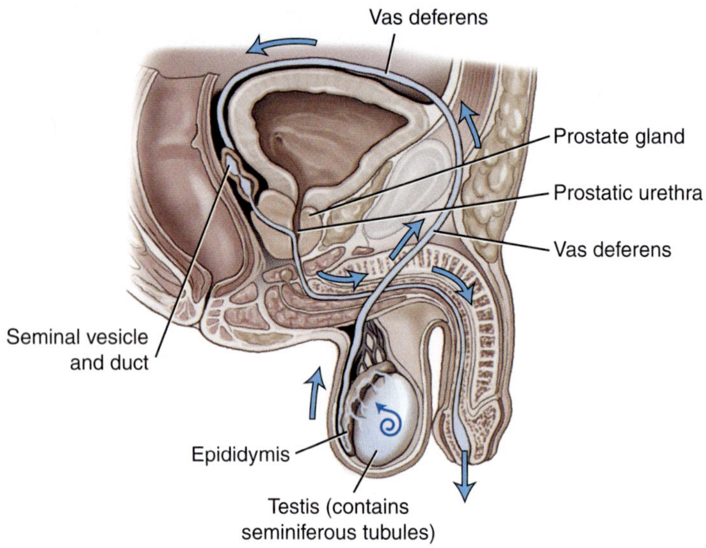

FIGURE 7-2
Origination and transportation of sperm.

EXERCISE 1

Match the anatomic terms in the first column with the correct definitions in the second column. *To check your answers to the exercises in this chapter, go to Answers, p. 305, at the end of the chapter.*

_____ 1. epididymis
_____ 2. glans penis
_____ 3. penis
_____ 4. prepuce, or foreskin
_____ 5. prostate gland
_____ 6. scrotum
_____ 7. semen
_____ 8. seminal vesicles
_____ 9. seminiferous tubules
_____ 10. spermatic cord
_____ 11. testes
_____ 12. vas deferens
_____ 13. genitalia
_____ 14. sperm
_____ 15. testosterone

a. sac in which the testes are enclosed
b. structures in testes where the sperm originate
c. duct atop the testis that stores sperm, allows it to mature, and carries it to the vas deferens
d. reproductive organs (male or female)
e. male organ of copulation
f. encircles upper end of urethra
g. glands that open into the vas deferens
h. primary male sex organs
i. large tip at end of male organ of copulation
j. the male germ cell
k. fold of skin at tip of penis
l. comprises sperm and secretions
m. male sex hormone
n. encloses the vas deferens with other anatomic structures
o. duct that carries sperm to the urethra

WORD PARTS

Word parts you need to learn to complete this chapter are listed on the following pages. The exercises at the end of each list help you learn their definitions and spellings.

Use the flashcards accompanying this text or electronic flashcards to assist you in memorizing the word parts for this chapter.

To use electronic flashcards, go to http://evolve.elsevier.com. Refer to p. 18 for your Evolve Access Information. Select Flashcards, Chapter 7.

Combining Forms of the Male Reproductive System

Combining Form	Definition
balan/o	glans penis
epididym/o	epididymis
orchid/o, orchi/o, orch/o, test/o	testis, testicle
prostat/o	prostate gland
vas/o	vessel, duct
vesicul/o	seminal vesicle

EXERCISE 2

Write the definitions of the following combining forms.

1. test/o ____________________
2. vas/o ____________________
3. balan/o ____________________
4. prostat/o ____________________
5. orch/o ____________________
6. vesicul/o ____________________
7. orchi/o ____________________
8. epididym/o ____________________
9. orchid/o ____________________

EXERCISE FIGURE A

Fill in the blanks with combining forms for this diagram of the male reproductive system. *To check your answers, go to p. 305.*

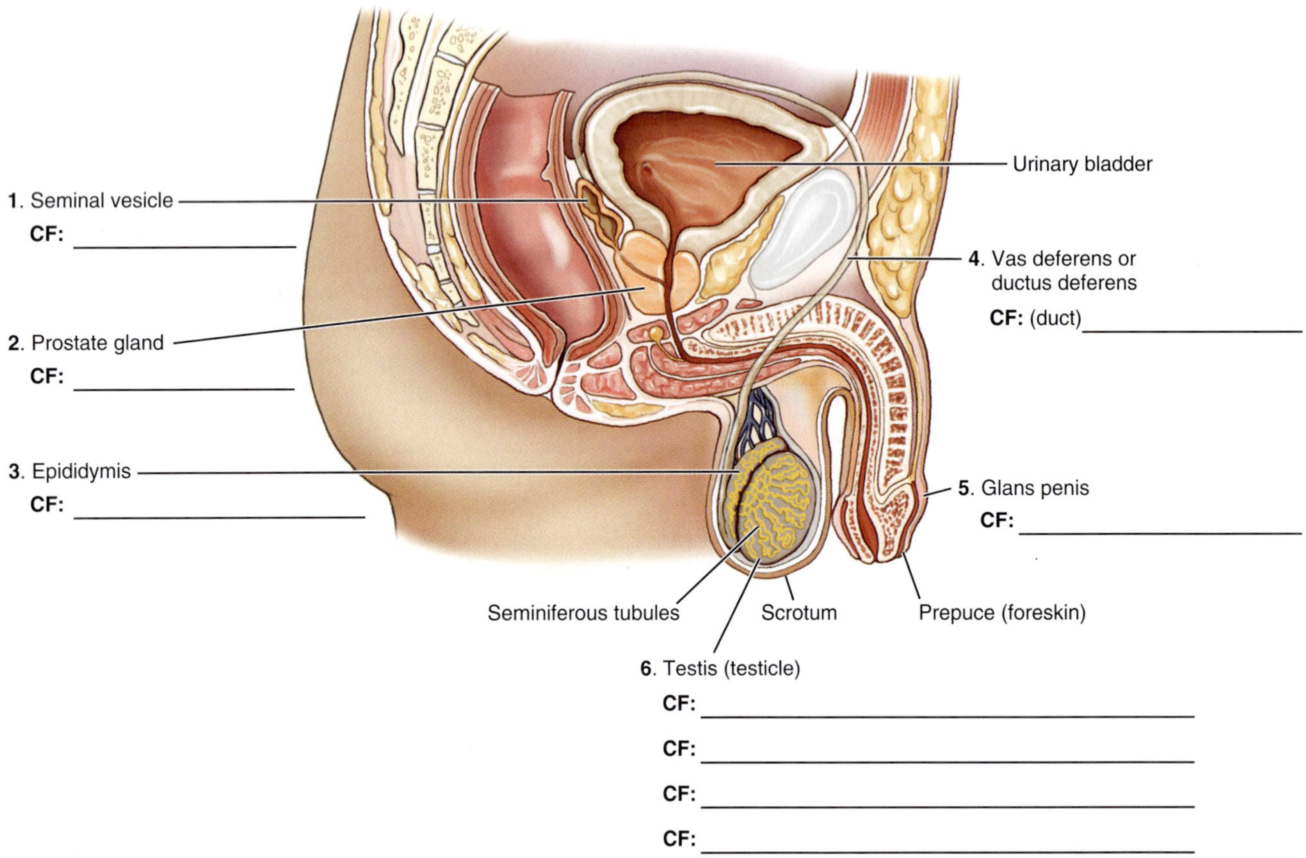

EXERCISE 3

Write the combining form for each of the following terms.

1. vessel, duct ____________
2. prostate gland ____________
3. glans penis ____________
4. seminal vesicle ____________
5. epididymis ____________
6. testicle, or testis
   a. ____________
   b. ____________
   c. ____________
   d. ____________

Combining Forms Commonly Used with Male Reproductive System Terms

Combining Form	Definition
andr/o	male
sperm/o, spermat/o	spermatozoon (*pl.* spermatozoa), sperm (Figure 7-3)

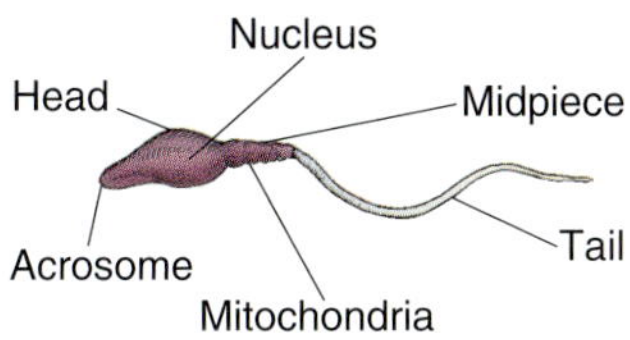

FIGURE 7-3
Spermatozoon, or sperm. In normal ejaculation there may be as many as 300 to 500 million sperm.

EXERCISE 4

Write the definition of the following combining forms.

1. sperm/o ______________
2. andr/o ______________
3. spermat/o ______________

EXERCISE 5

Write the combining form for each of the following.

1. spermatozoon, sperm a. ______________ b. ______________
2. male ______________

Suffix

Suffix	Definition
-ism	state of

Refer to **Appendix A** and **Appendix B** for alphabetized word parts and their meanings.

EXERCISE 6

Write the definition for the suffix.

1. –ism ______________

EXERCISE FIGURE B

Fill in the blanks with word parts to label the diagram.

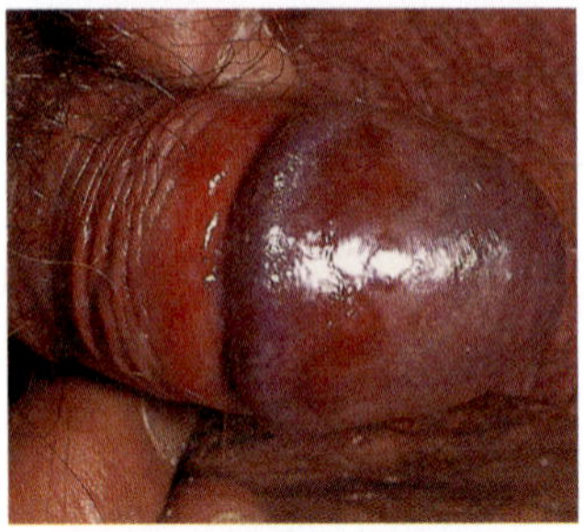

glans penis / inflammation

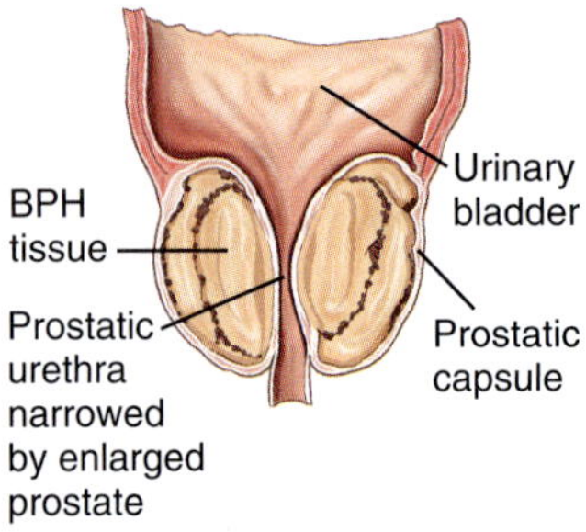

FIGURE 7-4
Benign prostatic hyperplasia grows inward, causing narrowing of the urethra.

BENIGN PROSTATIC HYPERPLASIA AND BENIGN PROSTATIC HYPERTROPHY

As the male ages, the prostate gland may undergo tissue changes called **prostatic hyperplasia**, which is the abnormal increase in the number of cells. The result is an enlarged prostate gland, referred to as **prostatic hypertrophy. Benign prostatic hyperplasia** is the correct term for the pathologic process, but **benign prostatic hypertrophy** is also currently used to describe this condition. As the gland enlarges, it causes narrowing of the urethra, which interferes with the passage of urine. Symptoms include frequency of urination, nocturia, urinary retention, and incomplete emptying of the bladder.

MEDICAL TERMS

The terms you need to learn to complete this chapter are listed below. The exercises following each list will help you learn the definition and the spelling of each word.

Disease and Disorder Terms

Built from Word Parts

The following terms are built from word parts you have already learned and can be translated literally to find their meanings. Further explanation of terms beyond the definition of their word parts, if needed, is included in parentheses.

Term	Definition
anorchism (an-OR-kizm)	state of absence of testis (unilateral or bilateral)
balanitis (*bal*-a-NĪ-tis)	inflammation of the glans penis (Exercise Figure B)
balanorrhea (*bal*-a-nō-RĒ-a)	discharge from the glans penis
benign prostatic hyperplasia (BPH) (be-NĪN) (pros-TAT-ik) (*hī*-per-PLĀ-zha)	excessive development pertaining to the prostate gland (nonmalignant enlargement of the prostate gland) (Figure 7-4)
cryptorchidism (krip-TOR-ki-*diz-m*)	state of hidden testes. (During fetal development, testes are located in the abdominal area near the kidneys. Before birth they move down into the scrotal sac. Failure of the testes to descend from the abdominal cavity into the scrotum before birth results in cryptorchidism, or undescended testicles.) (Exercise Figure C)
epididymitis (*ep*-i-*did*-i-MĪ-tis)	inflammation of an epididymis
orchiepididymitis (*or*-kē-*ep*-i-*did*-i-MĪ-tis)	inflammation of the testis and epididymis
orchitis, orchiditis, or testitis (or-KĪ-tis) (or-ki-DĪ-tis) (tes-TĪ-tis)	inflammation of the testis or testicle
prostatitis (pros-ta-TĪ-tis)	inflammation of the prostate gland
prostatocystitis (*pros*-ta-tō-sis-TĪ-tis)	inflammation of the prostate gland and the bladder
prostatolith (pros-TAT-ō-lith)	stone in the prostate gland
prostatorrhea (pros-ta-tō-RĒ-a)	discharge from the prostate gland
prostatovesiculitis (*pros*-ta-tō-ves-*ik*-ū-LĪ-tis)	inflammation of the prostate gland and seminal vesicles

EXERCISE 7

Practice saying aloud each of the disease and disorder terms built from word parts on p. 276.

To hear the terms, go to http://evolve.elsevier.com. Refer to p. 18 for your Evolve Access Information. Select Exercises & Review, Chapter 7, Chapter Exercises, Pronunciation.

☐ Place a check mark in the box when you have completed this exercise.

EXERCISE FIGURE C

Fill in the blanks to label the diagram.

1

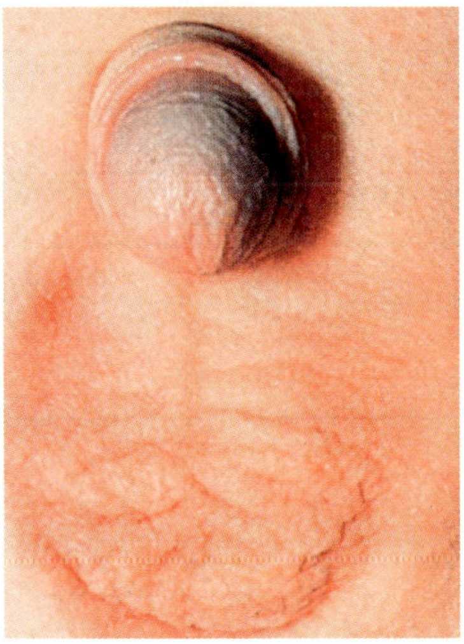

2

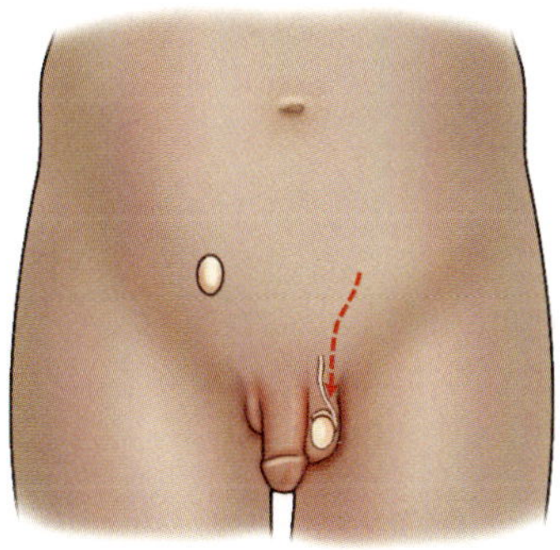

1. ________ / ________ / ________
hidden / testis / state of

2. The *arrow* shows the path the testis takes in its descent to the scrotal sac before birth.

CAM TERM

Herbal therapy uses plant-based remedies to promote health and healing. Studies have documented the efficacy of using a variety of herbs to address the symptoms of **benign prostatic hyperplasia** and the treatment and prevention of **prostate cancer.**

EXERCISE 8

Analyze and define the following disease and disorder terms.

1. prostatolith ________________
2. balanitis ________________
3. a. orchitis ________________
   b. orchiditis ________________
   c. testitis ________________
4. prostatovesiculitis ________________
5. prostatocystitis ________________
6. orchiepididymitis ________________
7. prostatorrhea ________________
8. epididymitis ________________
9. (benign) prostatic hyperplasia ________________
10. cryptorchidism ________________
11. balanorrhea ________________
12. prostatitis ________________
13. anorchism ________________

EXERCISE 9

Build disease and disorder terms for the following definitions with the word parts you have learned.

1. inflammation of the prostate gland and urinary bladder ______ WR / CV / WR / S
2. stone in the prostate gland ______ WR / CV / WR
3. inflammation of the testis
   a. ______ WR / S
   b. ______ WR / S
   c. ______ WR / S
4. (a nonmalignant) excessive development pertaining to the prostate gland

   benign ______ WR / S ______ P / S(WR)
5. state of hidden testes ______ WR / WR / S
6. inflammation of the prostate gland and seminal vesicles ______ WR / CV / WR / S
7. state of absence of testis ______ P / WR / S
8. inflammation of the prostate gland ______ WR / S
9. inflammation of the testis and the epididymis ______ WR / WR / S
10. discharge from the glans penis ______ WR / CV / S
11. inflammation of an epididymis ______ WR / S
12. inflammation of the glans penis ______ WR / S
13. discharge from the prostate gland ______ WR / CV / S

EXERCISE 10

Spell each of the disease and disorder terms built from word parts on p. 276 by having someone dictate them to you.

To hear and spell the terms, go to http://evolve.elsevier.com. Refer to p. 18 for your Evolve Access Information. Select Exercises & Review, Chapter 7, Chapter Exercises, Spelling.

☐ Place a check mark in the box if you have completed this exercise online.

1. ______________________
2. ______________________
3. ______________________
4. ______________________
5. ______________________
6. ______________________
7. ______________________
8. ______________________
9. ______________________
10. ______________________
11. ______________________
12. ______________________
13. ______________________
14. ______________________
15. ______________________

ERECTILE DYSFUNCTION (ED)

Oral therapies, such as sildenafil (Viagra), vardenafil (Levitra), and tadalafil (Cialis) are currently first-line treatment for erectile dysfunction and work by relaxing smooth muscle cells and, as such, increasing the flow of blood in the genital area. Second-line treatment includes penile self-injectable drugs and vacuum devices. Surgical implantation of a penile prosthesis is available for men who cannot use or who have not responded to other treatments.

Disease and Disorder Terms

Not Built from Word Parts

In some of the following terms, you may recognize word parts you have already learned; however, the full meaning of the terms cannot be discerned by the definition of their word parts.

Term	Definition
erectile dysfunction (ED) (e-REK-tīl) (dis-FUNK-shun)	the inability of the male to attain or maintain an erection sufficient to perform sexual intercourse (formerly called **impotence**)
hydrocele (HĪ-drō-sēl)	scrotal swelling caused by a collection of fluid (Figure 7-5)
phimosis (fi-MŌ-sis)	a tightness of the prepuce (foreskin of the penis) that prevents its retraction over the glans penis; it may be congenital or a result of balanitis. Circumcision is the usual treatment (Figure 7-6).
priapism (PRĪ-a-*piz-m*)	persistent abnormal erection of the penis accompanied by pain and tenderness
prostate cancer (PROS-tāt) (KAN-cer)	cancer of the prostate gland, usually occurring later in life (Table 7-1)
testicular cancer (tes-TIK-ū-ler) (KAN-cer)	cancer of the testicle, usually occurring in men 15 to 35 years of age

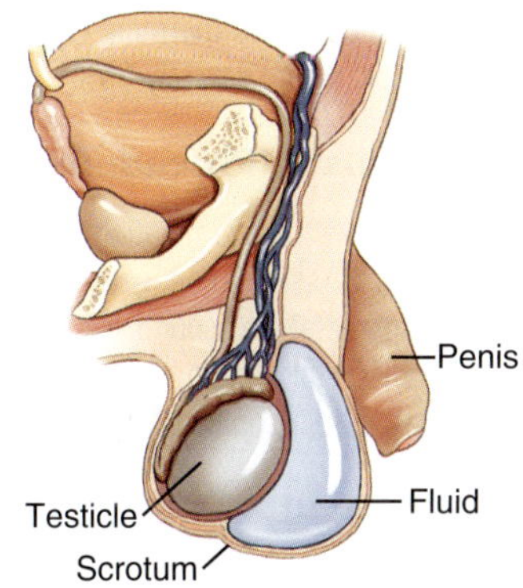

FIGURE 7-5
Hydrocele.

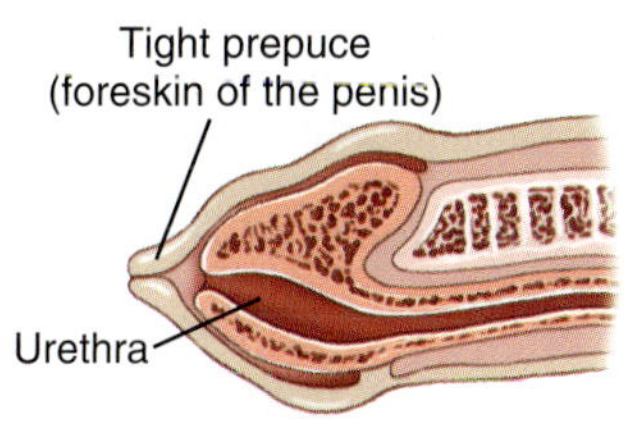

FIGURE 7-6
Phimosis. Cross section of the penis showing foreskin covering the opening.

Disease and Disorder Terms—*cont'd*

Not Built from Word Parts

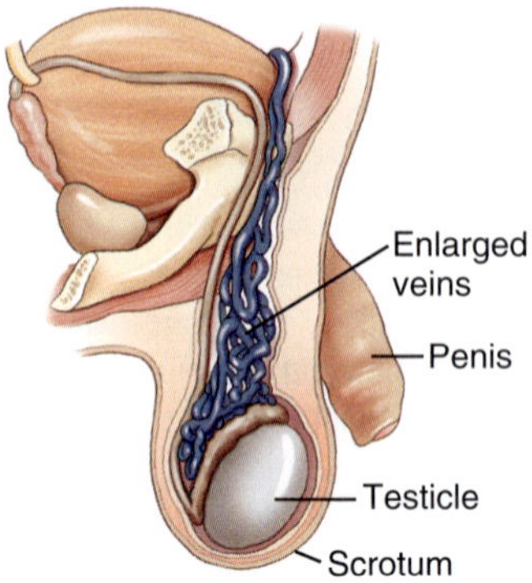

FIGURE 7-7
Varicocele.

Term	Definition
testicular torsion (tes-TIK-ū-ler) (TOR-shun)	twisting of the spermatic cord causing decreased blood flow to the testis; occurs most often during puberty and often presents with a sudden onset of severe testicular or scrotal pain. Because of lack of blood flow to the testis, it is often considered a surgical emergency.
varicocele (VAR-i-kō-*sēl*)	enlarged veins of the spermatic cord (Figure 7-7)

TABLE 7-1

Prostate Cancer

Prostate cancer is the most commonly diagnosed cancer in men and the second most common cause of cancer death among men in the United States. Approximately 95% of all cancers of the prostate are adenocarcinomas, arising from epithelial cells.

Diagnostic Procedures

1. Digital rectal examination (DRE)
2. Prostate-specific antigen (PSA)
3. Transrectal ultrasound
4. Transrectal ultrasonically guided biopsy
5. Magnetic resonance imaging with endorectal surface coil

Treatment

Treatment depends on the stage of the prostate cancer, the age of the patient, and choices of treatment by the patient and his physician. Options include the following:

1. **Radical prostatectomy (RP)**, which may be performed by retropubic or perineal routes, laparoscopically, or with the use of robotic-assisted devices
2. **Radiation therapy**, which may be performed with an external beam or with radioactive seeds (brachytherapy)
3. **Bilateral orchidectomy** or **hormonal therapy** to reduce the production of testosterone, which fuels the growth of prostate cancer
4. **Chemotherapy**, treating cancer with drugs
5. **Watchful waiting**, with the intent to pursue active therapy on disease progression

Progression of Prostate Cancer

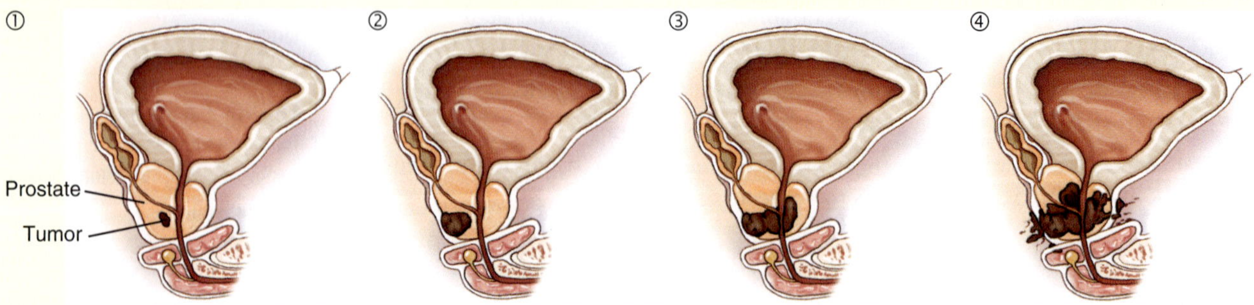

EXERCISE 11

Practice saying aloud each of the disease and disorder terms not built from word parts on pp. 279-280.

To hear the terms, go to http://evolve.elsevier.com. Refer to p. 18 for your Evolve Access Information. Select Exercises & Review, Chapter 7, Chapter Exercises, Pronunciation.

☐ Place a check mark in the box when you have completed this exercise.

EXERCISE 12

Fill in the blanks with the correct terms.

1. Another way of referring to cancer of the testicle is ________________ ________________.
2. A tightness of the prepuce is called ________________.
3. The condition of having enlarged veins of the spermatic cord is known medically as a(n) ________________.
4. A scrotal swelling caused by a collection of fluid is called a(n) ________________.
5. Cancer of the prostate gland is called ________________ ________________.
6. Inability of the man to attain or maintain an erection is called ________________ ________________.
7. Persistent abnormal erection is called ________________.
8. ________________ ________________ is the twisting of the spermatic cord.

EXERCISE 13

Match the terms in the first column with the correct definitions in the second column.

_____ 1. varicocele	a.	scrotal swelling caused by a collection of fluid
_____ 2. phimosis	b.	inability to attain or maintain an erection
_____ 3. testicular cancer	c.	a condition that prevents the retraction of the prepuce
_____ 4. erectile dysfunction	d.	enlarged veins of the spermatic cord
_____ 5. hydrocele	e.	cancer of the testicle
_____ 6. prostate cancer	f.	cancer of the prostate gland
_____ 7. testicular torsion	g.	stone in the prostate gland
_____ 8. priapism	h.	persistent abnormal erection
	i.	twisting of the spermatic cord

EXERCISE 14

Spell each of the disease and disorder terms not built from word parts on pp. 279-280 by having someone dictate them to you.

To hear and spell the terms, go to http://evolve.elsevier.com. Refer to p. 18 for your Evolve Access Information. Select Exercises & Review, Chapter 7, Chapter Exercises, Spelling.

☐ Place a check mark in the box if you have completed this exercise online.

1. ______________________
2. ______________________
3. ______________________
4. ______________________
5. ______________________
6. ______________________
7. ______________________
8. ______________________

Surgical Terms

Built from Word Parts

The following terms are built from word parts you have already learned and can be translated literally to find their meanings. Further explanation of terms beyond the definitions of their word parts, if needed, is included in parentheses.

Term	Definition
balanoplasty (BAL-a-nō-*plas*-tē)	surgical repair of the glans penis
epididymectomy (*ep*-i-*did*-i-MEK-to-mē)	excision of an epididymis
orchidectomy, orchiectomy (*or*-kid-EK-to-mē), (*or*-kē-EK-to-mē)	excision of the testis (bilateral orchidectomy also is called **castration**)
orchidopexy, orchiopexy (OR-kid-ō-pek-sē), (OR-kē-ō-pek-sē)	surgical fixation of a testicle (performed to bring undescended testicle[s] into the scrotum)
orchidotomy, orchiotomy (*or*-kid-OT-o-mē), (*or*-kē-OT-o-mē)	incision into a testis
orchioplasty (OR-kē-ō-*plas*-tē)	surgical repair of a testis
prostatectomy (*pros*-ta-TEK-to-mē)	excision of the prostate gland
prostatocystotomy (*pros*-tat-ō-sis-TOT-o-mē)	incision into the prostate gland and bladder
prostatolithotomy (*pros*-tat-ō-li-THOT-o-mē)	incision into the prostate gland to remove a stone
prostatovesiculectomy (*pros*-tat-ō-ves-*ik*-ū-LEK-to-mē)	excision of the prostate gland and seminal vesicles

Term	Definition
vasectomy (va-SEK-to-mē)	excision of a duct (partial excision of the vas deferens bilaterally, resulting in male sterilization) (Exercise Figure D)
vasovasostomy (*vas*-ō-vā-ZOS-to-mē)	creation of artificial openings between ducts (the severed ends of the vas deferens are reconnected in an attempt to restore fertility in men who have had a vasectomy)
vesiculectomy (ve-*sik*-ū-LEK-to-mē)	excision of the seminal vesicle(s)

EXERCISE FIGURE D

Fill in the blanks to label the diagram.

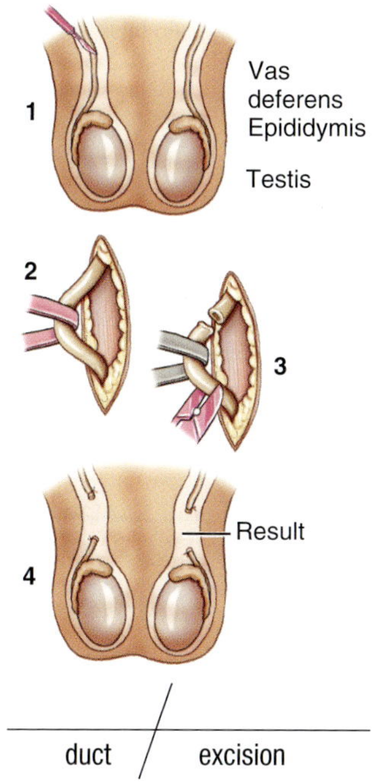

1. incision is made into the covering of the vas deferens
2. vas deferens is exposed
3. segment of vas deferens is excised
4. vas deferens is repositioned and skin is sutured

EXERCISE 15

Practice saying aloud each of the surgical terms built from word parts on these two pages.

To hear the terms, go to http://evolve.elsevier.com. Refer to p. 18 for your Evolve Access Information. Select Exercises & Review, Chapter 7, Chapter Exercises, Pronunciation.

☐ Place a check mark in the box when you have completed this exercise.

EXERCISE 16

Analyze and define the following surgical terms.

1. vasectomy ______________________
2. prostatocystotomy ______________________
3. orchidotomy, orchiotomy ______________________
4. epididymectomy ______________________
5. orchidopexy, orchiopexy ______________________
6. prostatovesiculectomy ______________________
7. orchioplasty ______________________
8. vesiculectomy ______________________
9. prostatectomy ______________________
10. balanoplasty ______________________
11. vasovasostomy ______________________
12. orchidectomy, orchiectomy ______________________
13. prostatolithotomy ______________________

EXERCISE 17

Build surgical terms for the following definitions by using the word parts you have learned.

1. excision of the testis
   a. ______ WR / S ______
   b. ______ WR / S ______
2. surgical repair of the glans penis ______ WR /CV/ S ______
3. incision into the prostate gland and bladder ______ WR /CV/ WR /CV/ S ______
4. excision of the seminal vesicle(s) ______ WR / S ______
5. incision into the prostate gland to remove a stone ______ WR /CV/ WR /CV/ S ______
6. incision into a testis
   a. ______ WR /CV/ S ______
   b. ______ WR /CV/ S ______
7. excision of the epididymis ______ WR / S ______
8. surgical repair of a testis ______ WR /CV/ S ______
9. excision of the prostate gland ______ WR / S ______
10. excision of a duct (partial excision of the vas deferens) ______ WR / S ______
11. excision of the prostate gland and seminal vesicles ______ WR /CV/ WR / S ______
12. surgical fixation of a testicle
    a. ______ WR /CV/ S ______
    b. ______ WR /CV/ S ______
13. creation of artificial openings between the severed ends of the vas deferens ______ WR /CV/ WR /CV/ S ______

EXERCISE 18

Spell each of the surgical terms built from word parts on pp. 282-283 by having someone dictate them to you.

To hear and spell the terms, go to http://evolve.elsevier.com. Refer to p. 18 for your Evolve Access Information. Select Exercises & Review, Chapter 7, Chapter Exercises, Spelling.

☐ Place a check mark in the box if you have completed this exercise online.

1. ____________________ 9. ____________________
2. ____________________ 10. ____________________
3. ____________________ 11. ____________________
4. ____________________ 12. ____________________
5. ____________________ 13. ____________________
6. ____________________ 14. ____________________
7. ____________________ 15. ____________________
8. ____________________ 16. ____________________

Surgical Terms

Not Built from Word Parts

In some of the following terms, you may recognize word parts you have already learned; however, the full meaning of the terms cannot be discerned by the definition of their word parts.

Term	Definition
circumcision (*ser*-kum-SI-zhun)	surgical removal of the prepuce (foreskin) (Figure 7-8)
hydrocelectomy (*hī*-drō-sē-LEK-to-mē)	surgical removal of a hydrocele
radical prostatectomy (RP) (RAD-i-kel) (*pros*-ta-TEK-to-mē)	excision of the prostate gland with its capsule, seminal vesicles, vas deferens, and sometimes pelvic lymph nodes; performed by a retropubic or perineal approach, or laparoscopically; used to treat prostate cancer (Figure 7-9, *B* and 7-10)
suprapubic prostatectomy (*sū*-pra-PŪ-bik) (*pros*-ta-TEK-to-mē)	excision of the prostate gland through an abdominal incision made above the pubic bone and through an incision in the bladder; used to treat benign prostatic hyperplasia and prostate cancer (Figure 7-9, *A*) (also called **suprapubic transvesical prostatectomy**)

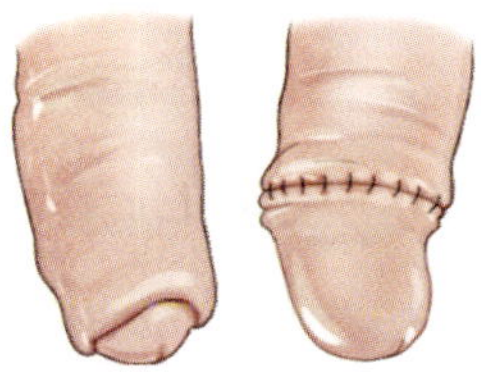

FIGURE 7-8
Circumcision.

Surgical Terms—*cont'd*

Not Built from Word Parts

Term	Definition
transurethral incision of the prostate gland (TUIP) (trans-ū-RĒ-thral) (in-SIZH-en) (PROS-tāt)	a surgical procedure that widens the urethra by making a few small incisions in the bladder neck and the prostate gland. No prostate tissue is removed. TUIP may be used instead of TURP when the prostate gland is less enlarged.
transurethral microwave thermotherapy (TUMT) (trans-ū-RĒ-thral) (MĪ-krō-wāv) (*ther*-mō-THER-a-pē)	a treatment that eliminates excess tissue present in benign prostatic hyperplasia by using heat generated by microwave
transurethral resection of the prostate gland (TURP) (trans-ū-RĒ-thral) (rē-SEK-shun) (PROS-tāt)	surgical removal of pieces of the prostate gland tissue by using a resectoscope inserted through the urethra. The capsule is left intact; usually performed when the enlarged prostate gland interferes with urination (Table 7-2).

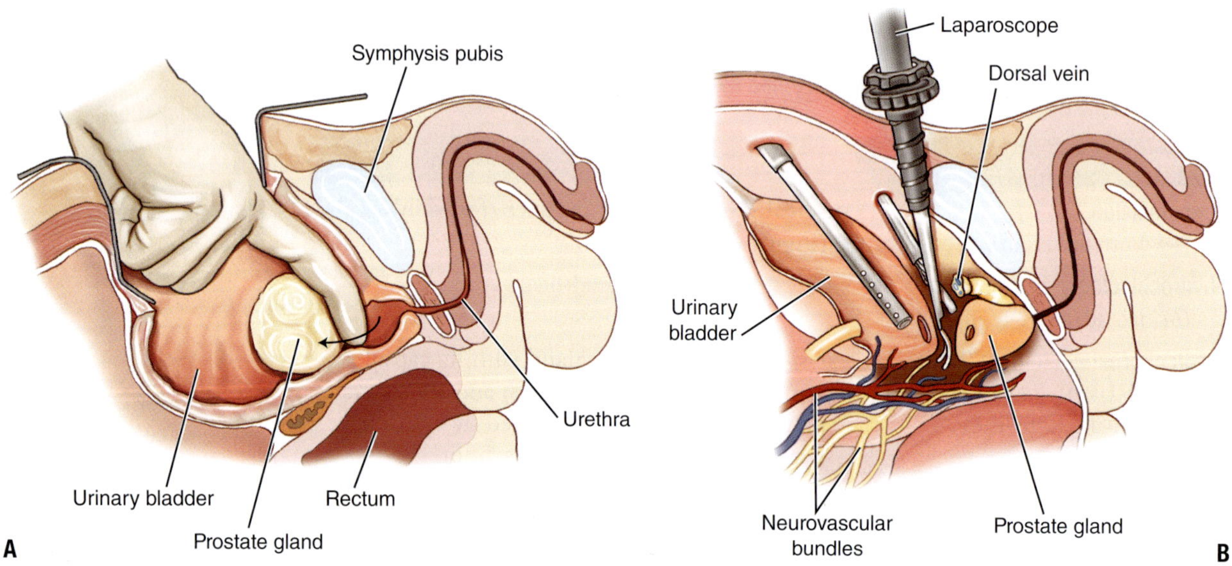

FIGURE 7-9

A, A large incision surgery. In suprapubic prostatectomy, the surgeon approaches the prostate gland through an incision in the urinary bladder and uses a finger to remove the hyperplastic tissue. A similar incision is used for radical retropubic prostectomy to treat cancer of the prostate. **B**, A small incision surgery. Laparoscopic radical prostatectomy and/or robotic-assisted prostatectomy is a new procedure used to treat early stages of prostate cancer.

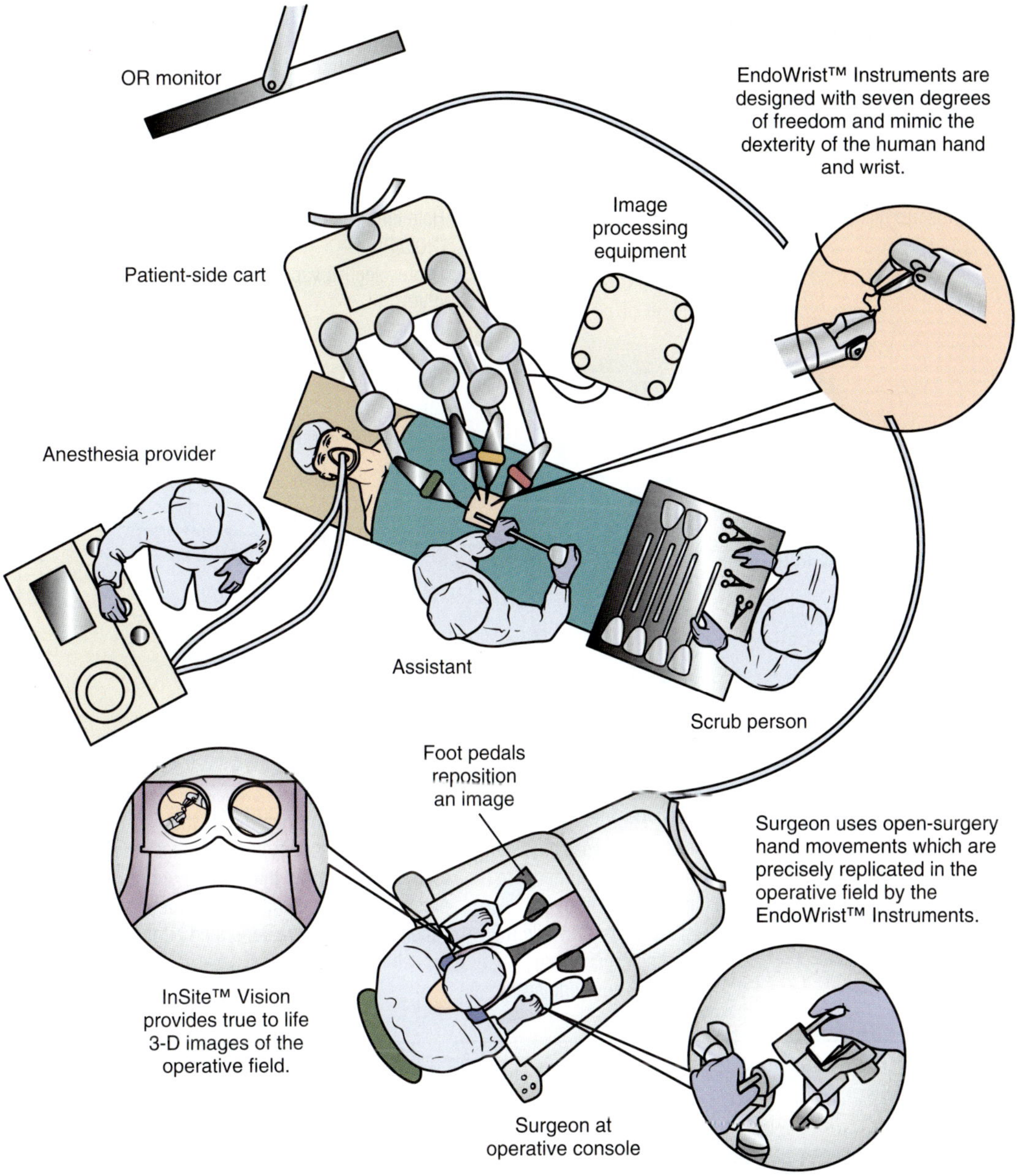

FIGURE 7-10
Operating room set-up for robotic-assisted laparoscopic radical prostatectomy (RALRP) with a da Vinci robotic system.

TABLE 7-2
Surgical Treatments for Benign Prostatic Hyperplasia

Incisional	Thermotherapy	Laser Prostatectomy
1. Transurethral resection of the prostate gland (TURP) 2. Prostatectomy 3. Transurethral incision of the prostate gland (TIP)	1. Transurethral microwave thermotherapy (TUMT) 2. Cooled Thermotherapy	1. Transurethral laser incision of the prostate gland (TULIP) 2. Holmium laser enucleation of the prostate gland (HOLEP) 3. Photoselective vaporization of the prostate gland (PVP)

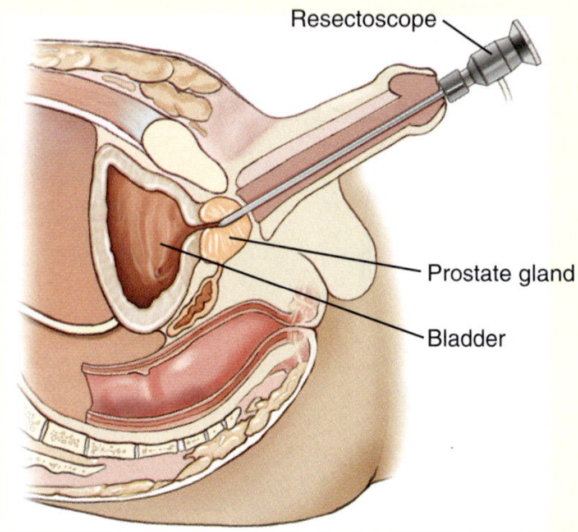

Transurethral resection of the prostate gland (TURP) uses a resectoscope inserted through the urethra to the prostate gland. The end of the instrument is equipped to remove pieces of the enlarged prostate gland to relieve bladder outlet obstruction.

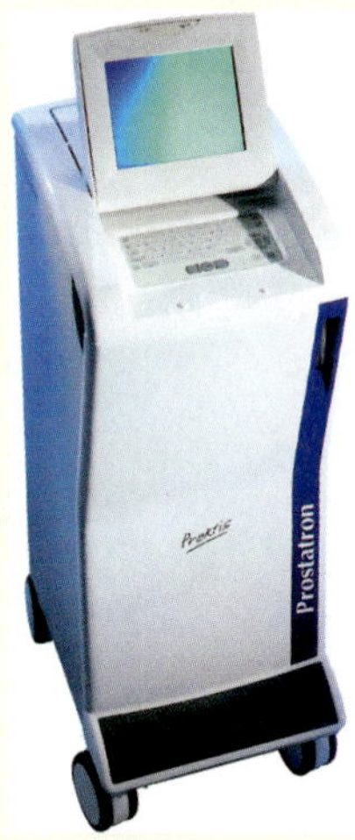

Cooled ThermoTherapy device delivers precise microwavable energy to heat and destroy prostate tissue while a cooling mechanism protects surrounding tissue.

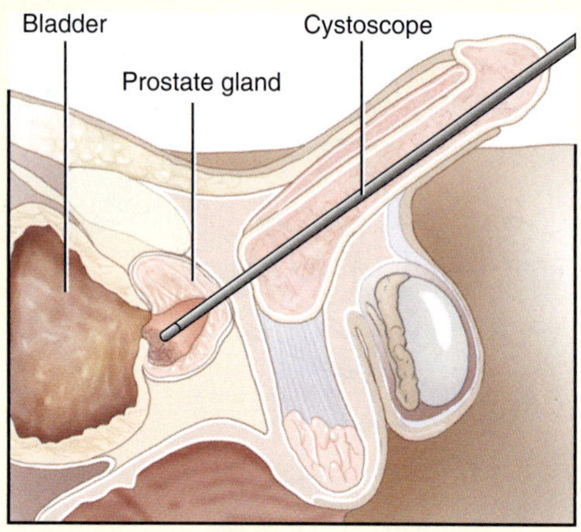

Photoselective vaporization of the prostate gland (PVP) uses a laser system operated through a cystoscope inserted through the urethra to the prostate gland. Overgrown prostate tissue is vaporized using heat generated by the laser.

EXERCISE 19

Practice saying aloud each of the surgical terms not built from word parts on pp. 285-286.

To hear the terms, go to http://evolve.elsevier.com. Refer to p. 18 for your Evolve Access Information. Select Exercises & Review, Chapter 7, Chapter Exercises, Pronunciation.

☐ Place a check mark in the box when you have completed this exercise.

EXERCISE 20

Fill in the blanks with the correct term.

1. The surgery performed to remove the prostate gland through the urinary bladder and an abdominal incision is ____________________ ____________________.
2. The surgical procedure performed to remove the prepuce is called a(n) ____________________.
3. The surgical removal of the prostate gland and surrounding structures, sometimes including pelvic lymph nodes, is called ____________________ ____________________.
4. Surgical removal of a hydrocele is ______________________________________.
5. ____________________ ____________________ ____________________ is a treatment for benign prostatic hyperplasia that uses heat generated by microwave.
6. A surgical procedure for benign prostatic hyperplasia that widens the urethra by making small incisions is called ____________________ ____________________ of the ____________________ ____________________.
7. Pieces of prostate gland tissue are removed with a resectoscope during the surgical procedure called ____________________ ____________________ of the ____________________ ____________________.

EXERCISE 21

Spell each of the surgical terms not built from word parts on pp. 285-286 by having someone dictate them to you.

To hear and spell the terms, go to http://evolve.elsevier.com. Refer to p. 18 for your Evolve Access Information. Select Exercises & Review, Chapter 7, Chapter Exercises, Spelling.

☐ Place a check mark in the box if you have completed this exercise online.

1. ______________________________
2. ______________________________
3. ______________________________
4. ______________________________
5. ______________________________
6. ______________________________
7. ______________________________

Diagnostic Terms

Not Built from Word Parts

In some of the following terms, you may recognize word parts you have already learned; however, the full meaning of the terms cannot be discerned by the definition of their word parts.

Term	Definition
DIAGNOSTIC IMAGING	
transrectal ultrasound (TRUS) (trans-REK-tal) (UL-tra-sound)	an ultrasound procedure used to diagnose prostate cancer. Sound waves are sent and received by a transducer in the form of a probe that is placed into the rectum. The sound waves are transformed into an image of the prostate gland.
LABORATORY	
prostate-specific antigen (PSA) (PROS-tāt) (spe-SIF-ik) (AN-ti-jen)	a blood test that measures the level of prostate-specific antigen in the blood. Elevated test results may indicate the presence of prostate cancer or excess prostate tissue, as found in benign prostatic hyperplasia.
semen analysis (SĒ-men) (a-NAL-i-sis)	microscopic observation of ejaculated semen, revealing the size, structure, and movement of sperm; used to evaluate male infertility and to determine the effectiveness of a vasectomy (also called **sperm count** and **sperm test**).
OTHER	
digital rectal examination (DRE) (DIJ-i-tal) (REK-tal) (eg-*zam*-i-NĀ-shun)	a physical examination in which the physician inserts a finger into the rectum and feels for the size and shape of the prostate gland through the rectal wall. Used to screen for BPH and cancer of the prostate. BPH usually presents as a uniform, nontender enlargement, whereas cancer usually presents as a stony hard nodule.

EXERCISE 22

Practice saying aloud each of the diagnostic terms not built from word parts above.

To hear the terms, go to http://evolve.elsevier.com. Refer to p. 18 for your Evolve Access Information. Select Exercises & Review, Chapter 7, Chapter Exercises, Pronunciation.

☐ Place a check mark in the box when you have completed this exercise.

EXERCISE 23

Fill in the blanks with the correct terms.

1. A physical examination in which the physician feels for the size and shape of the prostate gland through the rectal wall is called _________________ _________________ _________________.
2. A blood test that, when elevated, may indicate the presence of prostate cancer is called _________________ _________________ _________________.
3. A diagnostic ultrasound procedure used to obtain images of the prostate gland is called _________________ _________________.
4. A laboratory test for microscopic observation of ejaculated semen to evaluate male infertility is called _________________ _________________.

EXERCISE 24

Spell each of the diagnostic terms not built from word parts on p. 290 by having someone dictate them to you.

To hear and spell the terms, go to http://evolve.elsevier.com. Refer to p. 18 for your Evolve Access Information. Select Exercises & Review, Chapter 7, Chapter Exercises, Spelling.
☐ Place a check mark in the box if you have completed this exercise online.

1. _________________
2. _________________
3. _________________
4. _________________

Complementary Terms

Built from Word Parts

The following terms are built from word parts you have already learned and can be translated literally to find their meanings. Further explanation of terms beyond the definitions of their word parts, if needed, is included in parentheses.

Term	Definition
andropathy (an-DROP-a-thē)	disease of the male (specific to the male, such as testitis)
aspermia (a-SPER-mē-a)	condition of being without sperm (or semen or ejaculation)
oligospermia (*ol*-i-gō-SPER-mē-a)	condition of scanty sperm (in the semen; may contribute to infertility)
spermatolysis (*sper*-ma-TOL-i-sis)	dissolution (destruction) of sperm

ASPERMIA

condition of without sperm, may indicate the lack of production of spermatozoa, the lack of production of semen, or the lack of ejaculation of semen.

EXERCISE 25

Practice saying aloud each of the complementary terms built from word parts on p. 291.

To hear the terms, go to http://evolve.elsevier.com. Refer to p. 18 for your Evolve Access Information. Select Exercises & Review, Chapter 7, Chapter Exercises, Pronunciation.

☐ Place a check mark in the box when you have completed this exercise.

EXERCISE 26

Analyze and define the following complementary terms.

1. oligospermia ______________________________
2. andropathy ______________________________
3. spermatolysis ______________________________
4. aspermia ______________________________

EXERCISE 27

Build the complementary terms for the following definitions by using the word parts you have learned.

1. dissolution (destruction) of sperm
   ______ / ______ / ______
   WR / CV / S

2. condition of without spermatozoa (or semen or ejaculation)
   ______ / ______ / ______
   P / WR / S

3. disease of the male
   ______ / ______ / ______
   WR / CV / S

4. condition of scanty sperm (in the semen)
   ______ / ______ / ______ / ______
   WR / CV / WR / S

EXERCISE 28

Spell each of the complementary terms built from word parts on p. 291 by having someone dictate them to you.

To hear and spell the terms, go to http://evolve.elsevier.com. Refer to p. 18 for your Evolve Access Information. Select Exercises & Review, Chapter 7, Chapter Exercises, Spelling.

☐ Place a check mark in the box if you have completed this exercise online.

1. ______________________________
2. ______________________________
3. ______________________________
4. ______________________________

Complementary Terms

Not Built from Word Parts

In some of the following terms, you may recognize word parts you have already learned; however, the full meaning of the terms cannot be discerned by the definition of their word parts.

Term	Definition
acquired immunodeficiency syndrome (AIDS) (*im*-ū-nō-de-FISH-en-sē) (SIN-drōm)	a disease that affects the body's immune system, transmitted by exchange of body fluid during the sexual act, reuse of contaminated needles, or receiving contaminated blood transfusions (also called **acquired immune deficiency syndrome**)
artificial insemination (ar-ti-FISH-al) (in-*sem*-i-NĀ-shun)	introduction of semen into the vagina by artificial means
azoospermia (ā-*zō*-a-SPUR-mē-a)	lack of live sperm in the semen
chlamydia (kla-MID-ē-a)	a sexually transmitted disease, sometimes referred to as a **silent STD** because many people are not aware they have the disease. Symptoms that occur when the disease becomes serious are painful urination and discharge from the penis in men and genital itching, vaginal discharge, and bleeding between menstrual periods in women. The causative agent is *C. trachomatis*.
coitus (KŌ-i-tus)	sexual intercourse between male and female (also called **copulation**)
condom (KON-dum)	cover for the penis worn during coitus to prevent conception and the spread of sexually transmitted disease
ejaculation (ē-*jak*-ū-LĀ-shun)	ejection of semen from the male urethra
genital herpes (JEN-i-tal) (HER-pēz)	sexually transmitted disease caused by *Herpesvirus hominis* type 2 (also called **herpes simplex virus**)
gonads (GŌ-nads)	male and female sex glands
gonorrhea (gon-ō-RĒ-a)	contagious, inflammatory sexually transmitted disease caused by a bacterial organism that affects the mucous membranes of the genitourinary system
heterosexual (*het*-er-ō-SEK-shū-al)	person who is attracted to a member of the opposite sex
homosexual (*hō*-mō-SEK-shū-al)	person who is attracted to a member of the same sex

AZOOSPERMIA

the lack of live sperm in the semen, may be:

1) **obstructive**, caused by blocked vessels or ducts;

2) **nonobstructive**, caused by infection, lack of production of spermatozoa, or retrograde ejaculation where semen travels into the urinary bladder rather than exiting through the urethra.

Complementary Terms—*cont'd*

Not Built from Word Parts

Term	Definition
human immunodeficiency virus (HIV) (*im*-ū-nō-de-FISH-en-sē)	a type of retrovirus that causes AIDS. HIV infects T-helper cells of the immune system, allowing for opportunistic infections such as candidiasis, *Pneumocystis jiroveci* pneumonia, tuberculosis, and Kaposi sarcoma
human papillomavirus (HPV) (HŪ-man) (*pap*-i-LŌ-ma-*vī*-rus)	a prevalent sexually transmitted disease causing benign or cancerous growths in male and female genitals (also called **venereal warts**)
infertility (*in*-fer-TIL-i-tē)	reduced or absent ability to produce offspring
orgasm (ŌR-gazm)	climax of sexual stimulation
puberty (PŪ-ber-tē)	period when secondary sex characteristics develop and the ability to reproduce sexually begins
sexually transmitted disease (STD) (SEK-shū-al-ē) (TRANS-mi-ted) (di-ZĒZ)	diseases, such as syphilis, gonorrhea, and genital herpes, transmitted during sexual contact (also called **venereal disease** and **sexually transmitted infection [STI]**)
sterilization (*stār*-i-li-ZĀ-shun)	process that renders an individual unable to produce offspring
syphilis (SIF-i-lis)	chronic infection caused by the bacterium *Treponema pallidum*, which usually is transmitted by sexual contact, may be acquired in utero, or (less often) contracted through direct contact with infected tissue. If untreated, the infection usually progresses through three clinical stages with a latent period. The initial local infection quickly becomes systemic with widespread dissemination of the bacterium (Figure 7-11).
trichomoniasis (*trik*-ō-mō-NĪ-a-sis)	a sexually transmitted disease caused by a one-cell organism, *Trichomonas*. It infects the genitourinary tract. Men may be asymptomatic or may develop urethritis, an enlarged prostate gland, or epididymitis. Women have vaginal itching, dysuria, and vaginal or urethral discharge.

HUMAN PAPILLOMAVIRUS

infection in women is thought to be a major cause of cervical cancer.

LIST OF MALE AND FEMALE SEXUALLY TRANSMITTED DISEASES

- acquired immunodeficiency syndrome
- human immunodeficiency virus infections
- syphilis
- genital herpes
- venereal warts (human papillomavirus)
- gonorrhea
- chlamydia
- trichomoniasis
- cytomegalovirus infections

VENEREAL

is derived from **Venus**, the goddess of love. In ancient times it was noted that the disease was part of the misfortunes of love.

Refer to **Appendix D** for pharmacology terms.

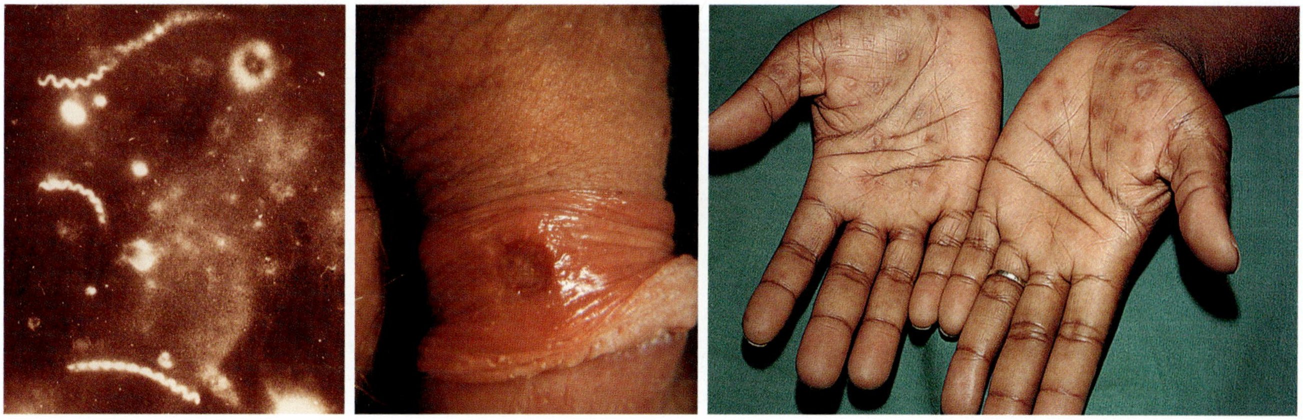

A B C

FIGURE 7-11
Syphilis. A) *Treponema pallidum*, organism responsible for syphilis viewed microscopically; B) Primary syphilis, depiciting a syphilitic chancre. C) Secondary syphilis, depicting rash on palms of hands.

EXERCISE 29

Practice saying aloud each of the complementary terms not built from word parts on pp. 293-294.

To hear the terms, go to http://evolve.elsevier.com. Refer to p. 18 for your Evolve Access Information. Select Exercises & Review, Chapter 7, Chapter Exercises, Pronunciation.

☐ Place a check mark in the box when you have completed this exercise.

EXERCISE 30

Write the definitions of the following complementary terms.

1. puberty ____________________
2. orgasm ____________________
3. gonorrhea ____________________
4. homosexual ____________________
5. coitus ____________________
6. genital herpes ____________________
7. heterosexual ____________________
8. syphilis ____________________
9. ejaculation ____________________
10. gonads ____________________
11. sexually transmitted disease ____________________
12. sterilization ____________________
13. human papillomavirus ____________________
14. acquired immunodeficiency syndrome ____________________
15. trichomoniasis ____________________
16. artificial insemination ____________________
17. chlamydia ____________________
18. condom ____________________

19. infertility ______________________________

20. human immunodeficiency virus ______________________________

21. azoospermia ______________________________

EXERCISE 31

Match the terms in the first column with their correct definitions in the second column.

_____ 1. coitus

_____ 2. ejaculation

_____ 3. human papillomavirus

_____ 4. gonads

_____ 5. genital herpes

_____ 6. gonorrhea

_____ 7. heterosexual

_____ 8. orgasm

_____ 9. condom

_____ 10. azoospermia

a. male and female sex glands

b. climax of sexual stimulation

c. one who is attracted to a member of the opposite sex

d. STD caused by *Herpesvirus hominis* type 2

e. ejection of semen

f. lack of live sperm in the semen

g. sexual intercourse between man and woman

h. venereal warts

i. contagious and inflammatory STD

j. cover for the penis worn during coitus

k. one who is attracted to a member of the same sex

EXERCISE 32

Match the terms in the first column with their correct definitions in the second column.

_____ 1. homosexual

_____ 2. STD

_____ 3. sterilization

_____ 4. syphilis

_____ 5. puberty

_____ 6. AIDS

_____ 7. trichomoniasis

_____ 8. artificial insemination

_____ 9. chlamydia

_____ 10. HIV

_____ 11. infertility

a. abbreviation for diseases such as syphilis, gonorrhea, and genital herpes

b. a disease that affects the body's immune system

c. a type of retrovirus that causes AIDS

d. a chronic infection that can be transmitted by sexual contact or acquired in utero

e. introduction of semen into the vagina by means other than intercourse

f. one who is attracted to members of the same sex

g. a prevalent STD caused by a bacterium, *C. trachomatis* (silent STD)

h. process rendering an individual unable to produce offspring

i. an STD caused by a one-cell organism, *Trichomonas*

j. period when the ability to sexually reproduce begins

k. reduced or absent ability to produce offspring

EXERCISE 33

Spell each of the complementary terms not built from word parts on pp. 293-294 by having someone dictate them to you.

To hear and spell the terms, go to http://evolve.elsevier.com. Refer to p. 18 for your Evolve Access Information. Select Exercises & Review, Chapter 7, Chapter Exercises, Spelling.
☐ Place a check mark in the box if you have completed this exercise online.

1. ____________________
2. ____________________
3. ____________________
4. ____________________
5. ____________________
6. ____________________
7. ____________________
8. ____________________
9. ____________________
10. ____________________
11. ____________________
12. ____________________
13. ____________________
14. ____________________
15. ____________________
16. ____________________
17. ____________________
18. ____________________
19. ____________________
20. ____________________
21. ____________________

Abbreviations

AIDS	acquired immunodeficiency syndrome
BPH	benign prostatic hyperplasia
DRE	digital rectal examination
ED	erectile dysfunction
HIV	human immunodeficiency virus
HPV	human papillomavirus
PSA	prostate-specific antigen
RP	radical prostatectomy
STD	sexually transmitted disease
TRUS	transrectal ultrasound
TUIP	transurethral incision of the prostate
TUMT	transurethral microwave thermotherapy
TURP	transurethral resection of the prostate

Refer to **Appendix C** for a complete list of abbreviations.

EXERCISE 34

Write the meaning of the abbreviations in the following sentences.

1. The physician performed a **DRE** ____________________

    ____________________ ____________________on the patient to assist in diagnosing **BPH**

    ____________________ ____________________

    ____________________. Surgical treatments

    for BPH include prostatectomy, **TURP** ____________________

    ____________________ of the ____________________ gland, **TUMT**

    ____________________ ____________________

    ____________________, and **TUIP** ____________________

    ____________________ of the ____________________ gland.

2. **AIDS** ____________________ ____________________

    ____________________ is an **STD** ____________________

    ____________________ ____________________. **HIV**

    ____________________ ____________________

    ____________________ is a type of retrovirus that causes AIDS. **HPV**

    ____________________ ____________________ is an STD that causes female and male venereal warts.

3. **PSA** ____

    ____________________ is a laboratory test used to diagnose cancer of the prostate.

4. **RP** ____________________ ____________________ is a surgical procedure to treat prostate cancer.

5. **ED** ____________________ ____________________ was formerly referred to as impotence.

6. **TRUS** ____________________ ____________________, used in the diagnosis of prostate cancer, provides imaging of the prostate gland and is used as a guide for biopsy of the prostate.

PRACTICAL APPLICATION

EXERCISE 35 *Interact with Medical Documents*

A. Complete the emergency department report by writing the medical terms in the blanks. Use the list of definitions with the corresponding numbers.

University Hospital and Medical Center
4700 North Main Street • Wellness, Arizona 54321 • (987) 555-3210

PATIENT NAME: Andrew Nguyen **CASE NUMBER:** 19504-MRSS
DATE OF BIRTH: 07/27/19XX **DATE OF ADMISSION:** 08/23/20XX

Emergency Department Report

CHIEF COMPLAINT: Severe lower abdominal pain and the inability to void for the past 12 hours.

PRESENT ILLNESS: Andrew Nguyen is a 75-year-old Asian American man who came into the emergency department at 3 AM stating that he was in great pain and could not urinate. He had not been seen by a physician for several years but claimed to be in good health except for "a little high blood pressure." The patient reports urinary frequency, 1. ____________________ x 2, hesitancy, intermittency, and diminished force and caliber of the urinary stream. He also has postvoid dribbling and the sensation of not having completely emptied the bladder. Earlier today, he had 2. ____________________ at the end of urination.

MEDICATION ALLERGIES: None

CURRENT MEDICATIONS: Benadryl 25 mg at bedtime.

PHYSICAL EXAM: Temperature, 98.6. Blood pressure, 140/90 mm Hg. Pulse, 98. Respirations, 24. Palpation of the abdomen shows a suprapubic mass approximately three fingerbreadths below the umbilicus, dull to percussion and slightly tender.

IMPRESSION: 3. ____________________ bladder distention caused by urinary outlet obstruction, probably from 4. __________ __________ __________.

PLAN:
Indwelling Foley catheter for relief of urinary obstruction.
5. ____________________ consult.

____
Eleanor Adams, MD

EA/mcm

1. night urination
2. blood in the urine
3. pertaining to urine
4. nonmalignant excessive development pertaining to the prostate gland (enlargement of the prostate gland)
5. study of the urinary tract

EXERCISE 35 *Interact with Medical Documents—cont'd*

B. Read the letter reviewing a patient's progress and answer the questions following it.

Michigan Oncology Group
44976 East Lincoln
Detroit, MI 97654

January 23, 20XX

Kathryn S. Marcus, MD
Internal Medicine Services
2301 North Brinkley
Detroit, MI 97654

RE: Brindley, John F.
DOB: 08/24/19XX

Dear Dr. Marcus:

It is now three years since he had brachytherapy using radioactive seeds for his T2a, Gleason 5 prostate cancer. He continues voiding uncomfortably with nocturia and a prostate obstructive score of 3.

His weight is stable at 209 pounds and blood pressure is 122/82 mm Hg. He has no adenopathy. DRE reveals a smooth prostate with no nodules and no suspicious areas. There is a slight asymmetry with greater prominence on the right side. The PSA remains 0.1 as of August 20, 20XX.

He is doing well and is likely cured of his cancer. He continues to experience some erectile dysfunction. I would like to continue seeing him on a yearly basis with a repeat PSA. He will continue seeing you as needed.

____
Joseph P. Potter, MD

JPP/bko

1. In addition to uncomfortable urination, the patient's symptoms include:
   a. pus in the urine
   b. excessive urine
   c. night urination
   d. blood in the urine

2. Brachytherapy using radioactive seeds were used to treat:
   a. benign prostatic hyperplasia
   b. prostate cancer
   c. erectile dysfunction

3. Which diagnostic test revealed "a smooth prostate"?
   a. transrectal ultrasound
   b. prostate-specific antigen
   c. digital rectal examination

4. Three years after treatment, the patient:
   a. appears to be cancer free
   b. shows disease progression
   c. has been recommended for a radical prostatectomy

EXERCISE 36 *Interpret Medical Terms*

To test your understanding of the terms introduced in this chapter, circle the words that correctly complete the sentences. The italicized words refer to the correct answer.

1. A *discharge from the glans penis* is referred to medically as (**balanitis, balanorrhea, balanorrhaphy**).
2. The surgical procedure circumcision is the removal of the *foreskin*, or (**glans penis, testes, prepuce**).
3. The surgery schedule indicated the patient was to undergo laparoscopic *excision of the prostate gland* (**epididymectomy, prostatectomy, prostatocystotomy**) with robotics.
4. The patient had a diagnosis of (**oligospermia, phimosis, impotence**), or a *narrowing of the opening of the prepuce*.
5. The operation for the surgical fixation of the testicle is (**orchidopexy, orchidotomy, orchioplasty**).
6. A *microscopic observation of ejaculated semen* (**prostate-specific antigen, transrectal ultrasound, semen analysis**) might be ordered after a(n) *excision of a duct (vas deferens)* (**vasovasotomy, vasectomy, varicocele**) to make sure sperm are not present in the semen.
7. The following is a *treatment for benign prostatic hyperplasia using heat* (**transurethral prostatectomy, suprapubic prostatectomy, transurethral microwave thermotherapy**).
8. *State of hidden testicles* (**testitis, anorchism, cryptorchidism**) is an associated risk factor for the development of *cancer of the testicle* (**testicular torsion, testicular cancer, prostate cancer**).
9. Upon diagnosis of an intratesticular mass, a radical inguinal *excision of the testes* (**orchiectomy, prostatectomy, vasectomy**) is recommended as a diagnostic and therapeutic procedure.
10. The term meaning *reduced or absent ability to produce offspring* (**erectile dysfunction, sterilization, infertility**) does not mean complete inability to create offspring as does the term sterility.
11. *Condition of scanty sperm (in semen)* (**aspermia, oligospermia**) and *lack of live sperm in semen* (**azoospermia, spermatolysis**) are terms frequently used in relation to male infertility.

EXERCISE 37 Read Medical Terms in Use

Practice pronunciation of the terms by reading the following medical document. Use the pronunciation key following the medical term to assist you in saying the word.

To hear these terms, go to http://evolve.elsevier.com. Refer to p. 18 for your Evolve Access Information. Select Exercises & Review, Chapter 7, Chapter Exercises, Read Medical Terms in Use.

A 62-year-old man was found to have an elevated **prostate-specific antigen** (PROS-tāt) (spe-SIF-ik) (AN-ti-jen) test during a routine physical examination. At the age of 42 years he underwent a **vasectomy** (va-SEK-to-mē). The patient denies having nocturia or any significant change in his urinary stream. **Digital rectal examination** (DIJ-i-tal) (REK-tal) (eg-*zam*-i-NĀ-shun) revealed a mildly enlarged prostate gland with a 1.0 cm nodule of the right lobe. The urologist performed a **transrectal ultrasound** (trans-REK-tal) (UL-tra-sound) and biopsy. A diagnosis of adenocarcinoma of the prostate was made. The patient elected to undergo a **suprapubic prostatectomy** (sū-pra-PŪ-bik) (*pros*-ta-TEK-to-mē). Urinary incontinence complicated his postoperative course but this lasted for only 3 months. No **erectile dysfunction** (e-REK-tīl) (dis-FUNK-shun) was reported. His prognosis for full recovery should be excellent.

EXERCISE 38 Comprehend Medical Terms in Use

Test your comprehension of the terms in the previous medical document by circling the correct answer.

1. Before being diagnosed with cancer of the prostate the patient had surgery for:
   a. sterilization
   b. excision of the seminal vesicle
   c. removal of the prepuce
   d. repair of the glans penis

2. The patient chose which of the following types of treatment for prostate cancer?
   a. radiation
   b. chemotherapy
   c. surgery
   d. hormonal therapy

3. After surgery the patient:
   a. had absence of sperm
   b. had persistent abnormal erection
   c. had a narrowing of the opening of the prepuce of the glans penis
   d. was able to have an erection

4. Using word parts you have already learned, write the definition of terms used in this document from previous chapters.

   a. urin/ary ____________________

   b. ur/o/logist ____________________

   c. bi/opsy ____________________

   d. dia/gno/sis ____________________

   e. aden/o/carcin/oma ____________________

CHAPTER REVIEW

ONLINE CHAPTER REVIEW

To access the Evolve website, go to http://evolve.elsevier.com. Refer to p. 18 for your Evolve Access Information. Select Exercises & Review, Chapter 7, then select Chapter Exercises, Practice Activities, Animations, or Games. Place a check mark in the box when you have completed an exercise or activity, watched an animation, or played a game. Have fun!

Chapter Exercises

Exercises in this section of your Evolve resources correlate to exercises in your textbook. You may have completed them as you worked through the chapter.

- ☐ Pronunciation
- ☐ Spelling
- ☐ Read Medical Terms in Use

Practice Activities

Practice in study mode, then test your learning in assessment mode. Keep track of your scores from assessment mode if you wish.

	SCORE
☐ Picture It	______
☐ Define World Parts	______
☐ Build Medical Terms	______
☐ World Shop	______
☐ Define Medical Terms	______
☐ Use it	______
☐ Hear It and Type It: Clinical Vignettes	______

Animations

- ☐ Benign Prostatic Hyperplasia
- ☐ Retropubic Prostatectomy
- ☐ Testicular Torsion
- ☐ Transurethral Resection of the Prostate Gland

Games

- ☐ Name that World Part
- ☐ Term Storm
- ☐ Term Explorer
- ☐ Termbusters
- ☐ Medical Millionaire
- ☐ Crossword Puzzles

REVIEW OF WORD PARTS

Can you define and spell the following word parts?

Combining Forms

andr/o
balan/o
epididym/o
orch/o
orchi/o
orchid/o
prostat/o
sperm/o
spermat/o
test/o
vas/o
vesicul/o

Suffix

-ism

REVIEW OF TERMS

Can you define, pronounce, and spell the following terms *built from word parts*?

Diseases and Disorders

anorchism
balanitis
balanorrhea
benign prostatic hyperplasia (BPH)
cryptorchidism
epididymitis
orchiepididymitis
orchitis, orchiditis, or testitis
prostatitis
prostatocystitis
prostatolith
prostatorrhea
prostatovesiculitis

Surgical

balanoplasty
epididymectomy
orchidectomy, orchiectomy
orchidopexy, orchiopexy
orchidotomy, orchiotomy
orchioplasty
prostatectomy
prostatocystotomy
prostatolithotomy
prostatovesiculectomy
vasectomy
vasovasostomy
vesiculectomy

Complementary

andropathy
aspermia
oligospermia
spermatolysis

Can you define, pronounce, and spell the following terms *not built from word parts*?

Diseases and Disorders

erectile dysfunction (ED)
hydrocele
phimosis
priapism
prostate cancer
testicular cancer
testicular torsion
varicocele

Surgical

circumcision
hydrocelectomy
radical prostatectomy (RP)
suprapubic prostatectomy
transurethral incision of the prostate gland (TUIP)
transurethral microwave thermotherapy (TUMT)
transurethral resection of the prostate gland (TURP)

Diagnostic

digital rectal examination (DRE)
prostate-specific antigen (PSA)
semen analysis
transrectal ultrasound (TRUS)

Complementary

acquired immunodeficiency syndrome (AIDS)
artificial insemination
azoospermia
chlamydia
coitus
condom
ejaculation
genital herpes
gonads
gonorrhea
heterosexual
homosexual
human immunodeficiency virus (HIV)
human papillomavirus (HPV)
infertility
orgasm
puberty
sexually transmitted disease (STD)
sterilization
syphilis
trichomoniasis

ANSWERS

Exercise figures

Exercise Figure

A. 1. seminal vesicle: vesicul/o
2. prostate gland: prostat/o
3. epididymis: epididym/o
4. vas deferens or ductus deferens: vas/o
5. glans penis: balan/o
6. testis: orchid/o, orchi/o, orch/o, test/o

Exercise Figure

B. balan/itis

Exercise Figure

C. crypt/orchid/ism

Exercise Figure

D. vas/ectomy

Exercise 1

1. c
2. i
3. e
4. k
5. f
6. a
7. l
8. g
9. b
10. n
11. h
12. o
13. d
14. j
15. m

Exercise 2

1. testis, testicle
2. vessel, duct
3. glans penis
4. prostate gland
5. testis, testicle
6. seminal vesicle
7. testis, testicle
8. epididymis
9. testis, testicle

Exercise 3

1. vas/o
2. prostat/o
3. balan/o
4. vesicul/o
5. epididym/o
6. a. orchid/o
   b. orchi/o
   c. orch/o
   d. test/o

Exercise 4

1. spermatozoon, sperm
2. male
3. spermatozoon, sperm

Exercise 5

1. a. sperm/o
   b. spermat/o
2. andr/o

Exercise 6

1. state of

Exercise 7

Pronunciation Exercise

Exercise 8

1. WR CV WR
   prostat/o/lith
   CF
   stone in the prostate gland
2. WR S
   balan/itis
   inflammation of the glans penis
3. a. WR S
   orch/itis
   b. WR S
   orchid/itis
   c. WR S
   test/itis
   inflammation of the testis
4. WR CV WR S
   prostat/o/vesicul/itis
   CF
   inflammation of the prostate gland and seminal vesicles
5. WR CV WR S
   prostat/o/cyst/itis
   CF
   inflammation of the prostate gland and bladder
6. WR WR S
   orchi/epididym/itis
   inflammation of the testis and epididymis
7. WR CV S
   prostat/o/rrhea
   CF
   discharge from the prostate gland
8. WR S
   epididym/itis
   inflammation of an epididymis
9. WR S P S(WR)
   (benign) prostat/ic hyper/plasia
   excessive development pertaining to the prostate gland
10. WR WR S
    crypt/orchid/ism
    state of hidden testis
11. WR CV S
    balan/o/rrhea
    CF
    discharge from the glans penis
12. WR S
    prostat/itis
    inflammation of prostate gland
13. P WR S
    an/orch/ism
    state of absence of testis

Exercise 9

1. prostat/o/cyst/itis
2. prostat/o/lith
3. a. orchid/itis
   b. orch/itis
   c. test/itis
4. (benign) prostat/ic hyper/plasia
5. crypt/orchid/ism
6. prostat/o/vesicul/itis
7. an/orch/ism
8. prostat/itis
9. orchi/epididym/itis
10. balan/o/rrhea
11. epididym/itis
12. balan/itis
13. prostat/o/rrhea

Exercise 10

Spelling Exercise; see text p. 276.

Exercise 11

Pronunciation Exercise

Exercise 12

1. testicular cancer
2. phimosis
3. varicocele
4. hydrocele
5. prostate cancer
6. erectile dysfunction
7. priapism
8. testicular torsion

Exercise 13

1. d
2. c
3. e
4. b
5. a
6. f
7. i
8. h

Exercise 14

Spelling Exercise; see text pp. 279-280.

Exercise 15
Pronunciation Exercise

Exercise 16
1. WR S
vas/ectomy
excision of a duct
2. WR CV WR CV S
prostat/o/cyst/o/tomy
CF CF
incision into the prostate gland and bladder
3. a. WR CV S
orchid/o/tomy
CF
b. WR CV S
orchi/o/tomy
CF
incision into a testis
4. WR S
epididym/ectomy
excision of an epididymis
5. a. WR CV S
orchid/o/pexy
CF
b. WR CV S
orchi/o/pexy
CF
surgical fixation of a testicle
6. WR CV WR S
prostat/o/vesicul/ectomy
CF
excision of the prostate gland and seminal vesicles
7. WR CV S
orchi/o/plasty
CF
surgical repair of a testis
8. WR S
vesicul/ectomy
excision of the seminal vesicle(s)
9. WR S
prostat/ectomy
excision of the prostate gland
10. WR CV S
balan/o/plasty
CF
surgical repair of the glans penis
11. WR CV WR CV S
vas/o/vas/o/stomy
CF CF
creation of artificial openings between ducts
12. a. WR S
orchid/ectomy
b. WR S
orchi/ectomy
excision of the testis
13. WR CV WR CV S
prostat/o/lith/o/tomy
CF CF
incision into prostate gland to remove a stone

Exercise 17
1. a. orchid/ectomy
b. orchi/ectomy
2. balan/o/plasty
3. prostat/o/cyst/o/tomy
4. vesicul/ectomy
5. prostat/o/lith/o/tomy
6. a. orchid/o/tomy
b. orchi/o/tomy
7. epididym/ectomy
8. orchi/o/plasty
9. prostat/ectomy
10. vas/ectomy
11. prostat/o/vesicul/ectomy
12. a. orchid/o/pexy
b. orchi/o/pexy
13. vas/o/vas/o/stomy

Exercise 18
Spelling Exercise; see text pp. 282-283.

Exercise 19
Pronunciation Exercise

Exercise 20
1. suprapubic prostatectomy
2. circumcision
3. radical prostatectomy
4. hydrocelectomy
5. transurethral microwave thermotherapy
6. transurethral incision (of the) prostate gland
7. transurethral resection (of the) prostate gland

Exercise 21
Spelling Exercise; see text 289.

Exercise 22
Pronunciation Exercise

Exercise 23
1. digital rectal examination
2. prostate-specific antigen
3. transrectal ultrasound
4. semen analysis

Exercise 24
Spelling Exercise; see text p. 290.

Exercise 25
Pronunciation Exercise

Exercise 26
1. WR CV WR S
olig/o/sperm/ia
CF
condition of scanty sperm
2. WR CV S
andr/o/pathy
CF
disease of the male
3. WR CV S
spermat/o/lysis
CF
dissolution of sperm
4. P WR S
a/sperm/ia
condition of without sperm

Exercise 27
1. spermat/o/lysis
2. a/sperm/ia
3. andr/o/pathy
4. olig/o/sperm/ia

Exercise 28
Spelling Exercise; see text p. 291.

Exercise 29
Pronunciation Exercise

Exercise 30
1. period when secondary sex characteristics develop and the ability to sexually reproduce begins
2. climax of sexual stimulation
3. contagious, inflammatory sexually transmitted disease
4. person who is attracted to a member of the same sex
5. sexual intercourse between male and female
6. sexually transmitted disease caused by the *herpesvirus hominis* type 2
7. person who is attracted to a member of the oppostite sex
8. chronic infection caused by bacterium that can be transmitted by sexual contact, acquired in utero, or by contact with infected tissue
9. ejection of semen from the male urethra
10. male and female sex glands
11. a disease transmitted during sexual contact
12. process rendering an individual unable to produce offspring

13. an STD causing growths on the male and female genitalia
14. a disease transmitted by exchange of body fluids during the sexual act, reuse of contaminated needles, or contaminated blood transfusions
15. STD caused by a one-cell organism, *Trichomonas*; it affects the genitourinary system
16. introduction of semen into the vagina by artificial means
17. STD caused by bacterium, *C. trachomatis*
18. a cover for the penis worn during coitus
19. reduced or absent ability to produce offspring
20. a type of retrovirus that causes AIDS
21. lack of live sperm in semen

Exercise 31

1. g
2. e
3. h
4. a
5. d
6. i
7. c
8. b
9. j
10. f

Exercise 32

1. f
2. a
3. h
4. d
5. j
6. b
7. i
8. e
9. g
10. c
11. k

Exercise 33

Spelling Exercise; see text pp. 293-294.

Exercise 34

1. digital rectal examination; benign prostatic hyperplasia; transurethral resection (of the) prostate; transurethral microwave thermotherapy; transurethral incision (of the) prostate
2. acquired immunodeficiency syndrome; sexually transmitted disease; human immunodeficiency virus; human papillomavirus
3. prostate-specific antigen
4. radical prostatectomy
5. erectile dysfunction
6. transrectal ultrasound

Exercise 35

A. 1. nocturia
2. hematuria
3. urinary
4. benign prostatic hyperplasia
5. urology

B. 1. c
2. b
3. c
4. a

Exercise 36

1. balanorrhea
2. prepuce
3. prostatectomy
4. phimosis
5. orchidopexy
6. semen analysis; vasectomy
7. transurethral microwave thermotherapy
8. cryptorchidism; testicular cancer
9. orchiectomy
10. infertility
11. oligospermia; azoospermia

Exercise 37

Reading Exercise

Exercise 38

1. a
2. c
3. d
4. a. pertaining to urine
   b. a physician who studies and treats diseases of the urinary tract
   c. view of life
   d. state of complete knowledge
   e. cancerous tumor of glandular tissue

Chapter 8

Female Reproductive System

OUTLINE

OBJECTIVES

Upon completion of this chapter you will be able to:

1. Identify organs and structures of the female reproductive system.
2. Define and spell word parts related to the female reproductive system.
3. Define, pronounce, and spell disease and disorder terms related to the female reproductive system.
4. Define, pronounce, and spell surgical terms related to the female reproductive system.
5. Define, pronounce, and spell diagnostic terms related to the female reproductive system.
6. Define, pronounce, and spell complementary terms related to the female reproductive system.
7. Interpret the meaning of abbreviations related to the female reproductive system.
8. Interpret, read, and comprehend medical language in simulated medical statements and documents.

ANATOMY

Externally, the female reproductive system consists of the vulva, clitoris, and mammary glands. Internally, this system consists of the vagina, uterus, uterine tubes, and ovaries (Figures 8-1 and 8-2).

Function

The female reproductive system comprises external and internal organs, glands, and structures and is responsible for supporting conception and pregnancy. As the female matures throughout her lifespan, this system develops and changes based on the influence of hormones produced by the ovaries—estrogen and progesterone. These hormones are essential for sexual maturation, the menstrual cycle, and pregnancy. Estrogen is also important for the overall health of the female, affecting the structure and function of the integumentary, urinary, cardiac, musculoskeletal, and neurologic systems.

Internal Organs of the Female Reproductive System

Term	Definition
ovaries	pair of almond-shaped organs located in the pelvic cavity. Egg cells are formed and stored in the ovaries.
ovum (*pl.* ova)	female egg cell
graafian follicles	100,000 microscopic sacs that make up a large portion of the ovaries. Each follicle contains an immature ovum. Normally one graafian follicle develops to maturity monthly between puberty and menopause. It moves to the surface of the ovary and releases the ovum, which passes into the uterine tube.
uterine, or fallopian, tubes	pair of 5-inch (12 to 13 cm) tubes, attached to the uterus, that provide a passageway for the ovum to move from the ovary to the uterus
fimbria (*pl.* fimbriae)	finger-like projection at the free end of the uterine tube
uterus	pear-sized and pear-shaped muscular organ that lies in the pelvic cavity, except during pregnancy when it enlarges and extends up into the abdominal cavity. Its functions are menstruation, pregnancy, and labor.
endometrium	inner lining of the uterus
myometrium	muscular middle layer of the uterus
perimetrium	outer thin layer that covers the surface of the uterus
corpus, or body	large central portion of the uterus
fundus	rounded upper portion of the uterus
cervix (Cx)	narrow lower portion of the uterus
vagina	a 3-inch (7-8 cm) tube that connects the uterus to the outside of the body
hymen	fold of membrane found near the opening of the vagina
rectouterine pouch	pouch between the posterior wall of the uterus and the anterior wall of the rectum (also called **Douglas cul-de-sac**)

THE GRAAFIAN FOLLICLE

is named for Dutch anatomist Reinier de ***Graaf***, who discovered the sac in 1672.

THE FALLOPIAN TUBE

was named in honor of Gabriele Fallopius because he described it in his works. Fallopius also gave the ***vagina*** and the ***placenta*** their names.

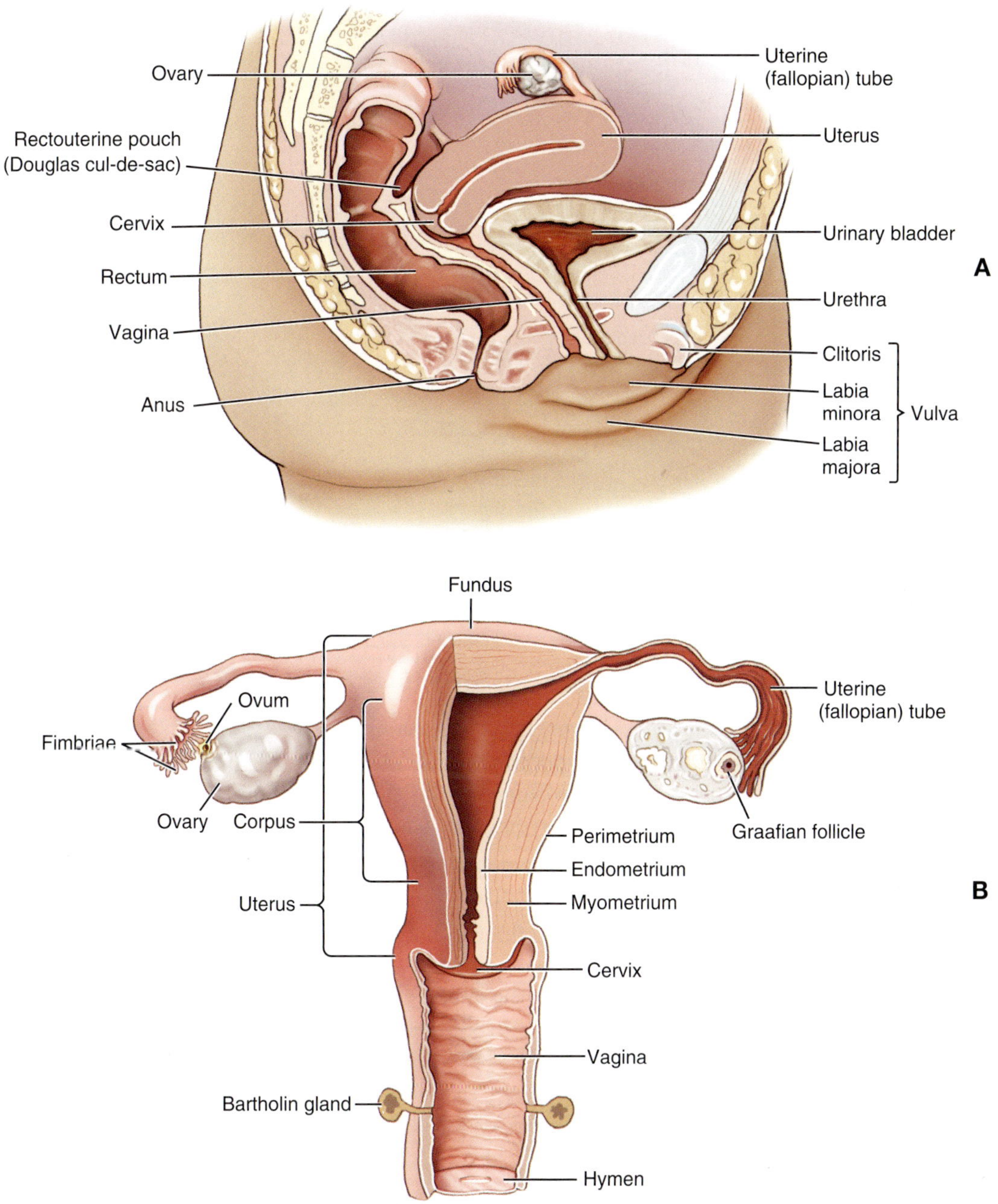

FIGURE 8-1
Female reproductive organs. **A,** Sagittal view **B,** Frontal view.

Glands of the Female Reproductive System

Term	Definition
Bartholin glands	pair of mucus-producing glands located on each side of the vagina and just above the vaginal opening
mammary glands, or breasts	pair of milk-producing glands of the female. Each breast consists of 15 to 20 divisions, or lobes (Figure 8-2).
mammary papilla	breast nipple
areola	pigmented area around the breast nipple

BARTHOLIN GLANDS

were described by Caspar Bartholin, a Danish anatomist, in 1675.

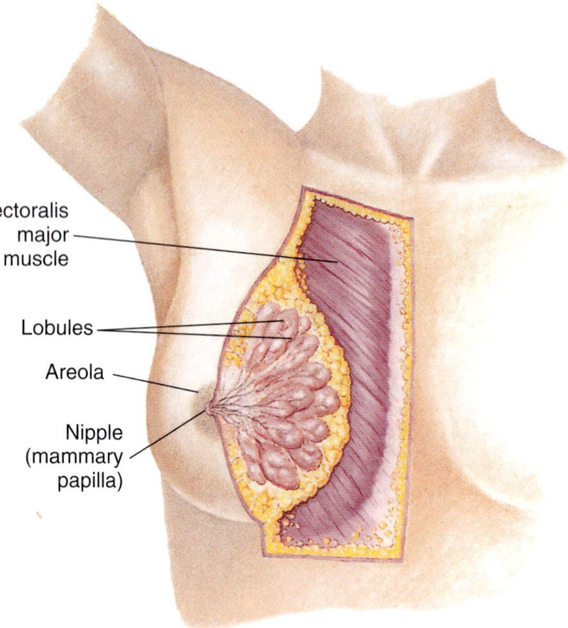

FIGURE 8-2
Female breast.

External Female Reproductive Structures

Term	Definition
vulva, or external genitalia	two pairs of lips (labia majora and labia minora) that surround the vagina
clitoris	highly erogenous erectile body located anterior to the urethra
perineum	pelvic floor in both the male and female. In females it usually refers to the area between the vaginal opening and the anus.

A & P Boosters
For students desiring more anatomy and physiology, go to http://evolve.elsevier.com. Refer to p. 18 for your Evolve Access Information. Select Exercises & Review, Chapter 8, A & P Booster.

EXERCISE 1

Match the definitions in the first column with the anatomic terms in the second column. *To check your answers to the exercises in this chapter, go to Answers, p. 357, at the end of the chapter.*

_____ 1. organs in which egg cells are formed	a. perimetrium
_____ 2. lower portion of the uterus	b. fundus
_____ 3. lining of the uterus	c. ovaries
_____ 4. upper portion of the uterus	d. perineum
_____ 5. pelvic floor	e. fimbriae
_____ 6. ends of uterine tubes	f. cervix
_____ 7. large central portion of the uterus	g. endometrium
_____ 8. layer that covers the uterus	h. corpus
_____ 9. muscle layer of the uterus	i. myometrium
	j. ovum

EXERCISE 2

Match the definitions in the first column with the anatomic terms in the second column.

_____ 1. connects the uterus to the outside of the body
_____ 2. mucus-producing glands located on each side of the vagina
_____ 3. breast
_____ 4. female egg cells
_____ 5. external genitals
_____ 6. passageway for ovum
_____ 7. pigmented area around the nipple
_____ 8. microscopic sacs in the ovaries
_____ 9. muscular organ
_____ 10. nipples
_____ 11. rectouterine pouch

a. ovary
b. vagina
c. Bartholin glands
d. mammary gland
e. vulva
f. uterine tube
g. areola
h. Douglas cul-de-sac
i. uterus
j. mammary papillae
k. ova
l. graafian follicles

WORD PARTS

Word parts you need to learn to complete this chapter are listed on the following pages. The exercises at the end of each list will help you learn their definitions and spellings.

Use the flashcards accompanying this text or the electronic flashcards to assist you in memorizing the word parts for this chapter.

To use electronic flashcards, go to http://evolve.elsevier.com. Refer to p. 18 for your Evolve Access Information. Select Flashcards, Chapter 8.

Combining Forms of the Female Reproductive System

Combining Form	Definition
arche/o	first, beginning
cervic/o	cervix
colp/o, vagin/o	vagina
culd/o	cul-de-sac
episi/o, vulv/o	vulva
gynec/o, gyn/o	woman
hymen/o	hymen
hyster/o, metr/o, metr/i (NOTE: the combining vowel *i* or *o* may be used with metr/.)	uterus

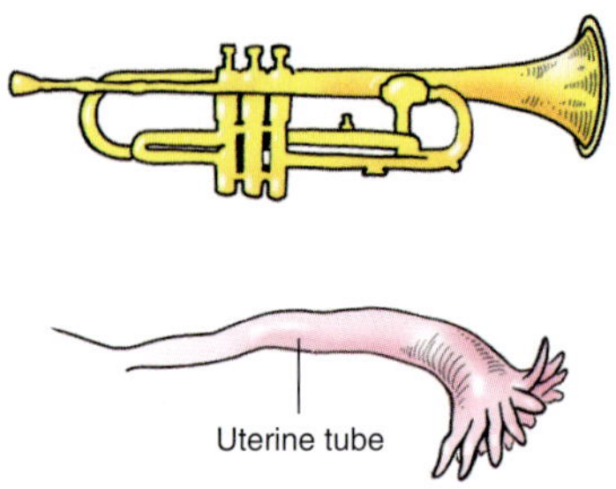

FIGURE 8-3
Salpinx is derived from the Greek term for trumpet. The term was used for the uterine tubes because of their trumpet-like shape.

Combining Forms of the Female Reproductive System—*cont'd*

Combining Form	Definition
mamm/o, mast/o	breast
men/o	menstruation
oophor/o	ovary
perine/o	perineum
salping/o	uterine tube (fallopian tube) (Figure 8-3)

EXERCISE FIGURE A

Fill in the blanks with combining forms in this diagram of the frontal view of the female reproductive system. *To check your ansers, go to p. 357.*

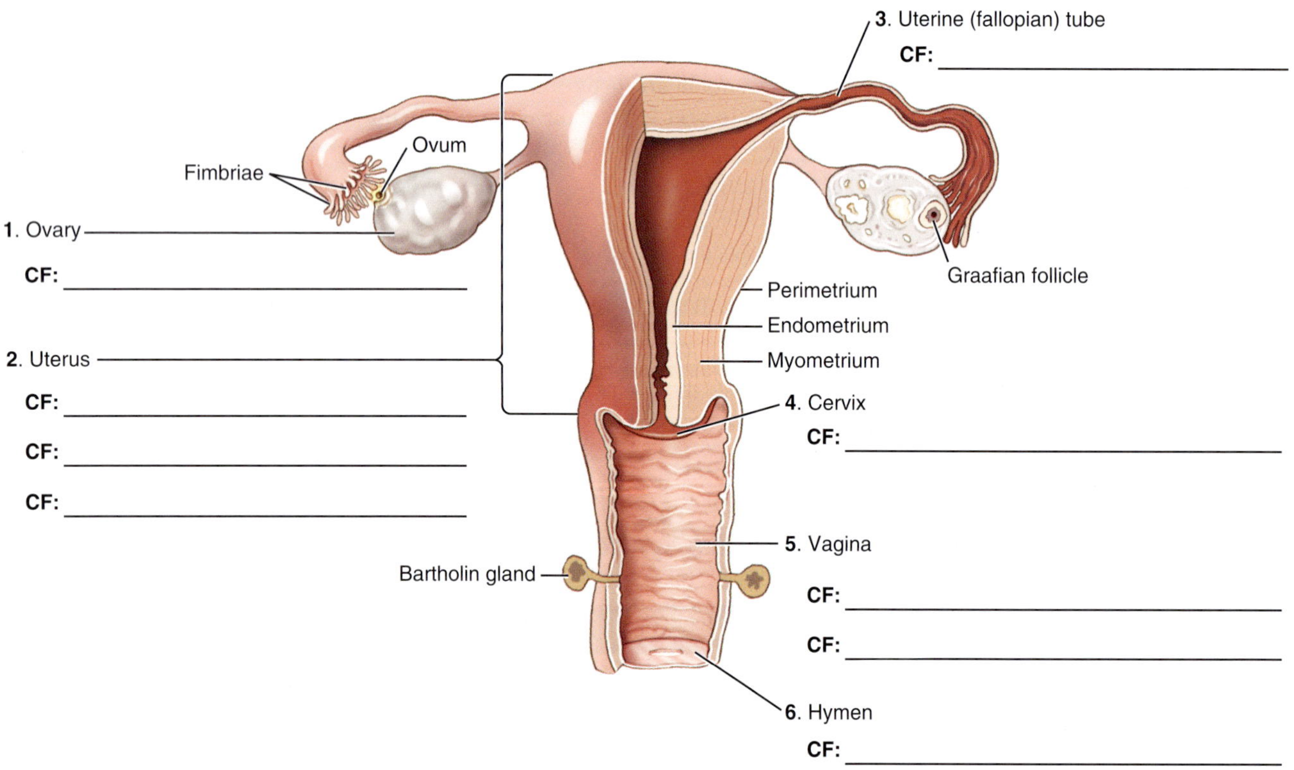

EXERCISE FIGURE B

Fill in the blanks with combining forms in this diagram showing the external reproductive organs.

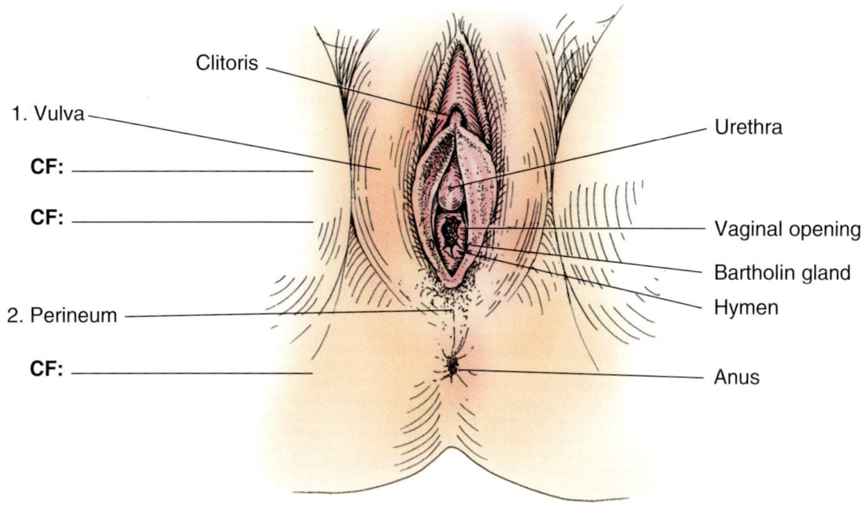

EXERCISE 3

Write the definitions of the following combining forms.

1. vagin/o ______________
2. oophor/o ______________
3. metr/o, metr/i ______________
4. gyn/o ______________
5. hymen/o ______________
6. hyster/o ______________
7. men/o ______________
8. episi/o ______________
9. cervic/o ______________
10. colp/o ______________
11. gynec/o ______________
12. mamm/o ______________
13. perine/o ______________
14. salping/o ______________
15. vulv/o ______________
16. mast/o ______________
17. arche/o ______________
18. culd/o ______________

EXERCISE 4

Write the combining form for each of the following terms.

1. vulva a. ___________ b. ___________
2. breast a ___________ b. ___________
3. menstruation ___________
4. ovary ___________
5. uterine tube ___________
6. perineum ___________
7. vagina a. ___________ b. ___________
8. uterus a. ___________ b. ___________ c. ___________
9. woman a. ___________ b. ___________
10. hymen ___________
11. cul-de-sac ___________
12. cervix ___________
13. first, beginning ___________

Prefix and Suffixes

Prefix	Definition
peri-	surrounding (outer)
Suffixes	**Definition**
-atresia	absence of a normal body opening; occlusion; closure
-salpinx (NOTE: for learning purposes *salpinx* and *atresia* are presented as suffixes.)	uterine tube (fallopian tube) (Figure 8-3)

ATRESIA

literally means **no perforation or hole.** It is composed of the Greek words **a,** meaning **without,** and **tresis,** meaning **perforation.** The term may be used alone, as in "atresia of the vagina," or combined with other word parts, as in "gynatresia," meaning closure of a part of the female genital tract, usually the vagina.

EXERCISE 5

Write the prefix or suffix for each of the following.

1. uterine tube ___________
2. surrounding ___________
3. absence of a normal body opening ___________

EXERCISE 6

Write the definitions of the following prefix and suffixes.

1. -salpinx ___________
2. peri- ___________
3. -atresia ___________

Refer to **Appendix A** and **Appendix B** for alphabetized word parts and their meanings.

MEDICAL TERMS

The terms you need to learn to complete this chapter are listed on the following pages. The exercises following each list will help you learn the definition and spelling of each word.

Disease and Disorder Terms

Built from Word Parts

The following terms are built from word parts you have already learned and can be translated literally to find their meanings. Further explanation of terms beyond the definition of their word parts, if needed, is included in parentheses.

Term	Definition
amenorrhea (a-*men*-ō-RĒ-a)	absence of menstrual discharge
Bartholin adenitis (BAR-tō-lin) (*ad*-e-NĪ-tis)	inflammation of a Bartholin gland (also called **bartholinitis**)
cervicitis (*ser*-vi-SĪ-tis)	inflammation of the cervix (see Figure 8-7)
colpitis, vaginitis (*kol*-PĪ-tis), (*vaj*-i-NĪ-tis)	inflammation of the vagina (see Figure 8-7)
dysmenorrhea (dis-*men*-ō-RĒ-a)	painful menstrual discharge
endocervicitis (*en*-dō-*ser*-vi-SĪ-tis)	inflammation of the inner (lining) of the cervix
endometritis (*en*-dō-mē-TRĪ-tis)	inflammation of the inner (lining) of the uterus (endometrium) (see Figure 8-7)
hematosalpinx (*hem*-a-tō-SAL-pinks)	blood in the uterine tube
hydrosalpinx (*hī*-drō-SAL-pinks)	water in the uterine tube (see Exercise Figure H, p. 339)
hysteratresia (*his*-ter-a-TRĒ-zha)	closure of the uterus (uterine cavity)
mastitis (*mas*-TĪ-tis)	inflammation of the breast
menometrorrhagia (*men*-ō-*met*-rō-RĀ-jea)	rapid flow of blood from the uterus at menstruation (and between menstrual cycles; increased amount)
menorrhagia (*men*-ō-RĀ-jea)	rapid flow of blood at menstruation (increased amount)
metrorrhagia (*mē*-trō-RĀ-jea)	rapid flow of blood from the uterus (between menstrual cycles)
myometritis (*mī*-o-me-TRĪ-tis)	inflammation of the uterine muscle (myometrium)
oligomenorrhea (*ol*-i-gō-*men*-ō-RĒ-a)	scanty menstrual flow (less often)
oophoritis (*ō*-of-o-RĪ-tis)	inflammation of the ovary

BARTHOLIN ADENITIS

Ever since I told a crowded room I had a Bavarian cyst [Bartholin adenitis] and not only did no one laugh, but two others had the same thing, I've been convinced that doctor and patient do not speak the same language. They speak Latin. We speak Reader's Digest.

Erma Bombeck, 1981

Disease and Disorder Terms—*cont'd*

Built from Word Parts

Term	Definition
perimetritis (*per*-i-me-TRĪ-tis)	inflammation surrounding the uterus (perimetrium)
pyosalpinx (*pī*-ō-SAL-pinks)	pus in the uterine tube
salpingitis (*sal*-pin-JĪ-tis)	inflammation of the uterine tube (Exercise Figure C and Figure 8-7)
salpingocele (sal-PING-gō-sēl)	hernia of the uterine tube
vulvovaginitis (*vul*-vō-*vaj*-i-NĪ-tis)	inflammation of the vulva and vagina

EXERCISE FIGURE C

Fill in the blanks to label the diagram.

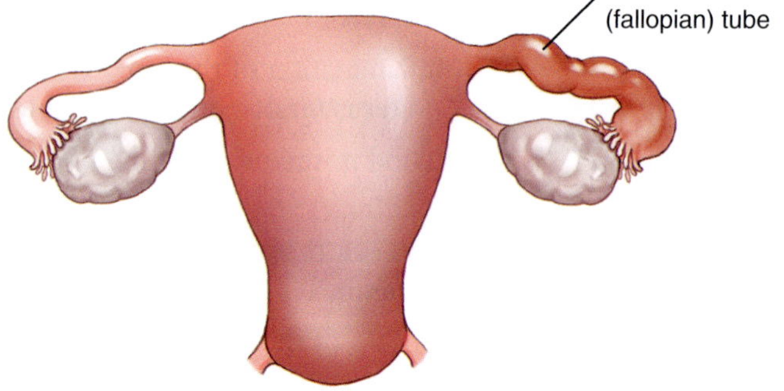

__________ / __________
uterine tube / inflammation

EXERCISE 7

Practice saying aloud each of the disease and disorder terms built from word parts on pp. 317-318 and above.

To hear the terms, go to http://evolve.elsevier.com. Refer to p. 18 for your Evolve Access Information. Select Exercises & Review, Chapter 8, Chapter Exercises, Pronunciation.

☐ Place a check mark in the box when you have completed this exercise.

EXERCISE 8

Analyze and define the following disease and disorder terms.

1. colpitis ______
2. cervicitis ______
3. hydrosalpinx ______
4. hematosalpinx ______
5. metrorrhagia ______
6. oophoritis ______
7. (Bartholin) adenitis ______
8. vulvovaginitis ______
9. salpingocele ______
10. menometrorrhagia ______
11. amenorrhea ______
12. dysmenorrhea ______
13. mastitis ______
14. perimetritis ______
15. myometritis ______
16. endometritis ______
17. endocervicitis ______
18. pyosalpinx ______
19. hysteratresia ______
20. salpingitis ______
21. vaginitis ______
22. menorrhagia ______
23. oligomenorrhea ______

EXERCISE 9

Build disease and disorder terms for the following definitions with the word parts you have learned.

1. inflammation of the breast ______ / ______ WR / S
2. rapid flow of blood from the uterus (between menstrual cycles) ______ / ______ / ______ WR / CV / S
3. inflammation of the uterine tube ______ / ______ WR / S
4. inflammation of the vulva and vagina ______ / ______ / ______ / ______ WR / CV / WR / S
5. absence of menstrual discharge ______ / ______ / ______ / ______ P / WR / CV / S
6. inflammation of the cervix ______ / ______ WR / S
7. inflammation of (Bartholin) gland Bartholin ______ / ______ WR / S
8. water in the uterine tube ______ / ______ / ______ WR / CV / S
9. painful menstrual discharge ______ / ______ / ______ / ______ P / WR / CV / S
10. blood in the uterine tube ______ / ______ / ______ WR / CV / S
11. inflammation of the vagina
    a. ______ / ______ WR / S
    b. ______ / ______ WR / S
12. rapid flow of blood from the uterus at menstruation (and between menstrual cycles) ______ / ______ / ______ / ______ / ______ WR / CV / WR / CV / S
13. inflammation of the ovary ______ / ______ WR / S
14. hernia of the uterine tube ______ / ______ / ______ WR / CV / S
15. inflammation surrounding the uterus (outer layer) ______ / ______ / ______ P / WR / S

16. inflammation of the inner (lining) of the uterus
_____ / _____ / _____
P / WR / S

17. inflammation of the inner (lining) of the cervix
_____ / _____ / _____
P / WR / S

18. inflammation of the uterine muscle
_____ / _____ / _____ / _____
WR / CV / WR / S

19. pus in the uterine tube
_____ / _____ / _____
WR / CV / S

20. closure of the uterus (uterine cavity)
_____ / _____
WR / S

21. scanty menstrual flow (less often)
_____ / _____ / _____ / _____ / _____
WR / CV / WR / CV / S

22. rapid flow of blood at menstruation (increased amount)
_____ / _____ / _____
WR / CV / S

EXERCISE 10

Spell each of the disease and disorder terms built from word parts on pp 317-318 by having someone dictate them to you.

To hear and spell the terms, go to http://evolve.elsevier.com. Refer to p. 18 for your Evolve Access Information. Select Exercises & Review, Chapter 8, Chapter Exercises, Spelling.
☐ Place a check mark in the box if you have completed this exercise online.

1. ____________________
2. ____________________
3. ____________________
4. ____________________
5. ____________________
6. ____________________
7. ____________________
8. ____________________
9. ____________________
10. ____________________
11. ____________________
12. ____________________
13. ____________________
14. ____________________
15. ____________________
16. ____________________
17. ____________________
18. ____________________
19. ____________________
20. ____________________
21. ____________________
22. ____________________
23. ____________________

Disease and Disorder Terms

Not Built from Word Parts

In some of the following terms, you may recognize word parts you have already learned; however, the full meaning of the terms cannot be discerned by the definition of their word parts.

Term	Definition
adenomyosis (*ad*-e-nō-mī-Ō-sis)	growth of endometrium into the muscular portion of the uterus
breast cancer (brest) (KAN-cer)	malignant tumor of the breast (Figure 8-4)
cervical cancer (SER-vi-kal) (KAN-cer)	malignant tumor of the cervix, which progresses from cellular dysplasia to carcinoma. Its cause is linked to human papillomavirus (HPV) infection.
endometrial cancer (*en*-dō-MĒ-trē-al) (KAN-cer)	malignant tumor of the endometrium (also called **uterine cancer**)
endometriosis (*en*-dō-*mē*-trē-Ō-sis)	abnormal condition in which endometrial tissue grows outside of the uterus in various areas in the pelvic cavity, including ovaries, uterine tubes, intestines, and uterus (Figure 8-5)

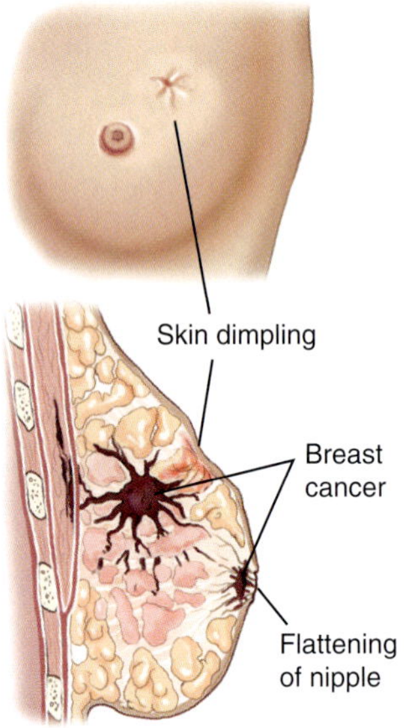

FIGURE 8-4
Clinical signs of breast cancer.

HPV VACCINE

The Food and Drug Administration (FDA) approved a vaccine for human papillomavirus (HPV) in 2006, directly impacting the prevention of **cervical cancer**. The vaccine is highly effective in protecting against a majority of forms of HPV as long as it is administered before a female becomes sexually active. Because vaccination is not 100% effective, annual cervical cancer screening (see **Pap smear**, p. 343) is strongly recommended.

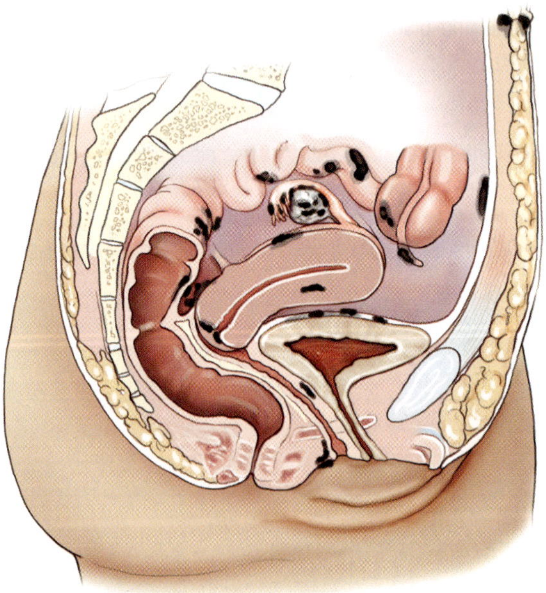

FIGURE 8-5
Endometriosis. Spots indicate common sites of endometrial deposits.

Term	Definition
fibrocystic breast disease (*fī*-brō-SIS-tik) (di-ZĒZ)	a disorder characterized by one or more benign cysts in the breast
fibroid tumor (FĪ-broyd) (TŪ-mor)	benign fibroid tumor of the uterine muscle (also called **myoma of the uterus** or **leiomyoma**) (Figure 8-6)
ovarian cancer (ō-VAR-ē-an) (KAN-cer)	malignant tumor of the ovary
pelvic inflammatory disease (PID) (PEL-vik) (in-FLAM-a-*tor*-ē) (di-ZĒZ)	inflammation of the female pelvic organs that can be caused by many different pathogens. If untreated, the infection may spread upward from the vagina, involving the uterus, uterine tubes, ovaries, and other pelvic organs. An ascending infection may result in infertility and, in acute cases, fatal septicemia (Figure 8-7).
prolapsed uterus (PRŌ-lapsd) (Ū-ter-us)	downward displacement of the uterus into the vagina (also called **hysteroptosis**) (Exercise Figure D)
toxic shock syndrome (TSS) (TOK-sik) (shok) (SIN-drōm)	a severe illness characterized by high fever, rash, vomiting, diarrhea, and myalgia, followed by hypotension and, in severe cases, shock and death; usually affects menstruating women using tampons; caused by *Staphylococcus aureus* and *Streptococcus pyogenes.*
vesicovaginal fistula (*ves*-i-kō-VAJ-i-nal) (FIS-tū-la)	abnormal opening between the bladder and the vagina (Exercise Figure E)

CAM TERM

Massage therapy is the manual manipulation of soft tissue, incorporating stroking, kneading, and percussion motions. Documented benefits of massage therapy during **breast cancer** treatment include reducing nausea and other side effects of chemotherapy and radiation, reducing anxiety and improving quality of life during treatment.

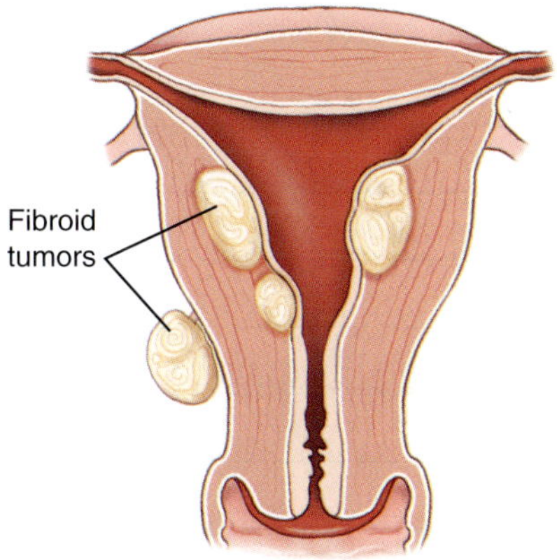

FIGURE 8-6
Fibroid tumors (also called myomas or leiomyomas).

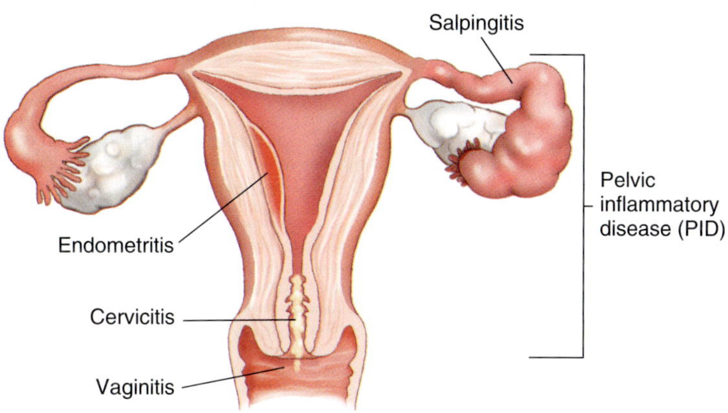

FIGURE 8-7
Ascending infection of the female reproductive system as seen in pelvic inflammatory disease.

EXERCISE FIGURE D

Fill in the blanks to complete labeling of the diagram.

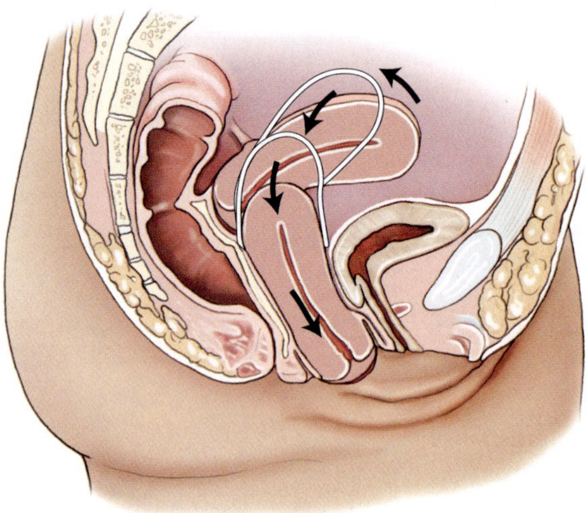

Prolapsed uterus or ______ / ___ / ______
uterus / cv / prolapse

EXERCISE FIGURE E

Fill in the blanks to complete labeling of the diagram.

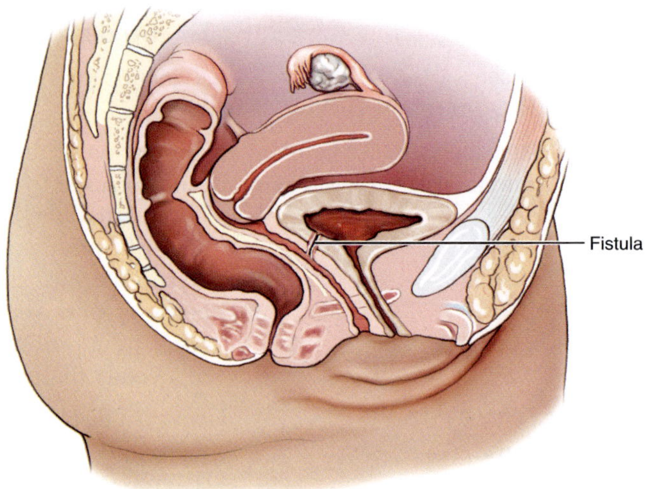

A ______ / ___ / ______ / ______ fistula
bladder / cv / vagina / pertaining to

EXERCISE 11

Practice saying aloud each of the disease and disorder terms not built from word parts on pp. 322-323.

To hear the terms, go to http://evolve.elsevier.com. Refer to p. 18 for your Evolve Access Information. Select Exercises & Review, Chapter 8, Chapter Exercises, Pronunciation.

☐ Place a check mark in the box when you have completed this exercise.

EXERCISE 12

Fill in the blanks with the correct definitions.

1. prolapsed uterus ______
2. pelvic inflammatory disease ______
3. vesicovaginal fistula ______
4. fibroid tumor ______
5. endometriosis ______
6. adenomyosis ______
7. toxic shock syndrome ______
8. fibrocystic breast disease ______
9. ovarian cancer ______
10. breast cancer ______

11. cervical cancer ______________________________
12. endometrial cancer ______________________________

EXERCISE 13

Write the term for each of the following.

1. abnormal opening between the bladder and the vagina ______________ ______________
2. benign tumor of the uterine muscle ______________ ______________
3. inflammation of the female pelvic organs ______________ ______________ ______________
4. downward displacement of the uterus into the vagina ______________ ______________
5. endometrial tissue in the pelvic cavity ______________________________
6. growth of endometrium into the muscular portion of the uterus ______________________________
7. affects menstruating women using tampons ______________ ______________ ______________
8. one or more benign cysts in the breast ______________ ______________ ______________
9. a malignant tumor of the breast ______________ ______________
10. also called uterine cancer ______________ ______________
11. malignant tumor of the ovaries ______________ ______________
12. malignant tumor of the cervix ______________ ______________

EXERCISE 14

Spell each of the disease and disorder terms not built from word parts on pp. 322-323 by having someone dictate them to you.

To hear and spell the terms, go to http://evolve.elsevier.com. Refer to p. 18 for your Evolve Access Information. Select Exercises & Review, Chapter 8, Chapter Exercises, Spelling.

☐ Place a check mark in the box if you have completed this exercise online.

1. ______________________ 7. ______________________
2. ______________________ 8. ______________________
3. ______________________ 9. ______________________
4. ______________________ 10. ______________________
5. ______________________ 11. ______________________
6. ______________________ 12. ______________________

ENDOSCOPIC SURGERY

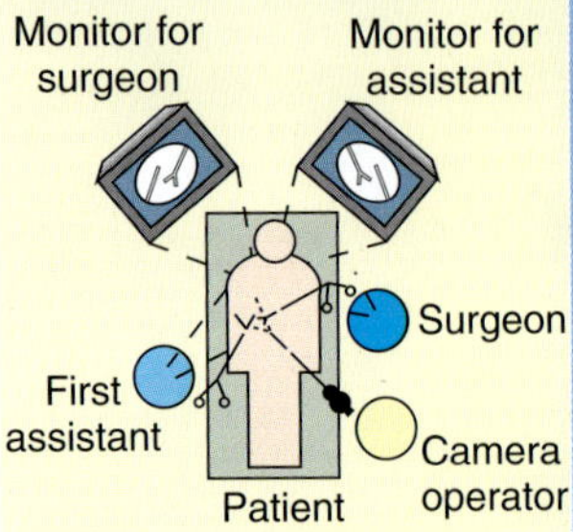

Operative setup for laparoscopic **hysterectomy**, a type of endoscopic surgery.

Endoscopic surgery includes the use of a slender, flexible fiberoptic **endoscope** that is inserted into a natural body cavity, such as the mouth, or other body areas through a small incision. Three or four other tiny incisions may be made to accommodate visualization equipment that projects the patient's internal organs and structures onto a television screen and to accommodate other instruments and devices needed to complete the surgery.

While endoscopic surgery results in less trauma and medical expense to the patient, large-incision surgery remains in use in certain clinical cases.

Other female reproductive system surgeries that may be performed endoscopically include **biopsies, myomectomy**, **oophorectomy**, and **tubal ligation** or **sterilization**.

Surgical Terms

Built from Word Parts

The following terms are built from word parts you have already learned and can be translated literally to find their meanings. Further explanation of terms beyond the definitions of their word parts, if needed, is included in parentheses.

Term	Definition
cervicectomy (*ser*-vi-SEK-to-mē)	excision of the cervix
colpoperineorrhaphy (kol-pō-*per*-i-nē-OR-a-fē)	suture of the vagina and perineum (performed to mend perineal vaginal tears)
colpoplasty (KOL-pō-*plas*-tē)	surgical repair of the vagina
colporrhaphy (kol-POR-a-fē)	suture of the vagina (wall of the vagina)
episioperineoplasty (e-*piz*-ē-ō-*per*-i-NĒ-o-*plas*-tē)	surgical repair of the vulva and perineum
episiorrhaphy (e-*piz*-ē-OR-a-fē)	suture of (a tear in) the vulva
hymenectomy (*hī*-men-EK-to-mē)	excision of the hymen
hymenotomy (*hī*-men-OT-o-mē)	incision of the hymen
hysterectomy (*his*-te-REK-to-mē)	excision of the uterus (Table 8-1) (Exercise Figure F)
hysteropexy (HIS-ter-ō-*pek*-sē)	surgical fixation of the uterus
hysterosalpingo-oophorectomy (*his*-ter-ō-sal-*ping*-gō-ō-*of*-o-REK-to-mē)	excision of the uterus, uterine tubes, and ovaries (Exercise Figure F)
mammoplasty (MAM-ō-*plas*-tē)	surgical repair of the breast (performed to enlarge or reduce in size, or to reconstruct after removal of a tumor) (Figure 8-8)
mastectomy (mas-TEK-tō-mē)	surgical removal of a breast (Table 8-2) (Figure 8-8)
mastopexy (MAS-tō-pek-sē)	surgical fixation of the breast (performed to lift sagging breast tissue or to create symmetry) (Figure 8-8)
oophorectomy (*ō*-of-o-REK-tō-mē)	excision of an ovary
perineorrhaphy (*per*-i-nē-OR-a-fē)	suture of (a tear in) the perineum
salpingectomy (*sal*-pin-JEK-to-mē)	excision of a uterine tube
salpingo-oophorectomy (sal-*ping*-gō-ō-*of*-o-REK-to-mē)	excision of the uterine tube and ovary (Exercise Figure F)
salpingostomy (*sal*-ping-GOS-to-mē)	creation of an artificial opening in a uterine tube (performed to restore patency)
vulvectomy (vul-VEK-to-mē)	excision of the vulva

TABLE 8-1
Types of Hysterectomies

Subtotal hysterectomy	Excision of the uterus, excluding cervix; rarely performed
Total hysterectomy	Excision of the uterus (abdominal, vaginal, or laparoscopic)
Panhysterectomy	Excision of the uterus, ovaries, and uterine tubes (abdominal)
Radical hysterectomy	Excision of the uterus, ovaries, uterine tubes; lymph nodes, upper portion of the vagina, and the surrounding tissues (abdominal)
Laparoscopic-assisted vaginal hysterectomy	Vaginal excision of the uterus with the use of the laparoscope to view the abdominopelvic cavity. Laparoscopic instruments are used to sever the ligaments that hold the uterus in place.

EXERCISE FIGURE F

Fill in the blanks to label the diagram.

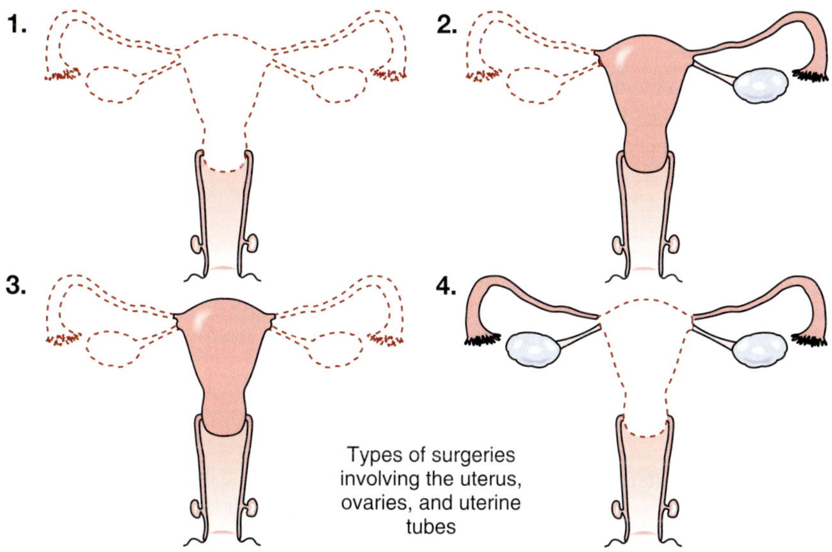

Types of surgeries involving the uterus, ovaries, and uterine tubes

1. ______ / ______ / ______ / ______ / ______ / ______.
uterus / cv / uterine tube / cv / ovary / excision

2. ______ / ______ / ______ / ______.
uterine tube / cv / ovary / excision

3. Bilateral ______ / ______ / ______ / ______.
uterine tube / cv / ovary / excision

4. ______ / ______.
uterus / excision

TYPES OF MAMMOPLASTY

- **Implant** uses a silicone or saline implant to create a breast.
- **Autologous** uses the patient's own tissue to reconstruct a breast.
- **TRAM** (transverse rectus abdominis muscle) **flap reconstruction** is most commonly used. Muscle and surrounding tissue is transferred from the abdomen to the chest to create a breast mound (Figure 8-8, *B*).

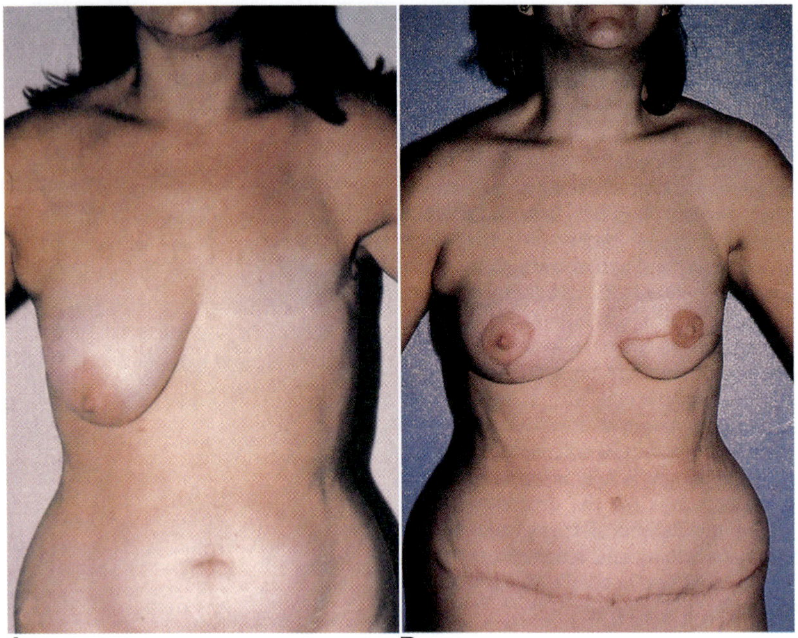

A B

FIGURE 8-8
Breast surgery and reconstruction. **A,** Left breast shows modified radical mastectomy scar. **B,** Left breast shows mammoplasty by TRAM reconstruction (note the extensive lower abdominal scar, repositioned navel, and recreated nipple) and right mastopexy.

TABLE 8-2
Types of Surgeries Performed to Treat Malignant Breast Tumors

Radical mastectomy	Removal of breast tissue, nipple, lymph nodes, and underlying chest wall muscle; also called *Halsted mastectomy* (rarely performed)
Modified radical mastectomy	Removal of breast tissue, nipple, and lymph nodes (Figure 8-8)
Simple mastectomy	Removal of breast tissue and nipple; also called *total mastectomy*
Subcutaneous mastectomy	Removal of breast tissue only, preserving the overlying skin, nipple and areola
Segmental mastectomy	Removal of a quadrant, or wedge, of breast tissue; also called *quadrantectomy*
Lumpectomy	Removal of the cancerous lesion along with a margin of surrounding healthy breast tissue; also called *partial mastectomy* or *breast-conserving surgery*

EXERCISE 15

Practice saying aloud each of the surgical terms built from word parts on p. 326.

To hear the terms, go to http://evolve.elsevier.com. Refer to p. 18 for your Evolve Access Information. Select Exercises & Review, Chapter 8, Chapter Exercises, Pronunciation.

☐ Place a check mark in the box when you have completed this exercise.

EXERCISE 16

Analyze and define the following surgical terms.

1. colporrhaphy ______
2. colpoplasty ______
3. episiorrhaphy ______
4. hymenotomy ______
5. hysteropexy ______
6. vulvectomy ______
7. perineorrhaphy ______
8. salpingostomy ______
9. salpingo-oophorectomy ______
10. oophorectomy ______
11. mastectomy ______
12. salpingectomy ______
13. cervicectomy ______
14. colpoperineorrhaphy ______
15. episioperineoplasty ______
16. hymenectomy ______
17. hysterosalpingo-oophorectomy ______
18. hysterectomy ______
19. mammoplasty ______
20. mastopexy ______

EXERCISE 17

Build surgical terms for the following definitions by using the word parts you have learned.

1. suture of the vagina ______ / ______ / ______
   WR / CV / S

2. excision of the cervix ______ / ______
   WR / S

3. suture of the vulva ______ / CV / ______
WR CV S

4. surgical repair of the vulva and perineum
WR CV WR CV S

5. surgical repair of the vagina
WR CV S

6. suture of the vagina and perineum
WR CV WR CV S

7. excision of the uterus, ovaries, and uterine tubes
WR CV WR CV WR S

8. surgical fixation of the uterus
WR CV S

9. excision of the hymen
WR S

10. incision of the hymen
WR CV S

11. excision of the uterus
WR S

12. excision of the ovary
WR S

13. surgical removal of a breast
WR S

14. excision of a uterine tube
WR S

15. suture of the perineum
WR CV S

16. excision of the uterine tube and ovary
WR CV WR S

17. creation of an artificial opening in the uterine tube
WR CV S

18. excision of the vulva
WR S

19. surgical repair of the breast
WR CV S

20. surgical fixation of the breast
WR CV S

EXERCISE 18

Spell each of the surgical terms built from word parts on p. 326 by having someone dictate them to you.

To hear and spell the terms, go to http://evolve.elsevier.com. Refer to p. 18 for your Evolve Access Information. Select Exercises & Review, Chapter 8, Chapter Exercises, Spelling.

☐ Place a check mark in the box if you have completed this exercise online.

1. ______	11. ______
2. ______	12. ______
3. ______	13. ______
4. ______	14. ______
5. ______	15. ______
6. ______	16. ______
7. ______	17. ______
8. ______	18. ______
9. ______	19. ______
10. ______	20. ______

Surgical Terms

Not Built from Word Parts

In some of the following terms, you may recognize word parts you have already learned; however, the full meaning of the terms cannot be discerned by the definition of their word parts.

Term	Definition
anterior and posterior colporrhaphy (A&P repair) (kol-POR-a-fē)	surgical repair of a weakened vaginal wall to correct a cystocele (protrusion of the bladder against the anterior wall of the vagina) and a rectocele (protrusion of the rectum against the posterior wall of the vagina) (Exercise Figure G)
conization (*kon*-i-ZĀ-shun)	the surgical removal of a cone-shaped area of the cervix; used in the treatment for noninvasive cervical cancer (also called **cone biopsy**)
dilation and curettage (D&C) (dī-LĀ-shun) (kū-re-TAHZH)	dilation (widening) of the cervix and scraping of the endometrium with an instrument called a *curette*. It is performed to diagnose disease, to correct bleeding, and to empty uterine contents, such as tissue remaining after a miscarriage (see Figure 8-9)

Dilation or dilatation are both used in the presentation of dilation and curettage. Dilation is the more common usage and is used in this text.

TYPES OF CONIZATION

- **LEEP** (loop electrosurgical excision procedure) uses a thin electric loop to excise a cone of cervical tissue.
- **Cryosurgery** (also called *cold knife conization*) and laser ablation are also used to treat abnormal cells.

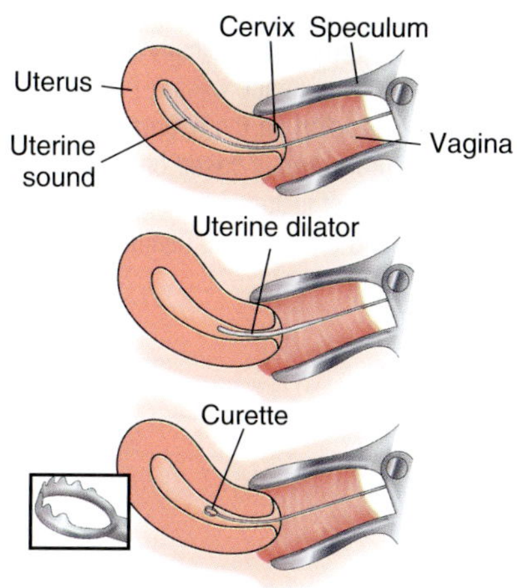

FIGURE 8-9
Dilation and curettage.

Surgical Terms—*cont'd*

Not Built from Word Parts

Term	Definition
endometrial ablation (*en*-dō-MĒ-trē-al) (ab-LĀ-shun)	a procedure to destroy or remove the endometrium by use of laser or thermal energy; used to treat abnormal uterine bleeding (Figure 8-10)
laparoscopy or laparoscopic surgery (*lap*-a-ROS-ko-pē) (*lap*-a-rō-SKOP-ik)	visual examination of the abdominal cavity, accomplished by inserting a laparoscope through a tiny incision near the umbilicus. It is used for surgical procedures such as tubal sterilization (closure of the uterine tubes), hysterectomy, oophorectomy, or biopsy of the ovaries. It may also be used to diagnose endometriosis. (Figure 8-13)
myomectomy (*mī*-ō-MEK-to-mē)	excision of a fibroid tumor (myoma) from the uterus
sentinel lymph node biopsy (SEN-tin-el) (limf) (nōd) (BĪ-op-sē)	an injection of blue dye and/or radioactive isotope used to identify the sentinel lymph node(s), the first in the axillary chain and most likely to contain metastasis of breast cancer. The nodes are removed and microscopically examined. If negative, no more nodes are removed (Figure 8-11).
stereotactic breast biopsy (*ster*-ē-ō-TAK-tik) (brest) (BĪ-op-sē)	a technique that combines mammography and computer-assisted biopsy to obtain tissue from a breast lesion (Figure 8-12)
tubal ligation (lī-GĀ-shun)	closure of the uterine tubes for sterilization by tying (ligation) (the broader term "tubal sterilization" includes cauterizing the cut ends) (also called **"tying of tubes"**) (Figure 8-13)
uterine artery embolization (UAE) (ū-ter-in) (AR-ter-ē) (*em*-be-li-ZĀ-shun)	minimally invasive procedure used to treat fibroids of the uterus by blocking arteries that supply blood to the fibroids. First, an arteriogram is used to identify the vessels. Once identified, tiny gelatin beads, about the size of grains of sand, are inserted into the vessels to create a blockage. The blockage stops the blood supply to the fibroids causing them to shrink.

ABLATION

is from the Latin **ablatum,** meaning **to carry away.** In surgery **ablation** means **removal** or **excision,** especially by cutting with laser or electrical energy.

TIPES OF BREART BIOPSY

- **Directed breast biopsy** uses mammography, sonography, or MRI radiographic images to guide a biopsy needle.
- **Surgical breast biopsy** involves making an incision to remove a palpable breast lesion (also called *open* or *incisional biopsy*).
- **Wire localization biopsy** combines both modalities and uses radiographic guidance to place a thin, flexible wire directly into a breast lesion. The lesion is removed surgically with the wire intact.

Deciding on the optimal procedure is based on how a breast lesion is best visualized and the patient's health and preferences.

EXERCISE FIGURE G

Fill in the blanks to complete the labeling of the diagrams.

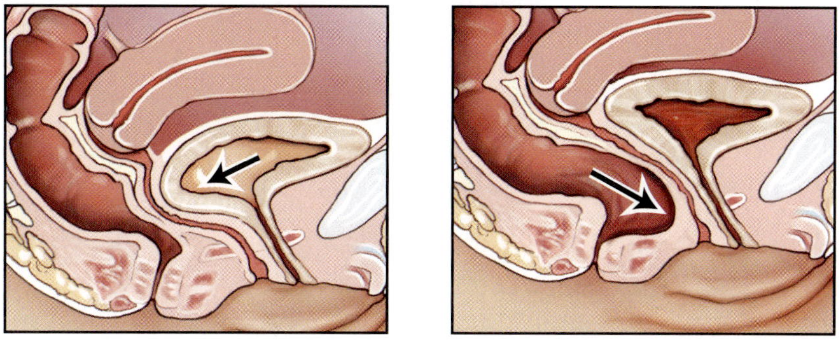

Anterior and posterior ________ / ____ / ________ corrects the conditions of:
vagina / cv / suturing

1. ________ / ____ / ________
bladder / cv / protrusion

2. Rectocele

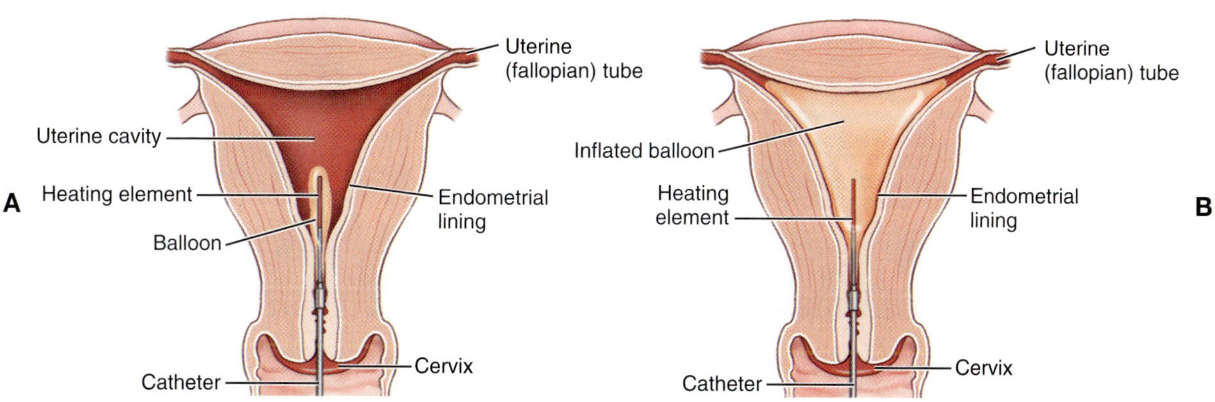

FIGURE 8-10
Endometrial ablation. **A,** The balloon catheter (deflated) is inserted through the cervix into the uterine cavity. **B,** The balloon is inflated with a solution of 5% dextrose and water and heated to 87°C for 8 minutes, ablating the endometrial lining.

SENTINEL LYMPH NODE BIOPSY

was first developed for patients with melanoma. It is now used to determine metastasis of breast cancer to the lymph nodes. Previously, surgeons would remove 10 to 20 lymph nodes to determine the spread of cancer, often causing lymphedema, which can lead to painful and permanent swelling of the arm. With sentinel lymph node biopsy, if negative, additional lymph nodes are not removed.

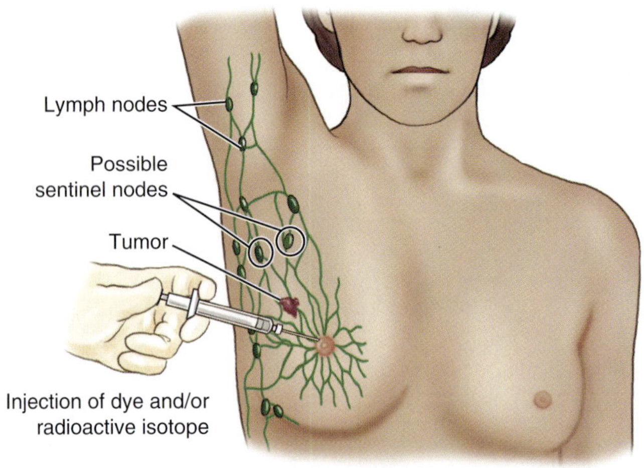

FIGURE 8-11
Preparation for sentinel lymph node biopsy.The process of identifying the sentinel node(s) is performed in the nuclear medicine department of radiology.The biopsy is performed in surgery.

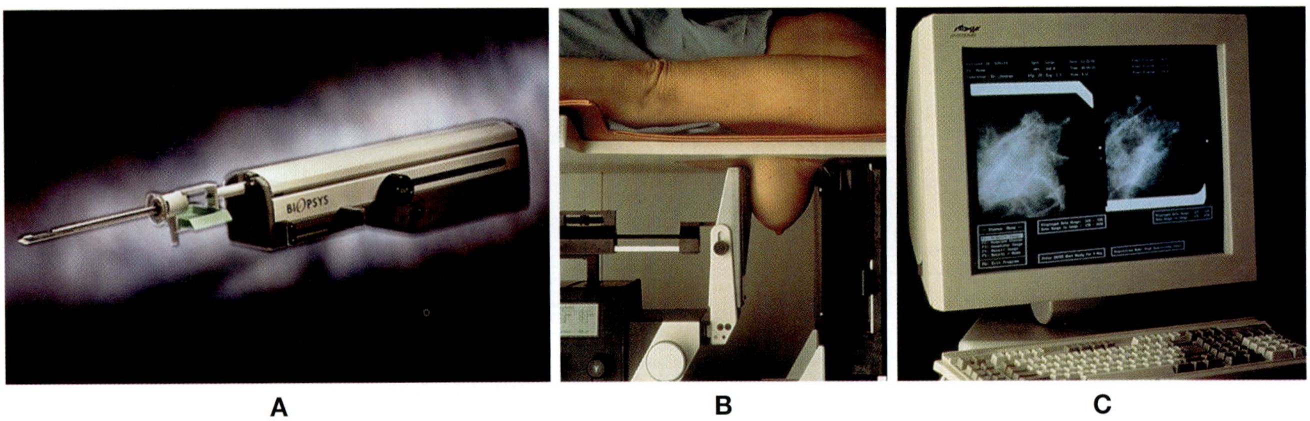

FIGURE 8-12
Stereotactic breast biopsy is the least invasive method of obtaining tissue to determine if a nonpalpable breast lesion is benign or malignant. Benefits include less pain and scarring, a shorter recovery time, and less expense than conventional surgery. The patient is placed prone on a special table with the breast suspended through an opening.The breast is placed in a mammography machine under the table. A digital mammogram is produced on a computer monitor to identify the exact location of the lesion. The biopsy instrument is guided by a radiologist or surgeon. Tissue obtained from the lesion is examined microscopically. **A,** The mammotome is used to obtain the specimen for biopsy. **B,** The patient is positioned for stereotactic breast biopsy. **C,** The mammogram appears digitally and is used to determine the placement of the biopsy needle.

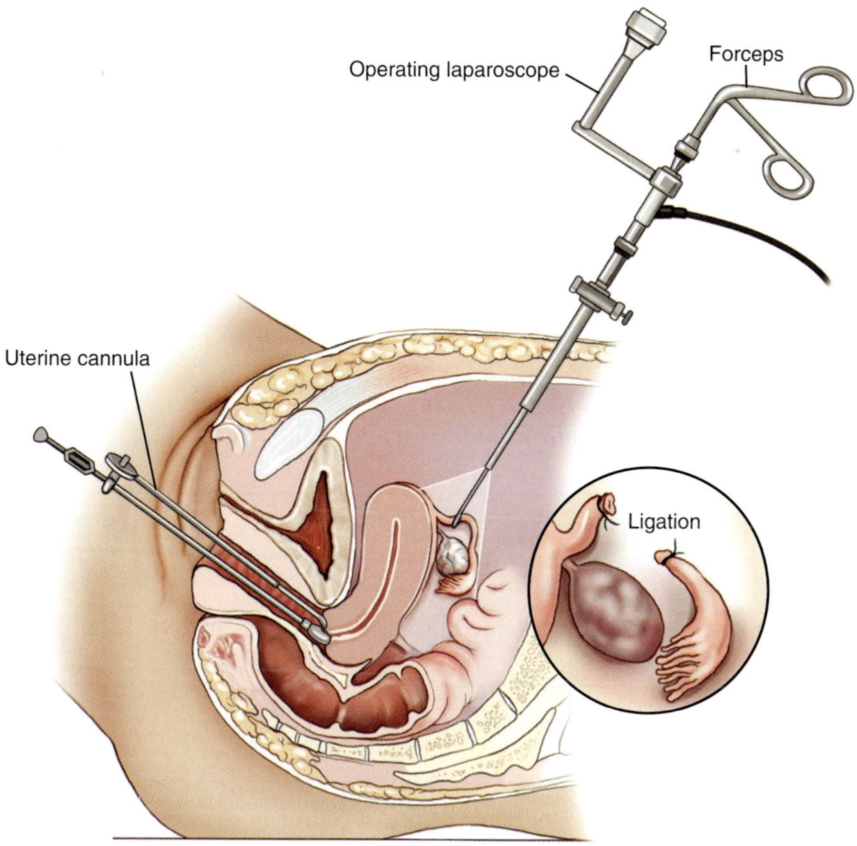

FIGURE 8-13
Laparoscopic tubal sterilization.

TUBAL STERILIZATION

is a form of permanent birth control, preventing pregnancy by cutting or blocking uterine tubes. In **tubal ligation**, which involves surgery, uterine tubes can be:

- cut and tied with surgical gut, cotton, silk, or wire
- cut and cauterized
- closed off with a clip, clamp, ring, or band

In **nonsurgical tubal sterilization**, uterine tubes are blocked by either:

- coils, Essure system
- plug, Adiana system

EXERCISE 19

Practice saying aloud each of the surgical terms not built from word parts on pp. 331-332.

To hear the terms, go to http://evolve.elsevier.com. Refer to p. 18 for your Evolve Access Information. Select Exercises & Review, Chapter 8, Chapter Exercises, Pronunciation.

☐ Place a check mark in the box when you have completed this exercise.

EXERCISE 20

Fill in the blanks with the correct term.

1. A procedure used for sterilization of the woman is ____________________ ____________________.
2. The surgery used to repair a cystocele and rectocele is a(n)________________ and ____________________ ____________________.
3. D&C is the abbreviation for __________________ and __________________.
4. __________________ __________________ __________________ is a technique used to obtain tissue from a breast lesion.
5. Excision of a fibroid tumor from the uterus is called ____.
6. A procedure to destroy endometrium by laser or thermal energy is called __________________ __________________.
7. A procedure used to treat uterine fibroids by blocking the blood supply is called __________________ __________________ __________________.
8. Surgical removal of a cone-shaped area of the cervix is called ____.
9. A procedure to identify metastasis of breast cancer in the axillary lymph nodes for biopsy is called __________________ __________________ __________________ __________________.
10. A surgical procedure performed through a tiny incision near the umbilicus is called __________________ or __________________ __________________.

EXERCISE 21

Match the surgical procedures in the first column with the corresponding organs in the second column. You may use the answers in the second column more than once.

_____ 1. dilation and curettage
_____ 2. laparoscopic surgery for sterilization
_____ 3. tubal ligation
_____ 4. anterior and posterior colporrhaphy repair
_____ 5. myomectomy
_____ 6. stereotactic breast biopsy
_____ 7. conization
_____ 8. endometrial ablation
_____ 9. sentinel lymph node biopsy
_____ 10. uterine artery embolization

a. uterine tubes
b. vagina
c. uterus
d. ovaries
e. vulva
f. mammary glands
g. lymph nodes

EXERCISE 22

Spell each of the surgical terms not built from word parts on pp. 331-332 by having someone dictate them to you.

To hear and spell the terms, go to http://evolve.elsevier.com. Refer to p. 18 for your Evolve Access Information. Select Exercises & Review, Chapter 8, Chapter Exercises, Spelling.
☐ Place a check mark in the box if you have completed this exercise online.

1. ______________________
2. ______________________
3. ______________________
4. ______________________
5. ______________________
6. ______________________
7. ______________________
8. ______________________
9. ______________________
10. ______________________

Diagnostic Terms

Built from Word Parts

The following terms are built from word parts you have already learned and can be translated literally to find their meanings. Further explanation of terms beyond the definitions of their word parts, if needed, is included in parentheses.

Term	Definition
DIAGNOSTIC IMAGING	
hysterosalpingogram (*his*-ter-ō-*sal*-PING-gō-gram)	radiographic image of the uterus and uterine tubes (after an injection of a contrast agent) (Exercise Figure H)
mammogram (MAM-ō-gram)	radiographic image of the breast (Figure 8-14)
mammography (ma-MOG-ra-fē)	radiographic imaging of the breast (also called **digital mammography** when images are obtained electronically and viewed on a computer) (Figure 8-14)
sonohysterography (SHG) (*son*-ō-*his*-ter-OG-ra-fē)	process of recording the uterus by use of sound (an ultrasound procedure)
ENDOSCOPY	
colposcope (KOL-pō-skōp)	instrument used for visual examination of the vagina (and cervix)
colposcopy (kol-POS-ko-pē)	visual examination (with a magnified view) of the vagina (and cervix)
culdoscope (KUL-dō-skōp)	instrument used for visual examination of Douglas cul-de-sac (rectouterine pouch)
culdoscopy (kul-DOS-ko-pē)	visual examination of Douglas cul-de-sac (rectouterine pouch) (Exercise Figure I)
hysteroscope (HIS-ter-ō-skōp)	instrument used for visual examination of the uterus (uterine cavity)
hysteroscopy (*his*-ter-OS-ko-pē)	visual examination of the uterus (uterine cavity)
OTHER	
culdocentesis (*kul*-dō-sen-TĒ-sis)	surgical puncture to remove fluid from Douglas cul-de-sac (rectouterine pouch) (Exercise Figure I)

SONOHYSTEROGRAPHY

is a technique for evaluating the uterine cavity. Saline solution is injected into the uterine cavity, followed by transvaginal sonography. It is used preoperatively to assess polyps, myomas, and adhesions.

ENDOSCOPY

dates back to the time of Hippocrates (460-375 BC), who mentions using a speculum to look into a rectum to see where it was affected. By the end of the nineteenth century, **cystoscopy, proctoscopy, laryngoscopy,** and **esophagoscopy** were well established. Use of the **endoscope** for surgery was not widely practiced in the United States until the 1970s when gynecologists started performing **laparoscopic tubal sterilization.** The first ectopic pregnancy was removed by laparoscopic surgery in 1973, the first **laparoscopic appendectomy** occurred in 1983, and the first laparoscopic **cholecystectomy** in 1989.

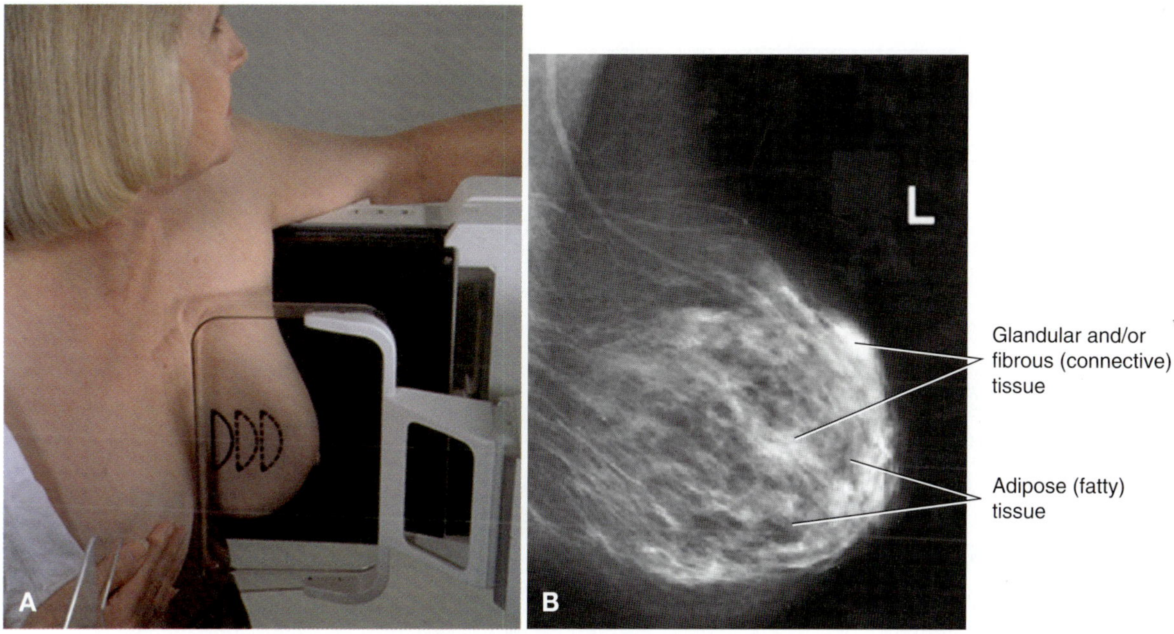

FIGURE 8-14
A, Mammography. **B,** Mammogram.

EXERCISE FIGURE H

Fill in the blanks to complete the labeling of the diagram.

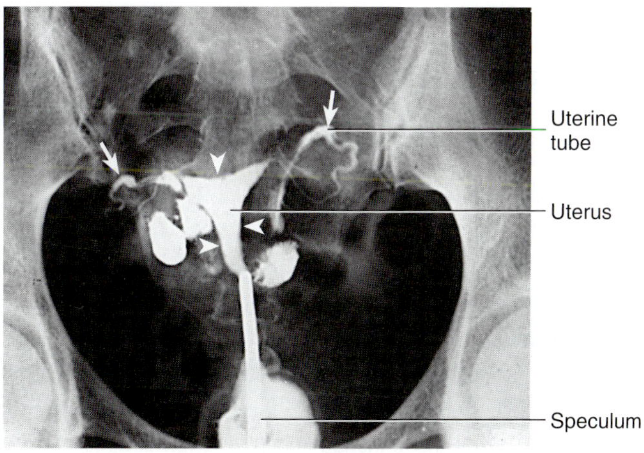

The ______ / ___ / ______ / ___ / ______
uterus / cv / uterine tube / cv / radiographic image

reveals ______ / ___ / ______
water / cv / uterine tube

Liquid contrast medium is injected through the vagina and is used to outline the uterus and uterine tubes before the radiographic image is made. This procedure usually is performed to determine whether obstructions exist in the uterine tubes causing infertility.

EXERCISE FIGURE I

Fill in the blanks to complete the labeling of the diagram.

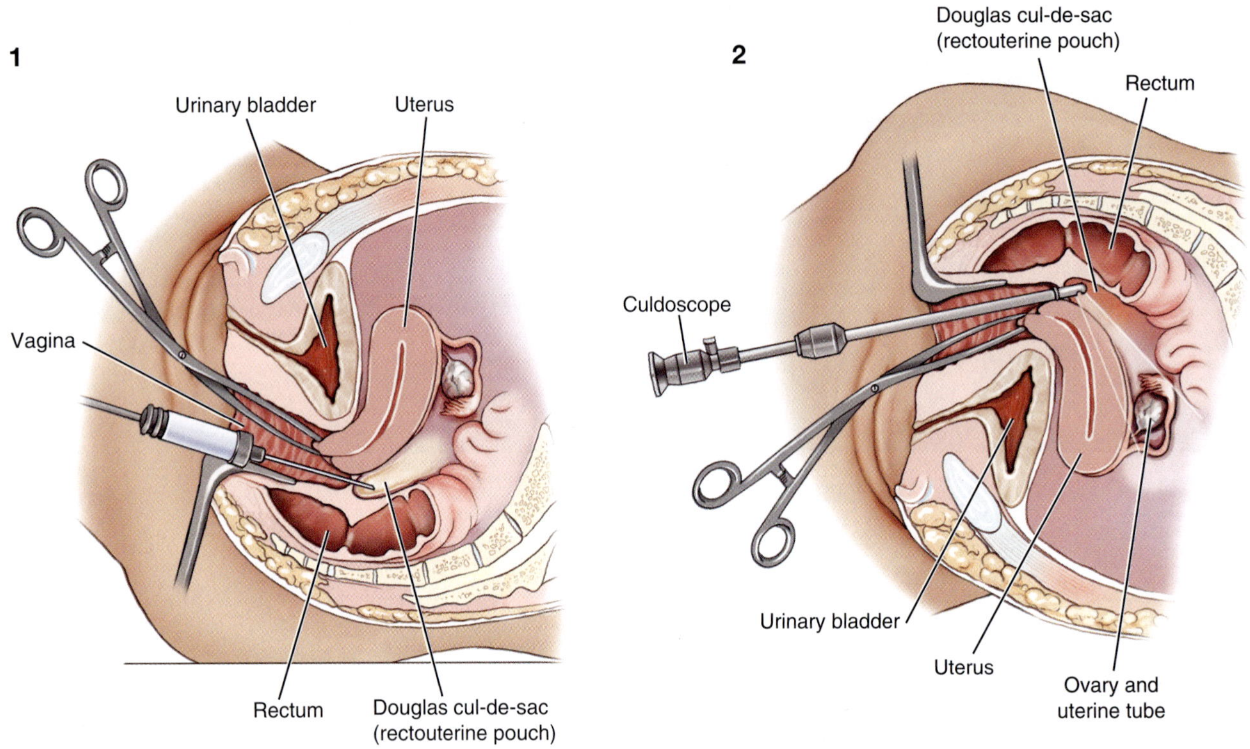

1. _____ / _____ / _____
cul-de-sac / cv / surgical procedure to remove fluid
is performed to remove pus or other fluid from the rectouterine pouch.

2. _____ / _____ / _____
cul-de-sac / cv / visual examination
is performed to view the pelvic cavity and organs.
It may be used to diagnose ectopic pregnancy.

EXERCISE 23

Practice saying aloud each of the diagnostic terms built from word parts on p. 338.

To hear the terms, go to http://evolve.elsevier.com. Refer to p. 18 for your Evolve Access Information. Select Exercises & Review, Chapter 8, Chapter Exercises, Pronunciation.

☐ Place a check mark in the box when you have completed this exercise.

EXERCISE 24

Analyze and define the following diagnostic terms.

1. colposcopy ______________________________
2. mammogram ______________________________
3. colposcope ______________________________
4. hysteroscopy ______________________________
5. hysterosalpingogram ______________________________
6. culdoscope ______________________________
7. culdoscopy ______________________________
8. culdocentesis ______________________________
9. mammography ______________________________
10. hysteroscope ______________________________
11. sonohysterography ______________________________

EXERCISE 25

Build diagnostic terms that correspond to the following definitions by using the word parts you have learned.

1. radiographic image of the uterus and uterine tubes
   ______ / ___ / ______ / ___ / ______
   WR / CV / WR / CV / S
2. visual examination of the vagina (and cervix)
   ______ / ___ / ______
   WR / CV / S
3. instrument used for visual examination of the vagina (and cervix)
   ______ / ___ / ______
   WR / CV / S
4. visual examination of the uterus
   ______ / ___ / ______
   WR / CV / S
5. radiographic image of the breast
   ______ / ___ / ______
   WR / CV / S
6. instrument used for visual examination of Douglas cul-de-sac
   ______ / ___ / ______
   WR / CV / S
7. visual examination of Douglas cul-de-sac
   ______ / ___ / ______
   WR / CV / S

8. surgical puncture to remove fluid from Douglas cul-de-sac ________ / ____ / ________
   WR / CV / S

9. instrument used for visual examination of the uterus ________ / ____ / ________
   WR / CV / S

10. radiographic imaging of the breast ________ / ____ / ________
    WR / CV / S

11. process of recording the uterus with sound ________ / ____ / ________ / ____ / ________
    WR / CV / WR / CV / S

EXERCISE 26

Spell each of the diagnostic terms built from word parts on p. 338 by having someone dictate them to you.

To hear and spell the terms, go to http://evolve.elsevier.com. Refer to p. 18 for your Evolve Access Information. Select Exercises & Review, Chapter 8, Chapter Exercises, Spelling.

☐ Place a check mark in the box if you have completed this exercise online.

1. ________________
2. ________________
3. ________________
4. ________________
5. ________________
6. ________________
7. ________________
8. ________________
9. ________________
10. ________________
11. ________________

Diagnostic Terms

Not Built from Word Parts

In some of the following terms, you may recognize word parts you have already learned; however, the full meaning of the terms cannot be discerned by the definition of their word parts.

Term	Definition
DIAGNOSTIC IMAGING	
transvaginal sonography (TVS) (trans-VAJ-i-nal) (so-NOG-ra-fē)	an ultrasound procedure that uses a transducer placed in the vagina to obtain images of the ovaries, uterus, cervix, uterine tubes, and surrounding structures; used to diagnose masses such as ovarian cysts or tumors, to monitor pregnancy, and to evaluate ovulation for the treatment of infertility (Figure 8-15)
LABORATORY	
CA-125 (cancer antigen-125 tumor marker) (C-Ā-125)	a blood test used in the detection of ovarian cancer. It is also used to monitor treatment and to determine the extent of the disease.
Pap smear (pap) (smēr)	a cytological study of cervical and vaginal secretions used to determine the presence of abnormal or cancerous cells; most commonly used to detect cancers of the cervix (also called **Papanicolaou** [*pap*-a-NIK kō-lā-oo] **smear** and **Pap test**) (Figure 8-16)

PAP SMEAR

is named after Dr. George N. Papanicolaou (1883–1962), a Greek physician practicing in the United States, who developed the cell smear method for the diagnosis of cancer in 1943. The test may be used for tissue specimen from any organ but is most commonly used on cervical and vaginal secretions. The Pap smear is 95% accurate in detecting cervical carcinoma. In 1966 a liquid-based screening system was approved by the Food and Drug Administration as an alternative for the conventional Pap smear. This system improves detection of squamous intraepithelial lesions.

A

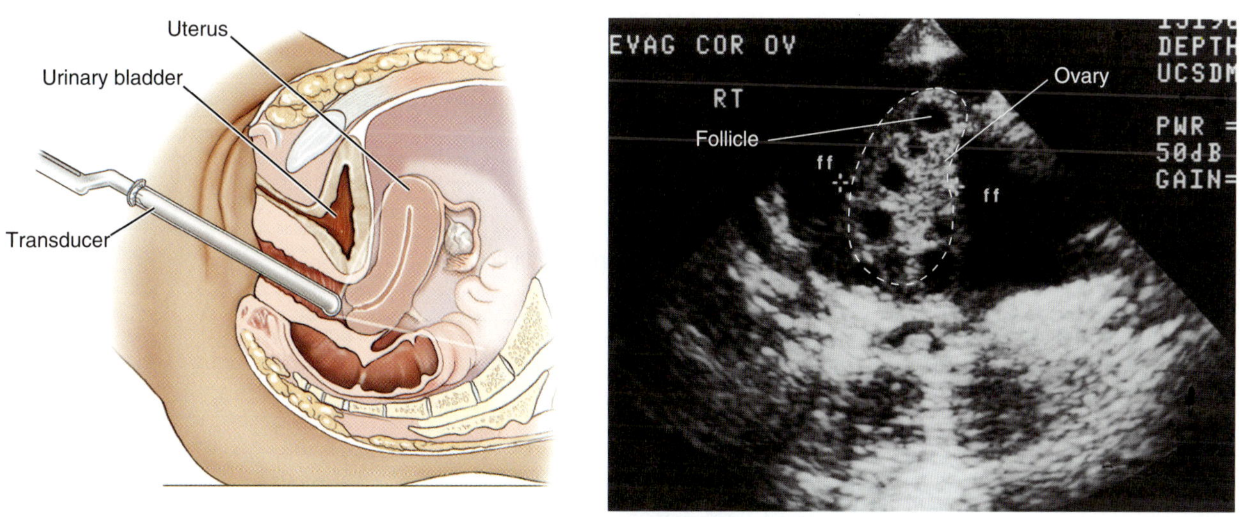

B

FIGURE 8-15
Transvaginal sonography. **A,** Transducer placed in the vagina. **B,** Transvaginal sagittal image of the right ovary with multiple follicles, showing free fluid surrounding the ovary.

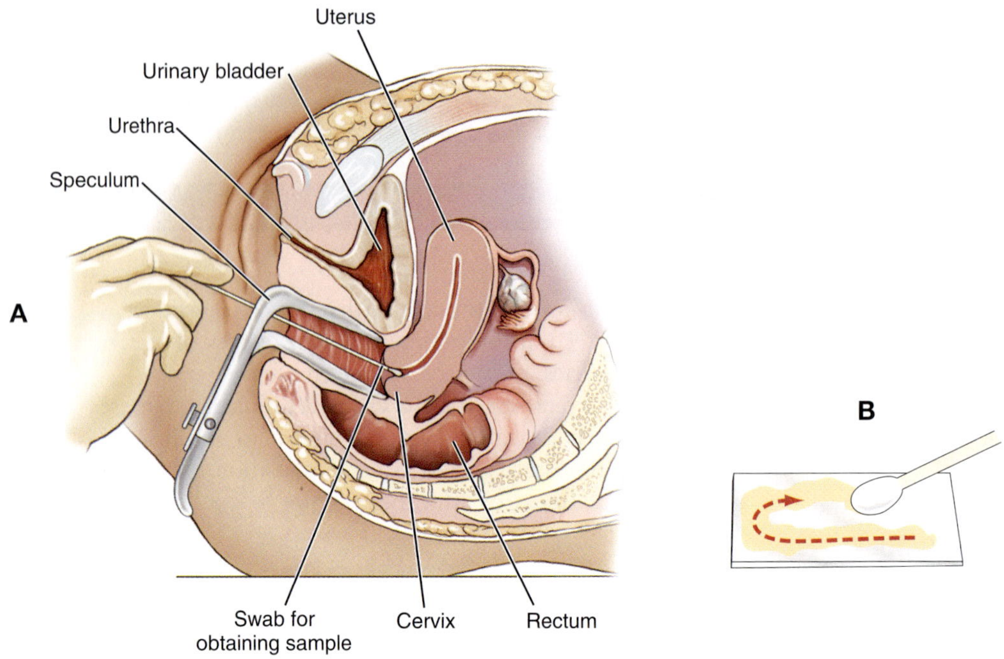

FIGURE 8-16
Pap smear. **A,** Obtaining the specimen. **B,** Transferring the specimen to a glass slide, where it will be stained and studied under a microscope in the laboratory.

EXERCISE 27

Practice saying aloud each of the diagnostic terms not built from word parts on p. 343.

To hear the terms, go to http://evolve.elsevier.com. Refer to p. 18 for your Evolve Access Information. Select Exercises & Review, Chapter 8, Chapter Exercises, Pronunciation.

☐ Place a check mark in the box when you have completed this exercise.

EXERCISE 28

Fill in the blanks with the correct definition.

1. Pap smear ______________________________
2. transvaginal sonography ______________________________
3. CA-125 ______________________________

EXERCISE 29

Write the term for each of the following.

1. study of cervical and vaginal secretions _______________ _______________
2. blood test used to detect ovarian cancer _______________
3. obtains images of the ovaries, uterus, cervix, uterine tubes, and surrounding structures _______________ _______________

EXERCISE 30

Spell each of the disease and disorder terms not built from word parts on p. 343 by having someone dictate them to you.

To hear and spell the terms, go to http://evolve.elsevier.com. Refer to p. 18 for your Evolve Access Information. Select Exercises & Review; Chapter 8, Chapter Exercises, Spelling.

☐ Place a check mark in the box if you have completed this exercise online.

1. ______________________
2. ______________________
3. ______________________

Complementary Terms

Built from Word Parts

The following terms are built from word parts you have already learned and can be translated literally to find their meanings. Further explanation of terms beyond the definition of their word parts, if needed, is included in parentheses.

Term	Definition
gynecologist (*gīn*-ek-OL-o-jist)	a physician who studies and treats diseases of women (female reproductive system)
gynecology (GYN) (*gīn*-ek-OL-o-jē)	study of women (a branch of medicine dealing with diseases of the female reproductive system)
gynopathic (*gīn*-ō-PATH-ik)	pertaining to diseases of women
leukorrhea (*lū*-kō-RĒ-a)	white discharge (from the vagina)
mastalgia (mas-TAL-ja)	pain in the breast
mastoptosis (*mas*-top-TŌ-sis)	sagging breast
menarche (me-NAR-kē)	beginning of menstruation (usually occurring between the ages of 11 and 16)
vaginal (VAJ-i-nal)	pertaining to the vagina
vulvovaginal (*vul*-vō-VAJ-i-nal)	pertaining to the vulva and vagina

EXERCISE 31

Practice saying aloud each of the complementary terms built from word parts above.

To hear the terms, go to http://evolve.elsevier.com. Refer to p. 18 for your Evolve Access Information. Select Exercises & Review, Chapter 8, Chapter Exercises, Pronunciation.

☐ Place a check mark in the box when you have completed this exercise.

EXERCISE 32

Analyze and define the following complementary terms.

1. gynecologist ____________________
2. gynecology ____________________
3. vulvovaginal ____________________
4. mastalgia ____________________
5. menarche ____________________
6. leukorrhea ____________________
7. gynopathic ____________________
8. mastoptosis ____________________
9. vaginal ____________________

EXERCISE 33

Build complementary terms that correspond to the following definitions by using the word parts you have learned.

1. white discharge (from the vagina) ______ WR / CV / ______ S
2. beginning of menstruation ______ WR / ______ WR
3. pain in the breast ______ WR / ______ S
4. pertaining to the vulva and vagina ______ WR / CV / ______ WR / ______ S
5. a physician who studies and treats diseases of women ______ WR / CV / ______ S
6. study of women (branch of medicine dealing with diseases of the female reproductive system) ______ WR / CV / ______ S
7. sagging breast ______ WR / CV / ______ S
8. pertaining to diseases of women ______ WR / CV / ______ WR / ______ S
9. pertaining to the vagina ______ WR / ______ S

EXERCISE 34

Spell each of the complementary terms built from word parts on p. 345 by having someone dictate them to you.

To hear and spell the terms, go to http://evolve.elsevier.com. Refer to p. 18 for your Evolve Access Information. Select Exercises & Review, Chapter 8, Chapter Exercises, Spelling.
☐ Place a check mark in the box if you have completed this exercise online.

1. ______________________
2. ______________________
3. ______________________
4. ______________________
5. ______________________
6. ______________________
7. ______________________
8. ______________________
9. ______________________

HORMONE REPLACEMENT THERAPY (HRT)

has decreased dramatically since 2002, following release of research data by the Women's Health Initiative, a trial conducted by the National Institutes of Health. This study demonstrated that women taking HRT had a significantly higher incidence of breast cancer, heart disease, and stroke. As a result, current practice recommendations state that menopausal women choosing HRT should take the lowest possible dose for the shortest amount of time.

Complementary Terms

Not Built from Word Parts

In some of the following terms, you may recognize word parts you have already learned; however, the full meaning of the terms cannot be discerned by the definition of their word parts.

Term	Definition
dyspareunia (*dis*-pa-RŪ-nē-a)	difficult or painful intercourse
fistula (FIS-tū-la)	abnormal passageway between two organs or between an internal organ and the body surface
hormone replacement therapy (HRT)	replacement of hormones, estrogen and/or progesterone, to treat symptoms associated with menopause
menopause (MEN-o-pawz)	cessation of menstruation, usually around the ages of 48 to 53 years
premenstrual syndrome (PMS) (prē-MEN-stroo-al) (SIN-drom)	a syndrome involving physical and emotional symptoms occurring in the 10 days before menstruation. Symptoms include nervous tension, irritability, mastalgia, edema, and headache. Its cause is not fully understood.
speculum (SPEK-ū-lum)	instrument for opening a body cavity to allow visual inspection (Figure 8-17)

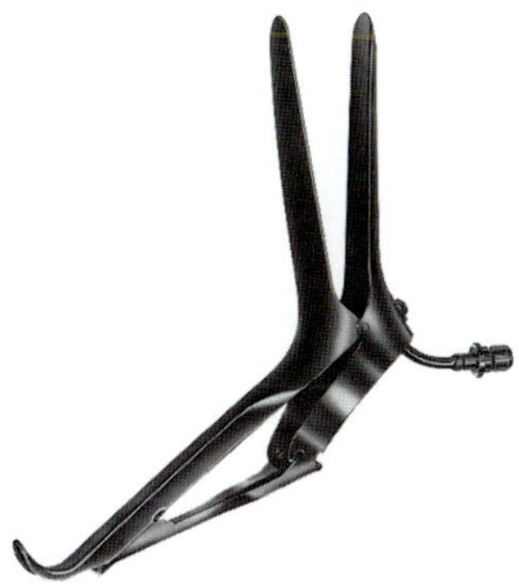

FIGURE 8-17
Vaginal speculum.

Refer to **Appendix D** for pharmacology terms related to the female reproductive system.

EXERCISE 35

Practice saying aloud each of the complementary terms not built from word parts on p. 347.

To hear the terms, go to http://evolve.elsevier.com. Refer to p. 18 for your Evolve Access Information. Select Exercises & Review, Chapter 8, Chapter Exercises, Pronunciation.

☐ Place a check mark in the box when you have completed this exercise.

EXERCISE 36

Write the definitions of the following terms.

1. menopause ______________________________
2. dyspareunia ______________________________
3. fistula ______________________________
4. premenstrual syndrome ______________________________
5. speculum ______________________________
6. hormone replacement therapy ______________________________

EXERCISE 37

Write the term for each of the following.

1. abnormal passageway ______________________________
2. painful intercourse ______________________________
3. cessation of menstruation ______________________________
4. syndrome involving physical and emotional symptoms ______________ ______________
5. instrument for opening a body cavity ______________________________
6. replacement of hormones to treat symptoms associated with menopause ______________ ______________ ______________

EXERCISE 38

Spell each of the complementary terms not built from word parts on p. 347 by having someone dictate them to you.

To hear and spell the terms, go to http://evolve.elsevier.com. Refer to p. 18 for your Evolve Access Information. Select Exercises & Review, Chapter 8, Chapter Exercises, Spelling.
☐ Place a check mark in the box if you have completed this exercise online.

1. ______________________ 4. ______________________
2. ______________________ 5. ______________________
3. ______________________ 6. ______________________

Abbreviations

A&P repair	anterior and posterior colporrhaphy
Cx	cervix
D&C	dilation and curettage
FBD	fibrocystic breast disease
GYN	gynecology
HRT	hormone replacement therapy
PID	pelvic inflammatory disease
PMS	premenstrual syndrome
SHG	sonohysterography
TAH/BSO	total abdominal hysterectomy/bilateral salpingo-oophorectomy
TSS	toxic shock syndrome
TVH	total vaginal hysterectomy
TVS	transvaginal sonography
UAE	uterine artery embolization

Refer to **Appendix C** for a complete list of abbreviations.

EXERCISE 39

Write the meaning for each of the abbreviations in the following sentences.

1. To repair a cystocele and rectocele the patient is scheduled in surgery for an **A&P repair** ________________ & ________________ ________________.
2. Following a **TAH/BSO** ________________ ________________ ________________ and ________________ ________________ the gynecologist prescribed **HRT** ________________ ________________ ________________ for the patient to take for 3 months after surgery.
3. **SHG** ________________ and **TVS** ________________ ________________ are diagnostic ultrasound procedures used to assist in diagnosing diseases and disorders of the female reproductive organs.
4. When performing a **TVH** ________________ ________________ ________________ the surgeon removes the uterus through the vagina without a surgical incision into the abdomen.
5. **D&C** ________________ & ________________ is the dilation of the **Cx** ________________ and scraping of the endometrium.
6. **FBD** ________________ ________________ ________________ is the most common breast problem of women in their 20s.
7. A female patient with probable **PID** ________________ ________________ ________________ was referred to the **GYN** ________________ clinic for evaluation and care.
8. The medical management of **PMS** ________________ ________________ emphasizes the relief of symptoms.
9. **UAE** ________________ ________________ ________________ offers a minimally invasive treatment option for some women with symptomatic fibroid tumors.

PRACTICAL APPLICATION

EXERCISE 40 *Interact with Medical Documents*

A. Complete the progress note by writing the medical terms in the blanks. Use the list of definitions with the corresponding numbers on the next page.

University Hospital and Medical Center
4700 North Main Street • Wellness, Arizona 54321 • (987) 555-3210

PATIENT NAME: Evelina Garcia **CASE NUMBER:** 234-5678BR
DOB:10/08/19XX **DATE:**11/17/20XX

SURGICAL PROGRESS NOTE:
Evelina Garcia is a 48-year-old Hispanic woman here for follow-up after a suspicious lesion in the left breast was discovered during routine 1. ____________________. Her husband and sister are present for this visit.

Family history is positive for breast 2. ____________________ in two maternal aunts, both under age 50 at diagnosis.

Past medical history includes 3. ____________________ for 4. ____________________ and 5. ____________________. She has been on 6. ____________________ since age 46 years.

The patient consented to a 7. ____________________ ____________________ ____________________.

The pathology report is as follows.

GROSS DESCRIPTION: Received in formalin are four, pink-tan, cylindrical fragments of fibroadipose tissue, which range from 0.8 to 1.3 cm in length, each with a 0.1-cm diameter. The specimen is entirely submitted in one cassette.

FINAL DIAGNOSIS: Mammary parenchyma, left breast guided needle biopsy: Infltrating, moderately differentiated ductal carcinoma with focal ductal carcinoma in situ, Grade 2, involving all four specimens. Lymphovascular invasion is identified.

Upon examination, the biopsy site reveals a 1-cm, healing surgical scar on the 8. ____________________ aspect of the left breast. The patient reports mild tenderness, alleviated with ibuprofen, but denies any signs or symptoms of infection.

Extensive education provided to patient and family regarding diagnosis and surgical treatment options. Patient states that she is interested in 9. ____________________ with immediate reconstruction. Due to presence of lymphovascular invasion, 10. ____________________ ____________________ ____________________ ____________________ will be scheduled at the time of definitive surgery.

Consultation appointments arranged through Breast Center with medical oncology and plastic surgery clinics within one week. Follow-up appointment scheduled for next week.

____
Meredith Woolridge, MD
MW/kpr

1. radiographic imaging of the breast
2. cancerous tumor
3. excision of the uterus
4. growth of endometrium into the muscular portion of the uterus
5. abnormal condition in which endometrial tissue occurs in various areas of the pelvic cavity
6. abbreviation for replacement of hormones to treat menopause
7. combines mammography and computer-assisted biopsy to obtain tissue from a breast lesion
8. pertaining to the middle and to (one) side
9. surgical removal of a breast
10. an injection of blue dye and/or radioactive isotope used to identify the first in the axillary chain and most likely to contain metastasis of breast cancer

B. Read the chart note and answer the questions following it.

47820 CARLSON, AKELAH

File Patient Navigate Custom Fields Help

Patient Chart | Lab | Rad | Notes | Documents | Rx | Scheduling | Images | Billing

Name: **CARLSON, Akelah** MR#: **47820** DOB: **2/15/19XX** Sex: **F**

CHART NOTE

ENCOUNTER DATE: 11/13/20XX

HISTORY: This 37-year-old gravida 2 para 2 African American woman was referred by her primary care provider. She complains of fullness in the pelvic region and menometrorrhagia. She admits to frequency and urgency of urination. Also, she complains of fatigue. The patient's last menstrual period was two weeks ago. Her mother was treated for ovarian cancer.

PHYSICAL EXAMINATION: Upon bimanual pelvic examination, an ill-defined mass was palpable on left lateral portion of the uterus.

DIAGNOSTIC STUDIES: Pap smear results showed normal cytology. CA-125 results were normal. Transvaginal sonography confirmed the presence of a pedunculated fibroid tumor. The uterine tubes and ovaries were normal.

IMPRESSION: Fibroid tumors.

RECOMMENDATION: We discussed the benefits of having a vaginal hysterectomy with bilateral salpingo-oophorectomy in view of her mother's history of ovarian cancer. The patient declined this approach because of the desire to have another child. A laparoscopic myomectomy is therefore recommended.

Electronically signed by: Elizabeth Fuller, MD 11/14/20XX 3:34 PM

EF/dlb

Start | Log On/Off | Print | Edit

1. The patient's symptoms include:
   a. absence of menstrual discharge
   b. scanty menstrual flow
   c. increased amount of menstrual flow during menses and bleeding between periods
   d. painful menstruation

2. The CA-125 diagnostic study was used to detect the presence of:
   a. ovarian cancer
   b. cervical cancer
   c. endometrial cancer
   d. endometriosis

3. The recommended procedure, a myomectomy, will entail the surgical excision of:
   a. a breast
   b. the uterus
   c. ovarian cancer
   d. a fibroid tumor

EXERCISE 41 *Interpret Medical Terms*

WEB LINK

For more information about breast health and the female reproductive system, visit the National Institutes of Health at ***www.health.nih.gov*** and click on Women's Health.

To test your understanding of the terms introduced in this chapter, circle the words that correctly complete the sentences. The italicized words refer to the correct answer.

1. The patient was diagnosed as having *painful menstruation*, or (**oligomenorrhea, dysmenorrhea, amenorrhea**).
2. *Inflammation of the inner lining of the uterus* is (**endocervicitis, endometritis, endometriosis**).
3. The patient is scheduled in surgery for a *salpingectomy*, which is the excision of the (**uterine tube, ovary, uterus**).
4. An *episiorrhaphy* is a (**suture of the vulva, discharge from the vulva, rapid discharge from the vulva**).
5. A *surgical procedure to reduce breast size* is called reduction (**mammogram, mammography, mammoplasty**).
6. A *hysterosalpingo-oophorectomy* is the excision of the (**uterus, uterine tubes, and ovaries; uterus, ovaries, and cervix; uterus, uterine tubes, and vagina**).
7. *Blood in the uterine tube* is called (**hematosalpinx, hydrosalpinx, pyosalpinx**).
8. *Endometrial tissue occurring in various areas of the pelvic cavity* is called (**adenomyosis, endometriosis, hysteratresia**).
9. The doctor requested a (**hysteroscope, colposcope, speculum**) *to open the vagina for visual examination.*
10. A severe illness *that may affect menstruating women after using tampons is* (**TVS, TSS, TVH**).
11. Cryosurgery, laser ablation, and LEEP are surgical *procedures performed to remove a cone-shaped area of the cervix* called (**colporrhaphy, conization, myomectomy**).

EXERCISE 42 *Read Medical Terms in Use*

Practice pronunciation of the terms by reading the following information on cancers of the female reproductive system. Use the pronunciation key following the medical terms to assist you in saying the words.

To hear these terms, go to http://evolve.elsevier.com. Refer to p. 18 for your Evolve Access Information. Select Exercises & Review, Chapter 8, Chapter Exercises, Read Medical Terms in Use.

CANCERS OF THE FEMALE REPRODUCTIVE SYSTEM

Breast Cancer

The breast is the second most common site of cancer in women. More than 80% of **breast cancer** (brest) (KAN-cer) is infiltrating ductal cancer (IDC), which originates in the mammary ducts. The rate of growth depends on hormonal influences. As long as the cancer remains in the duct, it is considered noninvasive and is called *ductal carcinoma in situ (DCIS)*.

Mammography (ma-MOG-ra-fē) is the most common method used for diagnosing cancer of the breast. Confirmation is done with a biopsy obtained by conventional surgery or guided breast biopsy, such as **stereotactic breast biopsy** (ster-ē-ō-TAK-tik) (brest) (BĪ-op-sē).Treatment may include lumpectomy, **mastectomy** (mas-TEK-to-mē),chemotherapy, radiation therapy, and hormonal therapy.

Cervical Cancer

In many regions of the world **cervical cancer** (SER-vi-kal) (KAN-cer) is the leading cause of death in women. Cervical cancer resembles a sexually transmitted disease, a feature that distinguishes it from other cancers. Abnormal **vaginal** (VAJ-i-nal) bleeding is the most common symptom. **Pap smear** followed by **colposcopy** (kol-POS-ko-pē) biopsy is used to diagnose this disease. Surgical treatment options are **conization** (*kon*-i-ZĀ-shun), such as LEEP, and **hysterectomy** (his-te-REK-to-mē). Chemotherapy and radiation therapy may also be used. A vaccine for human papillomavirus is now available and can be used for the prevention of cervical cancer.

Endometrial Cancer

Currently 75% of women diagnosed with **endometrial cancer** (en-dō-MĒ-trē-al) (KAN-cer) are postmenopausal. Inappropriate bleeding is the only warning sign; hence early diagnosis is common. Pelvic examination, Pap smear, and endometrial sampling are used to diagnose this disease. Treatment is **hysterosalpingo-oophorectomy** (*his*-ter-ō-sal-*ping*-gō-Ō-*of*-o-REK-to-mē), which may be followed by chemotherapy and radiation therapy. **Laparoscopic** (lap-a-RŌ-skop-ik)-assisted **vaginal hysterectomy** (VAJ-i-nal) (*his*-te-REK-to-mē) may also be used.

Ovarian Cancer

Ovarian cancer (ō-VAR-ē-an) (KAN-cer) is the sixth most common form of cancer in women. Early symptoms are often absent or associated with other problems; thus early diagnosis is uncommon. Early symptoms include abdominal discomfort and bloating; later stages include abdominal or pelvic pain and urinary or menstrual irregularities. **CA-125** and **transvaginal sonography** (trans-VAJ-i-nal) (so-NOG-ra-fē) are used in diagnosing this disease. Treatment is total abdominal **hysterectomy** (*his*-te-REK-to-mē) and bilateral **salpingo-oophorectomy** (sal-ping-gō-ō-*of*-o-REK-to-mē) and removal of as much additional involved tissue as possible.

Chemotherapy is usually prescribed, and in some instances, is followed a year later by a second-look **laparoscopy** (lap-a-ROS-ko-pē) to determine the presence or absence of the tumor.

EXERCISE 43 *Comprehend Medical Terms in Use*

Test your comprehension of the terms in the previous box by circling the correct answer.

1. Which of the following diagnostic tests would the physician use to diagnose ovarian cancer?
   a. colposcopy biopsy
   b. transvaginal sonography
   c. Pap smear
   d. mammography
2. T F Surgery is a treatment option for breast, cervical, endometrial, and ovarian cancer.
3. T F Excision of the uterus, uterine tubes, and ovaries is an accepted surgical treatment for both endometrial and ovarian cancer.
4. An instrument for visualization of the vagina is used to obtain a biopsy to confirm the diagnosis of cancer of the:
   a. ovary
   b. breast
   c. uterine tube
   d. cervix

CHAPTER REVIEW

ONLINE CHAPTER REVIEW

To access the Evolve website, go to http://evolve.elsevier.com. Refer to p. 18 for your Evolve Access Information. Select Exercises & Review, Chapter 3, then select Chapter Exercises, Practice Activities, Animations, or Games. Place a check mark in the box when you have completed an exercise or activity, watched an animation, or played a game. Have fun!

Chapter Exercises

Exercises in this section of your Evolve resources correlate to exercises in your textbook. You may have completed them as you worked through the chapter.

- ☐ Pronunciation
- ☐ Spelling
- ☐ Read Medical Terms in Use

Practice Activities

Practice in study mode, then test your learning in assessment mode. Keep track of your scores from assessment mode if you wish.

	SCORE
☐ Picture It	_______
☐ Define Word Parts	_______
☐ Build Medical Terms	_______
☐ Word Shop	_______
☐ Define Medical Terms	_______
☐ Use It	_______
☐ Hear It and Type It: Clinical Vignettes	_______

Animations

- ☐ Hysteroscope Insertion
- ☐ Hysteroscopy
- ☐ Ovarian Cysts
- ☐ Pelvic Inflammatory Disease

Games

- ☐ Name that Word Part
- ☐ Term Storm
- ☐ Term Explorer
- ☐ Termbusters
- ☐ Medical Millionaire
- ☐ Crossword Puzzle

REVIEW OF WORD PARTS

Can you define and spell the following word parts?

Combining Forms

arche/o
cervic/o
colp/o
culd/o
episi/o
gyn/o
gynec/o
hymen/o
hyster/o
mamm/o
mast/o
men/o
metr/i
metr/o
oophor/o
perine/o
salping/o
vagin/o
vulv/o

Prefix

peri-

Suffixes

-atresia
-salpinx

REVIEW OF TERMS

Can you build, analyze, define, pronounce, and spell the following terms *built from word parts?*

Diseases and Disorders

amenorrhea
Bartholin adenitis
cervicitis
colpitis
dysmenorrhea
endocervicitis
endometritis
hematosalpinx
hydrosalpinx
hysteratresia
mastitis
menometrorrhagia
menorrhagia
metrorrhagia
myometritis
oligomenorrhea
oophoritis
perimetritis
pyosalpinx
salpingitis
salpingocele
vaginitis
vulvovaginitis

Surgical

cervicectomy
colpoperineorrhaphy
colpoplasty
colporrhaphy
episioperineoplasty
episiorrhaphy
hymenectomy
hymenotomy
hysterectomy
hysteropexy
hysterosalpingo-oophorectomy
mammoplasty
mastectomy
mastopexy
oophorectomy
perineorrhaphy
salpingectomy
salpingo-oophorectomy
salpingostomy
vulvectomy

Diagnostic

colposcope
colposcopy
culdocentesis
culdoscope
culdoscopy
hysterosalpingogram
hysteroscope
hysteroscopy
mammogram
mammography
sonohysterography (SHG)

Complementary

gynecologist
gynecology (GYN)
gynopathic
leukorrhea
mastalgia
mastoptosis
menarche
vaginal
vulvovaginal

Can you define, pronounce, and spell the following terms *not built from word parts*?

Diseases and Disorders

adenomyosis
breast cancer
cervical cancer
endometrial cancer
endometriosis
fibrocystic breast disease (FBD)
fibroid tumor
ovarian cancer
pelvic inflammatory disease (PID)
prolapsed uterus
toxic shock syndrome (TSS)
vesicovaginal fistula

Surgical

anterior and posterior colporrhaphy (A&P repair)
conization
dilation and curettage (D&C)
endometrial ablation
laparoscopy
myomectomy
sentinel lymph node biopsy
stereotactic breast biopsy
tubal ligation
uterine artery embolization (UAE)

Diagnostic

CA-125
Pap smear
transvaginal sonography (TVS)

Complementary

dyspareunia
fistula
hormone replacement therapy (HRT)
menopause
premenstrual syndrome (PMS)
speculum

ANSWERS

Exercise figures

Exercise Figure

A. 1. ovary: oophor/o
2. uterus: hyster/o, metr/o, metr/i
3. uterine, or fallopian, tube: salping/o
4. cervix: cervic/o
5. vagina: colp/o, vagin/o
6. hymen: hymen/o

Exercise Figure

B. 1. vulva: episi/o, vulv/o
2. perineum: perine/o

Exercise Figure

C. salping/itis

Exercise Figure

D. hyster/o/ptosis

Exercise Figure

E. vesic/o/vagin/al

Exercise Figure

F. 1. hyster/o/salping/o/-oophor/ectomy
2. salping /o/-oophor/ectomy
3. (bilateral) salping/o/-oophor/ectomy
4. hyster/ectomy

Exercise Figure

G. colp/o/rrhaphy, cyst/o/cele

Exercise Figure

H. hyster/o/salping/o/gram, hydr/o/salpinx

Exercise Figure

I. 1. culd/o/centesis
2. culd/o/scopy

Exercise 1

1. c
2. f
3. g
4. b
5. d
6. e
7. h
8. a
9. i

Exercise 2

1. b
2. c
3. d
4. k
5. e
6. f
7. g
8. l
9. i
10. j
11. h

Exercise 3

1. vagina
2. ovary
3. uterus
4. woman
5. hymen
6. uterus
7. menstruation
8. vulva
9. cervix
10. vagina
11. woman
12. breast
13. perineum
14. uterine tube
15. vulva
16. breast
17. first, beginning
18. cul-de-sac

Exercise 4

1. a. episi/o
   b. vulv/o
2. a. mamm/o
   b. mast/o
3. men/o
4. oophor/o
5. salping/o
6. perine/o
7. a. vagin/o
   b. colp/o
8. a. metr/o
   b. metr/i
   c. hyster/o
9. a. gynec/o
   b. gyn/o
10. hymen/o
11. culd/o
12. cervic/o
13. arche/o

Exercise 5

1. -salpinx
2. peri-
3. -atresia

Exercise 6

1. uterine tube
2. surrounding
3. absence of a normal body opening, occlusion, closure

Exercise 7

Pronunciation Exercise

Exercise 8

1. WR S
   colp/itis
   inflammation of the vagina
2. WR S
   cervic/itis
   inflammation of the cervix
3. WR CV S
   hydr/o/salpinx
   CF
   water in the uterine tube
4. WR CV S
   hemat/o/salpinx
   CF
   blood in the uterine tube
5. WR CV S
   metr/o/rrhagia
   CF
   rapid flow of blood from the uterus (between menstrual cycles)
6. WR S
   oophor/itis
   inflammation of the ovary
7. WR S
   (Bartholin) aden/itis
   inflammation of (Bartholin) gland
8. WR CV WR S
   vulv/o/vagin/itis
   CF
   inflammation of the vulva and vagina
9. WR CV S
   salping/o/cele
   CF
   hernia of the uterine tube
10. WR CV WR CV S
    men/o/metr/o/rrhagia
    CF CF
    rapid flow of blood from the uterus at menstruation (and between menstrual cycles)
11. P WR CV S
    a/men/o/rrhea
    CF
    absence of menstrual discharge
12. P WR CV S
    dys/men/o/rrhea
    CF
    painful menstrual discharge
13. WR S
    mast/itis
    inflammation of the breast

14. P WR S
peri/metr/itis
inflammation surrounding the uterus (outer layer)
15. WR CV WR S
my/o/metr/itis
CF
inflammation of the uterine muscle
16. P WR S
endo/metr/itis
inflammation of the inner (lining) of the uterus
17. P WR S
endo/cervic/itis
inflammation of the inner (lining) of the cervix
18. WR CV S
py/o/salpinx
CF
pus in the uterine tube
19. WR S
hyster/atresia
closure of the uterus (uterine cavity)
20. WR S
salping/itis
inflammation of the uterine tube
21. WR S
vagin/itis
inflammation of the vagina
22. WR CV S
men/o/rrhagia
CF
rapid flow of blood at menstruation (increased amount)
23. WR CV WR CV S
olig/o/men/o/rrhea
CF CF
scanty menstrual flow (less often)

Exercise 9

1. mast/itis
2. metr/o/rrhagia
3. salping/itis
4. vulv/o/vagin/itis
5. a/men/o/rrhea
6. cervic/itis
7. (Bartholin) aden/itis
8. hydr/o/salpinx
9. dys/men/o/rrhea
10. hemat/o/salpinx
11. a. colp/itis
    b. vagin/itis
12. men/o/metr/o/rrhagia
13. oophor/itis
14. salping/o/cele
15. peri/metr/itis
16. endo/metr/itis
17. endo/cervic/itis
18. my/o/metr/itis
19. py/o/salpinx
20. hyster/atresia
21. olig/o/men/o/rrhea
22. men/o/rrhagia

Exercise 10

Spelling Exercise; see text pp. 317-318.

Exercise 11

Pronunciation Exercise

Exercise 12

1. downward displacement of the uterus into the vagina
2. inflammation of the female pelvic organs
3. abnormal opening between the bladder and vagina
4. benign fibroid tumor of the uterine muscle
5. abnormal condition in which endometrial tissue grows in various areas of the pelvic cavity
6. growth of endometrium into the muscular portion of the uterus
7. a severe illness characterized by high fever, vomiting, diarrhea, and myalgia
8. a disorder characterized by one or more benign cysts
9. malignant tumor of the ovary
10. malignant tumor of the breast
11. malignant tumor of the cervix
12. malignant tumor of the endometrium

Exercise 13

1. vesicovaginal fistula
2. fibroid tumor
3. pelvic inflammatory disease
4. prolapsed uterus
5. endometriosis
6. adenomyosis
7. toxic shock syndrome
8. fibrocystic breast disease
9. breast cancer
10. endometrial cancer
11. ovarian cancer
12. cervical cancer

Exercise 14

Spelling Exercise; see text pp. 322-323.

Exercise 15

Pronunciation Exercise

Exercise 16

1. WR CV S
colp/o/rrhaphy
CF
suture of the vagina
2. WR CV S
colp/o/plasty
CF
surgical repair of the vagina
3. WR CV S
episi/o/rrhaphy
CF
suture of the vulva (tear)
4. WR CV S
hymen/o/tomy
CF
incision of the hymen
5. WR CV S
hyster/o/pexy
CF
surgical fixation of the uterus
6. WR S
vulv/ectomy
excision of the vulva
7. WR CV S
perine/o/rrhaphy
CF
suture of the perineum (tear)
8. WR CV S
salping/o/stomy
CF
creation of an artificial opening in the uterine tube
9. WR CV WR S
salping/o/-oophor/ectomy
CF
excision of the uterine tube and ovary
10. WR S
oophor/ectomy
excision of an ovary
11. WR S
mast/ectomy
surgical removal of a breast
12. WR S
salping/ectomy
excision of a uterine tube
13. WR S
cervic/ectomy
excision of the cervix
14. WR CV WR CV S
colp/o/perine/o/rrhaphy
CF CF
suture of the vagina and perineum
15. WR CV WR CV S
episi/o/perine/o/plasty
CF CF
surgical repair of the vulva and perineum
16. WR S
hymen/ectomy
excision of the hymen

17. WR CV WR CV WR S
hyster/o/salping/o/-oophor/ectomy
CF CF
excision of the uterus, uterine tubes, and ovaries
18. WR S
hyster/ectomy
excision of the uterus
19. WR CV S
mamm/o/plasty
CF
surgical repair of the breast
20. WR CV S
mast/o/pexy
CF
surgical fixation of the breast

Exercise 17

1. colp/o/rrhaphy
2. cervic/ectomy
3. episi/o/rrhaphy
4. episi/o/perine/o/plasty
5. colp/o/plasty
6. colp/o/perine/o/rrhaphy
7. hyster/o/salping/o/-oophor/ectomy
8. hyster/o/pexy
9. hymen/ectomy
10. hymen/o/tomy
11. hyster/ectomy
12. oophor/ectomy
13. mast/ectomy
14. salping/ectomy
15. perine/o/rrhaphy
16. salping/o/-oophor/ectomy
17. salping/o/stomy
18. vulv/ectomy
19. mamm/o/plasty
20. mast/o/pexy

Exercise 18

Spelling Exercise; see text p. 326.

Exercise 19

Pronunciation Exercise

Exercise 20

1. tubal ligation
2. anterior and posterior colporrhaphy
3. dilation and curettage
4. stereotactic breast biopsy
5. myomectomy
6. endometrial ablation
7. uterine artery embolization
8. conization
9. sentinel lymph node biopsy
10. laparoscopy or laparoscopic surgery

Exercise 21

1. c	6. f
2. a	7. c
3. a	8. c
4. b	9. g
5. c	10. c

Exercise 22

Spelling Exercise; see text pp. 331-332.

Exercise 23

Pronunciation Exercise

Exercise 24

1. WR CV S
colp/o/scopy
CF
visual examination of the vagina
2. WR CV S
mamm/o/gram
CF
radiographic image of the breast
3. WR CV S
colp/o/scope
CF
instrument used for visual examination of the vagina
4. WR CV S
hyster/o/scopy
CF
visual examination of the uterus
5. WR CV WR CV S
hyster/o/salping/o/gram
CF CF
radiographic image of the uterus and uterine tubes
6. WR CV S
culd/o/scope
CF
instrument used for visual examination of the Douglas cul-de-sac
7. WR CV S
culd/o/scopy
CF
visual examination of the Douglas cul-de-sac
8. WR CV S
culd/o/centesis
CF
surgical puncture to remove fluid from the Douglas cul-de-sac
9. WR CV S
mamm/o/graphy
CF
radiographic imaging of the breast
10. WR CV S
hyster/o/scope
CF
instrument used for visual examination of the uterus
11. WR CV WR CV S
son/o/hyster/o/graphy
CF CF
process of recording the uterus with sound

Exercise 25

1. hyster/o/salping/o/gram
2. colp/o/scopy
3. colp/o/scope
4. hyster/o/scopy
5. mamm/o/gram
6. culd/o/scope
7. culd/o/scopy
8. culd/o/centesis
9. hyster/o/scope
10. mamm/o/graphy
11. son/o/hyster/o/graphy

Exercise 26

Spelling Exercise; see text p. 338.

Exercise 27

Pronunciation Exercise

Exercise 28

1. cytological study of cervical and vaginal secretions used to determine the presence of abnormal or cancerous cells
2. an ultrasound procedure that obtains images of the ovaries, uterus, cervix, and uterine tubes
3. a blood test used to detect and monitor treatment of ovarian cancer

Exercise 29

1. Pap smear
2. CA-125
3. transvaginal sonography

Exercise 30

Spelling Exercise; see text p. 343.

Exercise 31

Pronunciation Exercise

Exercise 32

1. WR CV S
gynec/o/logist
CF
a physician who studies and treats (diseases of) women

2. WR CV S
gynec/o/logy
CF
study of women (branch of medicine dealing with diseases of the female reproductive system)
3. WR CV WR S
vulv/o/vagin/al
CF
pertaining to the vulva and vagina
4. WR S
mast/algia
pain in the breast
5. WR WR
men/arche
beginning of menstruation
6. WR CV S
leuk/o/rrhea
CF
white discharge (from the vagina)
7. WR CV WR S
gyn/o/path/ic
CF
pertaining to diseases of women
8. WR CV S
mast/o/ptosis
CF
sagging breast
9. WR S
vagin/al
pertaining to the vagina

Exercise 33

1. leuk/o/rrhea
2. men/arche
3. mast/algia
4. vulv/o/vagin/al
5. gynec/o/logist
6. gynec/o/logy
7. mast/o/ptosis
8. gyn/o/path/ic
9. vagin/al

Exercise 34

Spelling Exercise; see text p. 345.

Exercise 35

Pronunciation Exercise

Exercise 36

1. cessation of menstruation
2. difficult or painful intercourse
3. abnormal passageway between two organs or between an internal organ and the body surface
4. a syndrome involving physical and emotional symptoms occurring during the 10 days before menstruation
5. instrument for opening a body cavity to allow for visual inspection
6. replacement of hormones to treat symptoms associated with menopause

Exercise 37

1. fistula
2. dyspareunia
3. menopause
4. premenstrual syndrome
5. speculum
6. hormone replacement therapy

Exercise 38

Spelling Exercise; see text p. 347.

Exercise 39

1. anterior; posterior colporrhaphy
2. total abdominal hysterectomy and bilateral salpingo-oophorectomy; hormone replacement therapy
3. sonohysterography and transvaginal sonography
4. total vaginal hysterectomy
5. dilation and curettage; cervix
6. fibrocystic breast disease
7. pelvic inflammatory disease; gynecology
8. premenstrual syndrome
9. uterine artery embolization

Exercise 40

A. 1. mammography
2. carcinoma
3. hysterectomy
4. adenomyosis
5. endometriosis
6. HRT
7. stereotactic breast biopsy
8. mediolateral
9. mastectomy
10. sentinel lymph node biopsy

Exercise 40

B. 1. c
2. a
3. d

Exercise 41

1. dysmenorrhea
2. endometritis
3. uterine tube
4. suture of the vulva
5. mammoplasty
6. uterus, uterine tubes, and ovaries
7. hematosalpinx
8. endometriosis
9. speculum
10. TSS
11. conization

Exercise 42

Reading Exercise

Exercise 43

1. b
2. *T*
3. *T*
4. d

NOTES

Chapter 9

Obstetrics and Neonatology

OUTLINE

OBJECTIVES

Upon completion of this chapter you will be able to:

1. Identify organs and structures relating to pregnancy.
2. Define and spell word parts related to obstetrics and neonatology.
3. Define, pronounce, and spell disease and disorder terms related to obstetrics and neonatology.
4. Define, pronounce, and spell surgical and diagnostic terms related to obstetrics.
5. Define, pronounce, and spell complementary terms related to obstetrics and neonatology.
6. Interpret the meaning of abbreviations related to obstetrics and neonatology.
7. Interpret, read, and comprehend medical language in simulated medical statements and documents.

ANATOMY

Obstetrics is the branch of medicine that deals with childbirth and the care of the mother before, during, and after birth. **Neonatology** is the branch of medicine that deals with the diagnosis and treatment of disorders of the newborn.

Terms Relating to Pregnancy

Term	Definition
gamete	mature germ cell, either sperm (male) or ovum (female)
ovulation	expulsion of a mature ovum from an ovary (Figure 9-1)
conception, or fertilization	beginning of pregnancy, when the sperm enters the ovum. Fertilization normally occurs in the uterine tubes (Figure 9-1).
zygote	cell formed by the union of the sperm and the ovum
embryo	unborn offspring in the stage of development from implantation of the zygote to the end of the eighth week of pregnancy. This period is characterized by rapid growth of the embryo.
fetus	unborn offspring from the beginning of the ninth week of pregnancy until birth (Figure 9-2)
gestation, pregnancy	development of a new individual from conception to birth
gestation period	duration of pregnancy; normally 38 to 42 weeks, which can be divided into three equal periods, called *trimesters*
implantation	embedding of the zygote in the uterine lining. The process normally begins about 7 days after fertilization and continues for several days (Figure 9-1).
placenta, or afterbirth	a structure that grows on the wall of the uterus during pregnancy and allows for nourishment of the unborn child (Figure 9-1)
amniotic, or amnionic, sac	membranous bag that surrounds the fetus before delivery (also called **bag of water**) (Figure 9-1)
chorion	outermost layer of the fetal membrane
amnion	innermost layer of the fetal membrane
amniotic, or amnionic, fluid	fluid within the amniotic sac, which surrounds the fetus

SKIN CHANGES THAT OCCUR THROUGHOUT PREGNANCY

- **striae gravidarum**: "stretch marks" occurring on the abdomen, breast, buttocks, and thighs from weakening of elastic tissues
- **linea nigra**: dark medial line extending from the pubis upward
- **chloasma**: hyperpigmentation of blotchy brown macules usually evenly distributed over the cheeks and forehead

A & P Booster
For students desiring more anatomy and physiology or to view animations, go to http://evolve.elsevier.com. Refer to p. 18 for your Evolve Access Information. Select A & P Booster, Chapter 9.

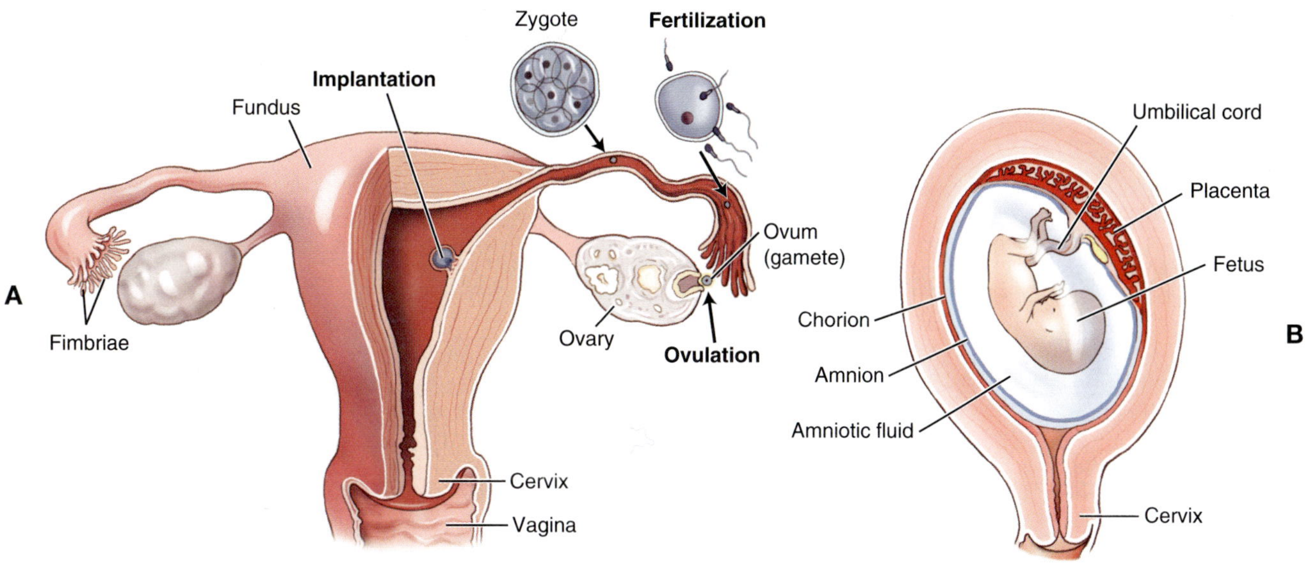

FIGURE 9-1
A, Ovulation, fertilization, and implantation. **B**, Development of the fetus.

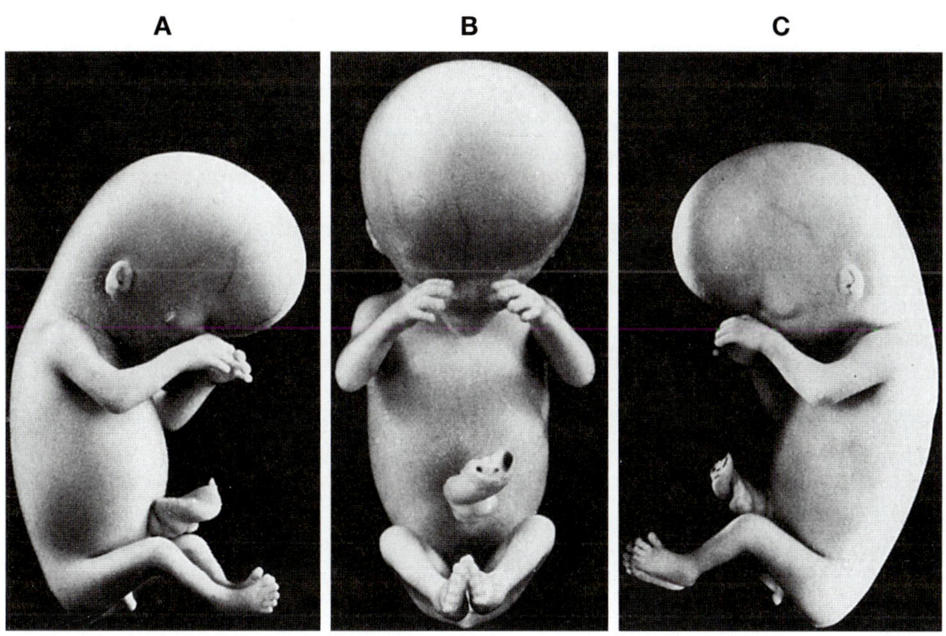

FIGURE 9-2
Human male fetus at 68 days (1.85 inches, 47 mm). **A**, Right. **B**, front. **C**, left.

EXERCISE 1

Fill in the blanks with the correct terms. *To check your answers to the exercises in this chapter, go to Answers, p. 401, at the end of the chapter.*

1. The expulsion of a mature ovum, or ________________, from an ovary is called ________________. When the male gamete enters the female gamete, ________________ occurs, and a(n) ________________ is formed. This marks the beginning of the ________________ period.
2. Once the zygote is implanted, it becomes a(n) ________________ until the end of the eighth week of gestation. The unborn offspring from the beginning of the ninth week until birth is called a(n) ________________.
3. The fetus is surrounded by a(n) ________________ sac, which has an outermost layer, called the ________________, and an innermost layer, called the ________________. This sac contains the ________________ fluid that surrounds the fetus.

WORD PARTS

Combining Forms of Obstetrics and Neonatology

Word parts you need to learn to complete this chapter are listed on the following pages. The exercises at the end of each list will help you learn their definitions and spelling.

Use the flashcards accompanying this text or electronic flashcards to assist you in memorizing the word parts for this chapter.

To use electronic flashcards, go to http://evolve.elsevier.com. Refer to p. 18 for your Evolve Access Information. Select Flashcards, Chapter 9.

Combining Form	Definition
amni/o, amnion/o	amnion, amniotic fluid
chori/o	chorion
embry/o	embryo, to be full (Figure 9-3)
fet/o, fet/i (NOTE: both *i* and *o* may be used as combining vowels with fet/)	fetus, unborn child
gravid/o	pregnancy
lact/o	milk
nat/o	birth
omphal/o	umbilicus, navel
par/o, part/o	bear, give birth to, labor, childbirth
puerper/o	childbirth

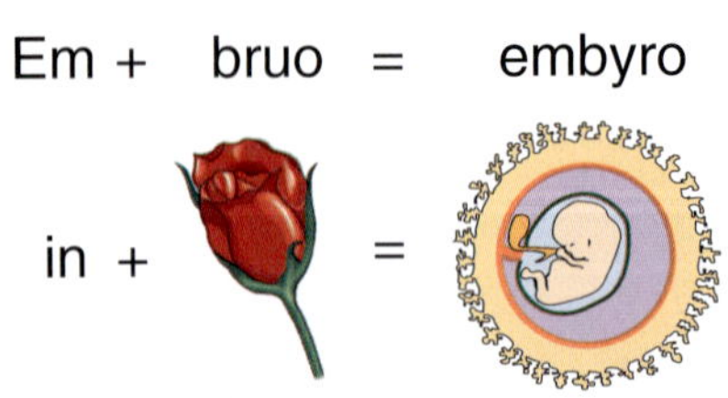

FIGURE 9-3
Embryo comes from the Greek *em*, meaning *in*, plus *bruo*, meaning to *bud* or *shoot*.

PUERPER

is made up of two Latin word roots: **puer**, meaning **child**, and per, meaning **through**.

EXERCISE FIGURE A

Fill in the blanks with combining forms in this diagram of fetal development. *To check your answers, go to p. 401.*

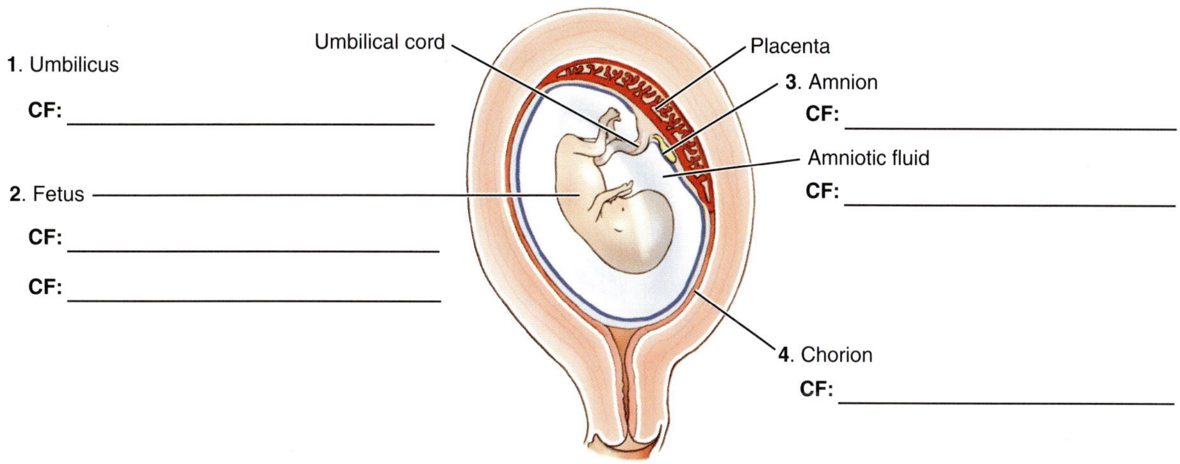

EXERCISE 2

Write the definitions of the following combining forms.

1. fet/o, fet/i ___
2. lact/o ___
3. par/o, part/o ___
4. omphal/o ___
5. amni/o, amnion/o ___
6. puerper/o ___
7. gravid/o ___
8. nat/o ___
9. chori/o ___
10. embry/o ___

EXERCISE 3

Write the combining form for each of the following terms.

1. milk ___
2. fetus a. ___
   b. ___
3. chorion ___
4. amnion, amniotic fluid a. ___
   b. ___
5. childbirth ___
6. bear, give birth to, labor, childbirth a. ___
   b. ___
7. pregnancy ___
8. embryo ___
9. birth ___
10. umbilicus, navel ___

Combining Forms Commonly Used in Obstetrics and Neonatology

Combining Form	Definition
cephal/o	head
esophag/o	esophagus (tube leading from the throat to the stomach) (see Figure 11-1)
pelv/o, pelv/i (NOTE: both *i* and *o* may be used as the combining vowel with pelv/)	pelvic bone, pelvis (see Chapter 14 Exercise Figure A and Exercise Figure B)
prim/i (NOTE: the combining vowel is *i*.)	first
pseud/o	false
pylor/o	pylorus (pyloric sphincter) (see Figure 11-2)
terat/o	malformations

TERAT/O

is translated literally as **monster**; however, in terms containing terat/o relating to obstetrics, terat/o refers to malformations or abnormal development.

EXERCISE 4

Write the definition of the following combining forms.

1. prim/i ____________________
2. pylor/o ____________________
3. cephal/o ____________________
4. esophag/o ____________________
5. pseud/o ____________________
6. pelv/o, pelv/i ____________________
7. terat/o ____________________

EXERCISE 5

Write the combining form for each of the following.

1. head ____________
2. pylorus ____________
3. false ____________
4. esophagus ____________
5. first ____________
6. malformations ____________
7. pelvic bone, pelvis a. ____________
   b. ____________

Prefixes

Prefix	Definition
ante-, pre-	before
micro-	small
multi-	many
nulli-	none
post-	after

EXERCISE 6

Write the definitions of the following prefixes.

1. post- ____________________
2. multi- ____________________
3. nulli- ____________________
4. micro- ____________________
5. ante- ____________________
6. pre- ____________________

EXERCISE 7

Write the prefix for each of the following definitions.

1. none ____________________
2. small ____________________
3. many ____________________
4. before a. ____________________
   b. ____________________
5. after ____________________

Suffixes

Suffix	Definition
-amnios	amnion, amniotic fluid
-cyesis	pregnancy
-e	noun suffix, no meaning
-is	noun suffix, no meaning
-partum	childbirth, labor
-rrhexis	rupture
-tocia	birth, labor
-um	noun suffix, no meaning
-us	noun suffix, no meaning

-RRHEXIS

is the last of the four **-rrh** suffixes to be learned. The other three introduced in earlier chapters are:
-rrhea—flow or discharge
-rrhagia—rapid flow (of blood)
-rrhaphy—suturing, repair

The noun suffix **-a**, introduced in Chapter 4, also has no meaning.

Refer to **Appendix A** and **Appendix B** for alphabetized word parts and their meanings.

EXERCISE 8

Write the definitions of the following suffixes.

1. -rrhexis ____________
2. -tocia ____________
3. -cyesis ____________
4. -partum ____________
5. -amnios ____________

EXERCISE 9

Write the suffix for each of the following definitions.

1. birth, labor ____________
2. rupture ____________
3. childbirth, labor ____________
4. pregnancy ____________
5. amnion, amniotic fluid ____________

EXERCISE 10

Write the noun suffixes introduced in this chapter that have no meaning.

1. ______________________
2. ______________________
3. ______________________
4. ______________________

MEDICAL TERMS

The terms you need to learn to complete this chapter are listed next. The exercises following each list will help you learn the definition and the spelling of each word.

Obstetric Disease and Disorder Terms

Built from Word Parts

The following terms are built from word parts you have already learned and can be translated literally to find their meanings. Further explanation of terms beyond the definition of their word parts, if needed, is included in parentheses.

Term	Definition
amnionitis (*am*-nē-ō-NĪ-tis)	inflammation of the amnion
chorioamnionitis (*kor*-ē-ō-*am*-nē-ō-NĪ-tis)	inflammation of the chorion and amnion
choriocarcinoma (*kor*-ē-ō-*kar*-si-NŌ-ma)	cancerous tumor of the chorion
dystocia (dis-TŌ-sha)	difficult labor
hysterorrhexis (*his*-ter-ō-REK-sis)	rupture of the uterus
oligohydramnios (*ol*-i-gō-hī-DRAM-nē-os)	scanty amnion water (less than the normal amount of amniotic fluid; 500 mL or less)
polyhydramnios (*pol*-ē-hī-DRAM-nē-os)	much amnion water (more than the normal amount of amniotic fluid; 2000 mL or more) (also called **hydramnios**)

CAM TERM

Acupuncture is the ancient practice of inserting very thin needles into acupoints just under the skin to treat disease, increase immune response, relieve pain, and restore health. Acupuncture has been found to be effective in **providing pain relief during labor.**

EXERCISE 11

Practice saying aloud each of the obstetric disease and disorder terms built from word parts on p. 371.

To hear the terms, go to http://evolve.elsevier.com. Refer to p. 18 for your Evolve Access Information. Select Exercises & Review, Chapter 9, Chapter Exercises, Pronunciation.

☐ Place a check mark in the box when you have completed this exercise.

EXERCISE 12

Analyze and define the following disease and disorder terms.

1. chorioamnionitis ______________________
2. choriocarcinoma ______________________
3. dystocia ______________________
4. amnionitis ______________________
5. hysterorrhexis ______________________
6. oligohydramnios ______________________
7. polyhydramnios ______________________

EXERCISE 13

Build disease and disorder terms for the following definitions by using the word parts you have learned.

1. cancerous tumor of the chorion ______ / ___ / ______ / ______
   WR / CV / WR / S
2. inflammation of the amnion ______ / ______
   WR / S
3. inflammation of the chorion and amnion ______ / ___ / ______ / ______
   WR / CV / WR / S
4. difficult labor ______ / ______
   P / S(WR)
5. rupture of the uterus ______ / ___ / ______
   WR / CV / S
6. scanty amnion water (less than normal amniotic fluid) ______ / ___ / ______ / ______
   WR / CV / WR / S
7. much amnion water (more than normal amniotic fluid) ______ / ______ / ______
   P / WR / S

EXERCISE 14

Spell each of the obstetric disease and disorder terms built from word parts on p. 371 by having someone dictate them to you.

To hear and spell the terms, go to http://evolve.elsevier.com. Refer to p. 18 for your Evolve Access Information. Select Exercises & Review, Chapter 9, Chapter Exercises, Spelling.
☐ Place a check mark in the box if you have completed this exercise online.

1. ______________________
2. ______________________
3. ______________________
4. ______________________
5. ______________________
6. ______________________
7. ______________________

Obstetric Disease and Disorder Terms

Not Built from Word Parts

In some of the following terms you may recognize word parts you have already learned; however, the full meaning of the terms cannot be discerned by the definition of their word parts.

Term	Definition
abortion (a-BŌR-shun)	termination of pregnancy by the expulsion from the uterus of an embryo before fetal viability, usually before 20 weeks of gestation
abruptio placentae (ab-RUP-shē-ō) (pla-SEN-tē)	premature separation of the placenta from the uterine wall (Figure 9-5, *A*)
eclampsia (e-KLAMP-sē-a)	severe complication and progression of preeclampsia characterized by convulsion (see *preeclampsia* on the next page). Eclampsia is a potentially life-threatening disorder.
ectopic pregnancy (ek-TOP-ik) (PREG-nan-sē)	pregnancy occurring outside the uterus, commonly in the uterine tubes (Figure 9-4)
placenta previa (pla-SEN-ta) (PRĒ-vē-a)	abnormally low implantation of the placenta on the uterine wall completely or partially covering the cervix. (Dilation of the cervix can cause separation of the placenta from the uterine wall, resulting in bleeding. With severe hemorrhage, a cesarean section may be necessary to save the mother's life.) (Figure 9-5, *B*)

TYPES OF ABORTION

Spontaneous abortion is the termination of pregnancy that occurs naturally. It is commonly referred to as *miscarriage.*
Induced abortion is the intentional termination of pregnancy by surgical or medical intervention.
Therapeutic abortion is an induced abortion performed because of health risks to the mother or for fetal disease.
Elective abortion is an induced abortion performed at the request of the woman.

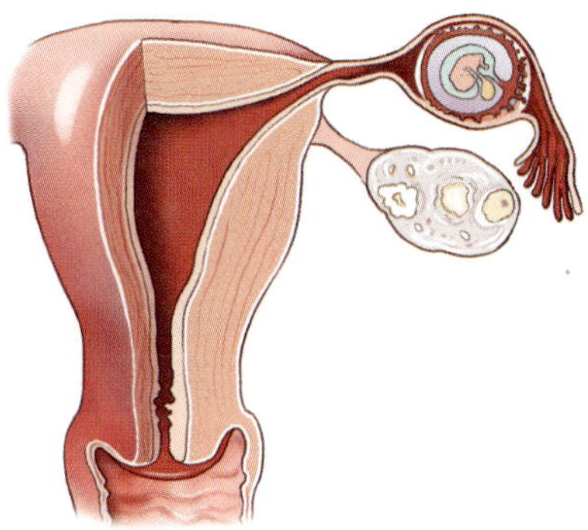

FIGURE 9-4
Ectopic pregnancy.

Obstetric Disease and Disorder Terms—*cont'd*

Not Built from Word Parts

Term	Definition
preeclampsia (prē-ē-KLAMP-sē-a)	abnormal condition encountered during pregnancy or shortly after delivery characterized by high blood pressure, edema, and proteinuria, but with no convulsions. The cause is unknown; if not successfully treated, the condition can progress to eclampsia. Eclampsia is the third most common cause of maternal death in the United States after hemorrhage and infection.

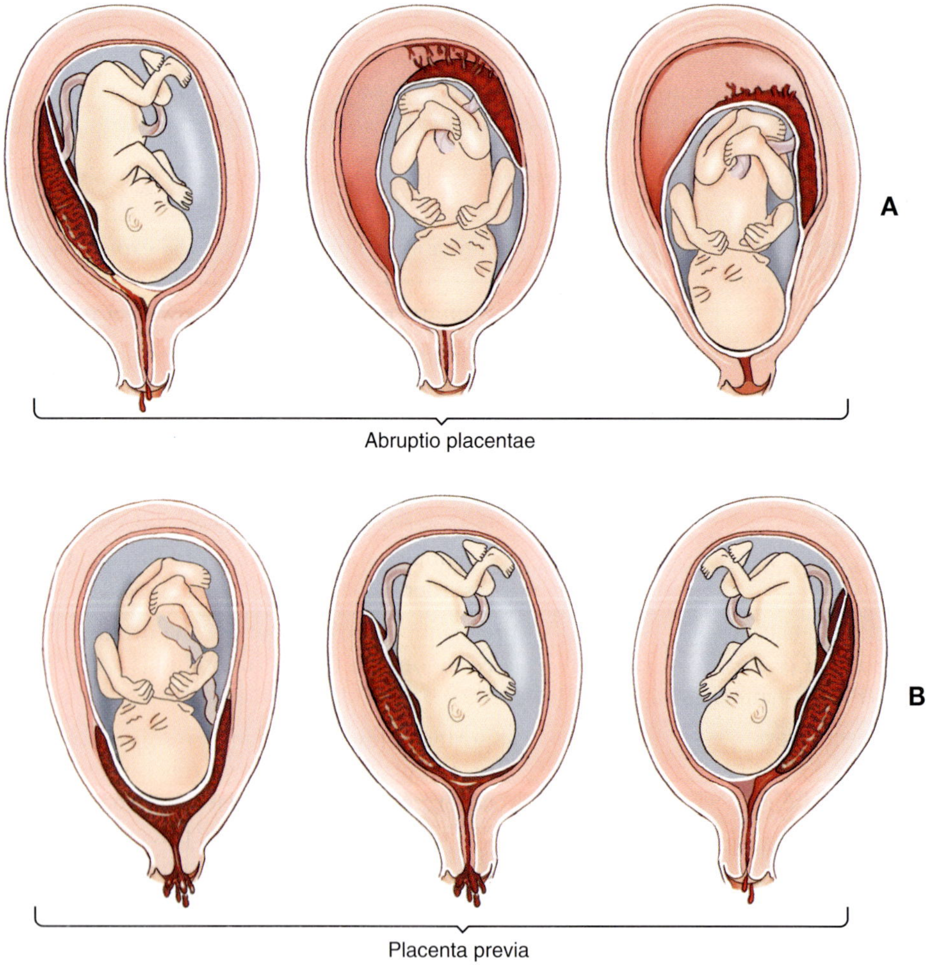

FIGURE 9-5

A, Various stages of abruptio placentae. **B,** Placenta previa.

EXERCISE 15

Practice saying aloud each of the obstetric disease and disorder terms not built from word parts on pp. 373-374.

To hear the terms, go to http://evolve.elsevier.com. Refer to p. 18 for your Evolve Access Information. Select Exercises & Review, Chapter 9, Chapter Exercises, Pronunciation.

☐ Place a check mark in the box when you have completed this exercise.

EXERCISE 16

Write the definitions of the following terms.

1. abruptio placentae ____________________
2. abortion ____________________
3. placenta previa ____________________
4. eclampsia ____________________
5. ectopic pregnancy ____________________
6. preeclampsia ____________________

EXERCISE 17

Write the term for each of the following definitions.

1. premature separation of the placenta from the uterine wall ____________________
2. severe complication and progression of preeclampsia ____________________
3. termination of pregnancy by the expulsion from the uterus of an embryo ____________________
4. pregnancy occurring outside the uterus ____________________
5. abnormally low implantation of the placenta on the uterine wall ____________________
6. characterized by high blood pressure, edema, and proteinuria, but with no convulsions ____________________

EXERCISE 18

Spell each of the obstetric disease and disorder terms not built from word parts on pp. 373-374 by having someone dictate them to you.

To hear and spell the terms, go to http://evolve.elsevier.com. Refer to p. 18 for your Evolve Access Information. Select Exercises & Review, Chapter 9, Chapter Exercises, Spelling.

☐ Place a check mark in the box if you have completed this exercise online.

1. ______________________
2. ______________________
3. ______________________
4. ______________________
5. ______________________
6. ______________________

Neonatology Disease and Disorder Terms

Built from Word Parts

The following terms are built from word parts you have already learned and can be translated literally to find their meanings. Further explanation of terms beyond the definition of their word parts, if needed, is included in parentheses.

Term	Definition
microcephalus (*mī*-krō-SEF-a-lus)	(fetus with a very) small head
omphalitis (*om*-fa-LĪ-tis)	inflammation of the umbilicus
omphalocele (OM-fal-ō-*sēl*)	herniation at the umbilicus (a part of the intestine protrudes through the abdominal wall at birth) (Exercise Figure B)
pyloric stenosis (pī-LOR-ik) (ste-NŌ-sis)	narrowing pertaining to the pyloric sphincter. (Congenital pyloric stenosis occurs in 1 of every 200 newborns.)
tracheoesophageal fistula (*trā*-kē-ō-ē-*sof*-a-jĒ-al) (FIS-tū-la)	abnormal passageway pertaining to the esophagus and the trachea (between the esophagus and trachea)

EXERCISE 19

Practice saying aloud each of the neonatology disease and disorder terms built from word parts above.

To hear the terms, go to http://evolve.elsevier.com. Refer to p. 18 for your Evolve Access Information. Select Exercises & Review, Chapter 9, Chapter Exercises, Pronunciation.

☐ Place a check mark in the box when you have completed this exercise.

EXERCISE FIGURE B

Fill in the blanks to label the diagram.

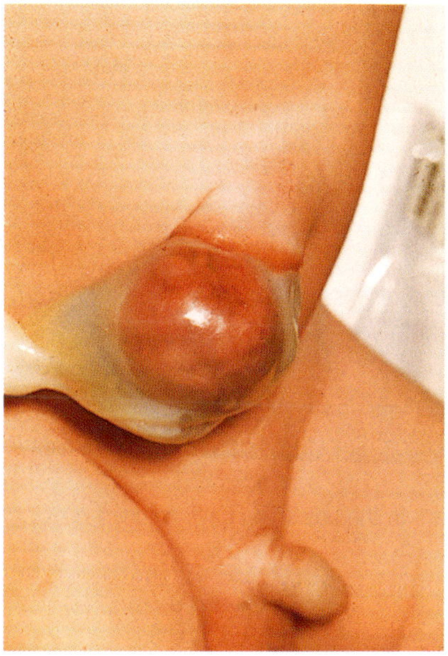

_____ umbilicus / cv / _____ herniation

EXERCISE 20

Analyze and define the following disease and disorder terms.

1. pyloric (stenosis) ____________________
2. omphalocele ____________________
3. omphalitis ____________________
4. microcephalus ____________________
5. tracheoesophageal (fistula) ____________________

EXERCISE 21

Build disease and disorder terms for the following definitions by using the word parts you have learned.

1. hernia at the umbilicus ______ WR / CV / ______ S
2. (fetus with a very) small head ______ P / ______ WR / ______ S
3. (narrowing) pertaining to the pyloric sphincter ______ WR / ______ S stenosis

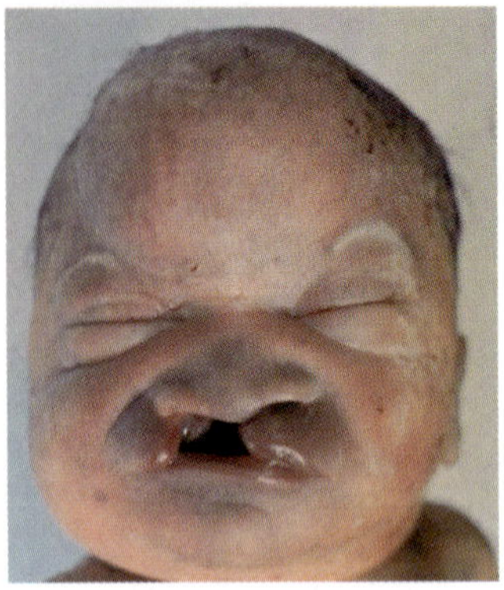

FIGURE 9-6
Cleft lip and palate.

4. abnormal passageway pertaining to the esophagus and the trachea (between the esophagus and trachea) ______ / ______ / ______ / ______ fistula
WR / CV / WR / S

5. inflammation of the umbilicus ______ / ______
WR / S

EXERCISE 22

Spell each of the neonatology disease and disorder terms built from word parts on p. 376 by having someone dictate them to you.

To hear and spell the terms, go to http://evolve.elsevier.com. Refer to p. 18 for your Evolve Access Information. Select Exercises & Review, Chapter 9, Chapter Exercises, Spelling.
☐ Place a check mark in the box if you have completed this exercise online.

1. ______________________
2. ______________________
3. ______________________
4. ______________________
5. ______________________

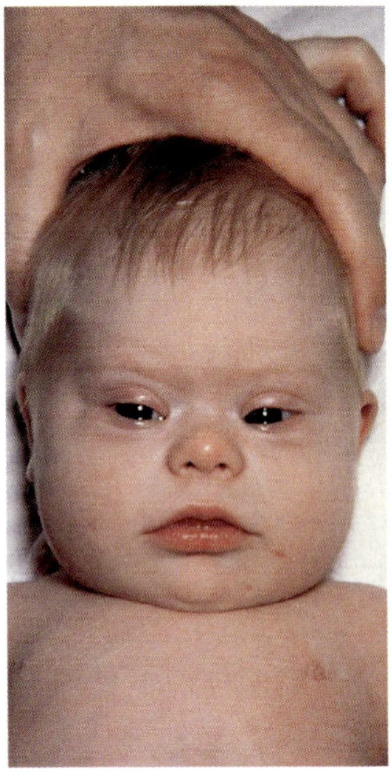

FIGURE 9-7
Down syndrome.

Neonatology Disease and Disorder Terms

Not Built from Word Parts

In some of the following terms you may recognize word parts you have already learned; however, the full meaning of the terms cannot be discerned by the definition of their word parts.

Term	Definition
cleft lip and palate (kleft) (lip) (PAL-at)	congenital split of the lip and roof of the mouth (*cleft* indicates a fissure) (Figure 9-6)
Down syndrome (down) (SIN-drōm)	genetic condition characterized by varying degrees of mental retardation and multiple defects (formerly called **mongolism**) (Figure 9-7)
erythroblastosis fetalis (e-*rith*-rō-blas-TŌ-sis) (fē-TAL-is)	condition of the newborn characterized by hemolysis of the erythrocytes. The condition is usually caused by incompatibility of the infant's and mother's blood, occurring when the mother's blood is Rh negative and the infant's blood is Rh positive.
esophageal atresia (e-*sof*-a-JĒ-al) (a-TRĒ-zha)	congenital absence of part of the esophagus. Food cannot pass from the baby's mouth to the stomach (Figure 9-8).

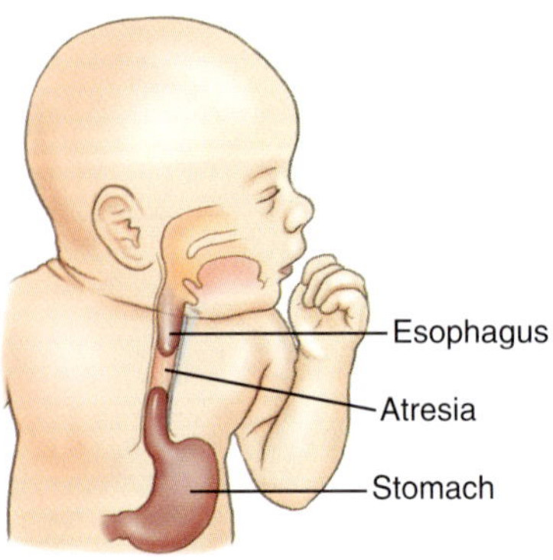

FIGURE 9-8
Esophageal atresia.

Term	Definition
fetal alcohol syndrome (FAS) (FĒ-tal) (AL-kō-hol) (SIN-drōm)	a condition caused by excessive alcohol consumption by the mother during pregnancy. Various birth defects may present, including central nervous system dysfunction and malformations of the skull and face.
gastroschisis (gas-TROS-ki-sis)	a congenital fissure of the abdominal wall not at the umbilicus. Enterocele, protrusion of the intestine, is usually present (Figure 9-9).
respiratory distress syndrome (RDS) (RES-pi-ra-*tōr*-ē) (di-STRESS) (SIN-drōm)	a respiratory complication in the newborn, especially in premature infants. In premature infants RDS is caused by normal immaturity of the respiratory system resulting in compromised respiration (formerly called **hyaline membrane disease**).
spina bifida (SPĪ-na) (BIF-i-da)	congenital defect in the vertebral column caused by the failure of the vertebral arch to close. If the meninges protrude through the opening the condition is called **meningocele**. Protrusion of both the meninges and spinal cord is called **meningomyelocele**. Both terms are covered in Chapter 15 (Figure 9-10).

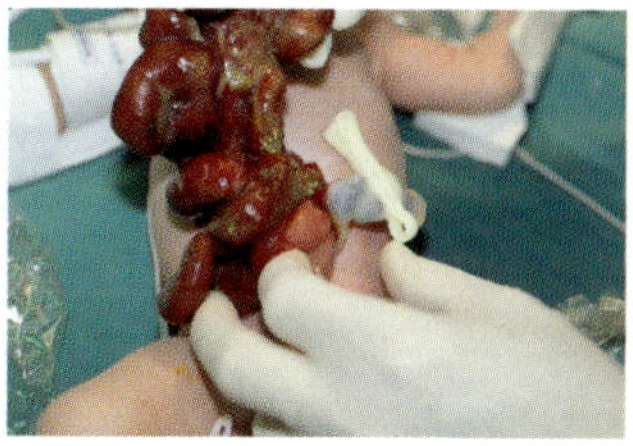

FIGURE 9-9
Gastroschisis.

BIRTHMARKS

are benign discolorations in the neonate's skin. Common birthmarks include **Mongolian spots**, which are bluish-black areas of hyperpigmentation often found on the lower back or buttocks of darker-skinned neonates, and **hemangiomas**, which are various benign vascular tumors or stains that cause reddish discoloration and/or malformations of the skin surface.

EXERCISE 23

Practice saying aloud each of the neonatology disease and disorder terms not built from word parts found on pp. 378-379.

To hear the terms, go to http://evolve.elsevier.com. Refer to p. 18 for your Evolve Access Information. Select Exercises & Review, Chapter 9, Chapter Exercises, Pronunciation.

☐ Place a check mark in the box when you have completed this exercise.

EXERCISE 24

Match the terms in the first column with their correct definitions in the second column.

_____ 1. Down syndrome	a. defect of the vertebral column
_____ 2. cleft lip and palate	b. respiratory complication
_____ 3. spina bifida	c. split of the lip and roof of the mouth
_____ 4. erythroblastosis fetalis	d. caused by incompatibility of the infant's and the mother's blood
_____ 5. fetal alcohol syndrome	e. congenital fissure of the abdominal wall
_____ 6. respiratory distress syndrome	f. genetic condition characterized by mental retardation
_____ 7. esophageal atresia	g. congenital absence of part of the esophagus
_____ 8. gastroschisis	h. causes various birth defects, including central nervous system dysfunction

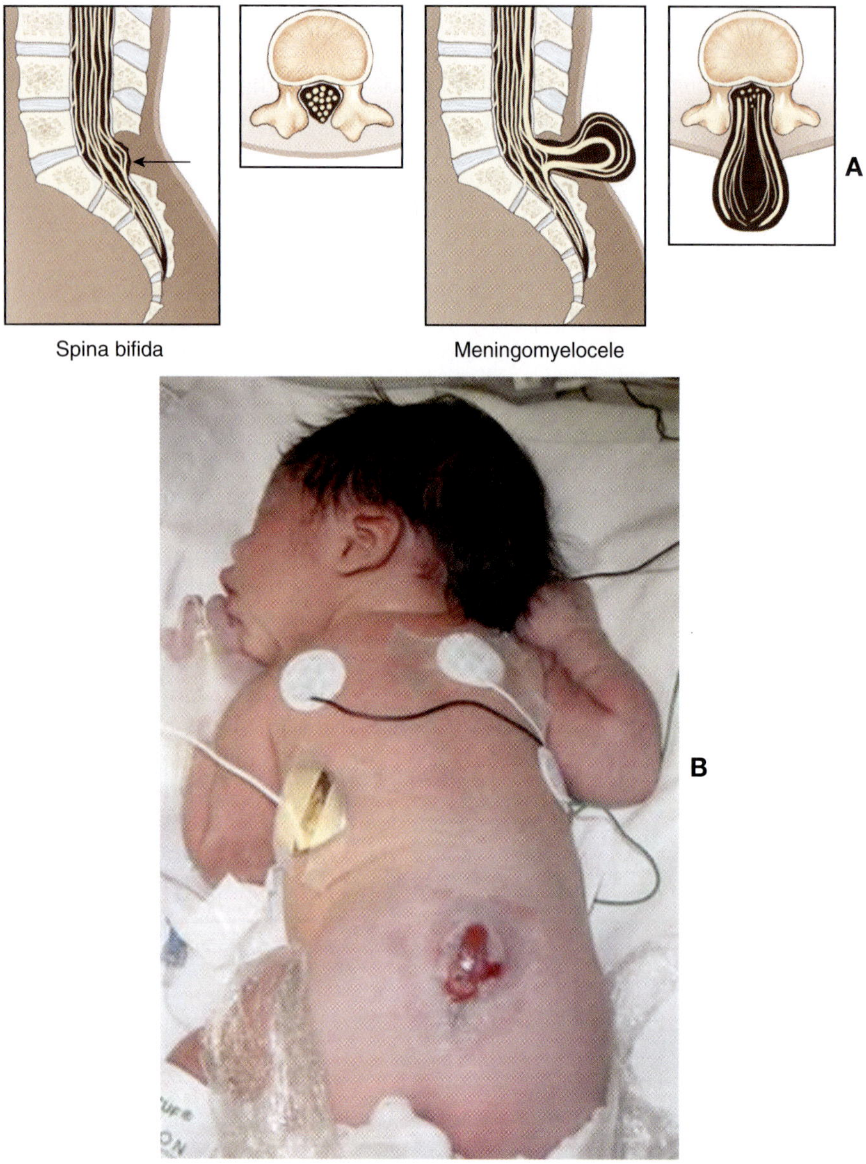

FIGURE 9-10
A, Drawings of spina bifida and meningomyelocele. **B,** Photograph of meningomyelocele.

EXERCISE 25

Spell each of the neonatal disease and disorder terms not built from word parts on pp. 378-379 by having someone dictate them to you.

To hear and spell the terms, go to http://evolve.elsevier.com. Refer to p. 18 for your Evolve Access Information. Select Exercises & Review, Chapter 9, Chapter Exercises, Spelling.
☐ Place a check mark in the box if you have completed this exercise online.

1. ______________________
2. ______________________
3. ______________________
4. ______________________
5. ______________________
6. ______________________
7. ______________________
8. ______________________

Obstetric Surgical Terms

Built from Word Parts

The following terms are built from word parts you have already learned and can be translated literally to find their meanings. Further explanation of terms beyond the definition of their word parts, if needed, is included in parentheses.

Term	Definition
amniotomy (*am*-nē-OT-o-mē)	incision into the amnion (rupture of the fetal membrane to induce labor; a special hook is generally used to make the incision)
episiotomy (e-*piz*-ē-OT-o-mē)	incision of the vulva (perineum) (sometimes performed during delivery) (also called **perineotomy**) (Figure 9-11)

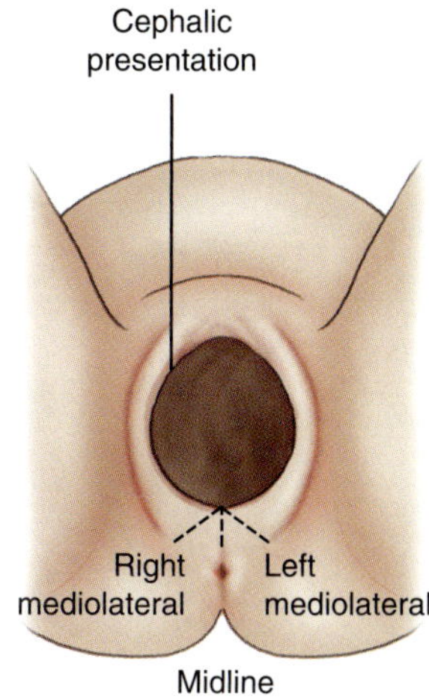

FIGURE 9-11 Episiotomies.

Obstetric Diagnostic Terms

Built from Word Parts

Term	Definition
DIAGNOSTIC IMAGING	
pelvic sonography (PEL-vik) (so-NOG-ra-fē)	pertaining to the pelvis, process of recording sound (pelvic ultrasound is used extensively to evaluate the fetus and pregnancy) (also called **pelvic ultrasonography, pelvic ultrasound,** and **obstetric ultrasonography**) (Figure 9-12)
OTHER	
amniocentesis (*am*-nē-ō-sen-TĒ-sis)	surgical puncture to aspirate amniotic fluid (the needle is inserted through the abdominal and uterine walls, using ultrasound to guide the needle. The fluid is used for the assessment of fetal health and maturity to aid in diagnosing fetal abnormalities.) (Figure 9-13).
amnioscope (AM-nē-ō-*skōp*)	instrument used for visual examination of the amniotic fluid (and the fetus)
amnioscopy (*am*-nē-OS-ko-pē)	visual examination of amniotic fluid (and the fetus)

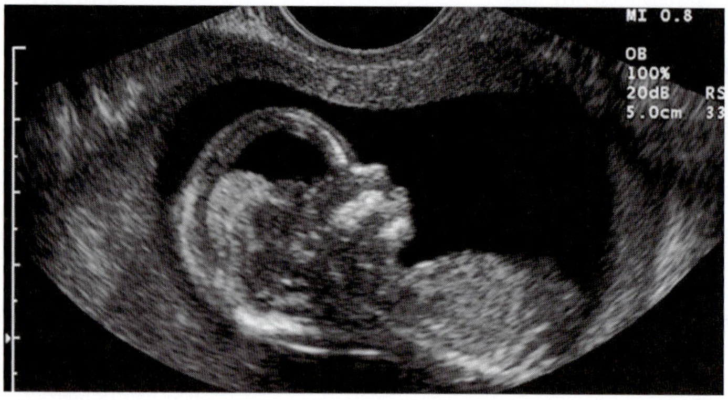

FIGURE 9-12
Pelvic ultrasound image showing a fetal profile. Some specific uses are to: (1) diagnose early abnormal pregnancy, (2) determine the age of the fetus, (3) measure fetal growth, and (4) determine fetal position.

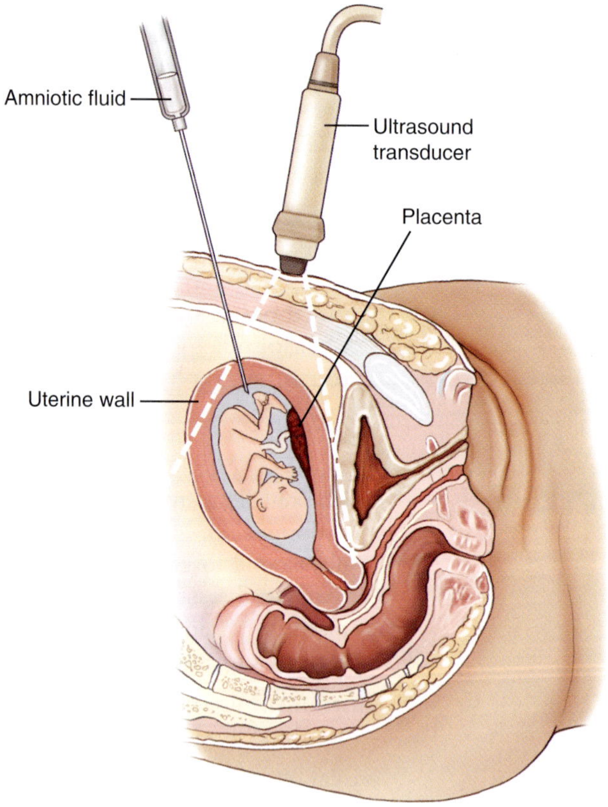

FIGURE 9-13
Amniocentesis. Ultrasound is used to guide the needle through the abdominal and uterine walls.

EXERCISE 26

Practice saying aloud each of the obstetric surgical and diagnostic terms built from word parts on p. 381.

To hear the terms, go to http://evolve.elsevier.com. Refer to p. 18 for your Evolve Access Information. Select Exercises & Review, Chapter 9, Chapter Exercises, Pronunciation.

☐ Place a check mark in the box when you have completed this exercise.

EXERCISE 27

Analyze and define the following obstetric surgical and diagnostic terms.

1. episiotomy ______________________
2. amniotomy ______________________
3. amnioscope ______________________
4. pelvic sonography ______________________
5. amniocentesis ______________________
6. amnioscopy ______________________

EXERCISE 28

Build obstetric surgical and diagnostic terms for the following definitions by using the word parts you have learned.

1. incision into the amnion ______ / ______ / ______ (WR / CV / S)
2. incision of the vulva ______ / ______ / ______ (WR / CV / S)
3. visual examination of the amniotic fluid (and fetus) ______ / ______ / ______ (WR / CV / S)
4. surgical puncture to aspirate amniotic fluid ______ / ______ / ______ (WR / CV / S)
5. instrument used for visual examination of the amniotic fluid (and fetus) ______ / ______ / ______ (WR / CV / S)
6. pertaining to the pelvis, process of recording sound ______ / ______ (WR / S)
   ______ / ______ / ______ (WR / CV / S)

EXERCISE 29

Spell each of the obstetric surgical and diagnostic terms built from word parts on p. 381 by having someone dictate them to you.

To hear and spell the terms, go to http://evolve.elsevier.com. Refer to p. 18 for your Evolve Access Information. Select Exercises & Review, Chapter 9, Chapter Exercises, Spelling.

☐ Place a check mark in the box if you have completed this exercise online.

1. ______________________
2. ______________________
3. ______________________
4. ______________________
5. ______________________
6. ______________________

Obstetric and Neonatal Complementary Terms

Built from Word Parts

The following terms are built from word parts you have already learned and can be translated literally to find their meanings. Further explanation of terms beyond the definition of their word parts, if needed, is included in parentheses.

Term	Definition
amniochorial (*am*-nē-ō-KOR-ē-al)	pertaining to the amnion and chorion
amniorrhea (*am*-nē-ō-RĒ-a)	discharge (escape) of amniotic fluid
amniorrhexis (*am*-nē-ō-REK-sis)	rupture of the amnion
antepartum (*an*-tē-PAR-tum)	before childbirth (reference to the mother)
embryogenic (*em*-brē-ō-JEN-ik)	producing an embryo
embryoid (EM-brē-oyd)	resembling an embryo
fetal (FĒ-tal)	pertaining to the fetus
gravida (GRAV-i-da)	pregnant (woman); (a woman who is or has been pregnant, regardless of pregnancy outcome)
gravidopuerperal (*grav*-i-dō-pū-ER-per-al)	pertaining to pregnancy and childbirth (from delivery until reproductive organs return to normal)
intrapartum (*in*-tra-PAR-tum)	within (during) labor and childbirth
lactic (LAK-tik)	pertaining to milk
lactogenic (*lak*-tō-JEN-ik)	producing milk (by stimulation)
lactorrhea (*lak*-tō-RĒ-a)	(spontaneous) discharge of milk
multigravida (*mul*-ti-GRAV-i-da)	many pregnancies (a woman who has been pregnant two or more times)
multipara (multip) (mul-TIP-a-ra)	many births (a woman who has given birth to two or more viable offspring)
natal (NĀ-tal)	pertaining to birth
neonate (NĒ-ō-nāt)	new birth (an infant from birth to 4 weeks of age) (synonymous with **newborn [NB]**) (Exercise Figure C)
neonatologist (*nē*-ō-nā-TOL-o-jist)	physician who studies and treats disorders of the newborn
neonatology (*nē*-ō-nā-TOL-o-jē)	study of the newborn (branch of medicine that deals with diagnosis and treatment of disorders in newborns)

Term	Definition
nulligravida (*nul*-li-GRAV-i-da)	no pregnancies (a woman who has never been pregnant)
nullipara (nu-LIP-a-ra)	no births (a woman who has not given birth to a viable offspring)
para (PAR-a)	birth (a woman who has given birth to an offspring, viable or stillborn)
postnatal (pōst-NĀ-tal)	pertaining to after birth (reference to the newborn)
postpartum (pōst-PAR-tum)	after childbirth (reference to the mother)
prenatal (prē-NĀ-tal)	pertaining to before birth (reference to the newborn)
primigravida (prī-mi-GRAV-i-da)	first pregnancy (a woman in her first pregnancy)
primipara (primip) (*prī*-MIP-a-ra)	first birth (a woman who has given birth to an offspring after the point of viability—20 weeks)
pseudocyesis (*sū*-dō-sī-Ē-sis)	false pregnancy (a woman who believes she is pregnant—this may be a psychological condition or related to underlying pathology, such as a uterine tumor)
puerpera (pū-ER-per-a)	childbirth (a woman who has just given birth)
puerperal (pū-ER-per-al)	pertaining to (immediately after) childbirth
teratogen (TER-a-tō-jen)	any agent producing malformations (in the developing embryo). Teratogens include chemical agents such as drugs, alcohol, viruses, x-rays, and environmental factors.
teratogenic (*ter*-a-tō-JEN-ik)	producing malformations (in the developing embryo)
teratology (*ter*-a-TOL-o-jē)	study of malformations (usually in regard to malformations caused by teratogens on the developing embryo)

APGAR SCORE

Developed in 1952 by Virginia Apgar, MD, the Apgar score provides a basic framework for rapid neonatal assessment by health care providers at 1 minute and 5 minutes after birth. Five vital criteria (**heart rate, respiration, muscle tone, response to stimulation**, and **color**) are assessed and scored on a 0 to 2 scale. The score is totaled, with a 5-minute Apgar score of 7 to 10 considered normal. The Apgar score is used only for quickly reporting a neonate's status and does not predict future health outcomes.

EXERCISE FIGURE C

Fill in the blanks to label the diagram.

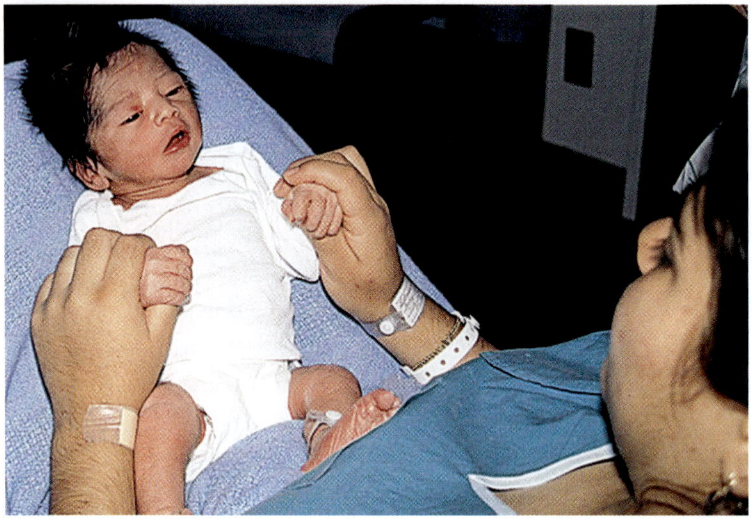

_____ / _____ / e
new / birth /

Terms Relating to Mother and Newborn

	Before Birth	After Birth
Mother	antepartum	postpartum
Newborn	prenatal	postnatal

Comparing Terms with gravid/o and par/o

gravid/o—pregnant	par/o—birth
nulli/gravid/a—no pregnancies	nulli/par/a—no births
primi/gravid/a—first pregnancy	primi/par/a—first birth
multi/gravid/a—many pregnancies	multi/par/a—many births

EXERCISE 30

Practice saying aloud each of the complementary terms built from word parts on pp. 384-385.

To hear the terms, go to http://evolve.elsevier.com. Refer to p. 18 for your Evolve Access Information. Select Exercises & Review, Chapter 9, Chapter Exercises, Pronunciation.

☐ Place a check mark in the box when you have completed this exercise.

EXERCISE 31

Analyze and define the following obstetric and neonatal complementary terms.

1. puerpera ______________________________
2. amniorrhexis ______________________________
3. antepartum ______________________________
4. pseudocyesis ______________________________
5. prenatal ______________________________
6. lactic ______________________________
7. lactorrhea ______________________________
8. amniorrhea ______________________________
9. multipara ______________________________
10. embryogenic ______________________________
11. embryoid ______________________________
12. fetal ______________________________
13. gravida ______________________________
14. amniochorial ______________________________
15. multigravida ______________________________
16. lactogenic ______________________________
17. natal ______________________________
18. gravidopuerperal ______________________________
19. neonatology ______________________________
20. nullipara ______________________________
21. para ______________________________
22. primigravida ______________________________
23. postpartum ______________________________
24. neonate ______________________________
25. primipara ______________________________
26. puerperal ______________________________
27. nulligravida ______________________________
28. intrapartum ______________________________
29. teratogen ______________________________
30. postnatal ______________________________
31. teratology ______________________________
32. neonatologist ______________________________
33. teratogenic ______________________________

EXERCISE 32

Build the complementary terms for the following definitions by using the word parts you have learned.

1. pertaining to the amnion and chorion
   ______ WR / CV / WR / S
2. before childbirth (reference to the mother)
   ______ P / WR / S
3. producing an embryo
   ______ WR / CV / S
4. pertaining to the fetus
   ______ WR / S
5. pertaining to before birth (reference to the newborn)
   ______ P / WR / S
6. pertaining to milk
   ______ WR / S
7. (spontaneous) discharge of milk
   ______ WR / CV / S
8. discharge (escape) of amniotic fluid
   ______ WR / CV / S
9. false pregnancy
   ______ WR / CV / S
10. the production of milk (by stimulation)
    ______ WR / CV / S
11. rupture of the amnion
    ______ WR / CV / S
12. resembling an embryo
    ______ WR / S
13. pregnant (woman)
    ______ WR / S
14. pertaining to pregnancy and childbirth
    ______ WR / CV / WR / S
15. many births
    ______ P / WR / S
16. pertaining to birth
    ______ WR / S
17. new birth (an infant from birth to 4 weeks of age)
    ______ P / WR / S

18. study of the newborn
    _____ / _____ / _____ / _____
    P / WR / CV / S

19. no births
    _____ / _____ / _____
    P / WR / S

20. birth
    _____ / _____
    WR / S

21. first pregnancy
    _____ / _____ / _____ / _____
    WR / CV / WR / S

22. after childbirth (reference to the mother)
    _____ / _____ / _____
    P / WR / S

23. first birth
    _____ / _____ / _____ / _____
    WR / CV / WR / S

24. many pregnancies
    _____ / _____ / _____
    P / WR / S

25. pertaining to (immediately after) childbirth
    _____ / _____
    WR / S

26. no pregnancies
    _____ / _____ / _____
    P / WR / S

27. any agent producing malformations
    _____ / _____ / _____
    WR / CV / S

28. childbirth
    _____ / _____
    WR / S

29. within (during) labor and childbirth
    _____ / _____ / _____
    P / WR / S

30. producing malformations
    _____ / _____ / _____
    WR / CV / S

31. physician who studies and treats disorders of the newborn
    _____ / _____ / _____ / _____
    P / WR / CV / S

32. pertaining to after birth (reference to the newborn)
    _____ / _____ / _____
    P / WR / S

33. study of malformations
    _____ / _____ / _____
    WR / CV / S

EXERCISE 33

Spell each of the complementary terms built from word parts on pp. 384-385 by having someone dictate them to you.

To hear and spell the terms, go to http://evolve.elsevier.com. Refer to p. 18 for your Evolve Access Information. Select Exercises & Review, Chapter 9, Chapter Exercises, Spelling.

☐ Place a check mark in the box if you have completed this exercise online.

1. ______________________
2. ______________________
3. ______________________
4. ______________________
5. ______________________
6. ______________________
7. ______________________
8. ______________________
9. ______________________
10. ______________________
11. ______________________
12. ______________________
13. ______________________
14. ______________________
15. ______________________
16. ______________________
17. ______________________
18. ______________________
19. ______________________
20. ______________________
21. ______________________
22. ______________________
23. ______________________
24. ______________________
25. ______________________
26. ______________________
27. ______________________
28. ______________________
29. ______________________
30. ______________________
31. ______________________
32. ______________________
33. ______________________

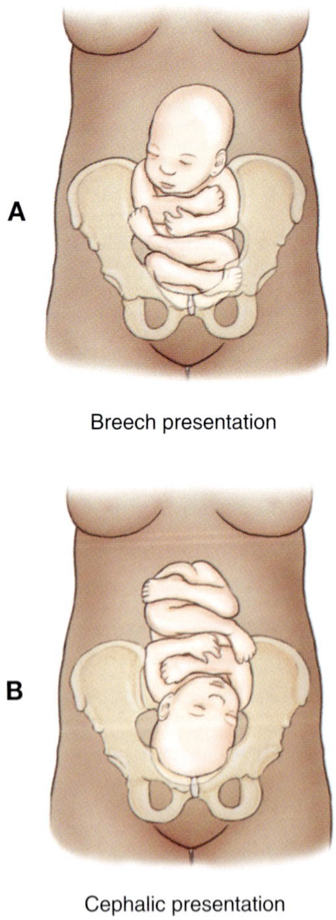

FIGURE 9-14
A, Breech presentation.
B, Cephalic presentation.

Obstetric and Neonatal Complementary Terms

Not Built from Word Parts

In some of the following terms you may recognize word parts you have already learned; however, the full meaning of the terms cannot be discerned by the definition of their word parts.

Term	Definition
breech presentation (brēch)	birth position in which the buttocks, feet, or knees emerge first (Figure 9-14, *A*)
cephalic presentation (se-FAL-ik)	birth position in which any part of the head emerges first. It is the most common presentation (Figure 9-14, *B*).
cesarean section (CS, C-section) (se-ZĀR-ē-an) (SEK-shun)	the birth of a baby through an incision in the mother's abdomen and uterus (may also be spelled **caesarean**)

Term	Definition
colostrum (k-LOS-trem)	thin, milky fluid secreted by the breast during pregnancy and during the first days after birth before lactation begins
congenital anomaly (kon-JEN-i-tal) (a-NOM-a-lē)	abnormality present at birth; often discovered before birth by ultrasonography and/or amniocentesis
in vitro fertilization (IVF) (in VĒ-trō) (*fer*-ti-li-ZĀ-shun)	a method of fertilizing human ova outside the body and placing the zygote into the uterus; used when infertility is present (Figure 9-15)
lactation (lak-TĀ-shun)	the secretion of milk
lochia (LŌ-kē-a)	vaginal discharge after childbirth
meconium (me-KŌ-nē-um)	first stool of the newborn (greenish-black)
midwife (MID-wīf)	an individual who practices midwifery
midwifery (MID-wif-rē)	the practice of assisting in childbirth
obstetrician (*ob*-ste-TRISH-an)	physician who specializes in obstetrics
obstetrics (OB) (ob-STET-riks)	medical specialty dealing with pregnancy, childbirth, and puerperium
parturition (*par*-tū-RISH-un)	act of giving birth
premature infant (PRĒ-ma-tur) (IN-fent)	infant born before completing 37 weeks of gestation (also called **preterm infant**)
puerperium (*pū*-er-PĒ-rē-um)	period from delivery until the reproductive organs return to normal (approximately 6 weeks)
quickening (KWIK-en-ing)	the first feeling of movement of the fetus in utero by the pregnant woman. It usually occurs between 16 and 20 weeks of gestation.
stillborn (STIL-born)	born dead

Refer to **Appendix D** for pharmacology terms related to obstetrics and neonatology.

CESAREAN SECTION (C-SECTION)

The origin of this term has no relation to the birth of Julius Caesar, as is commonly believed. One suggested etymology is that from 715 to 672 BC it was Roman law that the operation be performed on dying women in the last few months of pregnancy in the hope of saving the child. At that time the operation was called a ***caeso matris utero***, which means **the cutting of the mother's uterus**.

INFERTILITY

Managing infertility, a condition estimated by the CDC to affect approximately 12% of the U.S. reproductive-age population, has many options. They include medications to stimulate ova production and procedures to provide artificial insemination. Techniques that artificially combine *both* ova and sperm are referred to as *assisted reproductive technology* (**ART**).

MIDWIFERY

Midwives who practice midwifery supervise pregnancy, labor, delivery, and puerperium. They assist with delivery independently, care for the newborn, and obtain medical assistance as necessary. A midwife may or may not be a registered nurse. Education, certification, and licensure vary by state and country.

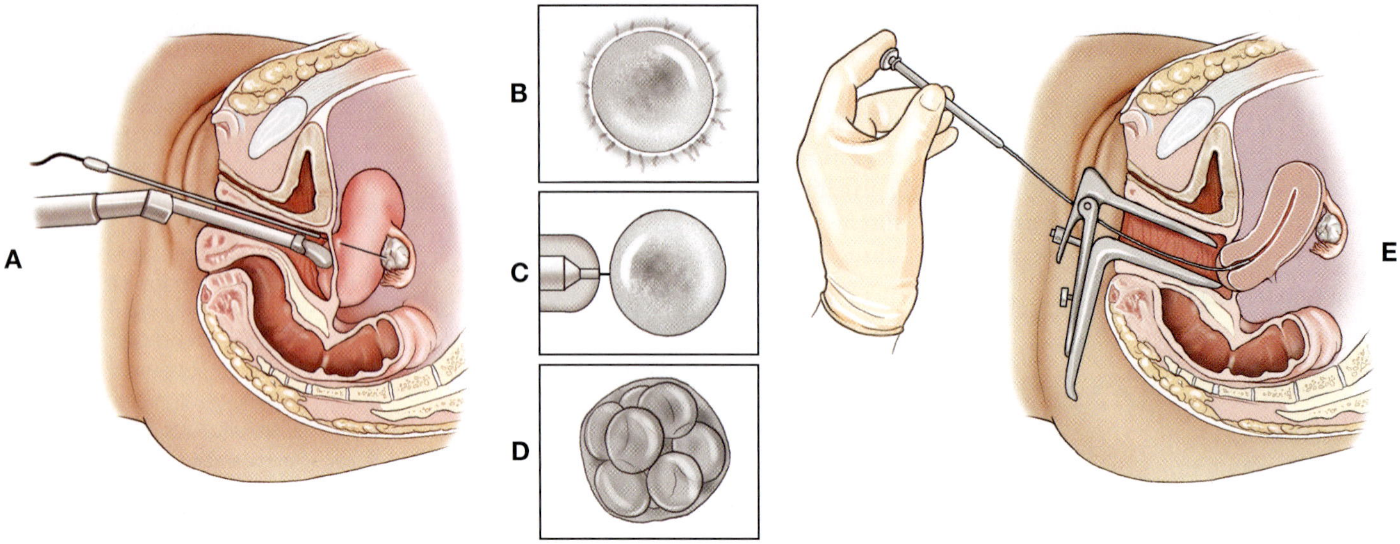

FIGURE 9-15

In vitro fertilization (IVF). After ovarian stimulation, ova are retrieved from the ovary by ultrasound-guided transvaginal needle aspiration **(A).** The ova are fertilized outside the body in a dish with spermatozoa obtained from semen **(B).** A technique using a single sperm called intracytoplasmic sperm injection may also be used **(C).** After 48 hours the fertilized ova (zygotes) **(D)** are injected into the uterus for implantation **(E).** The first pregnancy after in vitro fertilization was reported more than 3 decades ago. Since then **assisted reproductive technology (ART)** has achieved hundreds of thousands of pregnancies worldwide.

EXERCISE 34

Practice saying aloud each of the complementary terms not built from word parts on pp. 390-391.

To hear the terms, go to http://evolve.elsevier.com. Refer to p. 18 for your Evolve Access Information. Select Exercises & Review, Chapter 9, Chapter Exercises, Pronunciation.

☐ Place a check mark in the box when you have completed this exercise.

EXERCISE 35

Match the definitions in the first column with the correct terms in the second column.

	Definition		Term
______	1. vaginal discharge	a.	lochia
______	2. medical specialty	b.	obstetrician
______	3. abnormality present at birth	c.	premature infant
______	4. period after delivery	d.	meconium
______	5. giving birth	e.	obstetrics
______	6. physician specializing in obstetrics	f.	parturition
______	7. buttocks, feet, or knees first	g.	puerperium
______	8. first stool	h.	cesarean section
______	9. born before completing 37 weeks of gestation	i.	congenital anomaly
______	10. birth through an abdominal and uterine incision	j.	breech presentation

EXERCISE 36

Match the definitions in the first column with the correct terms in the second column.

	Definition	Term
______	1. assisting in childbirth	a. quickening
______	2. one who assists in childbirth	b. lactation
______	3. secretion of milk	c. cephalic presentation
______	4. head first	d. colostrum
______	5. born dead	e. midwife
______	6. movement of the fetus	f. stillborn
______	7. secreted before lactation	g. in vitro fertilization
______	8. method of fertilizing ova outside the body	h. midwifery

EXERCISE 37

Write the definitions of the following terms.

1. meconium ________________________________
2. obstetrics ________________________________
3. premature infant ________________________________
4. lochia ________________________________
5. puerperium ________________________________
6. parturition ________________________________

7. obstetrician ______________________________
8. congenital anomaly ______________________________
9. breech presentation ______________________________
10. cesarean section ______________________________
11. quickening ______________________________
12. lactation ______________________________
13. cephalic presentation ______________________________
14. colostrum ______________________________
15. midwife ______________________________
16. stillborn ______________________________
17. midwifery ______________________________
18. in vitro fertilization ______________________________

EXERCISE 38

Spell each of the complementary terms not bult from word parts on pp. 390-391 by having someone dictate them to you.

To hear and spell the terms, go to http://evolve.elsevier.com. Refer to p. 18 for your Evolve Access Information. Select Exercises & Review, Chapter 9, Chapter Exercises, Spelling.

☐ Place a check mark in the box if you have completed this exercise online.

1. ____________	10. ____________
2. ____________	11. ____________
3. ____________	12. ____________
4. ____________	13. ____________
5. ____________	14. ____________
6. ____________	15. ____________
7. ____________	16. ____________
8. ____________	17. ____________
9. ____________	18. ____________

Abbreviations

CS, C-section	cesarean section
DOB	date of birth
EDD	expected (estimated) date of delivery
FAS	fetal alcohol syndrome
IVF	in vitro fertilization
LMP	last menstrual period
multip	multipara
NB	newborn
OB	obstetrics
primip	primipara
RDS	respiratory distress syndrome
VBAC	vaginal birth after cesarean section

Refer to **Appendix C** for a complete list of abbreviations.

EXERCISE 39

Write the definition of the following abbreviations.

1. OB ____________________
2. EDD __________ __________ of __________
3. LMP __________ __________ __________
4. DOB __________ __________ __________
5. NB ____________________
6. multip ____________________
7. C/S, C-section __________ __________
8. VBAC ______ ______ ______ ______ ______
9. RDS __________ __________ __________
10. primip ____________________
11. FAS __________ __________ __________
12. IVF __________ __________ __________

LAMAZE

is a method of psychophysical preparation for childbirth started in the 1950s by a French obstetrician, Fernand Lamaze. The method requires classes and practice before and coaching during labor and delivery.

PRACTICAL APPLICATION

EXERCISE 40 *Interact with Medical Documents*

A. Complete the progress note by writing the medical terms in the blanks. Use the list of definitions with the corresponding numbers.

University Hospital and Medical Center

4700 North Main Street • Wellness, Arizona 54321 • (987) 555-3210

PATIENT NAME: Gloria Cisneros **CASE NUMBER:** 17432-OBN

DATE OF BIRTH: 08/26/19XX **DATE:** 09/23/20XX

PROGRESS NOTE

HISTORY: Gloria Cisneros is a 24-year-old married Latina 1. ________________ 3, and 2. ________________ 2 who is here today with her husband. Her 3. ________________ is 1 week from today. She has received 4. ________________ care here at the Medical Center Obstetrics Clinic since her second month of pregnancy. This 5. ________________ has been uncomplicated with no spotting, albuminuria, hypertension, edema, or glycosuria. Patient has attended Lamaze classes with her husband.

PHYSICAL EXAM: Her breasts are enlarged. She has gained 2 pounds since her last visit and she has gained 25 pounds throughout her pregnancy. Her current weight is 164 pounds. Her cervix is 1 cm dilated. Routine 6. ________________ reveals a single 7. ________________ low in the pelvis in the 8. ________________.

PLAN: Patient will return to clinic once a week until delivery.

____

Heather Strom, MD

HS/mcm

1. pregnant (woman)
2. birth
3. abbreviation for expected delivery date
4. pertaining to before birth (reference to the newborn)
5. development of a new individual from conception to birth
6. pertaining to the pelvis, process of recording sound
7. unborn offspring from the ninth week of pregnancy
8. birth position in which any part of the head emerges first

EXERCISE 40 *Interact with Medical Documents—cont'd*

B. Read the following radiology report and answer the questions following it.

053447 SMITH, EMMA

File Patient Navigate Custom Fields Help

Patient Chart | Lab | Rad | Notes | Documents | Rx | Scheduling | Images | Billing

Name: **SMITH, EMMA** MR#: **053447** Sex: **F**
DOB:

RADIOLOGY REPORT

04/17/20XX

PATIENT NAME: Emma Smith NUMBER: 053447

REFERRING PHYSICIAN: Joseph Plains, MD

INDICATIONS: Lower abdominal pain

EXAMINATION: Pelvic sonography

HISTORY: Thirty-two-year-old primip with menstrual irregularity and abdominal pain. History of pelvic inflammatory disease and spontaneous abortion x1.

FINDINGS: Sagittal and transverse images reveal an extrauterine sac containing a fetus in the left uterine tube. Cystic mass (hematoma) is evident in the rectouterine pouch. No fetal heart activity is noted.

OPINION: Ectopic pregnancy, left uterine tube.

A.W. Tyat, MD

AWT/ogo

Start | Log On/Off | Print | Edit

1. The patient has:
   a. been pregnant two or more times
   b. given birth to two or more viable offspring
   c. borne one viable offspring
   d. never been pregnant
2. T F The patient has experienced one abortion
3. T F Radiographic images were used to determine the findings.

EXERCISE 41 *Interpret Medical Terms*

To test your understanding of the terms introduced in this chapter, circle the words that correctly complete the sentences. The italicized words refer to the correct answer.

1. The premature infant was diagnosed as having *respiratory distress syndrome*, a disease of the (**umbilicus, erythrocytes, lungs**).
2. Because of inadequate uterine contractions, the patient was experiencing *difficult labor*, or (**dysphasia, dystocia, dysuria**).
3. Down syndrome was diagnosed prenatally by laboratory analysis of *amniotic fluid aspirated by surgical puncture*, or (**amniocentesis, amnioscopy, amnioscope**).

4. The word that means *before childbirth* (reference to the mother) is (**intrapartum, antepartum, postpartum**).
5. *Nulligravida* is a woman who (**has never been pregnant, has not given birth**).
6. *Multipara* is a woman who has (**given birth to two or more viable offspring, been pregnant two or more times**).
7. *Primigravida* is a woman (**in her first pregnancy, who has given birth to one child**).
8. The word that means the *act of giving birth* is (**parturition, puerperium, gravidopuerperal**).
9. *Rupture of the uterus* is called (**hysterorrhaphy, hysterorrhexis, hysteroptosis**).
10. Excessive alcohol intake during pregnancy may result in is *producing malformations* or (**quickening, colostrum, teratogenic**) changes to the fetus.

WEB LINK

For more information about obstetrics, visit The American College of Obstetricians and Gynecologists at ***http://www.acog.org/***. Additional information regarding assistive reproductive technology (ART) can be found at the Centers for Disease Control and Prevention website at ***http://www.cdc.gov/ART/***.

EXERCISE 42 *Read Medical Terms in Use*

Practice pronunciation of the terms by reading the following medical document. Use the pronunciation key following the medical term to assist you in saying the words.

To hear these terms, go to http://evolve.elsevier.com. Refer to p. 18 for your Evolve Access Information. Select Exercises & Review, Chapter 9, Chapter Exercises, Read Medical Terms in Use.

Jane Anne is a 34-year-old **gravida** (GRAV-i-da) 2 **para** (PAR-a) 1 woman. Her LMP was April 20, 20XX. The EDD is January 2, 20XX. The **obstetrician** (*ob*-ste-TRISH-an) prescribed folic acid to prevent **spina bifida** (SPĪ-na) (BIF-i-da). The patient's first pregnancy was complicated by **preeclampsia** (prē-ē-KLAMP-sē-a) and a **breech** (brēch) **presentation,** which required a **cesarean section** (se-ZĀR-ē-an) (SEK-shun). **Pelvic sonography** (PEL-vik) (so-NOG-ra-fē) showed a single female fetus with normal development. She went on to deliver a healthy baby by VBAC 3 days before her expected delivery date.

EXERCISE 43 *Comprehend Medical Terms in Use*

Test your comprehension of terms in the above medical document by circling the correct answer.

1. T F Jane Anne has been pregnant twice and has given birth once.
2. The obstetrician prescribed folic acid to prevent congenital:
   a. split of the lip and roof of the mouth
   b. mental retardation
   c. absence of part of the esophagus
   d. defect of the vertebral column
3. During her first pregnancy the patient had:
   a. abnormally low implantation of the placenta on the uterine wall
   b. high blood pressure, edema, and proteinuria
   c. premature separation of the placenta from the uterine wall
   d. convulsions and coma
4. T F The fetal presentation of the patient's first pregnancy was cephalic.

CHAPTER REVIEW

CHAPTER REVIEW ON EVOLVE

To access the Evolve website, go to http://evolve.elsevier.com. Refer to p. 18 for your Evolve Access Information. Select Exercises & Review, Chapter 3, then select Chapter Exercises, Practice Activities, Animations, or Games. Place a check mark in the box when you have completed an exercise or activity, watched an animation, or played a game. Have fun!

Chapter Exercises

Exercises in this section of your Evolve resources correlate to exercises in your textbook. You may have completed them as you worked through the chapter.

- ☐ Pronunciation
- ☐ Spelling
- ☐ Read Medical Terms in Use

Practice Activities

Practice in study mode, then test your learning in assessment mode. Keep track of your scores from assessment mode if you wish.

	SCORE
☐ Picture It	_____
☐ Define Word Parts	_____
☐ Build Medical Terms	_____
☐ Word Shop	_____
☐ Define Medical Terms	_____
☐ Use It	_____
☐ Hear It and Type It: Clinical Vignettes	_____

Animations

- ☐ Abruptio Placentae (placental abruption)
- ☐ Breech Presentation Exam
- ☐ Breech Delivery Arms
- ☐ Breech Delivery Face
- ☐ Dystocia Delivery
- ☐ Ectopic Pregnancy
- ☐ Placenta Previa

Games

- ☐ Name that Word Part
- ☐ Term Storm
- ☐ Term Explorer
- ☐ Termbusters
- ☐ Medical Millionaire
- ☐ Crossword Puzzle

REVIEW OF WORD PARTS

Can you define and spell the following word parts?

Combining Forms

amni/o
amnion/o
cephal/o
chori/o
embry/o
esophag/o
fet/i
fet/o
gravid/o
lact/o
nat/o
omphal/o
par/o
part/o
pelv/i
pelv/o
prim/i
pseud/o
puerper/o
pylor/o
terat/o

Prefixes

ante-
micro-
multi-
nulli-
post-
pre-

Suffixes

-amnios
-cyesis
-e
-is
-partum
-rrhexis
-tocia
-um
-us

REVIEW OF TERMS

Can you build, analyze, define, pronounce, and spell the following terms *built from word parts?*

Diseases and Disorders (Obstetrics)

amnionitis
chorioamnionitis
choriocarcinoma
dystocia
hysterorrhexis
oligohydramnios
polyhydramnios

Diseases and Disorders (Neonatology)

microcephalus
omphalitis
omphalocele
pyloric stenosis
tracheoesophageal fistula

Surgical (Obstetrics)

amniotomy
episiotomy

Diagnostic (Obstetrics)

amniocentesis
amnioscope
amnioscopy
pelvic sonography

Complementary (Obstetrics and Neonatology)

amniochorial
amniorrhea
amniorrhexis
antepartum
embryogenic
embryoid
fetal
gravida
gravidopuerperal
intrapartum
lactic
lactogenic
lactorrhea
multigravida
multipara (multip)
natal
neonate
neonatologist
neonatology
nulligravida
nullipara
para
postnatal
postpartum
prenatal
primigravida
primipara (primip)
pseudocyesis
puerpera
puerperal
teratogen
teratogenic
teratology

Can you define, pronounce, and spell the following terms *not built from word parts?*

Diseases and Disorders (Obstetrics)

abortion
abruptio placentae
eclampsia
ectopic pregnancy
placenta previa
preeclampsia

Diseases and Disorders (Neonatology)

cleft lip and palate
Down syndrome
erythroblastosis fetalis
esophageal atresia
fetal alcohol syndrome (FAS)
gastroschisis
respiratory distress syndrome (RDS)
spina bifida

Complementary (Obstetrics and Neonatology)

breech presentation
cephalic presentation
cesarean section (CS, C-section)
colostrum
congenital anomaly
in vitro fertilization (IVF)
lactation
lochia
meconium
midwife
midwifery
obstetrician
obstetrics (OB)
parturition
premature infant
puerperium
quickening
stillborn

ANSWERS

Exercise Figures

Exercise Figure

A. 1. umbilicus: omphal/o
2. fetus: fet/o, fet/i
3. amnion, amniotic fluid: amni/o, amnion/o
4. chorion: chori/o

Exercise Figure

B. omphal/o/cele

Exercise Figure

C. neo/nat/e

Exercise 1

1. gamete; ovulation; fertilization; zygote; gestation
2. embryo; fetus
3. amniotic; chorion; amnion; amniotic

Exercise 2

1. fetus, unborn child
2. milk
3. bear, give birth to, labor, childbirth
4. umbilicus, navel
5. amnion, amniotic fluid
6. childbirth
7. pregnancy
8. birth
9. chorion
10. embryo, to be full

Exercise 3

1. lact/o
2. a. fet/o, b. fet/i
3. chori/o
4. a. amni/o, b. amnion/o
5. puerper/o
6. a. par/o, b. part/o
7. gravid/o
8. embry/o
9. nat/o
10. omphal/o

Exercise 4

1. first
2. pylorus
3. head
4. esophagus
5. false
6. pelvic bone, pelvis
7. malformations

Exercise 5

1. cephal/o
2. pylor/o
3. pseud/o
4. esophag/o
5. prim/i
6. terat/o
7. a. pelv/i, b. pelv/o

Exercise 6

1. after
2. many
3. none
4. small
5. before
6. before

Exercise 7

1. nulli-
2. micro-
3. multi-
4. a. ante-
b. pre-
5. post-

Exercise 8

1. rupture
2. birth, labor
3. pregnancy
4. childbirth, labor
5. amnion, amniotic fluid

Exercise 9

1. -tocia
2. -rrhexis
3. -partum
4. -cyesis
5. -amnios

Exercise 10

1. -e
2. -is
3. -us
4. -um

Answers may be in any order.

Exercise 11

Pronunciation Exercise

Exercise 12

1. WR CV WR S
chori/o/amnion/itis
CF
inflammation of the chorion and amnion
2. WR CV WR S
chori/o/carcin/oma
CF
cancerous tumor of the chorion
3. P S(WR)
dys/tocia
difficult labor
4. WR S
amnion/itis
inflammation of the amnion
5. WR CV S
hyster/o/rrhexis
CF
rupture of the uterus
6. WR CV WR S
olig/o/hydr/amnios
CF
scanty amnion water (less than the normal amount of amniotic fluid)
7. P WR S
poly/hydr/amnios
much amnion water (more than the normal amount of amniotic fluid)

Exercise 13

1. chori/o/carcin/oma
2. amnion/itis
3. chori/o/amnion/itis
4. dys/tocia
5. hyster/o/rrhexis
6. olig/o/hydr/amnios
7. poly/hydr/amnios

Exercise 14

Spelling Exercise; see text p. 371.

Exercise 15

Pronunciation Exercise

Exercise 16

1. premature separation of the placenta from the uterine wall
2. termination of pregnancy by the expulsion from the uterus of an embryo
3. abnormally low implantation of the placenta on the uterine wall
4. severe complication and progression of preeclampsia
5. pregnancy occurring outside the uterus
6. abnormal condition, encountered during pregnancy or shortly after delivery, of high blood pressure, edema, and proteinuria

Exercise 17

1. abruptio placentae
2. eclampsia
3. abortion
4. ectopic pregnancy
5. placenta previa
6. preeclampsia

Exercise 18

Spelling Exercise; see text pp. 373-374.

Exercise 19

Pronunciation Exercise

Exercise 20

1. WR S
pylor/ic (stenosis)
narrowing pertaining to the pyloric sphincter
2. WR CV S
omphal/o/cele
CF
hernia at the umbilicus
3. WR S
omphal/itis
inflammation of the umbilicus
4. P WR S
micro/cephal/us
(fetus with a very) small head
5. WR CV WR S
trache/o/esophag/eal (fistula)
CF
abnormal passageway pertaining to the esophagus and the trachea (between the esophagus and trachea)

Exercise 21

1. omphal/o/cele
2. micro/cephal/us
3. pylor/ic (stenosis)
4. trache/o/esophag/eal (fistula)
5. omphal/itis

Exercise 22

Spelling Exercise; see text p. 376.

Exercise 23

Pronunciation Exercise

Exercise 24

1. f
2. c
3. a
4. d
5. h
6. b
7. g
8. e

Exercise 25

Spelling Exercise; see text p. 378-379.

Exercise 26

Pronunciation Exercise

Exercise 27

1. WR CV S
episi/o/tomy
CF
incision of the vulva (perineum)
2. WR CV S
amni/o/tomy
CF
incision into the amnion (rupture of the fetal membrane to induce labor)
3. WR CV S
amni/o/scope
CF
instrument used for visual examination of amniotic fluid (and fetus)
4. WR S WR CV S
pelv/ic son/o/graphy
CF
pertaining to the pelvis, process of recording sound
5. WR CV S
amni/o/centesis
CF
surgical puncture to aspirate amniotic fluid
6. WR CV S
amni/o/scopy
CF
visual examination of amniotic fluid (and fetus)

Exercise 28

1. amni/o/tomy
2. episi/o/tomy
3. amni/o/scopy
4. amni/o/centesis
5. amni/o/scope
6. pelv/ic son/o/graphy

Exercise 29

Spelling Exercise; see text p. 381.

Exercise 30

Pronunciation Exercise

Exercise 31

1. WR S
puerper/a
childbirth
2. WR CV S
amni/o/rrhexis
CF
rupture of the amnion
3. P WR S
ante/part/um
before childbirth
4. WR CV S
pseud/o/cyesis
CF
false pregnancy
5. P WR S
pre/nat/al
pertaining to before birth
6. WR S
lact/ic
pertaining to milk
7. WR CV S
lact/o/rrhea
CF
(spontaneous) discharge of milk
8. WR CV S
amni/o/rrhea
CF
discharge (escape) of amniotic fluid
9. P WR S
multi/par/a
many births
10. WR CV S
embry/o/genic
CF
producing an embryo
11. WR S
embry/oid
resembling an embryo
12. WR S
fet/al
pertaining to the fetus
13. WR S
gravid/a
pregnant (woman)
14. WR CV WR S
amni/o/chori/al
CF
pertaining to the amnion and chorion
15. P WR S
multi/gravid/a
many pregnancies
16. WR CV S
lact/o/genic
CF
producing milk (by stimulation)
17. WR S
nat/al
pertaining to birth
18. WR CV WR S
gravid/o/puerper/al
CF
pertaining to pregnancy and childbirth
19. P WR CV S
neo/nat/o/logy
CF
study of the newborn
20. P WR S
nulli/par/a
no births
21. WR S
par/a
birth
22. WR CV WR S
prim/i/gravid/a
CF
first pregnancy

23. P WR S
post/part/um
after childbirth
24. P WR S
neo/nat/e
new birth (an infant from birth to 4 weeks of age, synonymous with newborn)
25. WR CV WR S
prim/i/par/a
CF
first birth
26. WR S
puerper/al
pertaining to (immediately after) childbirth
27. P WR S
nulli/gravid/a
no pregnancies
28. P WR S
intra/part/um
within (during) labor and childbirth
29. WR CV S
terat/o/gen
CF
any agent producing malformations (in the developing embryo)
30. P WR S
post/nat/al
pertaining to after birth
31. WR CV S
terat/o/logy
CF
study of malformations (in the developing embryo)
32. P WR CV S
neo/nat/o/logist
CF
physician who studies and treats disorders of the newborn
33. WR CV S
terat/o/genic
CF
producing malformations

Exercise 32
1. amni/o/chori/al
2. ante/part/um
3. embry/o/genic
4. fet/al
5. pre/nat/al
6. lact/ic
7. lact/o/rrhea
8. amni/o/rrhea
9. pseud/o/cyesis
10. lact/o/genic
11. amni/o/rrhexis
12. embry/oid
13. gravid/a
14. gravid/o/puerper/al
15. multi/par/a
16. nat/al
17. neo/nat/e
18. neo/nat/o/logy
19. nulli/par/a
20. par/a
21. prim/i/gravid/a
22. post/part/um
23. prim/i/par/a
24. multi/gravid/a
25. puerper/al
26. nulli/gravid/a
27. terat/o/gen
28. puerper/a
29. intra/part/um
30. terat/o/genic
31. neo/nat/o/logist
32. post/nat/al
33. terat/o/logy

Exercise 33
Spelling Exercise; see text Pp. 384-385.

Exercise 34
Pronunciation Exercise

Exercise 35

1. a	6. b
2. e	7. j
3. i	8. d
4. g	9. c
5. f	10. h

Exercise 36

1. h	5. f
2. e	6. a
3. b	7. d
4. c	8. g

Exercise 37
1. first stool of the newborn
2. medical specialty dealing with pregnancy, childbirth, and puerperium
3. infant born before completing 37 weeks of gestation
4. vaginal discharge after childbirth
5. period after delivery until the reproductive organs return to normal
6. act of giving birth
7. physician who specializes in obstetrics
8. abnormality present at birth
9. birth position in which the buttocks, feet, or knees emerge first
10. birth of a baby through an incision in the mother's abdomen and uterus
11. first feeling of movement of the fetus in utero by the pregnant woman
12. secretion of milk
13. birth position in which any part of the head emerges first
14. fluid secreted by the breast during pregnancy and after birth until lactation begins
15. an individual who practices midwifery
16. born dead
17. the practice of assisting in childbirth
18. a method of fertilizing human ova outside the body

Exercise 38
Spelling Exercise; see text pp. 390-391.

Exercise 39
1. obstetrics
2. expected (estimated) date of delivery
3. last menstrual period
4. date of birth
5. newborn
6. multipara
7. cesarean section
8. vaginal birth after cesarean section
9. respiratory distress syndrome
10. primapara
11. fetal alcohol syndrome
12. in vitro fertilization

Exercise 40
A.

1. gravida	5. gestation
2. para	6. pelvic sonography
3. EDD	7. fetus
4. prenatal	8. cephalic presentation

B.
1. c
2. *T*
3. *F*, sonography was used

Exercise 41
1. lungs
2. dystocia
3. amniocentesis
4. antepartum
5. has never been pregnant
6. given birth to two or more viable offspring
7. in her first pregnancy
8. parturition
9. hysterorrhexis
10. teratogenic

Exercise 42
Reading Exercise

Exercise 43
1. *T*
2. d
3. b
4. *F*, the fetal presentation was breech.

Chapter 10

Cardiovascular, Immune, Lymphatic Systems and Blood

OUTLINE

OBJECTIVES

Upon completion of this chapter you will be able to:

1. Identify the organs and structures of the cardiovascular and lymphatic systems and blood and the function of the immune system.
2. Define and spell word parts related to the cardiovascular and lymphatic systems and blood.
3. Define, pronounce, and spell disease and disorder terms related to the cardiovascular and lymphatic systems and blood.
4. Define, pronounce, and spell surgical terms related to the cardiovascular and lymphatic systems and blood.
5. Define, pronounce, and spell diagnostic terms related to the cardiovascular system and blood.
6. Define, pronounce, and spell complementary terms related to the cardiovascular, immune systems, and blood.
7. Interpret the meaning of abbreviations presented in the chapter.
8. Interpret, read, and comprehend medical language in simulated medical statements and documents.

ANATOMY

At first glance this may seem like an overabundance of material to cover in one chapter. It is a lot of material, but as you will see the systems have interactive functions, and learning the terms for these systems at the same time is beneficial.

The functions are interactive in many ways. The lymphatic and immune systems support each other by providing an immune response to invading microorganisms and foreign substances. The lymphatic system and blood share macrophages and lymphocytes. Lymph is drained into large veins of the cardiovascular system, and the cardiovascular system is responsible for circulating blood throughout the body.

Cardiovascular System

The cardiovascular system consists of the heart and a closed network of blood vessels composed of arteries, capillaries, and veins (Figure 10-1).

Function

The heart pumps blood containing oxygen and nutrients to body tissues through the arteries. The exchange of gases, nutrients, and waste between the blood and body tissue takes place in the capillaries. The blood carrying carbon dioxide and waste is carried from the tissues through veins to organs of excretion.

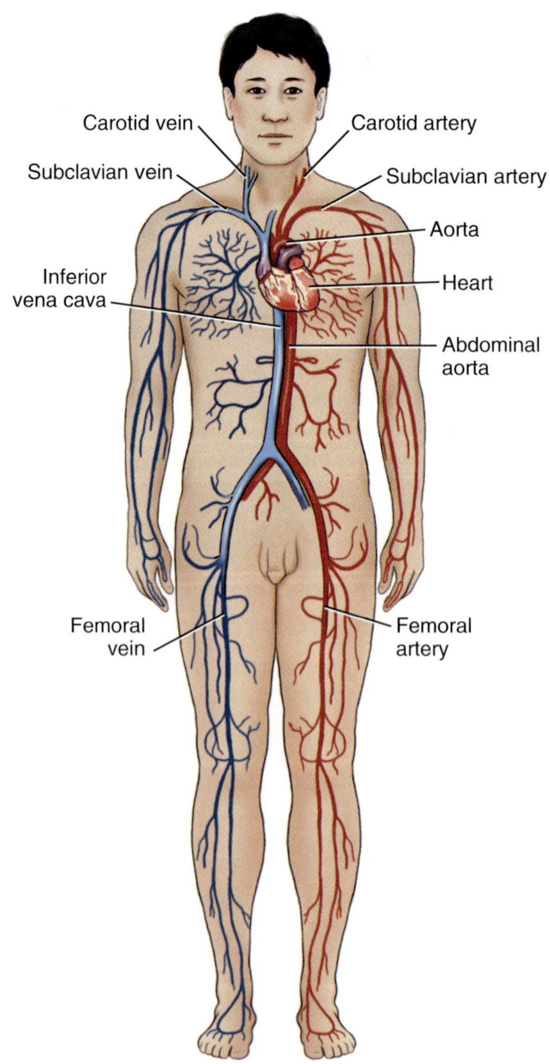

FIGURE 10-1
Cardiovascular system.

Structures of the Cardiovascular System

Term	Definition
heart	muscular cone-shaped organ the size of a fist, located behind the sternum (breast bone) and between the lungs. The pumping action of the heart circulates blood throughout the body (Figure 10-2). The heart consists of two upper chambers, the **right atrium** and the **left atrium** (*pl.* **atria**), and two lower chambers, the **right ventricle** and the **left ventricle** (*pl.* **ventricles**). The right atrium receives blood returning from the body through the veins; the left atrium receives blood from the lungs. The left ventricle pumps blood through the arteries from the heart back to the body tissue; the right ventricle pumps blood to the lungs. The **atrial septum** separates the atria and the **ventricular septum** separates the ventricles.
atrioventricular valves	Consist of the **tricuspid** and **mitral** valves, which lie between the right atrium and the right ventricle and the left atrium and left ventricle, respectively. Valves of the heart keep blood flowing in one direction.
semilunar valves	**pulmonary** and **aortic** valves located between the right ventricle and the pulmonary artery and between the left ventricle and the aorta, respectively.
pericardium	two-layer sac surrounding the heart, consisting of an external fibrous and an internal serous layer. The serous layer secretes a fluid that facilitates movement of the heart. It consists of two layers, one lining the fibrous pericardium and one covering the heart, called epicardium.
three layers of the heart	
epicardium	covers the heart
myocardium	middle, thick, muscular layer
endocardium	inner lining of the heart
blood vessels	tubelike structures that carry blood throughout the body (Figure 10-3)
arteries	blood vessels that carry blood away from the heart. All arteries, with the exception of the pulmonary artery, carry oxygen and other nutrients from the heart to the body cells. The **pulmonary artery**, in contrast, carries carbon dioxide and other waste products from the heart to the lungs.
arterioles	smallest arteries

Structures of the Cardiovascular System—*cont'd*

Term	Definition
aorta	largest artery in the body, originating at the left ventricle and descending through the thorax and abdomen
veins	blood vessels that carry blood back to the heart. All veins, with the exception of the pulmonary veins, carry blood containing carbon dioxide and other waste products. The pulmonary veins carry oxygenated blood from the lungs to the heart.
venules	smallest veins
venae cavae	largest veins in the body. The **inferior vena cava** carries blood to the heart from body parts below the diaphragm, and the **superior vena cava** returns the blood to the heart from the upper part of the body.
capillaries	microscopic blood vessels that connect arterioles with venules. Materials are passed between the blood and tissue through the capillary walls.

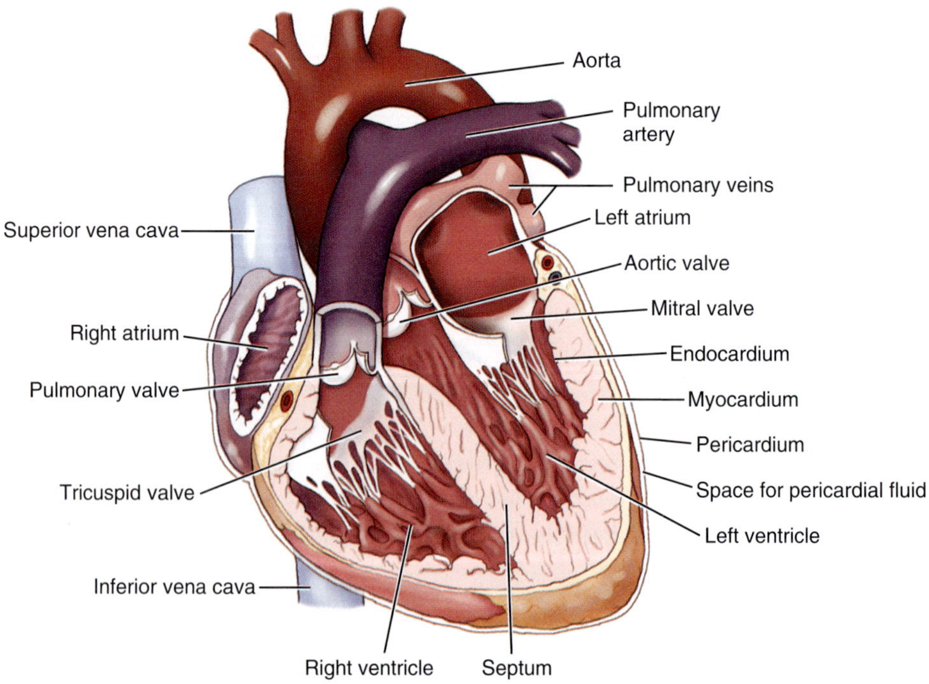

FIGURE 10-2
Interior of the heart.

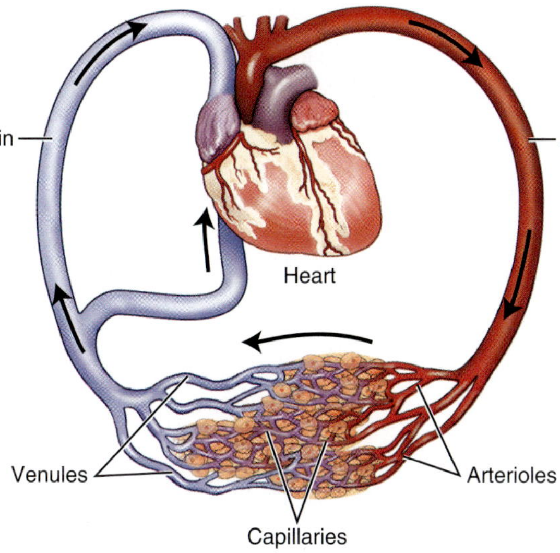

FIGURE 10-3
Types of blood vessels.

EXERCISE 1

Match the anatomic terms for the cardiovascular system in the first column with the correct definitions in the second column. *To check your answers to the exercises in this chapter, go to Answers, p. 477, at the end of the chapter.*

_____ 1. aorta
_____ 2. arteries
_____ 3. arterioles
_____ 4. atria
_____ 5. mitral valve
_____ 6. capillaries
_____ 7. endocardium
_____ 8. heart
_____ 9. atrioventricular valves

a. lies between the left atrium and left ventricle
b. pumps blood throughout the body
c. smallest arteries
d. inner lining of the heart
e. largest artery in the body
f. connect arterioles with venules
g. blood vessels that carry blood away from the heart
h. upper chambers of the heart
i. tricuspid and mitral valves

EXERCISE 2

Match the anatomic terms for the cardiovascular system in the first column with the correct definitions in the second column.

_____ 1. myocardium

_____ 2. pericardium

_____ 3. semilunar valves

_____ 4. atrial septum

_____ 5. tricuspid valve

_____ 6. veins

_____ 7. ventricles

_____ 8. venules

_____ 9. vena cava

a. carries blood back to the heart

b. two-layer sac that facilitates movement of the heart

c. smallest veins

d. separates the atria

e. lower chambers of the heart

f. largest vein in the body

g. located between the right ventricle and the pulmonary artery and between the left ventricle and the aorta

h. carries oxygenated blood away from the heart

i. located between the right atrium and the right ventricle

j. muscular layer of the heart

Blood

Function

The primary function of blood is to maintain internal balance in the body. Activities of the blood include **transportation** of nutrients, waste, oxygen, carbon dioxide, and hormones; **protection** provided by certain cells that protect the body against microorganisms; and **regulation** by controlling body temperature and maintaining fluid and electrolyte balance.

Composition of Blood

Term	Definition
blood	composed of **plasma** and **formed elements**, such as erythrocytes, leukocytes, and thrombocytes (platelets) (Figure 10-4)
plasma	clear, straw-colored, liquid portion of blood in which cells are suspended. Plasma is approximately 90% water and comprises approximately 55% of the total blood volume.
cells (formed elements)	
erythrocytes	red blood cells that carry oxygen. Erythrocytes develop in bone marrow.

Term	Definition
leukocytes	white blood cells that combat infection and respond to inflammation. There are five types of white blood cells (Figure 10-5).
platelets (thrombocytes)	one of the formed elements in the blood that is responsible for aiding in the clotting process
serum	clear, watery fluid portion of the blood that remains after a clot has formed

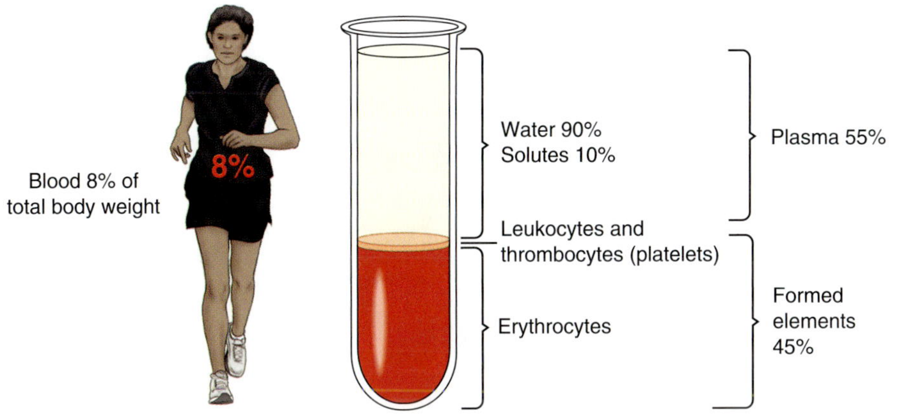

FIGURE 10-4
Composition of blood.

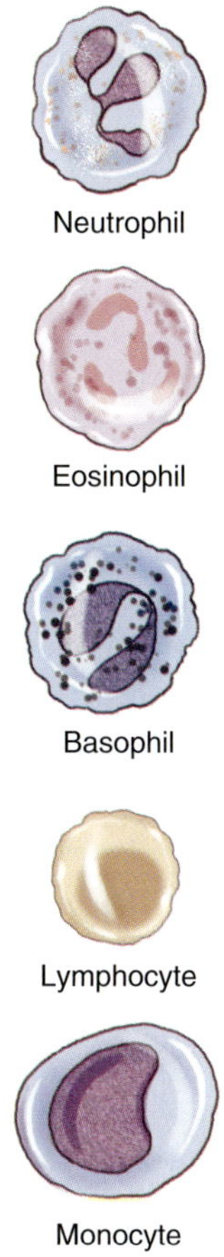

FIGURE 10-5
Types of leukocytes. Each leukocyte plays a different role in providing immune responses to pathogens, foreign agents, allergies, and abnormal body cells.

Lymphatic System

The lymphatic system consists of lymph transported through lymphatic vessels, lymph nodes, the spleen, and thymus gland.

Function

Three functions of the lymphatic system are to return excessive tissue fluid to the blood, absorb fats and fat-soluble vitamins from the small intestine and transport them to the blood, and provide defense against infection.

Collected interstitial fluid called lymph travels away from body tissue toward the heart and is drained into the cardiovascular system through ducts in the upper chest. Breathing and muscle action help propel lymph through the vessels (Figure 10-6).

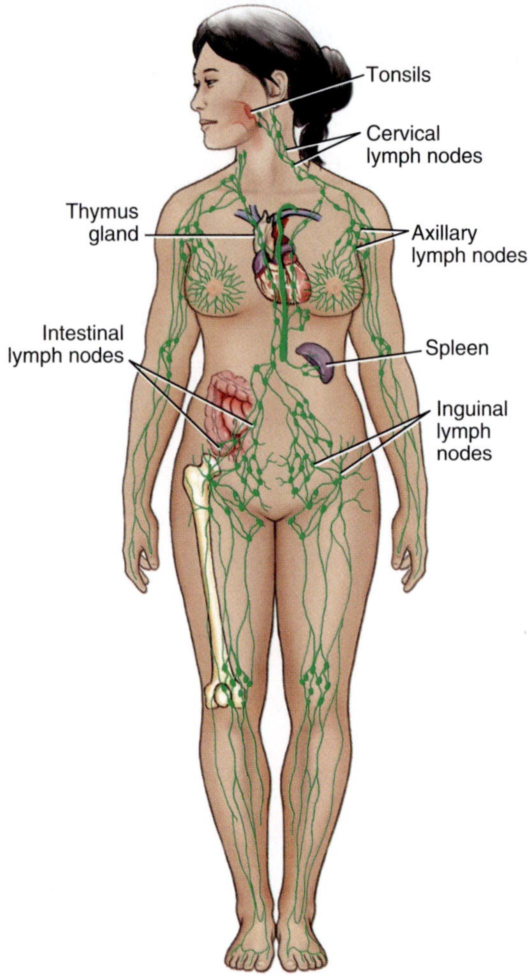

FIGURE 10-6
Lymphatic system.

Structures of the Lymphatic System

Term	Definition
lymph	transparent, colorless, tissue fluid that, on entering the lymphatic system, is called lymph. Lymph contains **lymphocytes** and **monocytes** and flows in a one-way direction to the heart. Lymph is similar to blood plasma.
lymphatic vessels	similar to veins, lymphatic vessels transport lymph from body tissues to the chest, where it enters the cardiovascular system. The vessels begin as capillaries spread throughout the body then merge into larger tubes that eventually become ducts in the chest. They provide a one-way flow for lymph gathered from the tissues to ducts in the chest, where lymph enters through veins into the circulatory system.

Term	Definition
lymph nodes	small, spherical bodies composed of lymphoid tissue. They may be singular or grouped together along the path of the lymph vessels. The nodes filter lymph to keep substances such as bacteria and other foreign agents from entering the blood. They also produce lymphocytes.
spleen	located in the left side of the abdominal cavity between the stomach and the diaphragm. In adulthood, the spleen is the largest lymphatic organ in the body. Blood, rather than lymph, flows through the spleen. Blood is cleansed of microorganisms in the spleen. The spleen stores blood and destroys worn out red blood cells.
thymus gland	one of the primary lymphatic organs, it is located anterior to the ascending aorta and posterior to the sternum between the lungs. It plays an important role in the development of the body's immune system, particularly from infancy to puberty. Around puberty the thymus gland atrophies so that most of the gland is connective tissue.

EXERCISE 3

Fill in the blanks with anatomic terms for blood and the lymphatic systems.

The function of the blood is to maintain internal balance in the body. The liquid portion of blood is called (1) _______________, in which (2) _______________, (3) _______________, and (4) _______________ are suspended. (5) _______________ aid in clotting blood; (6) _______________ is the clear liquid that remains after a clot is formed. The lymphatic system provides defense against infection. The lymphatic system is composed of the fluid (7) _______________; small spherical bodies (8) _______________ _______________, vessels for transporting lymph, the (9) _______________, which is the largest lymphatic organ; and the (10) _______________ gland.

Immune System

The immune system does not have its own organs and structures. Its function depends on organs and structures of other body systems, including the spleen, liver, intestinal tract, lymph nodes, and bone marrow.

Function

The immune system protects the body against pathogens (bacteria, fungi, and viruses), foreign agents that cause allergic reactions (e.g., peanuts) or toxins (e.g., insect bites), and abnormal body cells (e.g., cancer).

It has three lines of defense; the first is the prevention of foreign substances from entering the body. Unbroken skin and mucous membranes act as mechanical barriers. Ear wax and saliva act as chemical barriers.

If the first line of defense is penetrated by microorganisms, a second line of defense continues to battle disease. Second-line defenses include inflammation and fever plus phagocytosis, a process in which some of the white blood cells destroy the invading microorganisms. Also activated are protective proteins such as interferons, which fight viruses, and natural killer (NK) cells, which are effective against microorganisms and cancer cells (Figure 10-7).

Specific immunity, the third line of defense, provides protection against specific pathogens, such as the polio virus, by forming specific antibodies to fight against the infectious agent.

A & P Booster

For students desiring more anatomy and physiology, go to http://evolve.elsevier.com. Refer to p. 18 for your Evolve Access Information. Select A & P Booster, Chapter 10.

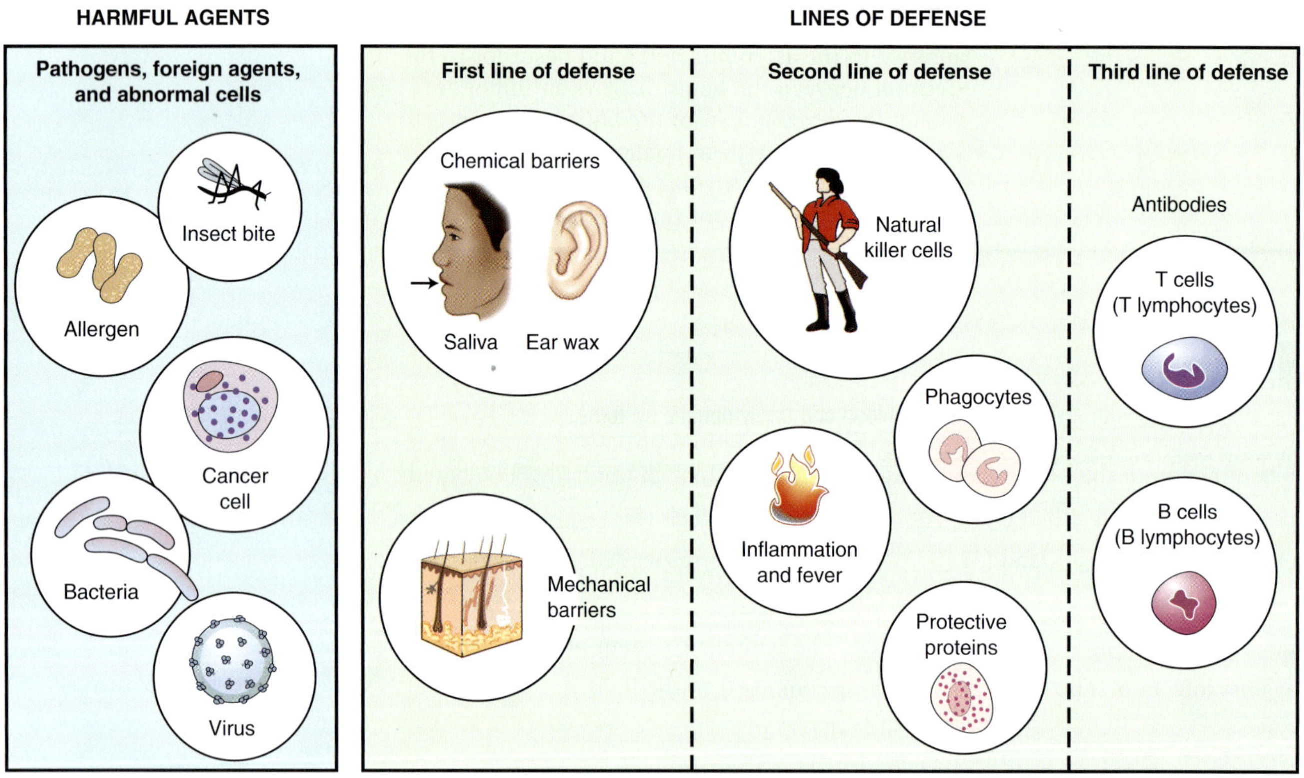

FIGURE 10-7

Three lines of defense provided by the immune system to protect the body against pathogens, foreign agents, and cancer.

EXERCISE 4

Complete the following exercise for the immune system.

1. The function of the immune system is to ______________________________ .

____

2. List five organs and structures from other body systems used by the immune system to carry out its function.

   a. ______________________________
   b. ______________________________
   c. ______________________________
   d. ______________________________
   e. ______________________________

3. The three lines of defense used by the immune system are:

   a. ______________________________
   b. ______________________________
   c. ______________________________

WORD PARTS

Word parts you need to learn to complete this chapter are listed on the following pages. The exercises at the end of each list will help you learn their definitions and spellings.

Use the flashcards accompanying this text or electronic flashcards to assist you in memorizing the word parts for this chapter.

To use the electronic flashcards, go to http://evolve.elsevier.com. Refer to p. 18 for your Evolve Access Information. Select Flashcards, Chapter 10.

Combining Forms of the Cardiovascular and Lymphatic Systems and Blood

Combining Form	Definition
angi/o	vessel (usually refers to blood vessel)
aort/o	aorta
arteri/o	artery
atri/o	atrium
cardi/o	heart
lymph/o	lymph, lymph tissue
lymphaden/o	lymph node
myel/o (NOTE: myel/o also means *spinal cord*; see Chapter 15)	bone marrow
phleb/o, ven/o	vein
plasm/o	plasma

VITAL AIR

It was believed in ancient times that arteries carried air. Vital air, or **pneuma,** did not allow blood in the arteries. A cut in an artery allowed vital air to escape and blood to replace it. The Greek **arteria,** meaning **windpipe,** was given for this reason.

VENTRICLE

Is derived from the Latin **venter,** meaning **little belly.** It was first applied to the belly and then to the stomach. Later it was extended to mean any small cavity in an organ or body.

Combining Forms of the Cardiovascular and Lymphatic Systems and Blood—*cont'd*

Combining Form	Definition
splen/o (NOTE: only one *e* in the word root for spleen)	spleen
thym/o	thymus gland
valv/o, valvul/o	valve
ventricul/o	ventricle

EXERCISE FIGURE A

Fill in the blanks with combining forms in this diagram of a cutaway section of the heart. *To check your answers, go to p. 477.*

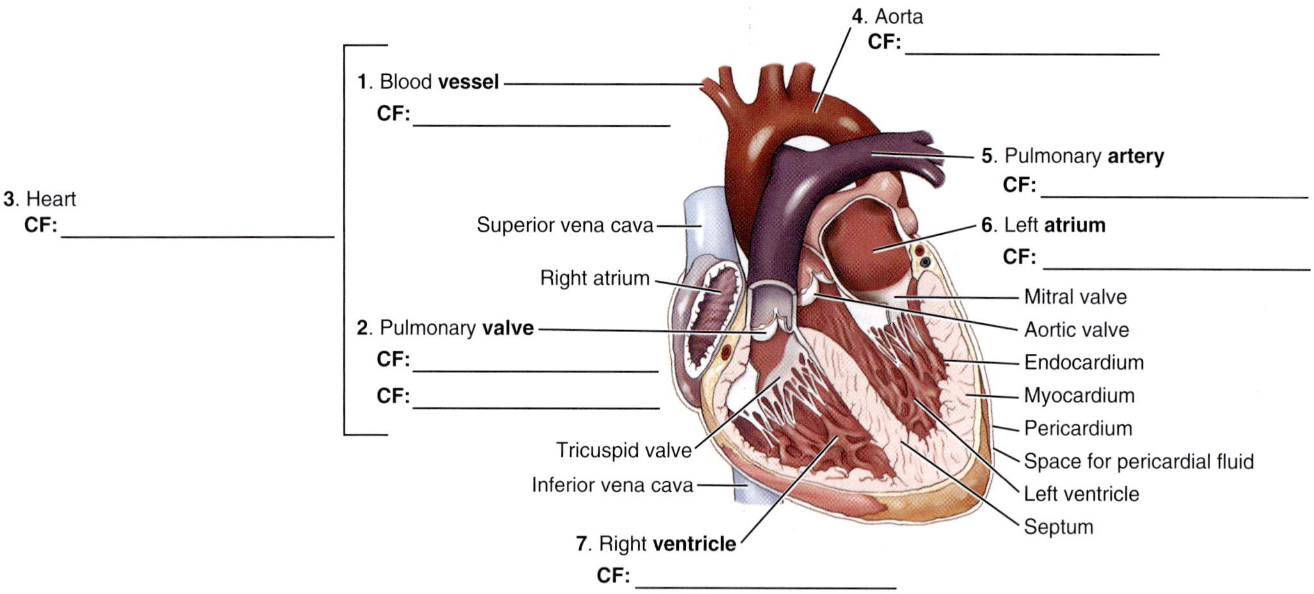

EXERCISE 5

Write the definitions of the following combining forms. *To check your answers, go to p. 477.*

1. cardi/o ____________
2. atri/o ____________
3. plasm/o ____________
4. angi/o ____________
5. ven/o ____________
6. aort/o ____________
7. valv/o ____________
8. splen/o ____________
9. thym/o ____________
10. phleb/o ____________
11. ventricul/o ____________
12. arteri/o ____________
13. valvul/o ____________
14. lymph/o ____________
15. lymphaden/o ____________
16. myel/o ____________

EXERCISE 6

Write the combining form for each of the following terms.

1. artery ______________
2. vein a. ______________ b. ______________
3. heart ______________
4. atrium ______________
5. ventricle ______________
6. lymph, lymph tissue ______________
7. aorta ______________
8. vessel (usually blood vessel) ______________
9. valve a. ______________ b. ______________
10. spleen ______________
11. plasma ______________
12. thymus gland ______________
13. lymph node ______________
14. bone marrow ______________

Combining Forms Commonly Used with the Cardiovascular and Lymphatic Systems and Blood Terms

Combining Form	Definition
ather/o	yellowish, fatty plaque
ech/o	sound
electr/o	electricity, electrical activity
isch/o	deficiency, blockage
therm/o	heat
thromb/o	clot

EXERCISE 7

Write the definition of the following combining forms.

1. ech/o ______________
2. thromb/o ______________
3. isch/o ______________
4. therm/o ______________
5. ather/o ______________
6. electr/o ______________

EXERCISE 8

Write the combining form for each of the following.

1. clot ________________
2. sound ________________
3. deficiency, blockage ________________
4. yellowish, fatty plaque ________________
5. heat ________________
6. electricity, electrical activity ________________

Prefix

Prefix	Definition
brady-	slow

Suffixes

Suffix	Definition
-ac	pertaining to
-apheresis	removal
-graph	instrument used to record; record
-penia	abnormal reduction in number
-poiesis	formation
-sclerosis	hardening

COMPARING -GRAPH, -GRAPHY, AND -GRAM

-graph is the instrument used to record, i.e., the machine, as in **telegraph** or **electrocardiograph** and also means record, as in **radiograph**.

-graphy is the process of recording, the act of setting down or registering a record, as in **photography** or **electroencephalography**.

-gram is the record (picture, radiographic image, or tracing), as in **telegram** or **electrocardiogram**.

Refer to **Appendix A** and **Appendix B** for alphabetical lists of word parts and their meanings.

EXERCISE 9

Write the definitions of the following prefix and suffixes.

1. brady- ______
2. -graph ______
3. -penia ______
4. -sclerosis ______
5. -apheresis ______
6. -poiesis ______
7. -ac ______

EXERCISE 10

Write the suffix or prefix for each of the following.

1. formation ______
2. pertaining to ______
3. hardening ______
4. instrument used to record; record ______
5. abnormal reduction in number ______
6. slow ______
7. removal ______

MEDICAL TERMS

The terms you need to learn to complete this chapter are listed below. The exercises following each list will help you learn the definition and the spelling of each word.

Disease and Disorder Terms

Built from Word Parts

The following terms are built from word parts you have already learned and can be translated literally to find their meanings. Further explanation of terms beyond the definition of their word parts, if needed, is included in parentheses.

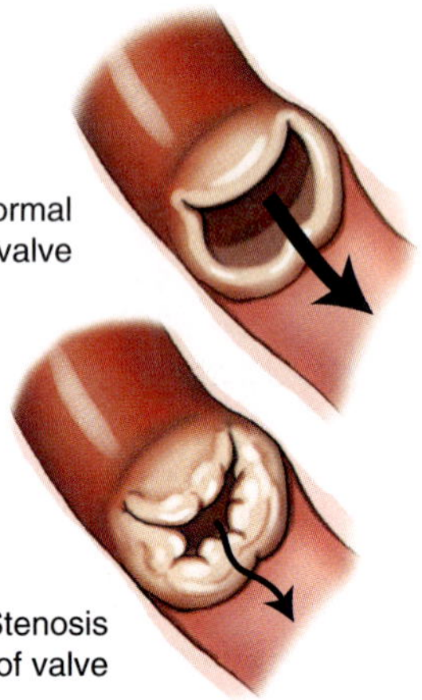

FIGURE 10-8 Aortic stenosis.

Term	Definition
CARDIOVASCULAR SYSTEM	
angioma (an-jē-Ō-ma)	tumor composed of blood vessels
angiostenosis (*an*-jē-ō-ste-NŌ-sis)	narrowing of a blood vessel
aortic stenosis (ā-OR-tik) (ste-NŌ-sis)	narrowing, pertaining to aorta (narrowing of the aortic valve) (Figure 10-8)
arteriosclerosis (ar-*tēr*-ē-ō-skle-RŌ-sis)	hardening of the arteries
atherosclerosis (*ath*-er-ō-skle-RŌ-sis)	hardening of fatty plaque (deposited on the arterial wall) (Exercise Figure B)
bradycardia (*brad*-ē-KAR-dē-a) (NOTE: the *i* in cardi/o has been dropped)	condition of a slow heart (rate less than 60 beats per minute)
cardiomegaly (*kar*-dē-ō-MEG-a-lē)	enlargement of the heart
cardiomyopathy (*kar*-dē-ō-mī-OP-a-thē)	disease of the heart muscle
endocarditis (*en*-dō-kar-DĪ-tis)	inflammation of the inner (lining) of the heart (particularly heart valves)
ischemia (is-KĒ-mē-a)	deficiency of blood (flow)
myocarditis (*mī*-ō-kar-DĪ-tis)	inflammation of the muscle of the heart
pericarditis (*per*-i-kar-DĪ-tis)	inflammation of the sac surrounding the heart (see Figure 10-13)
phlebitis (fle-BĪ-tis)	inflammation of a vein
polyarteritis (*pol*-ē-*ar*-te-RĪ-tis) (NOTE: the *i* in arteri/o has been dropped)	inflammation of many (sites in the) arteries

EXERCISE FIGURE B

Fill in the blanks to label the diagram.

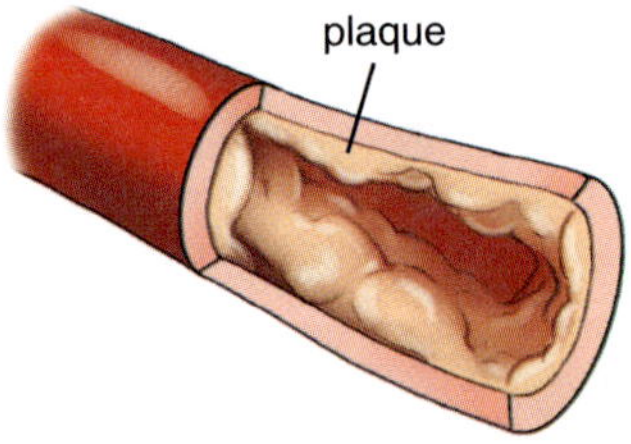

______ / ______ / ______
fatty plaque / cv / hardening

Term	Definition
tachycardia (*tak*-i-KAR-dē-a) (NOTE: the *i* in cardi/o has been dropped)	condition of a rapid heart (rate of more than 100 beats per min)
thrombophlebitis (*throm*-bō-fle-BĪ-tis)	inflammation of a vein associated with a clot
valvulitis (*val*-vū-LĪ-tis)	inflammation of a valve (of the heart)
BLOOD	
hematoma (*hē*-ma-TŌ-ma)	tumor of blood (collection of blood resulting from a broken blood vessel)
multiple myeloma (MUL-te-pl) (*mī*-e-LŌ-ma)	tumors of the bone marrow
pancytopenia (*pan*-sī-tō-PĒ-nē-a)	abnormal reduction of all (blood) cells
thrombosis (throm-BŌ-sis)	abnormal condition of a (blood) clot
thrombus (THROM-bus)	(blood) clot (attached to the interior wall of an artery or vein)
LYMPHATIC SYSTEM	
lymphadenitis (*lim*-fad-e-NĪ-tis)	inflammation of the lymph nodes
lymphadenopathy (lim-*fad*-e-NOP-a-thē)	disease of the lymph nodes (characterized by abnormal enlargement of the lymph nodes associated with an infection or malignancy)
lymphoma (lim-FŌ-ma)	tumor of lymphatic tissue (malignant)
splenomegaly (*splē*-nō-MEG-a-lē)	enlargement of the spleen
thymoma (thī-MŌ-ma)	tumor of the thymus gland

CAM TERM

Meditation is a mental practice focusing attention on a single activity such a breathing, an image, or a sound to calm and still the mind. Research has demonstrated the efficacy of using meditation to reduce heart rate and blood pressure, and to improve quality of life and clinical outcomes with various types of cardiovascular disease.

MULTIPLE MYELOMA

in the United States comprises approximately 10% of all blood malignancies. It most often occurs between 65 and 70 years of age. Most patients are asymptomatic until the disease is advanced. Symptoms and signs are varied and may include bone pain and fractures, infections, weight loss, anemia, and fatigue. Treatments include chemotherapy and stem cell transplantation. Multiple myeloma is seldom cured.

EMBOLUS, THROMBUS

An **embolus** circulates in the bloodstream until it becomes lodged in a vessel, whereas a **thrombus** is attached to the interior wall of a vessel. When a **thrombus** breaks away and circulates in the bloodstream, it becomes known as an **embolus.**

EXERCISE 11

Practice saying aloud each of the disease and disorder terms built from word parts on pp. 420-421.

To hear the terms, go to http://evolve.elsevier.com. Refer to p. 18 for your Evolve Access Information. Select Exercises & Review, Chapter 10, Chapter Exercises, Pronunciation.

☐ Place a check mark in the box when you have completed this exercise.

EXERCISE 12

Analyze and define the following terms.

1. endocarditis ______________________
2. bradycardia ______________________
3. cardiomegaly ______________________
4. arteriosclerosis ______________________
5. valvulitis ______________________
6. (multiple) myeloma ______________________
7. tachycardia ______________________
8. angiostenosis ______________________
9. thrombus ______________________
10. ischemia ______________________
11. pericarditis ______________________
12. aortic stenosis ______________________
13. thrombosis ______________________
14. atherosclerosis ______________________
15. myocarditis ______________________
16. angioma ______________________
17. thymoma ______________________
18. lymphoma ______________________
19. lymphadenitis ______________________
20. splenomegaly ______________________
21. hematoma ______________________

22. polyarteritis ______________________________
23. cardiomyopathy ______________________________
24. lymphadenopathy ______________________________
25. thrombophlebitis ______________________________
26. phlebitis ______________________________
27. pancytopenia ______________________________

EXERCISE 13

Build disease and disorder terms for the following definitions by using the word parts you have learned.

1. tumors of the bone marrow multiple ________ / ________ (WR / S)

2. enlargement of the heart ________ / CV / ________ (WR / CV / S)

3. deficiency of blood (flow) ________ / ________ (WR / S)

4. inflammation of the inner (layer) of the heart ________ / ________ / ________ (P / WR / S)

5. condition of slow heart rate ________ / ________ / ________ (P / WR / S)

6. hardening of the arteries ________ / CV / ________ (WR / CV / S)

7. abnormal condition of a (blood) clot ________ / ________ (WR / S)

8. inflammation of the muscle of the heart ________ / CV / ________ / ________ (WR / CV / WR / S)

9. narrowing of blood vessels ________ / CV / ________ (WR / CV / S)

10. condition of a rapid heart (rate) ________ / ________ / ________ (P / WR / S)

11. hardening of fatty plaque (deposited on the arterial wall) ________ / CV / ________ (WR / CV / S)

12. tumor composed of blood vessels
_______ / _______
WR / S

13. inflammation of a valve (of the heart)
_______ / _______
WR / S

14. narrowing, pertaining to the aorta (narrowing of the aortic valve)
_______ / _______ stenosis
WR / S

15. inflammation of the sac surrounding the heart
_______ / _______ / _______
P / WR / S

16. tumor of lymphatic tissue
_______ / _______
WR / S

17. tumor of the thymus gland
_______ / _______
WR / S

18. enlargement of the spleen
_______ /CV/ _______
WR /CV/ S

19. tumor (mass) of blood
_______ / _______
WR / S

20. inflammation of lymph nodes
_______ / _______
WR / S

21. disease of the heart muscle
_______ /CV/ _______ /CV/ _______
WR /CV/ WR /CV/ S

22. inflammation of many (sites in the) arteries
_______ / _______ / _______
P / WR / S

23. disease of the lymph nodes
_______ /CV/ _______
WR /CV/ S

24. inflammation of a vein associated with a clot
_______ /CV/ _______ / _______
WR /CV/ WR / S

25. inflammation of a vein
_______ / _______
WR / S

26. (blood) clot
_______ / _______
WR / S

27. abnormal reduction of all (blood) cells
_______ / _______ /CV/ _______
P / WR /CV/ S

EXERCISE 14

Spell each of the disease and disorder terms built from word parts on pp. 420-421 by having someone dictate them to you.

To hear and spell the terms, go to http://evolve.elsevier.com. Refer to p. 18 for your Evolve Access Information. Select Exercises & Review, Chapter 10, Chapter Exercises, Spelling.
☐ Place a check mark in the box if you have completed this exercise online.

1. ______________________ 15. ______________________
2. ______________________ 16. ______________________
3. ______________________ 17. ______________________
4. ______________________ 18. ______________________
5. ______________________ 19. ______________________
6. ______________________ 20. ______________________
7. ______________________ 21. ______________________
8. ______________________ 22. ______________________
9. ______________________ 23. ______________________
10. ______________________ 24. ______________________
11. ______________________ 25. ______________________
12. ______________________ 26. ______________________
13. ______________________ 27. ______________________
14. ______________________

Disease and Disorder Terms

Not Built from Word Parts

In some of the following terms, you may recognize word parts you have already learned; however, the full meaning of the terms cannot be discerned by the definition of their word parts.

Term	Definition
CARDIOVASCULAR SYSTEM	
acute coronary syndrome (ACS) (a-KŪT) (KOR-o-*nar*-ē) (SIN-drōm)	sudden symptoms of insufficient blood supply to the heart indicating **unstable angina** or **acute myocardial infarction**
aneurysm (AN-ū-rizm)	ballooning of a weakened portion of an arterial wall (Figure 10-9)
angina pectoris (an-JĪ-na) (PEK-to-ris)	chest pain, which may radiate to the left arm and jaw, that occurs when there is an insufficient supply of blood to the heart muscle

ACUTE CORONARY SYNDROME (ACS)

is an umbrella term used when a patient seeks care at an emergency care facility for symptoms of **acute angina** or **myocardial infarction not yet diagnosed.** Treatment includes rapid assessment to determine the diagnosis and treatment of symptoms to possibly minimize heart damage.

ANGINA PECTORIS

was believed by the ancients to be a disorder of the breast. The Latin **angere,** meaning **to throttle,** was used to represent the sudden pain and was added to **pectus,** meaning **breast.**

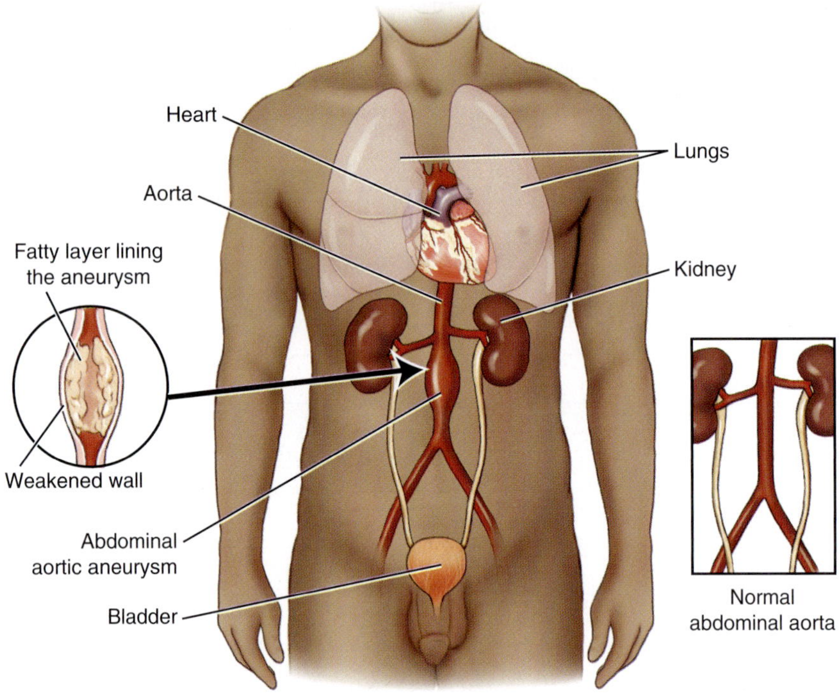

FIGURE 10-9
Abdominal aortic aneurysm. An abdominal aortic aneurysm (AAA) located in the abdominal area of the aorta, the main blood vessel that transports blood away from the heart. Surgery is the primary treatment for this most common site of aortic aneurysm. Because the success rate of surgery is much lower once the aneurysm has ruptured, more emphasis is being placed on early diagnosis. AAAs sometimes can be detected by physical examination but are more frequently detected by abdominal ultrasound. A newer procedure, called **endovascular stenting**, is performed through a puncture in the femoral artery, using a radiographic device called fluoroscopy. With this technique, a rigid graft can be placed within an aneurysm.

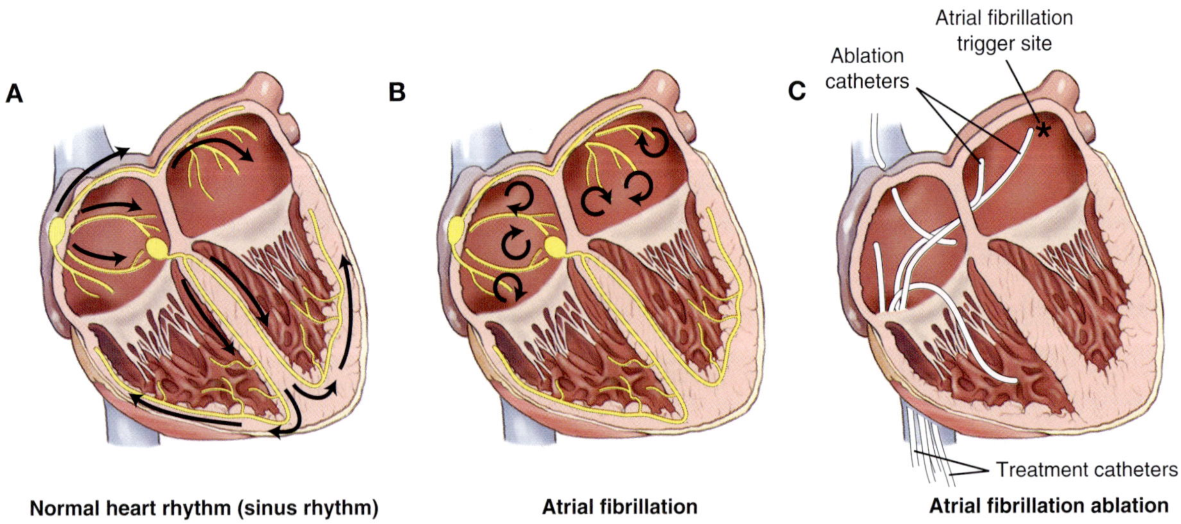

FIGURE 10-10
Atrial fibrillation. **A**, Normal heart rhythm. **B**, Atrial fibrillation showing chaotic, rapid electrical impulses. **C,** Atrial fibrillation ablation, which destroys the abnormal cells that trigger atrial fibrillation. Ablation is used to treat atrial fibrillation if drug therapy is not effective.

Disease and Disorder Terms—*cont'd*

Not Built from Word Parts

Term	Definition
arrhythmia (ā-RITH-mē-a)	any disturbance or abnormality in the heart's normal rhythmic pattern
atrial fibrillation (AFib) (Ā-trē-al) (fi-bri-LĀ-shun)	a cardiac arrhythmia characterized by chaotic, rapid electrical impulses in the atria. The atria quiver instead of contracting, causing irregular ventricular response and the ejection of a reduced amount of blood. The blood that remains in the atria becomes static, increasing the risk of clot formation, which may lead to a stroke. Two types of AFib are **paroxysmal atrial fibrillation (PAF),** which is intermittent, and **chronic atrial fibrillation,** which is sustained (Figure 10-10).
cardiac arrest (KAR-dē-ak) (a-REST)	sudden cessation of cardiac output and effective circulation, which requires cardiopulmonary resuscitation (CPR)
cardiac tamponade (KAR-dē-ak) (tam-po-NĀD)	acute compression of the heart caused by fluid accumulation in the pericardial cavity
coarctation of the aorta (*kō*-ark-TĀ-shun) (ā-OR-ta)	congenital cardiac condition characterized by a narrowing of the aorta (Figure 10-11)
congenital heart disease (kon-JEN-i-tal) (hart) (di-ZĒZ)	heart abnormality present at birth
congestive heart failure (CHF) (kon-JES-tiv) (hart) (fāl-ūr)	inability of the heart to pump enough blood through the body to supply the tissues and organs with nutrients and oxygen (also called **heart failure** [HF]). Coronary artery disease is a common cause of heart failure.
coronary artery disease (CAD) (KOR-o-*nar*-ē) (AR-te-rē) (di-ZĒZ)	a condition that reduces the flow of blood through the coronary arteries to the myocardium, denying the myocardial tissue of sufficient oxygen and nutrients to function fully; most often caused by coronary atherosclerosis
coronary occlusion (KOR-o-*nar*-ē) (o-KLŪ-zhun)	obstruction of an artery of the heart, usually from atherosclerosis. Coronary occlusion can lead to acute myocardial infarction.
deep vein thrombosis (DVT) (dēp) (vān) (throm-BŌ-sis)	condition of thrombus in a deep vein of the body. Most often occurs in the lower extremities. A clot can break off and travel to the lungs, causing a pulmonary embolism.

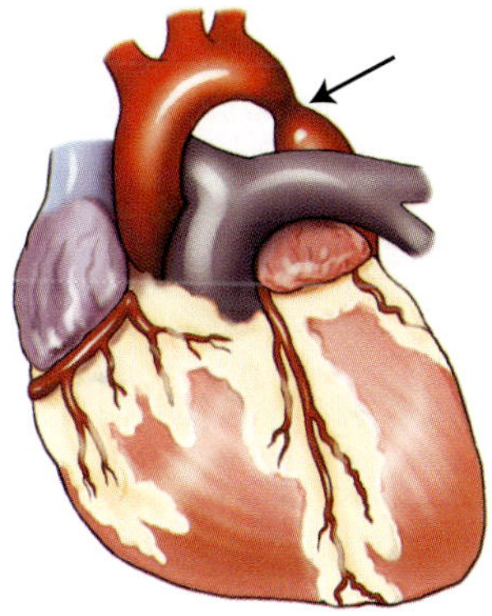

FIGURE 10-11
Coarctation of the aorta.

CORONARY

is derived from the Latin ***coronalis***, meaning ***crown*** or ***wreath***. It describes the arteries encircling the heart.

Disease and Disorder Terms—*cont'd*

Not Built from Word Parts

Term	Definition
hypertensive heart disease (HHD) (*hī*-per-TEN-siv) (hart) (di-ZĒZ)	disorder of the heart caused by persistent high blood pressure
intermittent claudication (*in*-ter-MIT-nt) (*klaw*-di-KĀ-shun)	pain and discomfort in calf muscles while walking; a condition seen in peripheral arterial disease.
mitral valve stenosis (MĪ-tral) (ste-NŌ-sis)	a narrowing of the mitral valve from scarring, usually caused by episodes of **rheumatic fever**
myocardial infarction (MI) (*mī*-ō-KAR-dē-al) (in-FARK-shun)	death (necrosis) of a portion of the myocardium caused by lack of oxygen resulting from an interrupted blood supply (also called **heart attack**)
peripheral arterial disease (PAD) (pe-RIF-er-al) (ar-TER-ē-al) (di-ZĒZ)	disease of the arteries in the arms and legs, resulting in narrowing or complete obstruction of the artery. This is caused most commonly by atherosclerosis, but occasionally by inflammatory diseases, emboli, or thrombus formation. The most common symptom of peripheral arterial disease is intermittent claudication. (also called **peripheral vascular disease [PVD]**).
rheumatic heart disease (rū-MAT-ik) (hart) (di-ZĒZ)	damage to the heart muscle or heart valves caused by one or more episodes of **rheumatic fever**
varicose veins (VAR-i-kōs) (vānz)	distended or tortuous veins usually found in the lower extremities (Figure 10-12)

RAYNAUD (rā-NŌ) PHENOMENON

is classified as a *peripheral arterial disease* (PAD). The condition was first described by Maurice Raynaud, a French physician, in 1862. Symptoms include intermittent, symmetric attacks of cyanosis and pallor of the distal ends of the fingers and toes often caused by exposure to cold temperature.

RHEUMATIC FEVER

is an inflammatory disease, usually occurring in children and young adults after an upper respiratory tract streptococcal infection.

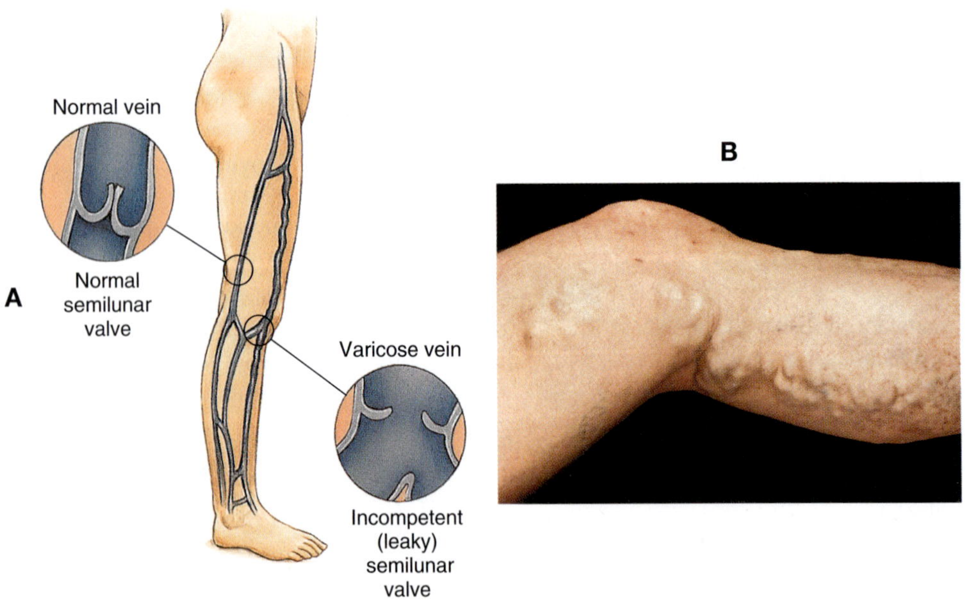

FIGURE 10-12
A, Normal and varicose veins. **B,** Appearance of varicose veins.

Varicose Veins and Current Treatment

Varicose veins usually occur in the superficial veins of the legs, which return approximately 15% of the blood back to the heart. One-way valves in the veins help move the blood upward. When these valves fail, or the veins lose their elasticity, the blood flows backward, pools, and forms varicose veins. Approximately 80 million Americans, mostly women, have varicose veins or small, shallow spider veins. Causes are heredity, obesity, pregnancy, illness, or injury. Ligation and stripping was previously considered the primary surgical procedure for treatment.

Current Treatment

Endovenous laser ablation—Closure of varicose veins by application of heat within the vein.

Ambulatory phlebectomy—Tiny punctures are made in the skin through which the varicose veins are pulled out. Local anesthetic is used, and the procedure is minimally invasive.

Sclerotherapy is the injection of a liquid or foam sclerosant solution into a varicose vein causing it to thrombose and close over a month or two. Sclerosants have been used in large and small veins. This therapy usually takes less than an hour and requires no anesthesia.

Laser or intense pulsed light—This noninvasive technique is used to remove spider veins. The light causes the veins to shrink and collapse.

Term	Definition
BLOOD	
anemia (a-NĒ-mē-a)	reduction in the number of red blood cells. Anemia may be caused by blood loss or decrease in the production or increase in the destruction of red blood cells.
embolus (*pl.* emboli) (EM-bō-lus) (EM-bo-lī)	blood clot or foreign material, such as air or fat, that enters the bloodstream and moves until it lodges at another point in the circulation
hemophilia (hē-mō-FIL-ē-a)	inherited bleeding disease most commonly caused by a deficiency of the coagulation factor VIII
leukemia (lū-KĒ-mē-a)	malignant disease characterized by excessive increase in abnormal white blood cells formed in the bone marrow
sepsis (SEP-sis)	a condition in which pathogenic microorganisms, usually bacteria, enter the bloodstream, causing a systemic inflammatory response to the infection (also called **septicemia**)
LYMPHATIC SYSTEM	
Hodgkin disease (HOJ-kin) (di-ZĒZ)	malignant disorder of the lymphatic tissue characterized by progressive enlargement of the lymph nodes, usually beginning in the cervical nodes
infectious mononucleosis (in-FEK-shus) (*mon*-ō-*nū*-klē-Ō-sis)	an acute infection caused by the Epstein-Barr virus characterized by swollen lymph nodes, sore throat, fatigue, and fever. The disease affects mostly young people and is usually transmitted by saliva.

COMMON TYPES OF ANEMIA

- **Acute blood loss anemia**—reduction in hemoglobin and hematocrit as a result of hemorrhage
- **Iron-deficiency anemia**—insufficient amount of iron in the body to produce hemoglobin; frequently caused by chronic blood loss
- **Pernicious anemia**—ineffective production of red blood cells from vitamin B_{12} deficiency
- **Hemolytic anemia**—reduced life of red blood cells (e.g., sickle cell anemia)
- **Anemia of chronic inflammation**—ineffective red blood cell production from chronic disease
- **Aplastic anemia**— resulting from bone marrow failure

SEPSIS OR SEPTICEMIA

can result when local infections such as **pneumonia** or **bladder infections** are untreated or treated with incomplete antibiotic therapy; the microorganism can enter the bloodstream, causing sepsis. Sepsis is the tenth most common cause of death in the United States. Patients in intensive care units or patients with impaired immune function are vulnerable to developing septicemia.

HODGKIN DISEASE

was first described in 1832 by Thomas Hodgkin, a pathologist at Guy's Hospital in London. In 1865 the name **Hodgkin's disease** was given to the condition by another English physician, Sir Samuel Wilks.

EXERCISE 15

Practice saying aloud each of the disease and disorder terms not built from word parts on pp. 425-429.

To hear the terms, go to http://evolve.elsevier.com. Refer to p. 18 for your Evolve Access Information. Select Exercises & Review, Chapter 10, Chapter Exercises, Pronunciation.

☐ Place a check mark in the box when you have completed this exercise.

EXERCISE 16

Fill in the blanks with the correct terms.

1. A congenital cardiac condition characterized by a narrowing of the aorta is called ________________ of the aorta.
2. A blood clot or foreign material that enters the bloodstream and moves until it lodges at another point in the circulation is called a(n) ________________.
3. Sudden cessation of cardiac output and effective circulation is referred to as a(n) ________________ ________________.
4. ________________ heart disease is the name given to a heart abnormality present at birth.
5. Veins that are distended or tortuous are called ________________ ________________.
6. Obstruction of an artery of the heart, usually from atherosclerosis, is called a(n) ________________ ________________.
7. ________________ is the name given to the ballooning of a weakened portion of an artery wall.
8. ________________ disease is the name given to a malignant disorder of lymphatic tissue characterized by enlarged lymph nodes.
9. ________________ ________________ ________________ is a condition most often caused by atherosclerosis.
10. ________________ ________________ is a cardiac condition characterized by chest pain caused by an insufficient blood supply to the cardiac muscle.
11. Death of a portion of myocardial muscle caused by lack of oxygen resulting from an interrupted blood supply is called a(n) ________________ ________________.

12. ________________ ________________ is a cardiac arrhythmia.

13. Any disturbance or abnormality in the heart's normal rhythmic pattern is called a(n) ________________.

14. A disorder of the heart caused by a persistently high blood pressure is called ________________ heart disease.

15. ________________ ________________ ________________ is the inability of the heart to pump enough blood through the body to supply tissues and organs.

16. ________________ ________________ ________________ is a disease of the arteries in the arms and legs resulting in narrowing or complete obstruction of an artery.

17. ________________ is an inherited bleeding disease most commonly caused by a deficiency of the coagulation factor VIII.

18. ________________ is a malignant disease in which the number of abnormal white blood cells formed in the bone marrow is excessively increased.

19. A reduction in the amount of hemoglobin in the red blood cells results in a condition known as ________________.

20. ________________ ________________ is an infection caused by the Epstein-Barr virus.

21. ________________ ________________ is a condition in which a patient has pain and discomfort in calf muscles while walking.

22. Acute compression of the heart caused by fluid accumulation in the pericardial cavity is known as ________________ ________________.

23. Episodes of rheumatic fever can cause ________________ ________________ ________________ and ________________ ________________ ________________.

24. ________________ ________________ ________________ usually occurs in the deep veins of the lower extremities.

25. ________________ ________________ ________________ is insufficient blood supply to the heart, indicating unstable angina or myocardial infarction.

26. ________________ is a systemic inflammatory response to an infection.

EXERCISE 17

Match the terms in the first column with the correct definitions in the second column.

_____ 1. anemia
_____ 2. aneurysm
_____ 3. angina pectors
_____ 4. arrhythmia
_____ 5. cardiac arrest
_____ 6. cardiac tamponade
_____ 7. coarctation of the aorta
_____ 8. congenital heart disease
_____ 9. congestive heart failure
_____ 10. coronary occlusion
_____ 11. intermittent claudication
_____ 12. deep vein thrombosis
_____ 13. coronary artery disease
_____ 14. peripheral arterial disease

a. sudden cessation of cardiac output and effective circulation
b. obstruction of an artery of the heart, usually from atherosclerosis
c. ballooning of a weak portion of an arterial wall
d. reduction of the amount of hemoglobin in the blood
e. any disturbance or abnormality in the heart's normal rhythmic pattern
f. chest pain occurring because of insufficient blood supply to the heart muscle
g. inability of the heart to pump enough blood through the body to supply tissues or organs
h. pain in calf muscles while walking
i. congenital cardiac condition with narrowing of the aorta
j. acute compression of the heart caused by fluid in the pericardial cavity
k. heart abnormality present at birth
l. clot in a deep vein
m. disease of the arteries in the arms and legs resulting in narrowing or complete obstruction of the artery
n. a condition that reduces the flow of blood through the coronary arteries

EXERCISE 18

Match the terms in the first column with the correct definitions in the second column.

_____ 1. embolus

_____ 2. atrial fibrillation

_____ 3. hemophilia

_____ 4. infectious mononucleosis

_____ 5. Hodgkin disease

_____ 6. hypertensive heart disease

_____ 7. leukemia

_____ 8. myocardial infarction

_____ 9. mitral valve stenosis

_____ 10. acute coronary syndrome

_____ 11. varicose veins

_____ 12. rheumatic heart disease

_____ 13. sepsis

a. inherited bleeding disease most commonly caused by a deficiency of the coagulation factor VIII

b. heart disorder brought on by persistent high blood pressure

c. distended or tortuous veins

d. excessive increase of abnormal white blood cells formed in the bone marrow

e. characterized by chaotic, rapid electrical impulses of the atria

f. systemic inflammatory response to an infection

g. symptoms indicating unstable angina or myocardial infarction

h. a disease that affects mostly young people; characterized by swollen lymph glands

i. blood clot or foreign material that enters the bloodstream and moves until it lodges at another point

j. malignant disorder of lymphatic tissue with enlargement of lymph nodes

k. death of a portion of myocardium caused by lack of oxygen resulting from an interrupted blood supply

l. narrowing of the valve between the left atrium and left ventricle

m. caused by episodes of rheumatic fever

EXERCISE 19

Spell each of the disease and disorder terms not built from word parts on pp. 425-429 by having someone dictate them to you.

To hear and spell the terms, go to http://evolve.elsevier.com. Refer to p. 18 for your Evolve Access Information. Select Exercises & Review, Chapter 10, Chapter Exercises, Spelling.

☐ Place a check mark in the box if you have completed this exercise online.

1. ______________________
2. ______________________
3. ______________________
4. ______________________
5. ______________________
6. ______________________
7. ______________________
8. ______________________
9. ______________________
10. ______________________
11. ______________________
12. ______________________
13. ______________________
14. ______________________
15. ______________________
16. ______________________
17. ______________________
18. ______________________
19. ______________________
20. ______________________
21. ______________________
22. ______________________
23. ______________________
24. ______________________
25. ______________________
26. ______________________
27. ______________________

PERCUTANEOUS CORONARY INTERVENTION (PCI)

includes a range of procedures, such as **coronary angioplasty** and **percutaneous transluminal coronary angioplasty** used to treat coronary artery disease. The procedure is usually performed by an invasive cardiologist.

Surgical Terms

Built from Word Parts

The following terms are built from word parts you have already learned and can be translated literally to find their meanings. Further explanation of terms beyond the definition of their word parts, if needed, is included in parentheses.

Term	Definition
CARDIOVASCULAR SYSTEM	
angioplasty (AN-jē-ō-*plas*-tē)	surgical repair of a blood vessel
atherectomy (ath-er-EK-to-mē)	excision of fatty plaque (from a blocked artery using a specialized catheter and a rotary cutter)
endarterectomy (*end*-ar-ter-EK-to-mē) (NOTE: the *o* from *endo-* is dropped for easier pronunciation)	excision within the artery (excision of plaque from the arterial wall). This procedure is usually named for the artery to be cleaned out, such as carotid endarterectomy, which means removal of plaque from the wall of the carotid artery (Exercise Figure C).

EXERCISE FIGURE C

Fill in the blanks to label the diagram.

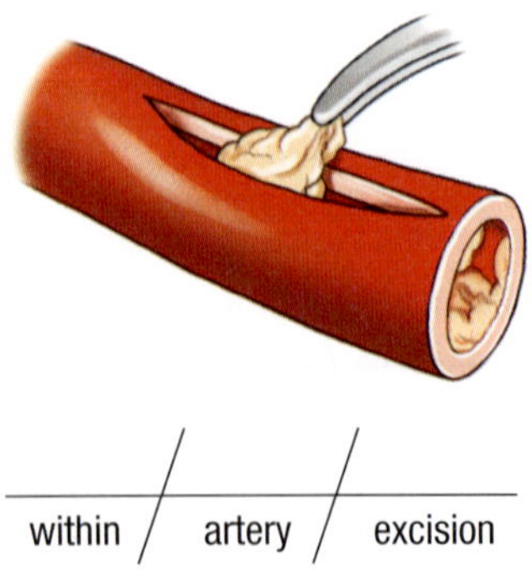

Term	Definition
pericardiocentesis (*per*-i-kar-dē-ō-sen-TĒ-sis)	surgical puncture to aspirate fluid from the sac surrounding the heart (pericardium) (used to remove fluid or air, usually to relieve cardiac tamponade) (Figure 10-13)
phlebectomy (fle-BEK-to-mē)	excision of a vein
phlebotomy (fle-BOT-o-mē)	incision into a vein (to remove blood or to give blood or intravenous fluids) (also called **venipuncture**)
valvuloplasty (VAL-vū-lō-*plas*-tē)	surgical repair of a valve (cardiac or venous)
LYMPHATIC SYSTEM	
splenectomy (splē-NEK-to-mē)	excision of the spleen
splenopexy (SPLĒ-nō-*peks*-ē)	surgical fixation of the spleen
thymectomy (thī-MEK-to-mē)	excision of the thymus gland

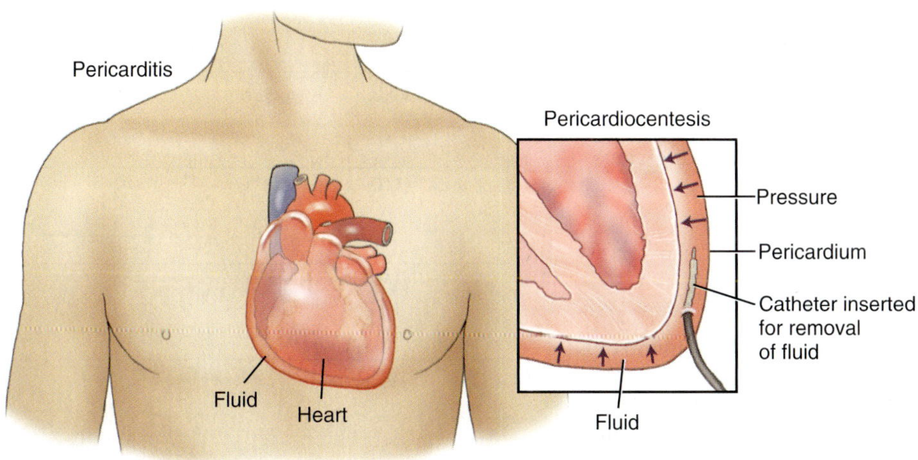

FIGURE 10-13
Pericarditis may produce excess fluid in the pericardium. If the fluid seriously affects the heart's ability to pump blood, pericardiocentesis may be performed to remove the fluid.

EXERCISE 20

Practice saying aloud each of the surgical terms built from word parts on these two pages.

To hear the terms, go to http://evolve.elsevier.com. Refer to p. 18 for your Evolve Access Information. Select Exercises & Review, Chapter 10, Chapter Exercises, Pronunciation.

☐ Place a check mark in the box when you have completed this exercise.

EXERCISE 21

Analyze and define the following surgical terms.

1. pericardiocentesis ____________________
2. thymectomy ____________________
3. angioplasty ____________________
4. splenopexy ____________________
5. valvuloplasty ____________________
6. endarterectomy ____________________
7. phlebotomy ____________________
8. splenectomy ____________________
9. phlebectomy ____________________
10. atherectomy ____________________

EXERCISE 22

Build surgical terms for the following definitions by using the word parts you have learned.

1. excision within the artery ______ / ______ / ______ (P / WR / S)
2. surgical fixation of the spleen ______ / ______ / ______ (WR / CV / S)
3. surgical repair of a valve ______ / ______ / ______ (WR / CV / S)
4. incision into a vein ______ / ______ / ______ (WR / CV / S)
5. excision of the thymus gland ______ / ______ (WR / S)
6. surgical puncture to aspirate fluid from the sac surrounding the heart ______ / ______ / ______ / ______ (P / WR / CV / S)
7. surgical repair of a blood vessel ______ / ______ / ______ (WR / CV / S)
8. excision of the spleen ______ / ______ (WR / S)
9. excision of a vein ______ / ______ (WR / S)
10. excision of fatty plaque ______ / ______ (WR / S)

EXERCISE 23

Spell each of the surgical terms built from word parts on pp. 434-435 by having someone dictate them to you.

To hear and spell the terms, go to http://evolve.elsevier.com. Refer to p. 18 for your Evolve Access Information. Select Exercises & Review, Chapter 10, Chapter Exercises, Spelling.
☐ Place a check mark in the box if you have completed this exercise online.

1. ______________________ 6. ______________________
2. ______________________ 7. ______________________
3. ______________________ 8. ______________________
4. ______________________ 9. ______________________
5. ______________________ 10. ______________________

Surgical Terms

Not Built from Word Parts

In some of the following terms, you may recognize word parts you have already learned; however, the full meaning of the terms cannot be discerned by the definition of their word parts.

Term	Definition
CARDIOVASCULAR SYSTEM	
aneurysmectomy (*an*-ū-riz-MEK-to-mē)	surgical excision of an aneurysm
atrial fibrillation ablation (Ā-tre-al) (fi-bri-LĀ-shun) (ab-LĀ-shun)	a procedure in which abnormal cells that trigger atrial fibrillation are destroyed by using radiofrequency energy (see Figure 10-7)
cardiac pacemaker (KAR-dē-ak) (PĀS-mā-kr)	battery-powered apparatus implanted under the skin with leads placed on the heart (See Figure 10-15, *A*) or in the chamber of the heart (Figure 10-15, *B*); used to treat an abnormal heart rhythm, usually one that is too slow, secondary to an abnormal sinus node.
coronary artery bypass graft (CABG) (KOR-o-*nar*-ē) (AR-te-rē) (BĪ-pas) (graft)	surgical technique to bring a new blood supply to heart muscle by detouring around blocked arteries (Figure 10-14)
coronary stent (KOR-o-*nar*-ē) (stent)	a supportive scaffold device placed in the coronary artery; used to prevent closure of the artery after angioplasty or atherectomy (Figure 10-16); used to treat an artery occluded by plaque.
embolectomy (*em*-bo-LEK-to-mē)	surgical removal of an embolus or clot, usually with a balloon catheter, inflating the balloon beyond the clot, then pulling the balloon back to the incision and bringing the clot with it

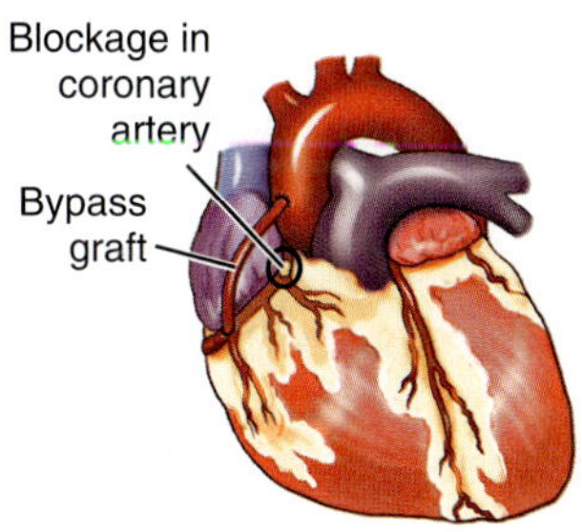

FIGURE 10-14
Coronary artery bypass graft.

STENT

is the name of a supporting device, such as a stiff cylinder or a mold, fashioned to anchor a graft. It is used to preserve dilation during healing or to provide support to keep a skin graft in place. Stent is not related to the term **stenosis**.

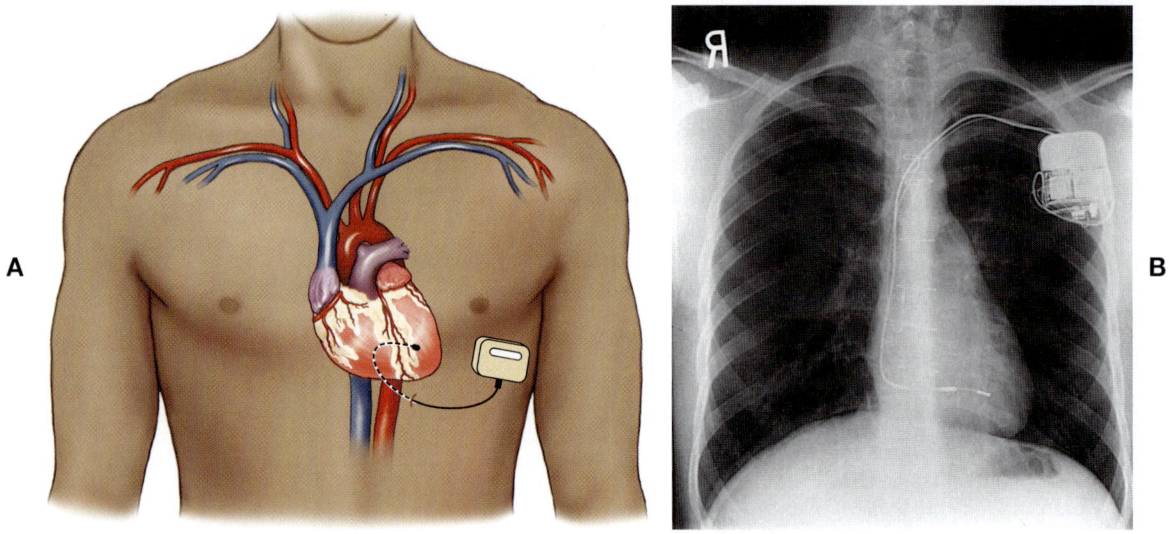

FIGURE 10-15
A, Cardiac pacemaker. The leads are implanted surgically on the epicardium through a thoracotomy. **B,** Chest radiograph of a patient with a cardiac pacemaker in which leads are implanted transvenously under fluoroscopic guidance. A pacemaker is used to treat irreversible complete heart block, which is caused by failure of the sinus node impulse to reach the ventricles.

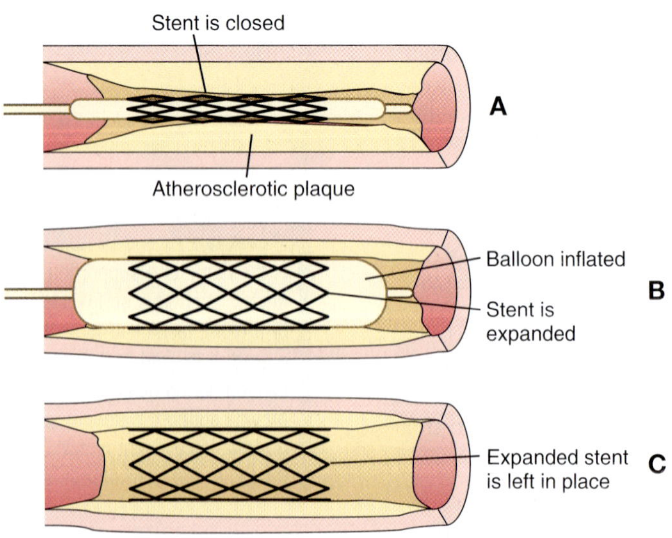

FIGURE 10-16
Coronary stent. **A,** Stent at the site of plaque formation. **B,** Inflated balloon and expanded stent. **C,** Stent with balloon removed.

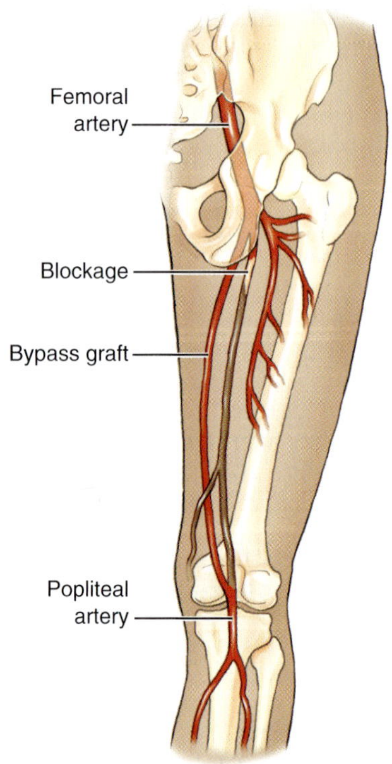

FIGURE 10-17
Femoropopliteal bypass.

Surgical Terms—*cont'd*

Not Built from Word Parts

Term	Definition
femoropopliteal bypass (*fem*-o-rō-pop-LIT-ē-al) (BĪ-pass)	surgery to establish an alternate route from femoral artery to popliteal artery to bypass an obstruction (Figure 10-17)
implantable cardiac defibrillator (ICD) (im-PLANT-a-bl) (KAR-dē-ak) (dē-FIB-ri-lā-tor)	a device implanted in the body that continuously monitors the heart rhythm. If life-threatening arrhythmias occur, the device delivers an electric shock to convert the arrhythmia back to a normal rhythm (Figure 10-18).
intracoronary thrombolytic therapy (in-tra-KOR-o-nar-ē) (*throm*-bō-LIT-ik) (THER-a-pē)	an injection of a medication either intravenously or intraarterially to dissolve blood clots in the coronary arteries
percutaneous transluminal coronary angioplasty (PTCA) (*per*-kū-TĀ-nē-us) (trans-LŪ-min-al) (KOR-o-*nar*-ē) (AN-jē-ō-*plas*-tē)	procedure in which a balloon is passed through a blood vessel into a coronary artery to the area where plaque is formed. Inflation of the balloon compresses the plaque against the vessel wall, expanding the inner diameter of the blood vessel, which allows the blood to circulate more freely (also called **balloon angioplasty**) (Figure 10-19).

Intracoronary Thrombolytic Therapy for Acute Myocardial Infarction

Intracoronary thrombolytic therapy is the administration of a medication that breaks blood clots apart (thrombolysis) before they become hardened. It is sometimes used in emergency departments (for acute myocardial infarction) and is administered immediately after the diagnosis is made. The drugs, such as streptokinase, tPA (alteplase), or recombinant tissue plasminogen activator (rtPA) (reteplase), are administered intravenously. Emergency **percutaneous transluminal coronary angioplasty** (PTCA) appears to be more effective than thrombolytic therapy for acute myocardial infarction. However, thrombolytic therapy can be administered in an emergency department when PTCA is not readily available.

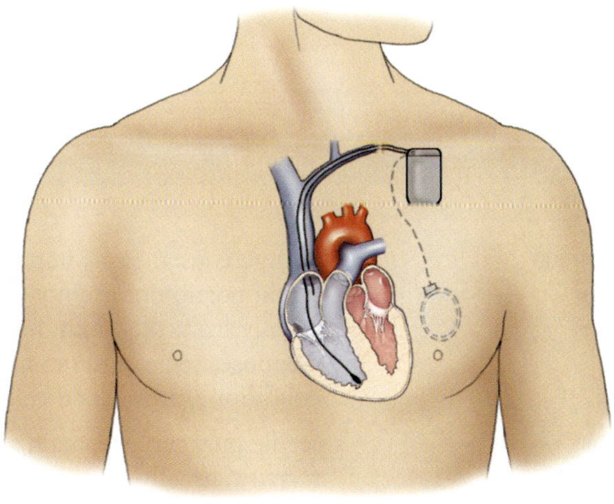

FIGURE 10-18
An implantable cardiac defibrillator.

CARDIAC RESYNCHRONIZATION THERAPY (CRT)

also called biventricular pacing, is the use of an implantable device, alone or in combination with an **ICD**, that provides simultaneous pacing of both ventricles of the heart. CRT is used in the treatment of severe congestive heart failure (see Figure 10-18)

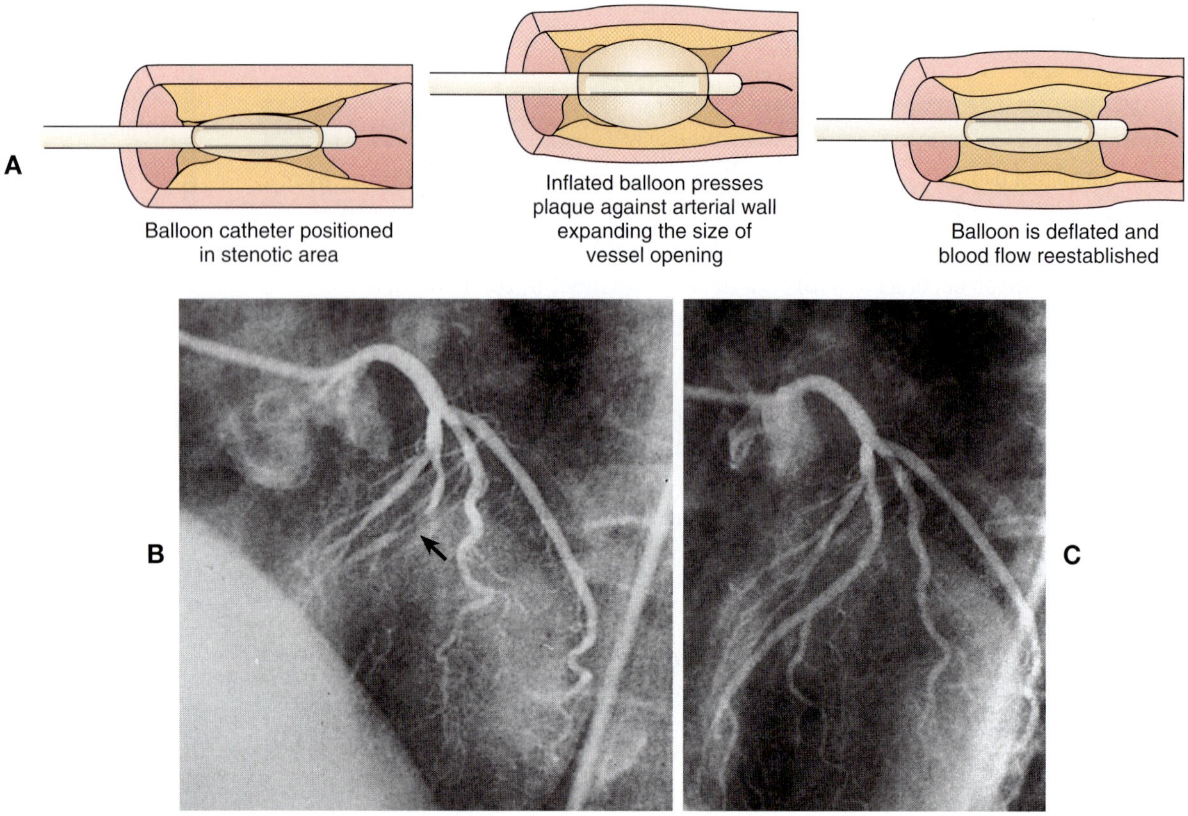

FIGURE 10-19
Percutaneous transluminal coronary angioplasty. **A,** Balloon dilation. **B,** Coronary arteriogram before PTCA. The *arrow* indicates the stenotic area, estimated at 95% minimum blood flow distal to the lesion. **C,** Coronary arteriogram after PTCA in the same patient. Blood flow is estimated to be 100%.

Peripheral Blood Stem Cell Transplant (PBSCT)

PBSCT is similar to **bone marrow transplant**. Stem cells are collected by apheresis, a process in which blood is removed from the patient or a matched donor and spun through a machine to harvest stem cells. The concentrated stem cells are given to the recipient by infusion. Both types of transplant are used to treat certain blood-related cancers and disorders, such as **leukemia** or **anemia**.

Surgical Terms—*cont'd*

Not Built from Word Parts

Term	Definition
BLOOD	
bone marrow aspiration (bōn) (MAR-ō) (*as*-pi-RĀ-shun)	a syringe is used to aspirate a sample of the liquid portion of the bone marrow, usually from the ilium, for study; used to diagnose, stage, and monitor disease and condition of the blood cells (Figure 10-20)
bone marrow biopsy (bōn) (MAR-ō) (BĪ-op-sē)	a needle puncture to obtain a sample of bone marrow, usually from the ilium, for study; used to diagnose, stage, and monitor disease and condition of the blood cells
bone marrow transplant (bōn) (MAR-ō) (TRANS-plant)	infusion of healthy bone marrow cells from a donor with matching cells and tissue to a recipient

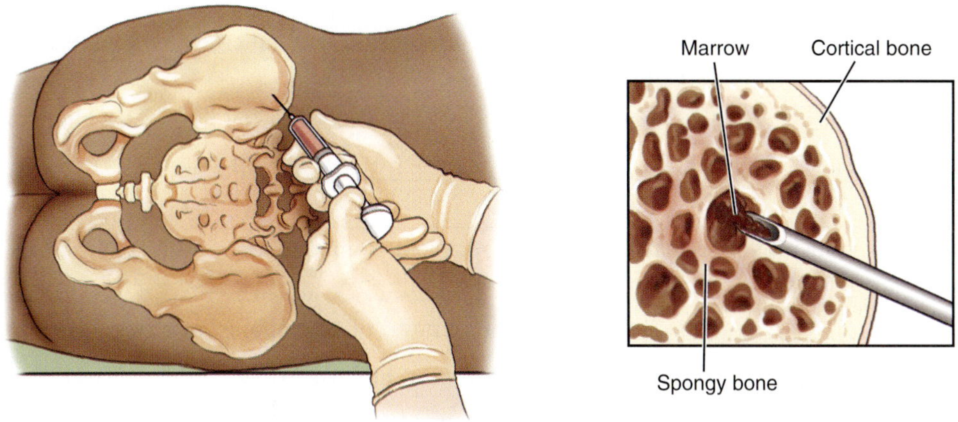

FIGURE 10-20
Bone marrow aspiration. Study of the bone marrow can be used to identify the presence of leukemia or other malignancies or to determine the cause of anemia.

BONE MARROW

is a spongy tissue found in the hollow part of the larger bones of the body. It is made up of both a solid and liquid portion. Stem cells within the bone marrow turn into platelets, red blood cells, and white blood cells. **Bone marrow aspiration** and **bone marrow biopsy** are both used to obtain specimens for study. Each provides complementary information about the condition of blood cells. Bone marrow aspiration is performed first if both are being performed on the patient. Information from both procedures is used for staging, monitoring, and diagnosing diseases and conditions of the blood such as **anemia**, **leukemia, lymphoma**, and **multiple myeloma**.

EXERCISE 24

Practice saying aloud each of the surgical terms not built from word parts on pp. 437-440.

To hear the terms, go to http://evolve.elsevier.com. Refer to p. 18 for your Evolve Access Information. Select Exercises & Review, Chapter 10, Chapter Exercises, Pronunciation.

☐ Place a check mark in the box when you have completed this exercise.

EXERCISE 25

1. The procedure used to treat atrial fibrillation using radiofrequency energy is called atrial fibrillation ________________.
2. The procedure in which a balloon is passed through a blood vessel into a coronary artery (where plaque is formed) to compress plaque against the vessel wall when the balloon is inflated is called ________________ ________________ ________________ ________________.
3. To regulate the heart rate, the physician may insert a(n) ________________ ________________ with leads on or in the patient's heart.
4. Bone marrow aspiration and biopsy are used to diagnose, stage, and monitor disease and conditions of the ________________ ________________.
5. The surgery performed to detour blood around a blocked artery so that a new blood supply can be given to heart muscles is called ________________ ________________ ________________ ________________.
6. The surgical excision of an aneurysm is called a(n) ________________.

7. A(n) ________________ ________________ is the name of the surgery performed to establish an alternate route from femoral artery to popliteal artery to bypass an obstruction.
8. An injection of a medication in a blocked coronary vessel to dissolve blood clots is called ________________ ________________ therapy.
9. ________________ ________________ ________________ is a procedure to transfuse bone marrow cells to a recipient from a donor with matching tissue and cells.
10. ________________ is the surgical removal of an embolus, or clot.
11. A supportive scaffold device used to prevent closure of a coronary artery is called a(n) ________________ ________________.
12. ________________ ________________ ________________ is used to treat life-threatening arrhythmias.

EXERCISE 26

Match the terms in the first column with their correct definitions in the second column.

______ 1. aneurysmectomy
______ 2. coronary artery bypass graft
______ 3. femoropopliteal bypass
______ 4. bone marrow aspiration
______ 5. cardiac pacemaker
______ 6. atrial fibrillation ablation
______ 7. percutaneous transluminal coronary angioplasty
______ 8. bone marrow biopsy
______ 9. bone marrow transplant
______ 10. intracoronary thrombolytic therapy
______ 11. embolectomy
______ 12. coronary stent
______ 13. implantable cardiac defibrillator

a. compressing plaque against a blood vessel wall by inflating a balloon passed through the blood vessel
b. use of medication to dissolve blood clots in a blocked coronary vessel
c. used to obtain a sample of bone marrow
d. apparatus implanted under the skin to regulate the heartbeat
e. a procedure using radiofrequency energy
f. monitors and corrects heart rhythms
g. supportive scaffold device placed in an artery
h. excision of a weakened, ballooning blood vessel wall
i. healthy bone marrow cells infused from a donor with matching tissues and cells into a recipient with leukemia
j. surgical removal of an embolus
k. surgical procedure to establish an alternate route from the femoral artery to the popliteal artery to bypass an obstruction
l. aspiration of a sample of the liquid portion of bone marrow
m. diverts blood flow past a blocked artery in the heart

EXERCISE 27

Spell each of the surgical terms not built from word parts on pp. 437-440 by having someone dictate them to you.

To hear and spell the terms, go to http://evolve.elsevier.com. Refer to p. 18 for your Evolve Access Information. Select Exercises & Review, Chapter 10, Chapter Exercises, Spelling.
☐ Place a check mark in the box if you have completed this exercise online.

1. ______________	8. ______________
2 ______________	9. ______________
3. ______________	10. ______________
4. ______________	11. ______________
5. ______________	12. ______________
6. ______________	13. ______________
7. ______________	

Diagnostic Terms

Built from Word Parts

The following terms are built from word parts you have already learned and can be translated literally to find their meanings. Further explanation of terms beyond the definition of their word parts, if needed, is included in parentheses.

Term	Definition
CARDIOVASCULAR SYSTEM	
Diagnostic Imaging	
angiography (*an*-jē-OG-ra-fē)	radiographic imaging of blood vessels (the procedure is named for the vessel to be studied, e.g., **femoral angiography** or **coronary angiography**) (Table 10-1)
angioscope (AN-jē-ō-skōp)	instrument used for visual examination (of the lumen) of a blood vessel
angioscopy (*an*-jē-OS-ko-pē)	visual examination (of the lumen) of a blood vessel
aortogram (ā-ŌR-to-gram)	radiographic image of the aorta (after an injection of contrast media)
arteriogram (ar-TĒR-ē-ō-gram)	radiographic image of an artery (after an injection of contrast media) (Figure 10-21)
venogram (VĒ-nō-gram)	radiographic image of a vein (after an injection of contrast media) (Figure 10-22)
venography (vē-NOG-ra-fē)	radiographic imaging of a vein (after an injection of contrast media)

TABLE 10-1

Types of Angiography

Coronary Artery Visualization

Coronary angiography, commonly called cardiac catheterization, is an **invasive procedure** in which a catheter is inserted into the coronary vessels, contrast media are injected, and images are recorded. It is considered the best technique for determining the percentage of blockage in the coronary arteries.

Coronary computed tomography angiography (CCTA) also called a ***heart scan*** is a noninvasive procedure used to assist in the diagnosis of coronary artery disease. Two types of scanners used are:

- **multislice spiral CT scanner (MSCT)** is capable of scanning multiple images during each gantry rotation. The scanner can produce images of a beating heart and detailed cross-sectional images of the arteries. The first 4-slice scanner was first used in the 1990s and is now a 64-slice scanner.
- **electronic beam CT scanner (EBCT)** uses an electron beam to create three-dimensional images of the heart. EBCT, developed in the early 1980s is faster than MSCT and produces an accurate **coronary artery calcification (CAC)** score, also called coronary calcium score **(CCS),** which is predictive of the presence of coronary artery stenosis as a result of the build up of plaque on the arterial wall; may be used as a screening test for CAD.

Other Vascular Visualization

Magnetic resonance angiography (MRA) is a **noninvasive procedure** that does not require catheterization or the injection of dye and uses specialized MR imaging to study vascular structures of the body. MRA may be chosen over CTA because there is no exposure to ionizing radiation and contrast media.

Computed tomography angiography (CTA) is a **noninvasive procedure** that uses a high-resolution CT system to study vascular structures of the body after the injection of intravenous contrast media.

Digital subtraction angiography (DSA) is a procedure in which an image is taken and stored in the computer, then contrast medium is injected. A second image is taken and stored in the computer. The computer compares the two images and subtracts the first image from the second, removing structures not being studied. DSA enables better visualization of the arteries than regular angiography (Figure 10-23).

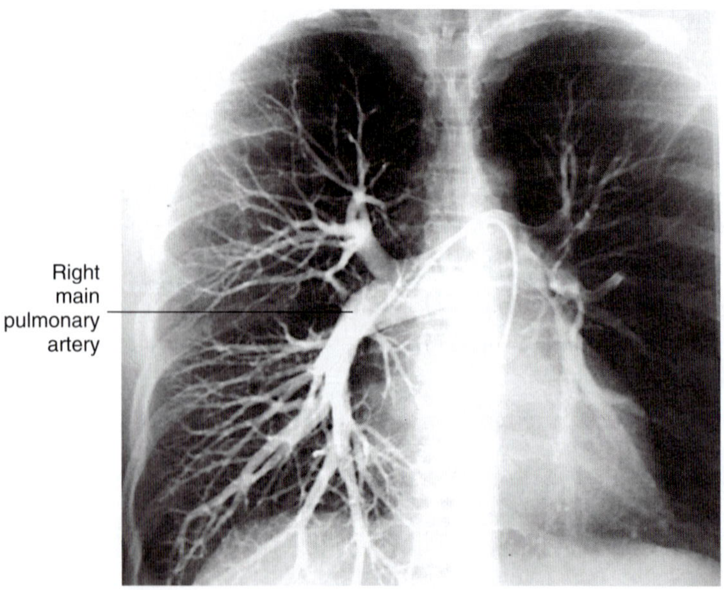

FIGURE 10-21
Arteriogram showing the right main pulmonary artery. This procedure (arteriography) is performed after injection of contrast material.

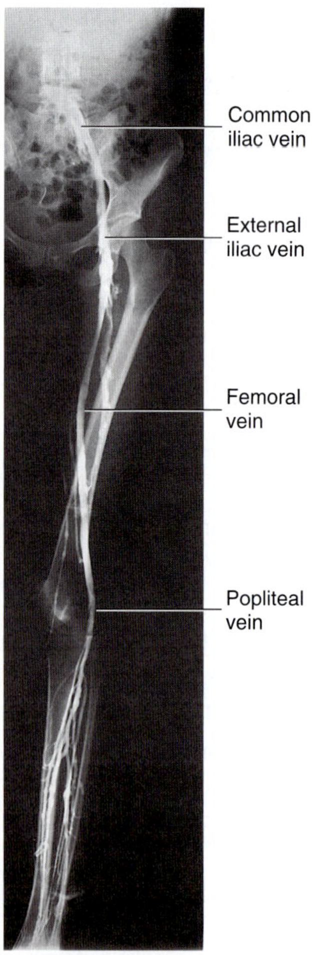

FIGURE 10-22
Normal venogram, lower left limb.

Diagnostic Terms—*cont'd*

Built from Word Parts

Term	Definition
Cardiovascular Procedures	
echocardiogram (ECHO) (*ek*-ō-KAR-dē-ō-gram)	record of the heart (structure and motion) using sound (used to detect valvular disease and evaluate heart function)
electrocardiogram (ECG, EKG) (ē-*lek*-trō-KAR-dē-ō-gram)	record of the electrical activity of the heart (Exercise Figure D)
electrocardiograph (ē-*lek*-trō-KAR-dē-ō-graf)	instrument used to record the electrical activity of the heart
electrocardiography (ē-*lek*-trō-*kar*-dē-OG-ra-fē)	process of recording the electrical activity of the heart

EXERCISE FIGURE D

Fill in the blanks to complete labeling of the diagram.

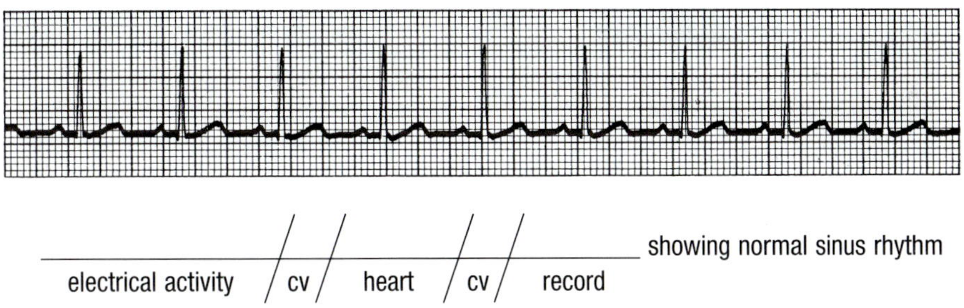

EXERCISE 28

Practice saying aloud each of the diagnostic terms built from word parts on pp. 443-445.

To hear the terms, go to http://evolve.elsevier.com. Refer to p. 18 for your Evolve Access Information. Select Exercises & Review, Chapter 10, Chapter Exercises, Pronunciation.

☐ Place a check mark in the box when you have completed this exercise.

EXERCISE 29

Analyze and define the following diagnostic terms.

1. electrocardiograph ______________________
2. venogram ______________________
3. angiography ______________________
4. echocardiogram ______________________
5. aortogram ______________________
6. electrocardiogram ______________________
7. arteriogram ______________________
8. electrocardiography ______________________
9. angioscopy ______________________
10. venography ______________________
11. angioscope ______________________

EXERCISE 30

Build diagnostic terms that correspond to the following definitions by using the word parts you have learned.

1. instrument used to record the electrical activity of the heart
   ______ / ___ / ______ / ___ / ______
   WR / CV / WR / CV / S

2. radiographic image of an artery (after an injection of contrast media)
   ______ / ___ / ______
   WR / CV / S

3. radiographic image of a vein (after an injection of contrast media)
   ______ / ___ / ______
   WR / CV / S

4. radiographic imaging of a blood vessel
   ______ / ___ / ______
   WR / CV / S

5. record of the electrical activity of the heart
   ______ / ___ / ______ / ___ / ______
   WR / CV / WR / CV / S

6. record of the heart (structure and motion) by using sound
_____ / _____ / _____ / _____ / _____
WR / CV / WR / CV / S

7. radiographic image of the aorta (after an injection of contrast media)
_____ / _____ / _____
WR / CV / S

8. process of recording the electrical activity of the heart
_____ / _____ / _____ / _____ / _____
WR / CV / WR / CV / S

9. visual examination (of the lumen) of a blood vessel
_____ / _____ / _____
WR / CV / S

10. radiographic imaging of a vein
_____ / _____ / _____
WR / CV / S

11. instrument used for visual examination (of the lumen) of a blood vessel
_____ / _____ / _____
WR / CV / S

EXERCISE 31

Spell each of the diagnostic terms built from word parts on pp. 443-445 by having someone dictate them to you.

To hear and spell the terms, go to http://evolve.elsevier.com. Refer to p. 18 for your Evolve Access Information. Select Exercises & Review, Chapter 10, Chapter Exercises, Spelling.

☐ Place a check mark in the box if you have completed this exercise online.

1. _____
2. _____
3. _____
4. _____
5. _____
6. _____
7. _____
8. _____
9. _____
10. _____
11. _____

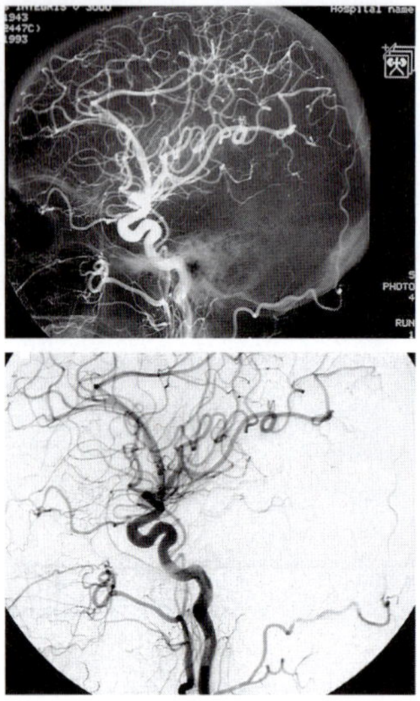

FIGURE 10-23
Digital subtraction angiography (DSA). **A,** Lateral digital **nonsubtracted** carotid artery. **B,** Lateral digital **subtracted** carotid artery. By removing unwanted anatomy, the image of the carotid artery is of high quality.

CHEMICAL STRESS TESTING

is the **use of drugs to simulate the stress of physical exercise** on the body. It is used to study patients who are unable to exercise.

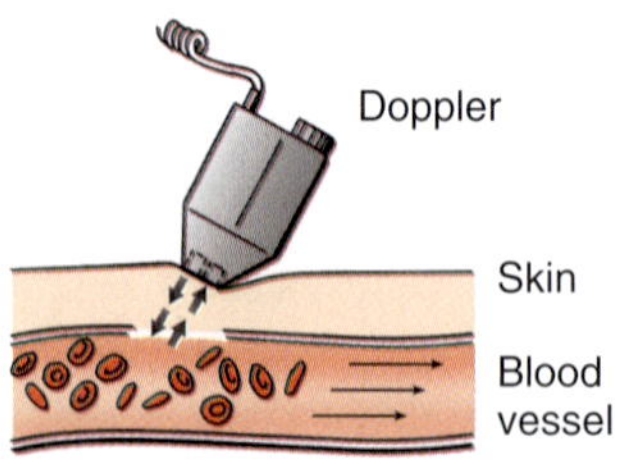

FIGURE 10-24
Doppler ultrasound showing the red blood cells reflecting sound.

Diagnostic Terms

Not Built from Word Parts

In some of the following terms, you may recognize word parts you have already learned; however, the full meaning of the terms cannot be discerned by the definition of their word parts.

Term	Definition
CARDIOVASCULAR SYSTEM	
Diagnostic Imaging	
digital subtraction angiography (DSA) (DIJ-i-tal) (sub-TRAK-shun) (*an*-jē-OG-ra-fē)	a process of digital radiographic imaging of the blood vessels that "subtracts" or removes structures not being studied (Figure 10-23 and Table 10-1)
Doppler ultrasound (DOP-ler) (UL-tra-sound)	a study that uses sound for detection of blood flow within the vessels; used to assess intermittent claudication, deep vein thrombosis, and other blood flow abnormalities (Figure 10-24)
exercise stress test (EK-ser-sīz) (stres) (test)	a study that evaluates cardiac function during physical stress by riding a bike or walking on a treadmill. **Electrocardiography, echocardiography,** and **nuclear medicine scanning** are three types of tests performed to measure cardiac function while exercising.
single-photon emission computed tomography (SPECT) (SING-el-fō-ton) (ē-MISH-on) (com-PŪ-td) (tō-MOG-ra-fē)	a nuclear medicine scan that visualizes the heart from several different angles. A radioactive tracer substance such as sestamibi or thallium is injected intravenously. The SPECT scanner creates images from the tracer absorbed by the body tissues. It is used to assess damage to cardiac tissue (Figure 10-25).

A

B

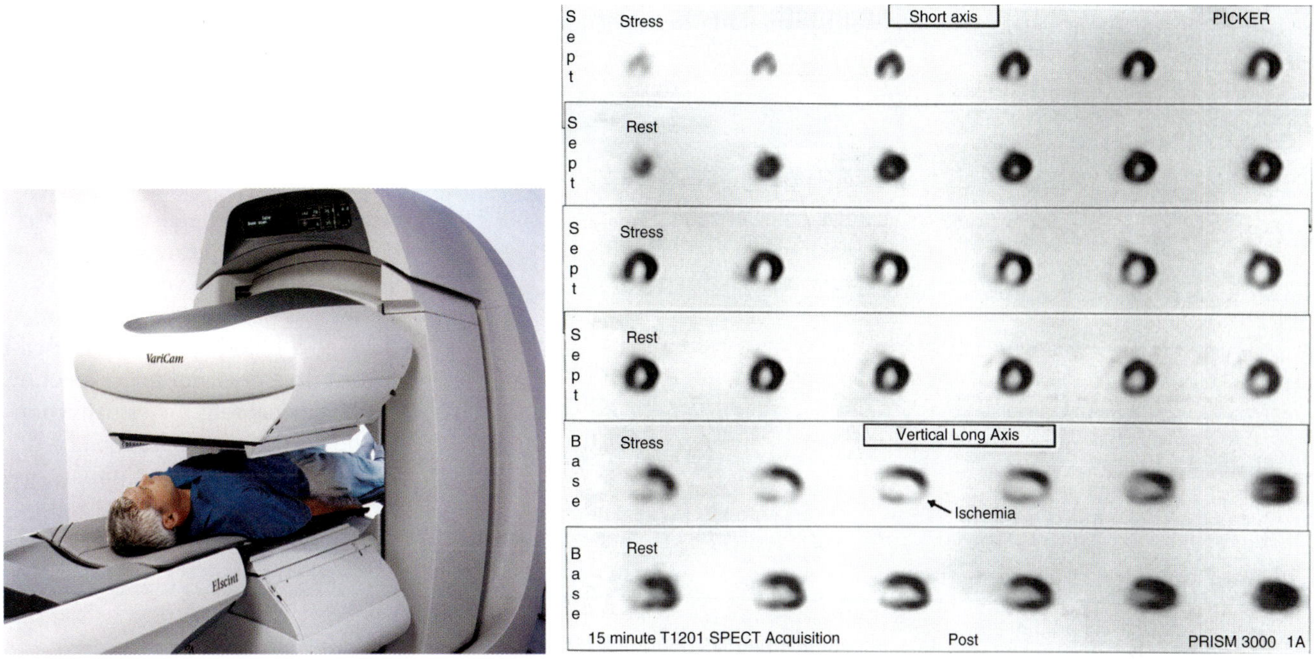

FIGURE 10-25
A, Single-photon emission computed tomography (SPECT) camera system. **B,** Thallium-201 myocardial perfusion scan comparing stress and redistribution (resting) images in various planes of the heart (short axis and long axis). A perfusion defect is identified in the stress images but not seen in the redistribution (rest) images. This finding is indicative of ischemia.

Term	Definition
thallium test (THĀL-ē-um) (test)	a nuclear medicine test used to diagnose coronary artery disease and assess revascularization after coronary artery bypass surgery. Thallium, a radioactive isotope, is injected into the body intravenously; a radiation detector is placed over the heart and images are recorded. Thallium is taken up by the normal myocardial cells, but not in ischemia or infarction. These areas are identified as "cold" spots on the images produced. Thallium testing can be performed when the patient is at rest or it can be part of a stress test.
transesophageal echocardiogram (TEE) (*trans*-e-*sof*-a-JĒ-al) (*ek*-ō-KAR-dē-ō-gram)	an ultrasound test that examines cardiac function and structure by using an ultrasound probe placed in the esophagus, which provides views of the heart structures

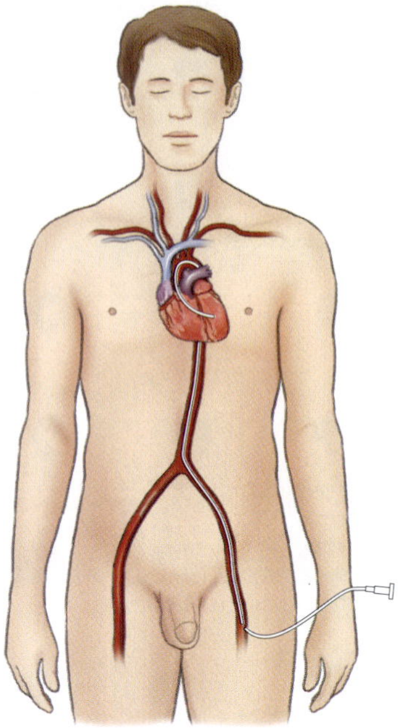

FIGURE 10-26
Cardiac catherization.

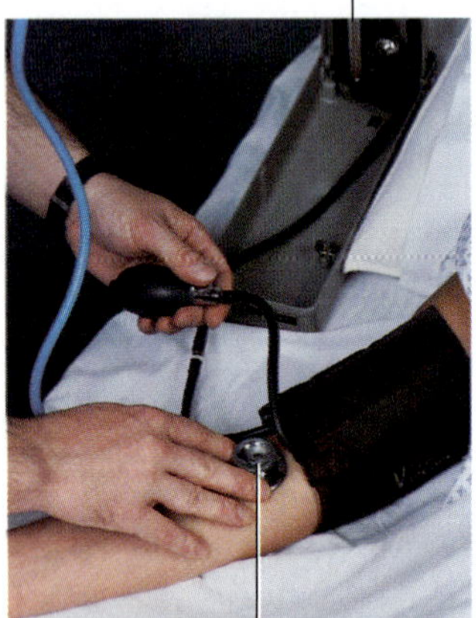

FIGURE 10-27
Measurement of blood pressure.

Diagnostic Terms—*cont'd*

Not Built from Word Parts

Term	Definition
Cardiovascular Studies	
cardiac catheterization (KAR-dē-ak) (*kath*-e-ter-i-ZĀ-shun)	an examination to determine the condition of the heart and surrounding blood vessels. A catheter is passed into the heart through a blood vessel and is used to record pressures and inject a contrast medium, enabling the visualization of the coronary arteries, great vessels, and the heart chambers; used most frequently to evaluate chest pain and coronary artery disease (also called **coronary angiography**) (Figure 10-26).
impedance plethysmography (IPG) (im-PĒD-ans) (*ple*-thiz-MOG-rā-fē)	measures venous flow of the extremities with a plethysmograph to detect clots by measuring changes in blood volume and resistance (impedance) in the vein; used to detect deep vein thrombosis
Other	
blood pressure (BP)	pressure exerted by the blood against the blood vessel walls. A blood pressure measurement written as systolic pressure (120) and diastolic pressure (80) is commonly recorded as 120/80 (Figure 10-27).
pulse (puls)	the rhythmic expansion of an artery that can be felt with a finger. The pulse is most commonly felt over the radial artery; however, the pulsations can be felt over a number of sites, including the femoral and carotid arteries.
sphygmomanometer (*sfig*-mō-ma-NOM-e-ter)	device used for measuring blood pressure (see Figure 10-27)

Term	Definition
Laboratory	
C-reactive protein (CRP) (rē-AK-tiv) (PRŌ-tēn)	a blood test to measure the amount of C-reactive protein in the blood, which, when elevated, indicates inflammation in the body. It is sometimes used in assessing the risk of cardiovascular disease.
creatine phosphokinase (CPK) (KRĒ-a-tin) (*fos*-fō-KĪ-nās)	a blood test used to measure the level of creatine phosphokinase, an enzyme of heart and skeletal muscle released into the blood after muscle injury or necrosis. The test is useful in evaluating patients with acute myocardial infarction.
homocysteine (*hō*-mō-SIS-tēn)	a blood test used to measure the amount of homocysteine in the blood. Homocysteine is an amino acid that, if elevated, may indicate an increased risk of cardiovascular disease.
lipid profile (LIP-id) (PRŌ-fīl)	a blood test used to measure the amount of lipids in a sample of blood. This test is used to evaluate the risk of developing cardiovascular disease and to monitor therapy of existing disease. Results provide levels of total cholesterol, high-density lipoprotein (HDL), low-density lipoprotein (LDL), very-low-density lipoprotein (VLDL), and triglycerides (Table 10-2).
troponin (TRŌ-po-nin)	a blood test that measures troponin, a heart muscle enzyme. Troponins are released into the blood approximately 3 hours after necrosis of the heart muscle and may remain elevated from 7 to 10 days. The test is useful in the diagnosis of a myocardial infarction.
BLOOD	
Laboratory	
coagulation time (kō-*ag*-ū-LĀ-shun)	blood test to determine the time it takes for blood to form a clot
complete blood count (CBC) and differential count (Diff)	basic blood screening that measures hemoglobin, hematocrit, red blood cell number and morphology (size and shape), leukocyte count, and white blood cell differential (types of white blood cells) and platelet count. The test is automated, thus done easily and rapidly, and provides a tremendous amount of information about the blood.

A BIOMARKER

is a naturally occurring substance of certain body cells that can be measured in the blood and used to aid in the diagnosis of various disorders. Troponin, creatinine phospho-kinase, homocysteine, and C-reactive protein are biomarkers, and elevated levels are used in diagnosing various disorders occurring in the body.

Diagnostic Terms—*cont'd*

Not Built from Word Parts

Term	Definition
hematocrit (HCT) (hē-MAT-o-crit)	a blood test to measure the volume of red blood cells. It is used in the diagnosis and evaluation of anemic patients.
hemoglobin (Hgb) (HĒ-mō-*glo*-bin)	blood test used to determine the concentration of oxygen-carrying components (hemoglobin) in red blood cells
prothrombin time (PT) (prō-THROM-bin)	blood test used to determine certain coagulation activity defects and to monitor anticoagulation therapy for patients taking Coumadin, an oral anticoagulant medication. (Activated partial thromboplastin time [PTT] is used to monitor anticoagulation therapy for patients taking heparin, an intravenous anticoagulant medication.)

PT/INR

stands for prothrombin time/international normalized ratio. Most institutions now, on the recommendation of the World Health Organization, report both absolute numbers and INR numbers, which provide uniform PT results to physicians worldwide.

TABLE 10-2

Understanding a Lipid Profile

Terms

Cholesterol—a compound important in the production of sex hormones, steroids, cell membranes, and bile acids. Cholesterol is produced by the body and contained in foods such as animal fats. Cholesterol is transported by lipoproteins.

High-density lipoprotein (HDL)—a type of lipoprotein that removes cholesterol from the tissues and transports it to the liver to be excreted in the bile. Elevated levels of HDL are considered protective against development of atherosclerosis, which may lead to coronary artery disease. HDL is often referred to as the "good" cholesterol.

Low-density lipoprotein (LDL)—a type of lipoprotein that transports cholesterol to the tissue and deposits it on the walls of the arteries. High levels of LDL are associated with the presence of atherosclerosis, which may lead to coronary artery disease. LDL is often referred to as the "bad" cholesterol.

Total cholesterol—the total amount of cholesterol contained in the HDL and LDL.

Triglycerides (TGs)—a form of fat in the blood. Triglycerides are synthesized in the liver and used to store energy. Test results are used to assess the risk of coronary artery disease.

Very-low-density lipoprotein (VLDL)—a type of lipoprotein that transports most of the triglycerides in the blood. Elevated levels of VLDL, to a lesser degree than LDL, indicate a risk for developing coronary artery disease.

Example of Lipid Profile Lab Report

Tests	Results	Flag	Normal Range
Cholesterol, total	188 mg/dL		100-199 mg/dL
Triglycerides	287 mg/dL	High	0-149 mg/dL
HDL cholesterol	50 mg/dL		40-59 mg/dL
VLDL cholesterol calc	57 mg/dL	High	5-40 mg/dL
LDL cholesterol calc	81 mg/dL		0-99 mg/dL

EXERCISE 32

Practice saying aloud each of the diagnostic terms not built from word parts on pp. 448-452.

To hear the terms, go to http://evolve.elsevier.com. Refer to p. 18 for your Evolve Access Information. Select Exercises & Review, Chapter 10, Chapter Exercises, Pronunciation.

☐ Place a check mark in the box when you have completed this exercise.

EXERCISE 33

Fill in the blanks with the correct terms.

1. A device for measuring blood pressure is called a(n) ____________________.
2. ________________ ________________ is a blood test that determines the time it takes for blood to form a clot.
3. ________________ ________________ ________________ and ________________ ________________ are the names of basic blood-screening tests.
4. A study that uses sound for detection of blood flow within blood vessels is called ________________ ________________.
5. Pressure exerted by blood against the blood vessel walls is called ________________ ________________.
6. A blood test used to determine certain coagulation activity defects and to monitor oral anticoagulation therapy is called ________________ ________________.
7. ____________________ ____________________ is a procedure in which a catheter is introduced into the heart to record pressures and enable the visualization of the heart chambers.
8. A blood test used to determine the oxygen-carrying component in the red blood cells is called ________________.
9. ____________________ ____________________ measures venous flow of the extremities.
10. A nuclear medicine test used to diagnose coronary artery disease is ________________ ________________.
11. ____________________ ____________________ is a test in which an ultrasound probe provides views of the heart structures from the esophagus.
12. A nuclear medicine test that visualizes the heart from different angles is called a(n) ________________ ________________ ________________ ________________.
13. ________________ ________________ ________________ evaluates cardiac function during physical stress.

14. A process of radiographic imaging of blood vessels that removes structures not being studied is called ________________ ________________ ________________.

15. A blood test to measure an enzyme of the heart released into the bloodstream after muscle injury is called ________________ ________________.

16. An elevated ________________ ________________ indicates inflammation in the body.

17. ________________ is the rhythmic expansion of an artery that can be felt with a finger.

18. ________________ is an amino acid that if elevated, indicates an increased risk of cardiovascular disease.

19. ________________ is a heart muscle enzyme released into the bloodstream approximately 3 hours after heart muscle necrosis.

20. ________________ ________________ is the name of the blood test that measures the amount of lipids in the blood.

21. A test of the red blood cells used in the diagnosis and evaluation of anemic patients is called ________________.

EXERCISE 34

Match the terms in the first column with their correct definition in the second column.

_____ 1. cardiac catheterization

_____ 2. complete blood count and differential count

_____ 3. coagulation time

_____ 4. hemoglobin

_____ 5. Doppler ultrasound

_____ 6. prothrombin time

_____ 7. sphygmomanometer

_____ 8. single-photon emission computed tomography

_____ 9. digital subtraction angiography

_____ 10. thallium test

_____ 11. transesophageal echocardiogram

a. device used for measuring blood pressure

b. digital radiographic imaging of blood vessels

c. test to determine certain coagulation activity defects

d. passage of a catheter into the heart to evaluate coronary artery disease

e. visualizes the heart from several different angles

f. used to assess revascularization after CABG

g. oxygen-carrying component of the red blood cell

h. basic blood-screening test

i. an ultrasound test that provides views of the heart from the esophagus

j. study in which sound is used to determine the flow of blood within the vessels

k. test to determine the number of red blood cells

l. determines the time it takes for blood to form a clot

EXERCISE 35

Match the terms in the first column with the correct definitions in the second column.

_____ 1. exercise stress test
_____ 2. impedance plethysmography
_____ 3. C-reactive protein
_____ 4. blood pressure
_____ 5. creatine phosphokinase
_____ 6. hematocrit
_____ 7. homocysteine
_____ 8. pulse
_____ 9. lipid profile
_____ 10. troponin

a. measures the volume and number of red blood cells
b. blood test to determine inflammation or risk of cardiovascular disease
c. measures cardiac function during physical stress
d. measures the level of an enzyme released into the blood after muscle injury
e. measures blood flow of the extremities
f. pressure exerted by blood against the blood vessel walls
g. measures the amount of an amino acid in the blood
h. measured most often over the radial artery
i. results provide levels of cholesterol, HDL, LDL, VLDL, and triglycerides
j. measures an enzyme released within hours after damage to the heart muscle

EXERCISE 36

Spell each of the diagnostic terms not built from word parts on pp. 448-452 by having someone dictate them to you.

To hear and spell the terms, go to http://evolve.elsevier.com. Refer to p. 18 for your Evolve Access Information. Select Exercises & Review, Chapter 10, Chapter Exercises, Spelling.
☐ Place a check mark in the box if you have completed this exercise online.

1. ______________________
2. ______________________
3. ______________________
4. ______________________

5. ______________________
6. ______________________
7. ______________________
8. ______________________
9. ______________________
10. ______________________
11. ______________________
12. ______________________
13. ______________________
14. ______________________
15. ______________________
16. ______________________
17. ______________________
18. ______________________
19. ______________________
20. ______________________
21. ______________________

Complementary Terms

Built from Word Parts

The following terms are built from word parts you have already learned and can be translated literally to find their meanings. Further explanation of terms beyond the definition of their word parts, if needed, is included in parentheses.

Term	Definition
CARDIOVASCULAR SYSTEM	
atrioventricular (AV) (*ā*-trē-ō-ven-TRIK-ū-ler)	pertaining to the atrium and ventricle
cardiac (KAR-dē-ak)	pertaining to the heart
cardiogenic (*kar*-dē-ō-JEN-ik)	originating in the heart
cardiologist (*kar*-dē-OL-o-jist)	physician who studies and treats diseases of the heart
cardiology (*kar*-dē-OL-o-jē)	study of the heart (a branch of medicine that deals with diseases of the heart and blood vessels)
hypothermia (*hī*-pō-THER-mē-a)	condition of (body) temperature that is below (normal) (sometimes induced for various surgical procedures, such as bypass surgery)
intravenous (IV) (*in*-tra-VĒ-nus)	pertaining to within the vein
phlebologist (fle-BOL-o-jist)	physician who studies and treats diseases of the veins
phlebology (fle-BOL-o-jē)	study of veins (a branch of medicine that deals with diseases of the veins)

ELECTROPHYSIOLOGIST

A cardiologist who specializes in the diagnosis and treatment of patients with arrhythmias.

Term	Definition
BLOOD	
hematologist (*hē*-ma-TOL-o-jist)	physician who studies and treats diseases of the blood
hematology (*hē*-ma-TOL-o-jē)	study of the blood (a branch of medicine that deals with diseases of the blood)
hematopoiesis (*hē*-ma-tō-poy-Ē-sis)	formation of blood (cells)
hemolysis (*hē*-MOL-i-sis)	dissolution of (red) blood (cells)
hemostasis (*hē*-mō-STĀ-sis)	stoppage of bleeding
myelopoiesis (*mī*-e-lō-poy-Ē-sis)	formation of bone marrow
plasmapheresis (*plaz*-ma-fe-RĒ-sis)	removal of plasma (from withdrawn blood)
thrombolysis (throm-BOL-i-sis)	dissolution of a clot

EXERCISE 37

Practice saying aloud each of the complementary terms built from word parts on these two pages.

To hear the terms, go to http://evolve.elsevier.com. Refer to p. 18 for your Evolve Access Information. Select Exercises & Review, Chapter 10, Chapter Exercises, Pronunciation.

☐ Place a check mark in the box when you have completed this exercise.

EXERCISE 38

Analyze and define the following complementary terms.

1. hypothermia ____________________
2. hematopoiesis ____________________
3. cardiology ____________________
4. cardiologist ____________________
5. hemolysis ____________________
6. hematologist ____________________
7. cardiac ____________________
8. hematology ____________________
9. plasmapheresis ____________________
10. hemostasis ____________________

11. cardiogenic ____________________
12. myelopoiesis ____________________
13. thrombolysis ____________________
14. atrioventricular ____________________
15. intravenous ____________________
16. phlebologist ____________________
17. phlebology ____________________

EXERCISE 39

Build the complementary terms for the following definitions by using the word parts you have learned.

1. study of the heart ______ / CV / ______ (WR / CV / S)
2. formation of blood (cells) ______ / CV / ______ (WR / CV / S)
3. condition of (body) temperature that is below (normal) ______ / ______ / ______ (P / WR / S)
4. dissolution of (red) blood (cells) ______ / CV / ______ (WR / CV / S)
5. removal of plasma (from withdrawn blood) ______ / ______ (WR / S)
6. physician who studies and treats diseases of the blood ______ / CV / ______ (WR / CV / S)
7. pertaining to the heart ______ / ______ (WR / S)
8. physician who studies and treats diseases of the heart ______ / CV / ______ (WR / CV / S)
9. study of the blood ______ / CV / ______ (WR / CV / S)
10. stoppage of bleeding ______ / CV / ______ (WR / CV / S)

11. formation of bone marrow ________ WR /CV/ ________ S

12. originating in the heart ________ WR /CV/ ________ S

13. dissolution of a clot ________ WR /CV/ ________ S

14. pertaining to the atrium and ventricle ________ WR /CV/ ________ WR / ________ S

15. pertaining to within the vein ________ P / ________ WR / ________ S

16. study of veins ________ WR /CV/ ________ S

17. physician who studies and treats diseases of the vein ________ WR /CV/ ________ S

EXERCISE 40

Spell each of the complementary terms built from word parts on pp. 456-457 by having someone dictate them to you.

To hear and spell the terms, go to http://evolve.elsevier.com. Refer to p. 18 for your Evolve Access Information. Select Exercises & Review, Chapter 10, Chapter Exercises, Spelling.

☐ Place a check mark in the box if you have completed this exercise online.

1. ________
2. ________
3. ________
4. ________
5. ________
6. ________
7. ________
8. ________
9. ________
10. ________
11. ________
12. ________
13. ________
14. ________
15. ________
16. ________
17. ________

Complementary Terms

Not Built from Word Parts

In some of the following terms, you may recognize word parts you have already learned; however, the full meaning of the terms cannot be discerned by the definition of their word parts.

Term	Definition
CARDIOVASCULAR SYSTEM	
cardiopulmonary resuscitation (CPR) (*kar*-dē-ō-PUL-mo-nar-ē) (rē-*sus*-i-TĀ-shun)	emergency procedure consisting of artificial ventilation and external cardiac massage
defibrillation (dē-*fib*-ri-LĀ-shun)	application of an electric shock to the myocardium through the chest wall to restore normal cardiac rhythm (Figure 10-28)
diastole (dī-AS-tō-lē)	phase in the cardiac cycle in which the ventricles relax between contractions (diastolic is the lower number of a blood pressure reading)
extracorporeal (*ek*-stra-kōr-POR-ē-al)	occurring outside the body. During open-heart surgery extracorporeal circulation occurs when blood is diverted outside the body to a heart-lung machine.
extravasation (ek-*strav*-a-SĀ-shun)	escape of blood from the blood vessel into the tissue
fibrillation (fi-bri-LĀ-shun)	rapid, quivering, noncoordinated contractions of the atria or ventricles
heart murmur (hart) (MER-mer)	a short-duration humming sound of cardiac or vascular origin
hypercholesterolemia (*hī*-per-k-*les*-ter-ol-Ē-mē-a)	excessive amount of cholesterol in the blood; associated with heightened risk of cardiovascular disease
hyperlipidemia (*hī*-per-*lip*-i-DĒ-mē-a)	excessive amount of fats (triglycerides and cholesterol) in the blood
hypertension (*hī*-per-TEN-shun)	blood pressure that is above normal (greater than 140/90)
hypertriglyceridemia (*hī*-per-trī-*glis*-er-rī-DĒ-mē-a)	excessive amount of triglycerides in the blood; associated with an increased risk of cardiovascular disease
hypotension (*hī*-pō-TEN-shun)	blood pressure that is below normal (less than 90/60)
lipids (LIP-ids)	fats and fatlike substances that serve as a source of fuel in the body and are an important constituent of cell structure
lumen (LŪ-men)	space within a tubular part or organ, such as the space within a blood vessel

Term	Definition
occlude (o-KLŪD)	to close tightly, to block
systole (SIS-tō-lē)	phase in the cardiac cycle in which the ventricles contract (systolic is the upper number of a blood pressure reading)
vasoconstrictor (*vās*-ō-kon-STRIK-tor)	agent or nerve that narrows the blood vessels
vasodilator (*vās*-ō-DĪ-lā-tor)	agent or nerve that enlarges the blood vessels
venipuncture (VEN-i-*punk*-chur)	puncture of a vein to remove blood, instill a medication, or start an intravenous infusion
BLOOD	
anticoagulant (*an*-tī-kō-AG-ū-lant)	agent that slows the blood clotting process
blood dyscrasia (blud) (dis-KRĀ-zha)	abnormal or pathologic condition of the blood
hemorrhage (HEM-o-rij)	rapid loss of blood, as in bleeding

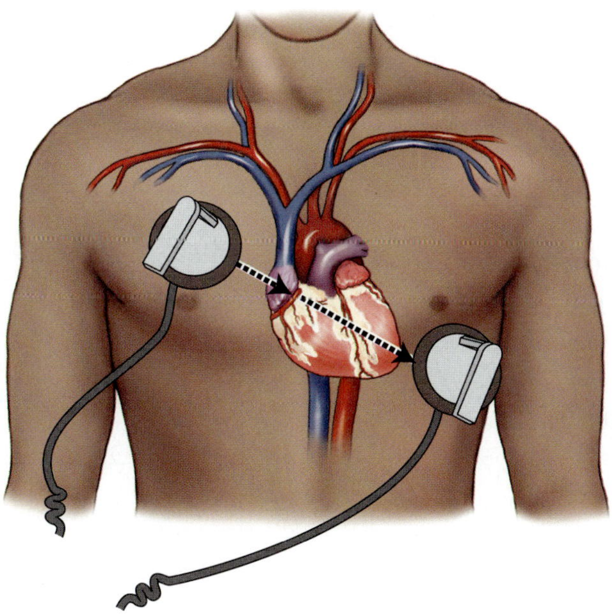

FIGURE 10-28
Placement of defibrillator paddles on the chest.

EXERCISE 41

Practice saying aloud each of the complementary terms not built from word parts on pp. 460-461.

To hear the terms, go to http://evolve.elsevier.com. Refer to p. 18 for your Evolve Access Information. Select Exercises & Review, Chapter 10, Chapter Exercises, Pronunciation.

☐ Place a check mark in the box when you have completed this exercise.

EXERCISE 42

Write the term for each of the following definitions.

1. agent that narrows the blood vessels ____________________
2. space within a tubelike structure ____________________
3. emergency procedure consisting of artificial ventilation and external cardiac massage __________ __________
4. phase in the cardiac cycle in which the ventricles relax ____________________
5. noncoordinated contractions of the atria or ventricles ____________________
6. blood pressure that is below normal ____________________
7. escape of blood from the blood vessel into the tissue ____________________
8. puncture of a vein to remove blood ____________________
9. phase in the cardiac cycle in which the ventricles contract ____________________
10. agent that enlarges the blood vessels ____________________
11. blood pressure that is above normal ____________________
12. to close tightly ____________________
13. excessive amount of triglycerides in the blood ____________________
14. excessive amount of fat in the blood ____________________
15. rapid loss of blood ____________________

16. excessive amount of cholesterol in the blood ____________________
17. pathologic condition of the blood __________ __________
18. a humming sound of cardiac or vascular origin __________ __________
19. occurring outside the body ____________________
20. fat and fat substances ____________________
21. used to restore normal cardiac rhythm ____________________
22. agent that slows the clotting process ____________________

EXERCISE 43

Write the definitions of the following terms.

1. lumen ____________________
2. extravasation ____________________
3. hypercholesterolemia ____________________
4. venipuncture ____________________
5. vasodilator ____________________
6. hypertension ____________________
7. cardiopulmonary resuscitation ____________________
8. systole ____________________
9. hypotension ____________________
10. vasoconstrictor ____________________
11. diastole ____________________
12. fibrillation ____________________
13. occlude ____________________
14. hyperlipidemia ____________________
15. hypertriglyceridemia ____________________
16. blood dyscrasia ____________________
17. hemorrhage ____________________
18. anticoagulant ____________________

19. extracorporeal ______________________
20. heart murmur ______________________
21. lipid ______________________
22. defibrillation ______________________

EXERCISE 44

Spell each of the complementary terms not built from word parts on pp. 460-461 by having someone dictate them to you.

To hear and spell the terms, go to http://evolve.elsevier.com. Refer to p. 18 for your Evolve Access Information. Select Exercises & Review, Chapter 10, Chapter Exercises, Spelling.
☐ Place a check mark in the box if you have completed this exercise online.

1. ____________	12. ____________
2. ____________	13. ____________
3. ____________	14. ____________
4. ____________	15. ____________
5. ____________	16. ____________
6. ____________	17. ____________
7. ____________	18. ____________
8. ____________	19. ____________
9. ____________	20. ____________
10. ____________	21. ____________
11. ____________	22. ____________

IMMUNE SYSTEM

Complementary Terms

Not Built From Word Parts

Term	Definition
allergen (AL-er-jen)	an environmental substance capable of producing an immediate hypersensitivity in the body (allergy). Common allergens are house dust, pollen, animal dander, and various foods.
allergist (AL-er-jist)	a physician who studies and treats allergic conditions

Term	Definition
allergy (AL-er-jē)	hypersensitivity to a substance, resulting in an inflammatory immune response
anaphylaxis (*an*-a-fe-LAK-sis)	an exaggerated, life-threatening reaction to a previously encountered antigen such as bee venom, peanuts, or latex. Symptoms range from mild, with patients experiencing hives or sneezing, to severe symptoms such as drop in blood pressure and blockage of the airway, which can lead to death within minutes (also called **anaphylactic shock**).
antibody (AN-ti-*bod*-ē)	a substance produced by lymphocytes that inactivates or destroys antigens (also called **immunoglobulins**)
antigen (AN-ti-jen)	a substance that triggers an immune response when introduced into the body. Examples of antigens are transplant tissue, toxins, and infectious organisms.
autoimmune disease (*aw*-to-i-MŪN) (di-ZĒZ)	a disease caused by the body's inability to distinguish its own cells from foreign bodies, thus producing antibodies that attack its own tissue. **Rheumatoid arthritis** and **systemic lupus erythematosus** are examples of autoimmune diseases.
immune (i-MŪN)	being resistant to specific invading pathogens
immunodeficiency (*im*-ū-nō-de-FISH-en-sē)	deficient immune response caused by the immune system dysfunction brought on by disease (HIV infection) or immunosuppressive drugs (prednisone)
immunologist (*im*-ū-NOL-o-jist)	a physician who studies and treats immune system disorders
immunology (*im*-ū-NOL-o-jē)	the branch of medicine dealing with immune system disorders
phagocytosis (*fā*-gō-sī-TŌ-sis)	a process in which some of the white blood cells destroy the invading microorganism and old cells
vaccine (vak-SĒN)	a suspension of inactivated microorganisms administered by injection, mouth, or nasal spray to prevent infectious diseases by inducing immunity

IMMUNITY

occurs in three ways:

- **natural immunity** between mother and child before birth and after birth through breast milk
- **active immunity** by the body producing antibodies in response to an infectious disease such as tuberculosis
- **artificial immunity** by receiving vaccinations to produce antibodies. Artificial immunity is used to prevent previously common diseases such as measles and mumps. In 2009, a new H1N1 influenza (swine flu) vaccine was released.

Refer to **Appendix D** for pharmacology terms related to the cardiovascular system and blood.

EXERCISE 45

Practice saying aloud each of the complementary terms not built from word parts on pp. 464-465.

To hear the terms, go to http://evolve.elsevier.com. Refer to p. 18 for your Evolve Access Information. Select Exercises & Review, Chapter 10, Chapter Exercises, Pronunciation.

☐ Place a check mark in the box when you have completed this exercise.

EXERCISE 46

Match the immune system terms in the first column with the phrases in the second column.

______	1. allergen	a.	deficient immune response
______	2. autoimmune disease	b.	a branch of medicine
______	3. immunologist	c.	administered by injection, nasal spray, or orally to prevent infectious diseases
______	4. antigen	d.	inactivates or destroys antigens
______	5. immune	e.	house dust, pollen, animal dander
______	6. allergist	f.	transplant tissue, toxin, infectious organisms
______	7. antibodies	g.	treats allergic conditions
______	8. immunodeficiency	h.	white blood cells destroy invading microorganisms
______	9. phagocytosis	i.	hypersensitivity to a substance
______	10. vaccine	j.	rheumatoid arthritis
______	11. allergy	k.	life-threatening reaction
______	12. immunology	l.	resistant to invading pathogens
______	13. anaphylaxis	m.	treats immune system disorders

EXERCISE 47

Spell each of the complementary terms not built from word parts on pp. 464-465 by having someone dictate them to you.

To hear and spell the terms, go to http://evolve.elsevier.com. Refer to p. 18 for your Evolve Access Information. Select Exercises & Review, Chapter 10, Chapter Exercises, Spelling.

☐ Place a check mark in the box if you have completed this exercise online.

1. ______________________
2. ______________________
3. ______________________
4. ______________________
5. ______________________
6. ______________________
7. ______________________
8. ______________________
9. ______________________
10. ______________________
11. ______________________
12. ______________________
13. ______________________

Abbreviations

ACS	acute coronary syndrome
AFib	atrial fibrillation
AV	atrioventricular
BP	blood pressure
CABG	coronary artery bypass graft
CAD	coronary artery disease
CBC and Diff	complete blood count and differential
CCU	coronary care unit
CHF	congestive heart failure
CPK	creatine phosphokinase
CPR	cardiopulmonary resuscitation
CRP	C-reactive protein
DSA	digital subtraction angiography
DVT	deep vein thrombosis
ECG, EKG	electrocardiogram
ECHO	echocardiogram
HCT	hematocrit
Hgb	hemoglobin

Abbreviations—*cont'd*

HHD	hypertensive heart disease
ICD	implantable cardiac defibrillator
IPG	impedance plethysmography
IV	intravenous
MI	myocardial infarction
PAD	peripheral arterial disease
PT	prothrombin time
PTCA	percutaneous transluminal coronary angioplasty
RBC	red blood cell (erythrocyte)
SPECT	single-photon emission computed tomography
TEE	transesophageal echocardiogram
WBC	white blood cell (leukocyte)

Refer to **Appendix C** for a complete list of abbreviations.

EXERCISE 48

Write the meaning of the abbreviation in the blanks.

1. **CAD** ______________ ______________ ______________ has received growing interest over the past 20 years. Diagnostic procedures for new patients usually begin with an exercise **ECG** ______________. Patients whose stress tests are borderline usually proceed to noninvasive imaging such as **SPECT** ______________ ______________ ______________ ______________ and stress **ECHO** ______________________________.
2. **DVT** ______________ ______________ ______________ is common in hospitalized patients. Early detection is important because DVT can result in death from a pulmonary embolism. Doppler ultrasound and **IPG** ______________ ______________ are two noninvasive diagnostic procedures used to diagnose DVT. MRI and venography may be used as well.
3. The **CBC** ______________ ______________ ______________ and differential count are a series of automated laboratory tests of the peripheral blood that provide a great deal of information about the blood and other body organs. Tests performed as part of the CBC are **RBC** ______________ ______________ ______________ count, **WBC** ______________ ______________ ______________ count and differential count, **Hgb** ______________, and **HCT** ______________.

4. Standard surgical treatment for CAD includes **CABG** ______________ ______________ ______________ ______________. There is a growth in the use of minimally invasive techniques to treat CAD, which include transmyocardial laser revascularization and **PTCA** ______________ ______________ ______________ ______________, atherectomy, and stent placement.
5. Hospitalized patients diagnosed with **MI** ______________ ______________ are cared for in the **CCU** ______________ ______________ ______________.
6. A sphygmomanometer is used to measure **BP** ______________ ______________.
7. Diagnosis used to indicate that a patient's heart is unable to pump enough blood through the body to supply tissues is **CHF** ______________ ______________ ______________.
8. If the patient's heart and/or lungs have ceased to function, the medical team must begin **CPR** ________________________ ________________________.
9. A patient with persistently elevated blood pressure is likely to be diagnosed with **HHD** ______________ ______________ ______________.
10. When scheduling blood tests for a patient on oral anticoagulant medication, the doctor is likely to include a **PT** ______________ ______________.
11. Any interruption of the conduction of electrical impulses from the atria to the ventricles is called **AV** ____ block.
12. The treatment of **ACS** ______________ ______________ ______________ is aimed at preventing thrombus formation and restoring blood flow to the occluded coronary artery.
13. Stopping smoking, exercising, and proper diet are important in the medical management of **PAD** ______________ ______________ ______________.
14. **DSA** ______________ ______________ ______________ is especially valuable in cardiac applications.
15. The physician ordered a **TEE** ______________ ______________ to examine the patient's heart structure and function.
16. Two blood tests used in assessing and evaluating cardiovascular diseases are **CRP** ______________ ______________ and **CPK** ______________ ______________.
17. A patient experiencing **AFib** ______________ ______________ may be referred to an electrophysiologist, a cardiology subspecialist.
18. An **ICD** ______________ ______________ ______________ delivers an electric shock to convert an arrhythmia back to normal rhythm.
19. The patient with dehydration was ordered **IV** ________________________ fluids by her physician.

PRACTICAL APPLICATION

EXERCISE 49 *Interact with Medical Documents*

A. Complete the inpatient progress note by writing the medical terms in the blanks. Use the list of definitions with the corresponding numbers on the next page.

University Hospital and Medical Center
4700 North Main Street • Wellness, Arizona 54321 • (987) 555-3210

PATIENT NAME: Josephine Willamett **CASE NUMBER:** 20922-CVR
DATE OF BIRTH: 01/14/19XX **DATE:** 04/07/20XX

INPATIENT PROGRESS NOTE

CHIEF COMPLAINT: Josephine Willamett is a 76-year-old African-American woman who was admitted to the hospital for recurrent chest pain.

HISTORY OF PRESENT ILLNESS: The patient has a long history of stable 1. ________________ ________________. She had a positive treadmill stress test in 1988. A 2. ________________ ________________ in 1998 showed reversible 3. ________________ . In May 1992 she underwent cataract surgery, and during her postoperative care she developed severe chest pain. An ECG at that time showed ischemic ST changes in the anterior leads. Subsequent coronary 4. ________________ revealed a 90% focal 5. ________________ left anterior descending coronary artery. The patient then underwent 6. ________________ of this lesion. The 90% stenosis was dilated to a 20% stenosis. The patient had an uncomplicated course.

Over the last 10 days the patient has had at least five episodes of chest pain, all relieved by rest or a single nitroglycerin tablet. She had an episode yesterday while gardening, which lasted almost 5 minutes before subsiding after a second nitroglycerin tablet. She went to her 7. ________________ office yesterday. 8. ________________ was performed, which showed marked T-wave inversion in the anterior leads, and she was immediately sent to this hospital for further evaluation. Atherogenic risk factors for her age include hypercholesterolemia and hypertension; she also smokes one pack of cigarettes per day. She is not a diabetic. Her family history reveals a brother who has had a coronary artery bypass graft.

PHYSICAL EXAM:
On exam today, blood pressure is 138/86. She has tachycardia with a pulse of 120. She is in no acute distress. Her lungs are clear and she has regular rhythm without a murmur. There is no edema or distention of neck veins.

CURRENT MEDICATIONS:
1. Lovastatin 20 mg with evening meal.
2. Enalapril 20 mg bid.
3. Nifedipine 10 mg tid.
4. Nitroglycerin 0.4 mg sublingual prn.

PLAN:
9. ________________ ________________ with possible coronary stent if necessary.
Serial ECGs, 10. ________________ ________________, and 11. ________________ will be obtained to rule out 12. ________________ ________________

____

Marguerite DeRouge, DO

MLD/mcm

1. chest pain, occurs when there is an insufficient supply of blood to the heart muscle
2. a nuclear medicine test used to determine blood flow to the myocardium
3. deficient supply of blood to the heart's blood vessels
4. radiographic imaging a blood vessel
5. narrowing
6. surgical repair of a blood vessel
7. physician who studies and treats diseases of the heart
8. process of recording electrical activity of the heart
9. introduction of a catheter into the heart by way of a blood vessel to determine coronary artery disease
10. an enzyme of heart and skeletal muscles
11. a blood test that measures the amount of a certain enzyme approximately 3 hours after necrosis of the heart muscle
12. death of a portion of the myocardial muscle caused by lack of oxygen resulting from an interrupted blood supply

B. Read the progress note and answer the questions following it.

063034 Kaveen, Nilay

File Patient Navigate Custom Fields Help

Patient Chart | Lab | Rad | Notes | Documents | Rx | Scheduling | Images | Billing

Name: **Kaveen, Nilay** MR#: **063034** DOB: **6/30/19XX** Sex: **Male**

PROGRESS NOTE

DATE: 03/07/20XX

INDICATIONS: This 85-year-old male presents with history of angina pectoris and hypertension. He has recently experienced profound weakness. Physical exam revealed blood pressure of 140/70 mm Hg and pulse of 40 beats/min. Auscultation of the heart revealed regular rhythm; no cardiac murmurs were audible. CPK and troponin levels were normal showing no evidence of an acute MI. The electrocardiogram revealed a low heart rate (37 beats/min) and complete heart block. The Holter monitor showed sustained bradycardia with a heart rate of 40 beats/min with a complete heart block. He was referred to an electrophysiologist for the implantation of a cardiac pacemaker.

Electronically signed by: Samantha Parker, MD, FACC 05/09/20XX 2:30 PM

Start | Log On/Off | Print | Edit

1. The patient had a history of (high or low) BP?
2. Cardiac murmur was ruled out by:
   a. diagnostic imaging test
   b. laboratory test
   c. stethoscope
3. An acute myocardial infarction was ruled out by:
   a. an EKG
   b. an ultrasound test
   c. a laboratory test
4. A cardiac pacemaker is used to:
   a. lower blood pressure
   b. regulate heart rate
   c. treat atrial fibrillation

EXERCISE 50 *Interpret Medical Terms*

To test your understanding of the terms introduced in this chapter, circle the words that correctly complete the sentences. The italicized words refer to the correct answer.

1. *Yellowish, fatty plaque within the arteries* is (**arteriosclerosis, atherosclerosis, aortosclerosis**).
2. *Inflammation of a vein associated with a clot* is called a (**thrombosis, phlebitis, thrombophlebitis**).
3. *Inflammation of the middle muscular layer of the heart is* (**endocarditis, myocarditis, pericarditis**).
4. Another name for a *heart attack* is (**myocardial infarction, coronary fibrillation, angina pectoris**).
5. The *surgical excision of a thickened artery interior* is an (**atherectomy, angioplasty, endarterectomy**).
6. An *acute infection caused by the Epstein-Barr virus* is (**anemia, infectious mononucleosis, rheumatic heart disease**).
7. *Reduction of body temperature to a level below normal* results in a condition called (**hypothermia, hypertension, hyperthermia**).
8. (**Impedance plethysmography, cardiac scan, aortogram**) is used to *determine if a patient has a blood clot in the femoral vein.*
9. *A humming sound* or (**hemorrhage, murmur, pulse**) originating *in the heart* is sometimes the result of many episodes of rheumatic fever, an inflammatory disease occurring in children.
10. The doctor uses an (**echocardiograph, electrocardiogram, angioscope**) to *visualize the blood vessel* and guide the laser beam to open blocked arteries; this procedure is called (**echocardiography, angioscopy**).
11. The following is *a nuclear medicine test used to diagnose coronary artery disease* (**coronary stent, thallium test, transesophageal echocardiogram**).
12. Each time *the patient came in contact with house dust she immediately began to sneeze and experienced rhinorrhea.* She visited a(n) (**allergist, immunologist, hematologist**) to seek relief from her symptoms.
13. Peanuts are an antigen that can trigger an *exaggerated life-threatening reaction* or (**allergen, anaphylaxis, allergies**).

EXERCISE 51 *Read Medical Terms in Use*

Practice pronunciation of terms by reading the following medical document. Use the pronunciation key following the medical terms to assist you in saying the word.

To hear these terms, go to http://evolve.elsevier.com. Refer to p. 18 for your Evolve Access Information. Select Exercises & Review, Chapter 10, Chapter Exercises, Read Medical Terms in Use.

A 55-year-old man presented to his doctor with pain in the calf and swelling in the left foot and ankle. Three days prior, the patient had completed trans-Pacific airline travel, spending several hours in a sitting position. He has a history of **varicose** (VAR-i-kōs) **veins** (vānz). No previous history of **hypertension** (*hī*-per-TEN-shun) or **thrombophlebitis** (*throm*-bō-fle-BĪ-tis) existed. Physical examination revealed an edematous left lower extremity and a tender calf. The pedal **pulse** (puls) was intact. A **Doppler ultrasound** (DOP-ler) (UL-tra-sound) was obtained, which revealed **deep vein thrombosis** (throm-BŌ-sis). The patient was hospitalized and subcutaneous low molecular weight heparin was begun. Concurrently, Coumadin was started and will continue for 6 months. The oral **anticoagulant** (*an*-tī-cō-AG-ū-lant) therapy will be monitored monthly by **prothrombin** (prō-THROM-bin) **time.**

EXERCISE 52 *Comprehend Medical Terms in Use*

Test your comprehension of the terms in the previous medical document by circling the correct answer.

1. T F A radiographic image was used to diagnose deep vein thrombosis.
2. The patient was diagnosed with:
   a. inflammation of the vein
   b. vascular inflammatory disorder
   c. a clot in a vein in the lower extremity
   d. a clot in the blood vessels of the heart
3. A blood test will be used to determine:
   a. bleeding time
   b. the time it takes for blood to form a clot
   c. the oxygen-carrying capacity of the red blood cell
   d. certain coagulation activity defects

WEB LINK

For additional information on heart disease, visit the **American Heart Association at *www.americanheart.org.***

CHAPTER REVIEW

ONLINE CHAPTER REVIEW

To access the Evolve website, go to http://evolve.elsevier.com. Refer to p. 18 for your Evolve Access Information. Select Exercises & Review, Chapter 10, then select Chapter Exercises, Practice Activities, Animations, or Games. Place a check mark in the box when you have completed an exercise or activity, watched an animation, or played a game. Have fun!

Chapter Exercises

Exercises in this section of your Evolve resources correlate to exercises in your textbook. You may have completed them as you worked through the chapter.

- ☐ Pronunciation
- ☐ Spelling
- ☐ Read Medical Terms in Use

Practice Activities

Practice in study mode, then test your learning in assessment mode. Keep track of your scores from assessment mode if you wish.

	SCORE
☐ Picture It	_____
☐ Define Word Parts	_____
☐ Build Medical Terms	_____
☐ Word Shop	_____
☐ Define Medical Terms	_____
☐ Use It	_____
☐ Hear It and Type It: Clinical Vignettes	_____

Animations

- ☐ Allergy
- ☐ Angioplasty
- ☐ Antibiotics
- ☐ Cardiac Ischemia and Arrhythmia
- ☐ Coronary Artery Bypass Graft
- ☐ Pericardiocentesis
- ☐ Phagocytosis
- ☐ PTCA
- ☐ Subaortic Stenosis and Echocardiography

Games

- ☐ Name that Word Part
- ☐ Term Storm
- ☐ Term Explorer
- ☐ Termbusters
- ☐ Medical Millionaire
- ☐ Crossword Puzzle

REVIEW OF WORD PARTS

Can you define and spell the following word parts?

Combining Forms

angi/o
aort/o
arteri/o
ather/o
atri/o
cardi/o
ech/o
electr/o
isch/o
lymph/o
lymphaden/o
myel/o
phleb/o
plasm/o
splen/o
therm/o
thromb/o
thym/o
valv/o
valvul/o
ven/o
ventricul/o

Prefixes

brady-

Suffixes

-ac
-apheresis
-graph
-penia
-poiesis
-sclerosis

REVIEW OF TERMS

Can you define, pronounce, and spell the following terms *built from word parts?*

Diseases and Disorders

Cardiovascular System
angioma
angiostenosis
aortic stenosis
arteriosclerosis
atherosclerosis
bradycardia
cardiomegaly
cardiomyopathy
endocarditis
ischemia
myocarditis
pericarditis
phlebitis
polyarteritis
tachycardia
thrombophlebitis
valvulitis

Blood
hematoma
multiple myeloma
pancytopenia
thrombosis
thrombus

Lymphatic System
lymphadenitis
lymphadenopathy
lymphoma
splenomegaly
thymoma

Surgical

Cardiovascular System
angioplasty
atherectomy
endarterectomy
pericardiocentesis
phlebectomy
phlebotomy
valvuloplasty

Lymphatic System
splenectomy
splenopexy
thymectomy

Diagnostic

Cardiovascular System
angiography
angioscope
angioscopy
aortogram
arteriogram
echocardiogram (ECHO)
electrocardiogram (ECG, EKG)
electrocardiograph
electrocardiography
venogram
venography

Complementary

Cardiovascular System
atrioventricular (AV)
cardiac
cardiogenic
cardiologist
cardiology
hypothermia
intravenous (IV)
phlebologist
phlebology

Blood
hematologist
hematology
hematopoiesis
hemolysis
hemostasis
myelopoiesis
plasmapheresis
thrombolysis

Can you define, pronounce, and spell the following terms *not built from word parts?*

Diseases and Disorders

Cardiovascular System

acute coronary syndrome (ACS)
aneurysm
angina pectoris
arrhythmia
atrial fibrillation (AFib)
cardiac arrest
cardiac tamponade
coarctation of the aorta
congenital heart disease
congestive heart failure (CHF)
coronary artery disease (CAD)
coronary occlusion
deep vein thrombosis (DVT)
hypertensive heart disease (HHD)
intermittent claudication
mitral valve stenosis
myocardial infarction (MI)
peripheral arterial disease (PAD)
rheumatic heart disease
varicose veins

Blood

anemia
embolus, *pl.* emboli
hemophilia
leukemia
sepsis

Lymphatic System

Hodgkin disease
infectious mononucleosis

Surgical

Cardiovascular System

aneurysmectomy
atrial fibrillation ablation
cardiac pacemaker
coronary artery bypass graft (CABG)
coronary stent
embolectomy
femoropopliteal bypass
implantable cardiac defibrillator (ICD)
intracoronary thrombolytic therapy
percutaneous transluminal coronary angioplasty (PTCA)

Blood

bone marrow aspiration
bone marrow biopsy
bone marrow transplant

Diagnostic

Cardiovascular System

blood pressure (BP)
cardiac catheterization
C-reactive protein (CRP)
creatine phosphokinase (CPK)
digital subtraction angiography (DSA)
Doppler ultrasound
exercise stress test
homocysteine
impedance plethysmography (IPG)
lipid profile
pulse
single-photon emission computed tomography (SPECT)
sphygmomanometer
thallium test
transesophageal echocardiogram (TEE)
troponin

Blood

coagulation time
complete blood count and differential (CBC and Diff)
hematocrit (HCT)
hemoglobin (Hgb)
prothrombin time (PT)

Complementary

Cardiovascular System

cardiopulmonary resuscitation (CPR)
defibrillation
diastole
extracorporeal
extravasation
fibrillation
heart murmur
hypercholesterolemia
hyperlipidemia
hypertension
hypertriglyceridemia
hypotension
lipids
lumen
occlude
systole
vasoconstrictor
vasodilator
venipuncture

Blood

anticoagulant
blood dyscrasia
hemorrhage

Immune System

allergen
allergist
allergy
anaphylaxis
antibodies
antigen
autoimmune disease
immune
immunodeficiency
immunologist
immunology
phagocytosis
vaccine

ANSWERS

Exercise Figures

Exercise Figure

A. 1. blood vessel: angi/o
2. valve: valv/o, valvul/o
3. heart: cardi/o
4. aorta: aort/o
5. artery: arteri/o
6. atrium: atri/o
7. ventricle: ventricul/o

Exercise Figure

B. ather/o/sclerosis

Exercise Figure

C. end/arter/ectomy

Exercise Figure

D. electr/o/cardi/o/gram

Exercise 1

1. e
2. g
3. c
4. h
5. a
6. f
7. d
8. b
9. i

Exercise 2

1. j
2. b
3. g
4. d
5. i
6. a
7. e
8. c
9. f

Exercise 3

1. plasma
2. erythrocytes
3. leukocytes
4. platelets
5. platelets
6. serum
7. lymph
8. lymph nodes
9. spleen
10. thymus

Exercise 4

1. protect the body against pathogens, foreign agents, and abnormal body cells
2. a. spleen
   b. liver
   c. intestinal tract
   d. lymph nodes
   e. bone marrow
3. a. prevention of foreign bodies from entering the body
   b. phagocytosis, inflammation, fever, and activation of protective proteins and natural killer cells
   c. forms specific antibodies to fight infectious agents

Exercise 5

1. heart
2. atrium
3. plasma
4. vessel
5. vein
6. aorta
7. valve
8. spleen
9. thymus gland
10. vein
11. ventricle
12. artery
13. valve
14. lymph, lymph tissue
15. lymph node
16. bone marrow

Exercise 6

1. arteri/o
2. a. phleb/o
   b. ven/o
3. cardi/o
4. atri/o
5. ventricul/o
6. lymph/o
7. aort/o
8. angi/o
9. a. valv/o
   b. valvul/o
10. splen/o
11. plasm/o
12. thym/o
13. lymphaden/o
14. myel/o

Exercise 7

1. sound
2. clot
3. deficiency, blockage
4. heat
5. yellowish, fatty plaque
6. electricity, electrical activity

Exercise 8

1. thromb/o
2. ech/o
3. isch/o
4. ather/o
5. therm/o
6. electr/o

Exercise 9

1. slow
2. instrument used to record; record
3. abnormal reduction in number
4. hardening
5. removal
6. formation
7. pertaining to

Exercise 10

1. -poiesis
2. -ac
3. -sclerosis
4. -graph
5. -penia
6. brady-
7. -apheresis

Exercise 11

Pronunciation Exercise

Exercise 12

1. P WR S
   endo/card/itis
   inflammation of the inner (lining) of the heart
2. P WR S
   brady/card/ia
   condition of slow heart (rate)
3. WR CV S
   cardi/o/megaly
   CF
   enlargement of the heart
4. WR CV S
   arteri/o/sclerosis
   CF
   hardening of the arteries
5. WR S
   valvul/itis
   CF
   inflammation of the valves of the heart

6. WR S
(multiple) myel/oma
tumors of the bone marrow

7. P WR S
tachy/card/ia
condition of a rapid heart (rate)

8. WR CV S
angi/o/stenosis
CF
narrowing of blood vessels

9. WR S
thromb/us
(blood) clot

10. WR S
isch/emia
deficiency of blood (flow)

11. P WR S
peri/card/itis
inflammation of the sac surrounding the heart

12. WR S
aort/ic stenosis
narrowing, pertaining to the aorta (narrowing of the aortic valve)

13. WR S
thromb/osis
abnormal condition of a (blood) clot

14. WR CV S
ather/o/sclerosis
CF
hardening of fatty plaque (deposited on the arterial wall)

15. WR CV WR S
my/o/card/itis
CF
inflammation of the muscle of the heart

16. WR S
angi/oma
tumor composed of blood vessels

17. WR S
thym/oma
tumor of the thymus gland

18. WR S
lymph/oma
tumor of lymphatic tissue

19. WR S
lymphaden/itis
inflammation of the lymph nodes

20. WR CV S
splen/o/megaly
CF
enlargement of the spleen

21. WR S
hemat/oma
tumor of blood

22. P WR S
poly/arter/itis
inflammation of many (sites in the) arteries

23. WR CV WR CV S
cardi/o/my/o/pathy
CF CF
disease of the heart muscle

24. WR CV S
lymphaden/o/pathy
CF
disease of the lymph nodes

25. WR CV WR S
thromb/o/phleb/itis
CF
inflammation of a vein associated with a clot

26. WR S
phleb/itis
inflammation of a vein

27. P WR CV S
pan/cyt/o/penia
CF
abnormal reduction of all (blood) cells

Exercise 13

1. myel/oma
2. cardi/o/megaly
3. isch/emia
4. endo/card/itis
5. brady/card/ia
6. arteri/o/sclerosis
7. thromb/osis
8. my/o/card/itis
9. angi/o/stenosis
10. tachy/card/ia
11. ather/o/sclerosis
12. angi/oma
13. valvul/itis
14. aort/ic (stenosis)
15. peri/card/itis
16. lymph/oma
17. thym/oma
18. splen/o/megaly
19. hemat/oma
20. lymphaden/itis
21. cardi/o/my/o/pathy
22. poly/arter/itis
23. lymphaden/o/pathy
24. thromb/o/phleb/itis
25. phleb/itis
26. thromb/us
27. pan/cyt/o/penia

Exercise 14

Spelling Exercise; see text pp. 420-421.

Exercise 15

Pronunciation Exercise

Exercise 16

1. coarctation
2. embolus
3. cardiac arrest
4. congenital
5. varicose veins
6. coronary occlusion
7. aneurysm
8. Hodgkin
9. coronary artery disease
10. angina pectoris
11. myocardial infarction
12. atrial fibrillation
13. arrhythmia
14. hypertensive
15. congestive heart failure
16. peripheral arterial disease
17. hemophilia
18. leukemia
19. anemia
20. infectious mononucleosis
21. intermittent claudication
22. cardiac tamponade
23. mitral valve stenosis and rheumatic heart disease
24. deep vein thrombosis
25. acute coronary syndrome
26. sepsis

Exercise 17

1. d
2. c
3. f
4. e
5. a
6. j
7. i
8. k
9. g
10. b
11. h
12. l
13. n
14. m

Exercise 18

1. i
2. e
3. a
4. h
5. j
6. b
7. d
8. k
9. l
10. g
11. c
12. m
13. f

Exercise 19

Spelling Exercise; see text pp. 425-429.

Exercise 20

Pronunciation Exercise

Exercise 21

1. P WR CV S
   peri/cardi/o/centesis
   CF
   surgical puncture to aspirate fluid from the sac surrounding the heart (pericardium)
2. WR S
   thym/ectomy
   excision of the thymus gland
3. WR CV S
   angi/o/plasty
   CF
   surgical repair of a blood vessel
4. WR CV S
   splen/o/pexy
   CF
   surgical fixation of the spleen
5. WR CV S
   valvul/o/plasty
   CF
   surgical repair of a valve
6. P WR S
   end/arter/ectomy
   excision within an artery
7. WR CV S
   phleb/o/tomy
   CF
   incision into a vein
8. WR S
   splen/ectomy
   excision of the spleen
9. WR S
   phleb/ectomy
   excision of a vein
10. WR S
   ather/ectomy
   excision of fatty plaque

Exercise 22

1. end/arter/ectomy
2. splen/o/pexy
3. valvul/o/plasty
4. phleb/o/tomy
5. thym/ectomy
6. peri/cardi/o/centesis
7. angi/o/plasty
8. splen/ectomy
9. phleb/ectomy
10. ather/ectomy

Exercise 23

Spelling Exercise; see text pp. 434-435.

Exercise 24

Pronunciation Exercise

Exercise 25

1. ablation
2. percutaneous transluminal coronary angioplasty
3. cardiac pacemaker
4. blood cells
5. coronary artery bypass graft
6. aneurysmectomy
7. femoropopliteal bypass
8. intracoronary thrombolytic
9. bone marrow transplant
10. embolectomy
11. coronary stent
12. implantable cardiac defibrillator

Exercise 26

1. h	8. c
2. m	9. i
3. k	10. b
4. l	11. j
5. d	12. g
6. e	13. f
7. a	

Exercise 27

Spelling Exercise; see text pp. 437-440.

Exercise 28

Pronunciation Exercise

Exercise 29

1. WR CV WR CV S
   electr/o/cardi/o/graph
   CF CF
   instrument used to record the electrical activity of the heart
2. WR CV S
   ven/o/gram
   CF
   radiographic image of the veins (after an injection of contrast medium)
3. WR CV S
   angi/o/graphy
   CF
   radiographic imaging of a blood vessel
4. WR CV WR CV S
   ech/o/cardi/o/gram
   CF CF
   record of the heart by using sound
5. WR CV S
   aort/o/gram
   CF
   radiographic image of the aorta (after an injection of contrast media)
6. WR CV WR CV S
   electr/o/cardi/o/gram
   CF CF
   record of the electrical activity of the heart
7. WR CV S
   arteri/o/gram
   CF
   radiographic image of an artery (after an injection of contrast media)
8. WR CV WR CV S
   electr/o/cardi/o/graphy
   CF CF
   process of recording the electrical activity of the heart
9. WR CV S
   angi/o/scopy
   CF
   visual examination of a blood vessel
10. WR CV S
   ven/o/graphy
   CF
   radiographic imaging a vein
11. WR CV S
   angi/o/scope
   CF
   instrument used for visual examination of a blood vessel

Exercise 30

1. electr/o/cardi/o/graph
2. arteri/o/gram
3. ven/o/gram
4. angi/o/graphy
5. electr/o/cardi/o/gram
6. ech/o/cardi/o/gram
7. aort/o/gram
8. electr/o/cardi/o/graphy
9. angi/o/scopy
10. ven/o/graphy
11. angi/o/scope

Exercise 31

Spelling Exercise; see text pp. 443-445.

Exercise 32

Pronunciation Exercise

Exercise 33

1. sphygmomanometer
2. coagulation time
3. complete blood count and differential count
4. Doppler ultrasound
5. blood pressure
6. prothrombin time
7. cardiac catheterization
8. hemoglobin
9. impedance plethysmography
10. thallium test
11. transesophageal echocardiogram
12. single-photon emission computed tomography
13. exercise stress test

14. digital subtraction angiography
15. creatine phosphokinase
16. C-reactive protein
17. pulse
18. homocysteine
19. troponin
20. lipid profile
21. hematocrit

Exercise 34

1. d
2. h
3. l
4. g
5. j
6. c
7. a
8. e
9. b
10. f
11. i

Exercise 35

1. c
2. e
3. b
4. f
5. d
6. a
7. g
8. h
9. i
10. j

Exercise 36

Spelling Exercise; see text pp. 448-452.

Exercise 37

Pronunciation Exercise

Exercise 38

1. P WR S
hypo/therm/ia
condition of (body) temperature that is below (normal)
2. WR CV S
hemat/o/poiesis
CF
formation of blood (cells)
3. WR CV S
cardi/o/logy
CF
study of the heart
4. WR CV S
cardi/o/logist
CF
physician who studies and treats diseases of the heart
5. WR CV S
hem/o/lysis
CF
dissolution of blood (cells)
6. WR CV S
hemat/o/logist
CF
physician who studies and treats diseases of the blood
7. WR S
cardi/ac
pertaining to the heart
8. WR CV S
hemat/o/logy
CF
study of the blood
9. WR S
plasm/apheresis
removal of plasma (from withdrawn blood)
10. WR CV S
hem/o/stasis
CF
stoppage of bleeding
11. WR CV S
cardi/o/genic
CF
originating in the heart
12. WR CV S
myel/o/poiesis
CF
formation of bone marrow
13. WR CV S
thromb/o/lysis
CF
dissolution of a clot
14. WR CV WR S
atri/o/ventricul/ar
CF
pertaining to the atrium and ventricle
15. P WR S
intra/ven/ous
pertaining to within the vein
16. WR CV S
phleb/o/logist
CF
physician who studies and treats disease of the veins
17. WR CV S
phleb/o/logy
CF
study of veins

Exercise 39

1. cardi/o/logy
2. hemat/o/poiesis
3. hypo/therm/ia
4. hem/o/lysis
5. plasm/apheresis
6. hemat/o/logist
7. cardi/ac
8. cardi/o/logist
9. hemat/o/logy
10. hem/o/stasis
11. myel/o/poiesis
12. cardi/o/genic
13. thromb/o/lysis
14. atri/o/ventricul/ar
15. intra/ven/ous
16. phleb/o/logy
17. phleb/o/logist

Exercise 40

Spelling Exercise; see text pp. 456-457.

Exercise 41

Pronunciation Exercise

Exercise 42

1. vasoconstrictor
2. lumen
3. cardiopulmonary resuscitation
4. diastole
5. fibrillation
6. hypotension
7. extravasation
8. venipuncture
9. systole
10. vasodilator
11. hypertension
12. occlude
13. hypertriglyceridemia
14. hyperlipidemia
15. hemorrhage
16. hypercholesterolemia
17. blood dyscrasia
18. heart murmur
19. extracorporeal
20. lipids
21. defibrillation
22. anticoagulant

Exercise 43

1. space within a tubelike structure
2. escape of blood from the blood vessel into the tissues
3. excessive amount of cholesterol in the blood
4. puncture of a vein to remove blood, start an intravenous infusion, or instill medication
5. agent or nerve that enlarges the blood vessels
6. blood pressure that is above normal
7. emergency procedure consisting of artificial ventilation and external cardiac massage
8. phase in the cardiac cycle in which ventricles contract
9. blood pressure that is below normal
10. agent or nerve that narrows blood vessels
11. cardiac cycle phase in which ventricles relax

12. rapid, quivering, noncoordinated contractions of the atria or ventricles
13. to close tightly
14. excessive amount of fat in the blood
15. excessive amount of triglycerides in the blood
16. abnormal or pathologic condition of the blood
17. rapid loss of blood
18. agent that slows down the clotting process
19. occurring outside the body
20. humming sound of cardiac or vascular origin
21. fats and fatlike substances that serve as a source of fuel in the body
22. application of electric shock to the myocardium to restore normal heart rhythm

Exercise 44
Spelling Exercise; see text pp. 460-461.

Exercise 45
Pronunciation Exercise

Exercise 46
1. e
2. j
3. m
4. f
5. l
6. g
7. d
8. a
9. h
10. c
11. i
12. b
13. k

Exercise 47
Spelling Exercise; see text pp. 464-465.

Exercise 48
1. coronary artery disease; electrocardiogram; single-photon emission computed tomography; echocardiogram
2. deep vein thrombosis; impedance plethysmography
3. complete blood count; red blood cell, white blood cell, hemoglobin, hematocrit
4. coronary artery bypass graft; percutaneous transluminal coronary angioplasty
5. myocardial infarction; coronary care unit
6. blood pressure
7. congestive heart failure
8. cardiopulmonary resuscitation
9. hypertensive heart disease
10. prothrombin time
11. atrioventricular
12. acute coronary syndrome
13. peripheral arterial disease
14. digital subtraction angiography
15. transesophageal echocardiogram
16. C-reactive protein, creatine phosphokinase
17. atrial fibrillation
18. implantable cardiac defibrillator
19. intravenous

Exercise 49
A. 1. angina pectoris
2. thallium test
3. ischemia
4. angiography
5. stenosis
6. angioplasty
7. cardiologist
8. electrocardiography
9. cardiac catheterization
10. creatine phosphokinase
11. troponin
12. myocardial infarction

B. 1. high
2. c
3. c
4. b

Exercise 50
1. atherosclerosis
2. thrombophlebitis
3. myocarditis
4. myocardial infarction
5. endarterectomy
6. infectious mononucleosis
7. hypothermia
8. impedance plethysmography
9. murmur
10. angioscope, angioscopy
11. thallium test
12. allergist
13. anaphylaxis

Exercise 51
Reading Exercise

Exercise 52
1. *F*, the diagnosis was made with an ultrasound procedure.
2. c
3. d

Chapter 11

Digestive System

OUTLINE

OBJECTIVES

Upon completion of this chapter you will be able to:

1. Identify organs and structures of the digestive system.
2. Define and spell word parts related to the digestive system.
3. Define, pronounce, and spell disease and disorder terms related to the digestive system.
4. Define, pronounce, and spell surgical terms related to the digestive system.
5. Define, pronounce, and spell diagnostic terms related to the digestive system.
6. Define, pronounce, and spell complementary terms related to the digestive system.
7. Interpret the meaning of abbreviations related to the digestive system.
8. Interpret, read, and comprehend medical language in simulated medical statements and documents.

ANATOMY

The digestive tract, also known as the **alimentary canal** or the **gastrointestinal tract** and abbreviated as **GI tract,** is a long continuous tube comprising the mouth, pharynx, esophagus, stomach, small intestine, large intestine, rectum, and anus. Accessory organs of the digestive tract are the salivary glands, liver, bile ducts, gallbladder, and pancreas (see Figures 11-1 through 11-5).

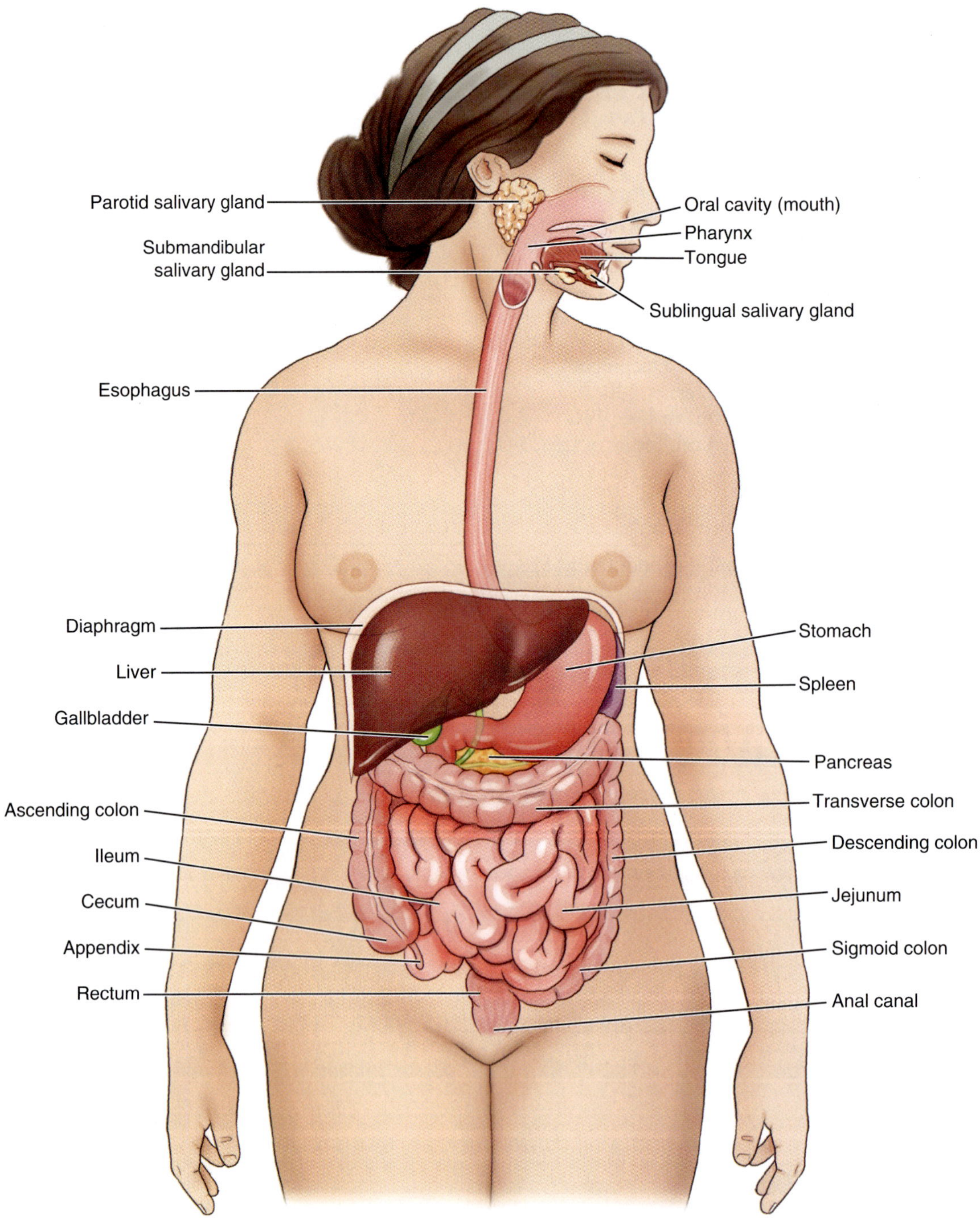

FIGURE 11-1
Organs of the digestive system.

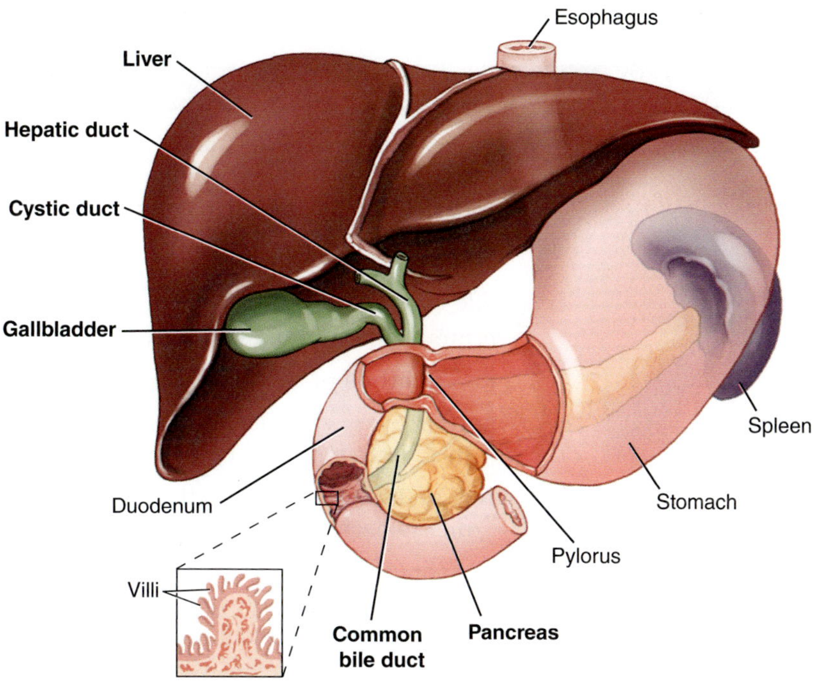

FIGURE 11-2
Accessory organs.

Function

Functions of the digestive tract are **ingestion,** the taking in of nutrients through the mouth; **digestion**, the mechanical and chemical breakdown of food for use by body cells; **absorption**, the transfer of digested food from the small intestine to the blood stream; and **elimination**, the removal of solid waste from the body.

Organs of the Digestive Tract

Term	Definition
mouth	opening through which food passes into the body; breaks food into small particles by mastication (chewing) and mixing with saliva (Figure 11-3)
tongue	consists mostly of skeletal muscle; attached in the posterior region of the mouth. It provides movement of food for mastication, directs food to the pharynx for swallowing, and is a major organ for taste and speech.
palate	separates the nasal cavity from the oral cavity
soft palate	posterior portion, not supported by bone
hard palate	anterior portion, supported by bone
uvula	soft V-shaped structure that extends from the soft palate; directs food into the throat
pharynx, throat	performs the swallowing action that passes food from the mouth into the esophagus
esophagus	10-inch (25 cm) tube that is a passageway for food extending from the pharynx to the stomach. **Peristalsis**, involuntary wavelike movements that propel food along the digestive tract, begins in the esophagus.

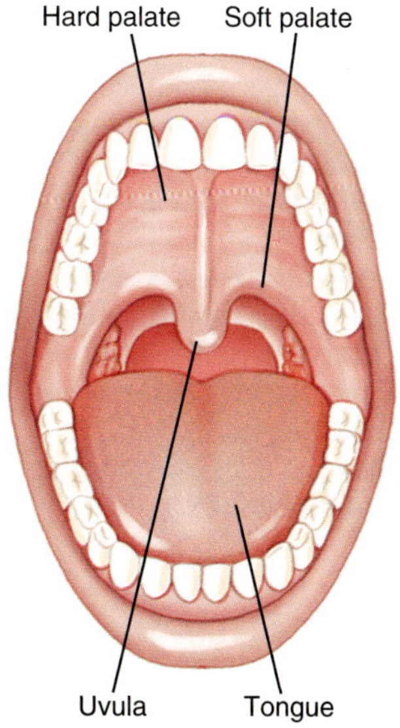

FIGURE 11-3
The oral cavity.

Organs of the Digestive Tract—*cont'd*

Term	Definition
stomach	J-shaped sac that mixes and stores food. It secretes chemicals for digestion and hormones for local communication control
cardia	area around the opening of the esophagus
fundus	uppermost domed portion of the stomach
body	central portion of the stomach
antrum	lower portion of the stomach
pylorus	portion of the stomach that connects to the small intestine
pyloric sphincter	ring of muscle that guards the opening between the stomach and the duodenum
small intestine	20-foot (6 m) canal extending from the pyloric sphincter to the large intestine. **Digestion** is completed in the small intestine. **Absorption**, the passage of the nutrients (end products of digestion) from the small intestine to the bloodstream, takes place through the **villi**, fingerlike projections that line the walls of the small intestine.
duodenum	first 10 to 12 inches (25 cm) of the small intestine
jejunum	second portion of the small intestine, approximately 8 feet (2.4 m) long
ileum	third portion of the small intestine, approximately 11 feet (3.3 m) long, which connects with the large intestine
large intestine	canal that is approximately 5 feet (1.5 m) long and extends from the ileum to the anus (Figure 11-4). **Absorption** of water and **elimination** of the solid waste products of digestion take place in the large intestine.
cecum	blind U-shaped pouch that is the first portion of the large intestine
colon	next portion of the large intestine. The colon is divided into four parts: ascending colon, transverse colon, descending colon, and sigmoid colon
rectum	remaining portion of the large intestine, approximately 8 to 10 inches (20 cm) long, extending from the sigmoid colon to the anus
anus	sphincter muscle (ringlike band of muscle fiber that keeps an opening tight) at the end of the digestive tract

DUODENUM

is derived from the Latin ***duodeni***, meaning ***12 each***, a reference to its length. It was named in 240 BC by a Greek physician.

Jejunum is derived from the Latin **jejunus**, meaning ***empty***; it was so named because the early anatomists always found it empty.

Ileum is derived from the Greek ***eilein***, meaning ***to roll***, a reference to the peristaltic waves that move food along the digestive tract. This term was first used in the early part of the seventeenth century.

Term	Definition
ACCESSORY ORGANS (see Figure 11-2)	
salivary glands	produce saliva, which flows into the mouth
liver	produces bile, which is necessary for the digestion of fats. The liver performs many other functions concerned with digestion and metabolism
bile ducts	passageways that carry bile: the **hepatic duct** is a passageway for bile from the liver, and the **cystic duct** carries bile from the gallbladder. They join to form the **common bile duct**, which conveys bile to the duodenum. Collectively, these passageways are referred to as the **biliary tract.**
gallbladder	small, saclike structure that stores bile
pancreas	produces pancreatic juice, which helps digest all types of food and secretes insulin for carbohydrate metabolism
OTHER STRUCTURES	
peritoneum	serous saclike lining of the abdominal and pelvic cavities
appendix	small pouch, which has no known function in digestion, attached to the cecum (also called **vermiform appendix**)
abdomen	portion of the body between the thorax and the pelvis

BILIARY SYSTEM

The liver, bile ducts, and gallbladder comprise the biliary system, which creates, transports, stores, and releases bile into the small intestine to facilitate the absorption of fat.

PANCREAS

is derived from the Greek **pan,** meaning **all,** and **krea,** meaning **flesh.** The pancreas was first described in 300 BC. It was so named because of its fleshy appearance.

A & P Booster
For students desiring more anatomy and physiology, go to http://evolve.elsever.com. Refer to p. 18 for your Evolve Access Information. Select A & P Booster, Chapter 11.

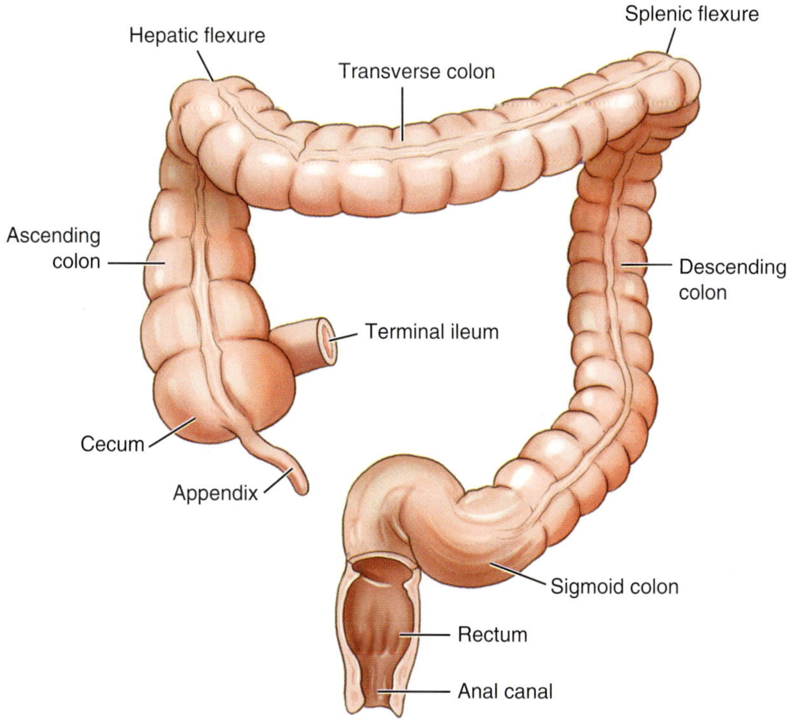

FIGURE 11-4
Anatomy of the large intestine.

EXERCISE 1

Fill in the blanks with the correct terms. *To check your answers to the exercises in this chapter, go to Answers, p. 544, at the end of the chapter.*

The digestive tract, also known as the (1) ____________________ ____________ and (2) ____________________ ____________, begins with the mouth, connects with the throat, or (3) ____________, and continues on to a 10-inch tube called the (4) ____________; this connects with the (5) ____________, a J-shaped sac that mixes and stores food. The small intestine, the next portion of the digestive tract, is made up of three portions. They are called the (6) ____________________, (7) ____________, and (8) ____________. The small intestine connects with the first portion of the large intestine, the (9) ____________, and then connects with the colon, which is divided into four parts called (10) ____________________ ____________, (11) ____________________ ____________, (12) ____________ ____________, and (13) ____________ ____________. The (14) ____________ extends from the sigmoid colon to the (15) ____________.

EXERCISE 2

Match the definitions in the first column with the correct terms in the second column.

______	1. lower portion of the stomach	a.	salivary glands
______	2. hangs from the roof of the mouth	b.	pancreas
______	3. produce saliva	c.	peritoneum
______	4. produces bile	d.	uvula
______	5. separates the nasal cavity from the oral cavity	e.	gallbladder
______	6. guards the opening between the stomach and the duodenum	f.	tongue
______	7. secretes insulin for carbohydrate metabolism	g.	abdomen
______	8. small pouch that has no function in digestion	h.	liver
______	9. lining of the abdominal and pelvic cavities	i.	appendix
______	10. portion of the body between the pelvis and thorax	j.	pyloric sphincter
______	11. stores bile	k.	fundus
______	12. uppermost domed portion of the stomach	l.	antrum
______	13. directs food to the pharynx for swallowing	m.	palate

WORD PARTS

Word parts you need to learn to complete this chapter are listed on the following pages. The exercises at the end of each list will help you learn their definitions and spellings.

Use the flashcards accompanying this text or electronic flashcards to assist you in memorizing the word parts for this chapter.

To use electronic flashcards, go to http://evolve.elsevier.com. Refer to p. 18 for your Evolve Access Information. Select Flashcards, Chapter 11.

Combining Forms of the Digestive Tract

Combining Form	Definition
an/o	anus
antr/o	antrum
cec/o	cecum
col/o, colon/o	colon (usually denoting the large intestine)
duoden/o	duodenum
enter/o	intestine (usually denoting the small intestine)
esophag/o (NOTE: *esophag/o* was covered in Chapter 9.)	esophagus
gastr/o	stomach
ile/o	ileum
jejun/o	jejunum
or/o, stomat/o	mouth
proct/o, rect/o	rectum
sigmoid/o	sigmoid colon

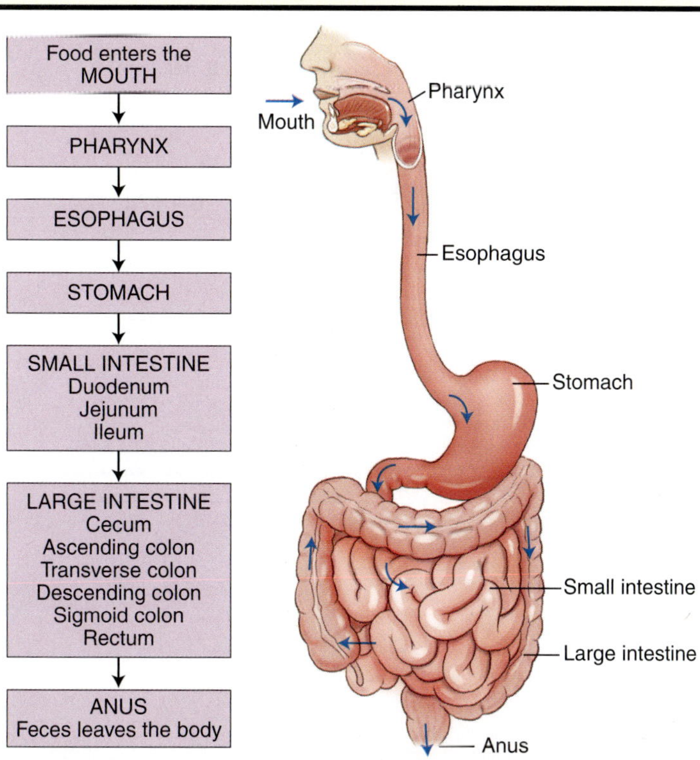

FIGURE 11-5
Pathway of food.

EXERCISE FIGURE A

Fill in the blanks with combining forms in this diagram of the digestive system. *To check your answers, go to p. 544.*

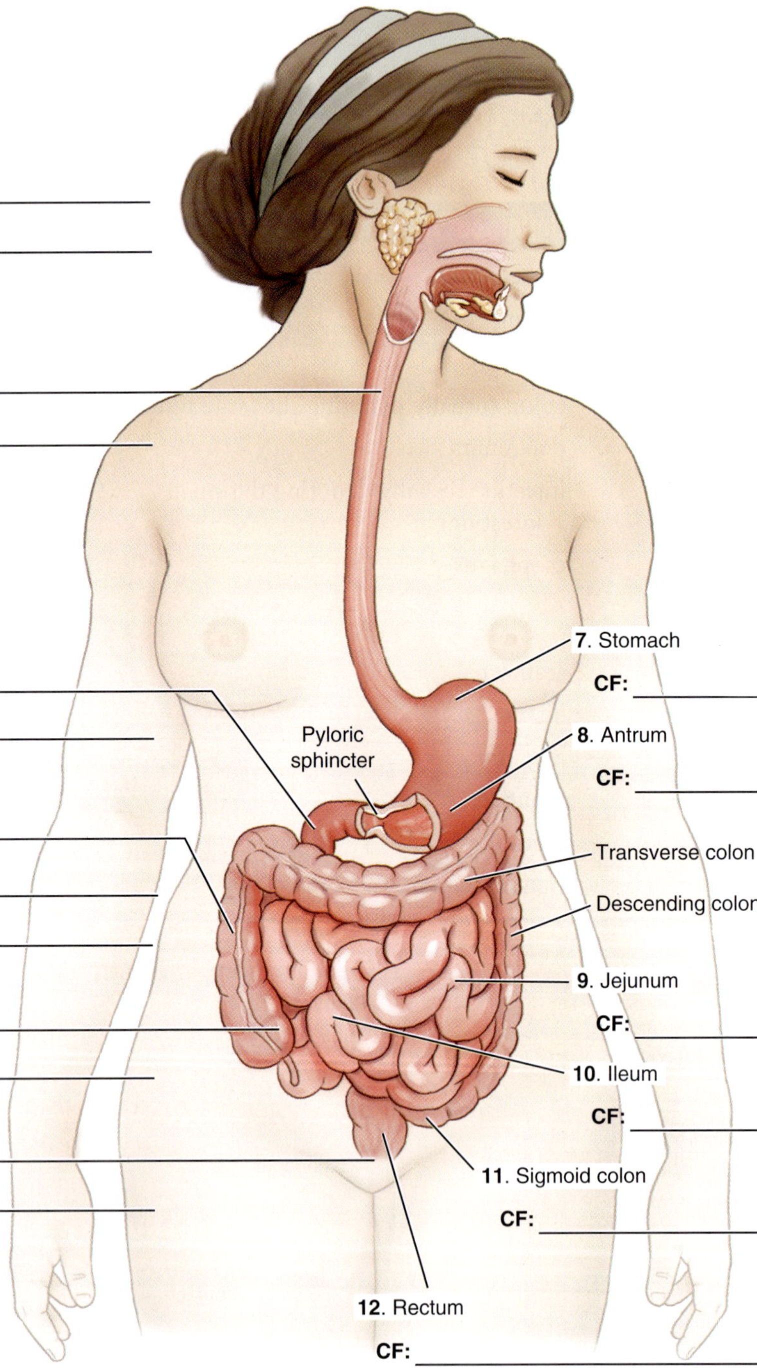

1. Mouth
   CF: ______________________
   CF: ______________________
2. Esophagus
   CF: ______________________
3. Duodenum
   CF: ______________________
4. Ascending **colon**
   CF: ______________________
   CF: ______________________
5. Cecum
   CF: ______________________
6. Anus
   CF: ______________________
7. Stomach
   CF: ______________________
8. Antrum
   CF: ______________________
9. Jejunum
   CF: ______________________
10. Ileum
   CF: ______________________
11. Sigmoid colon
   CF: ______________________
12. Rectum
   CF: ______________________
   CF: ______________________

EXERCISE 3

Write the definitions of the following combining forms.

1. proct/o ____________
2. gastr/o ____________
3. an/o ____________
4. cec/o ____________
5. ile/o ____________
6. stomat/o ____________
7. duoden/o ____________
8. col/o ____________
9. or/o ____________
10. enter/o ____________
11. rect/o ____________
12. antr/o ____________
13. esophag/o ____________
14. jejun/o ____________
15. sigmoid/o ____________ ____________
16. colon/o ____________

EXERCISE 4

Write the combining form for each of the following terms.

1. cecum ____________
2. stomach ____________
3. ileum ____________
4. jejunum ____________
5. sigmoid colon ____________
6. esophagus ____________
7. rectum a. ____________ b. ____________
8. intestine ____________
9. duodenum ____________
10. colon a. ____________ b. ____________
11. mouth a. ____________ b. ____________
12. anus ____________
13. antrum ____________

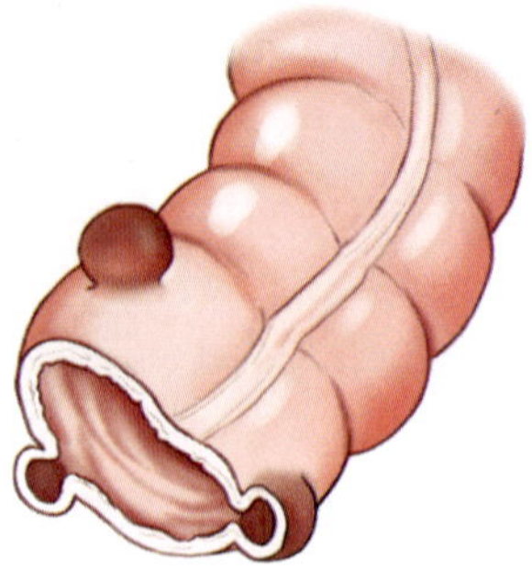

FIGURE 11-6
Diverticula of the large intestine.

HERNIA

The layman's term for hernia is **rupture.** Types include abdominal, hiatal or diaphragmatic, inguinal, and umbilical hernia.

Combining Forms of the Accessory Organs/Combining Forms Commonly Used with Digestive System Terms

Combining Form	Definition
abdomin/o, celi/o, lapar/o	abdomen (abdominal cavity)
append/o, appendic/o	appendix
cheil/o	lip
cholangi/o	bile duct
chol/e (NOTE: the combining vowel is *e*.)	gall, bile
choledoch/o	common bile duct
diverticul/o	diverticulum, or blind pouch, extending from a hollow organ (pl. diverticula) (Figure 11-6)
gingiv/o	gum
gloss/o, lingu/o	tongue
hepat/o	liver
herni/o	hernia, or protrusion of an organ through a membrane or cavity wall (Figure 11-7)
palat/o	palate
pancreat/o	pancreas
peritone/o	peritoneum
polyp/o	polyp, small growth
pylor/o (NOTE: *pylor/o* was covered in Chapter 9.)	pylorus, pyloric sphincter
sial/o	saliva, salivary gland
steat/o	fat
uvul/o	uvula

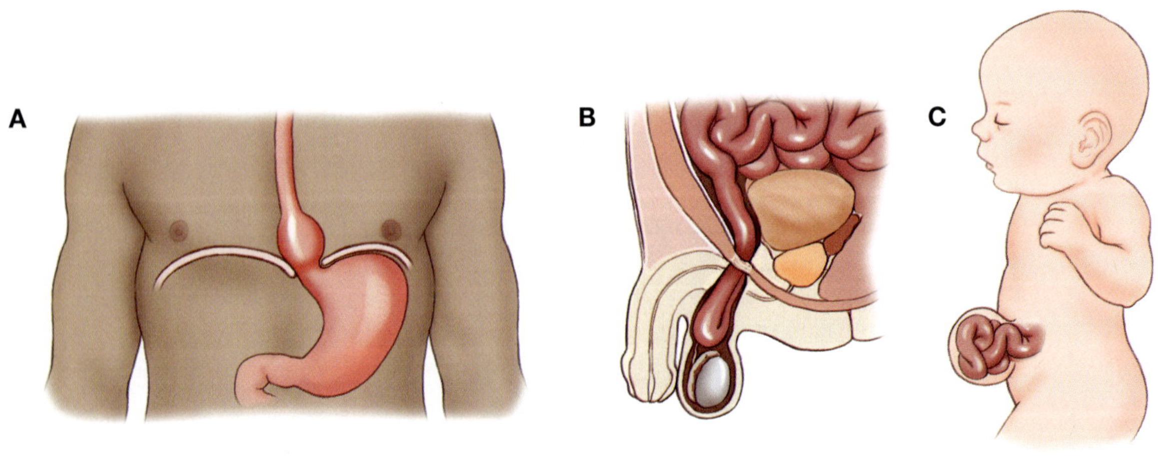

FIGURE 11-7
Types of hernias. **A**, Hiatal. **B**, Inguinal. **C**, Umbilical.

EXERCISE FIGURE B

Fill in the blanks with combining forms in this diagram of the digestive system and associated structures.

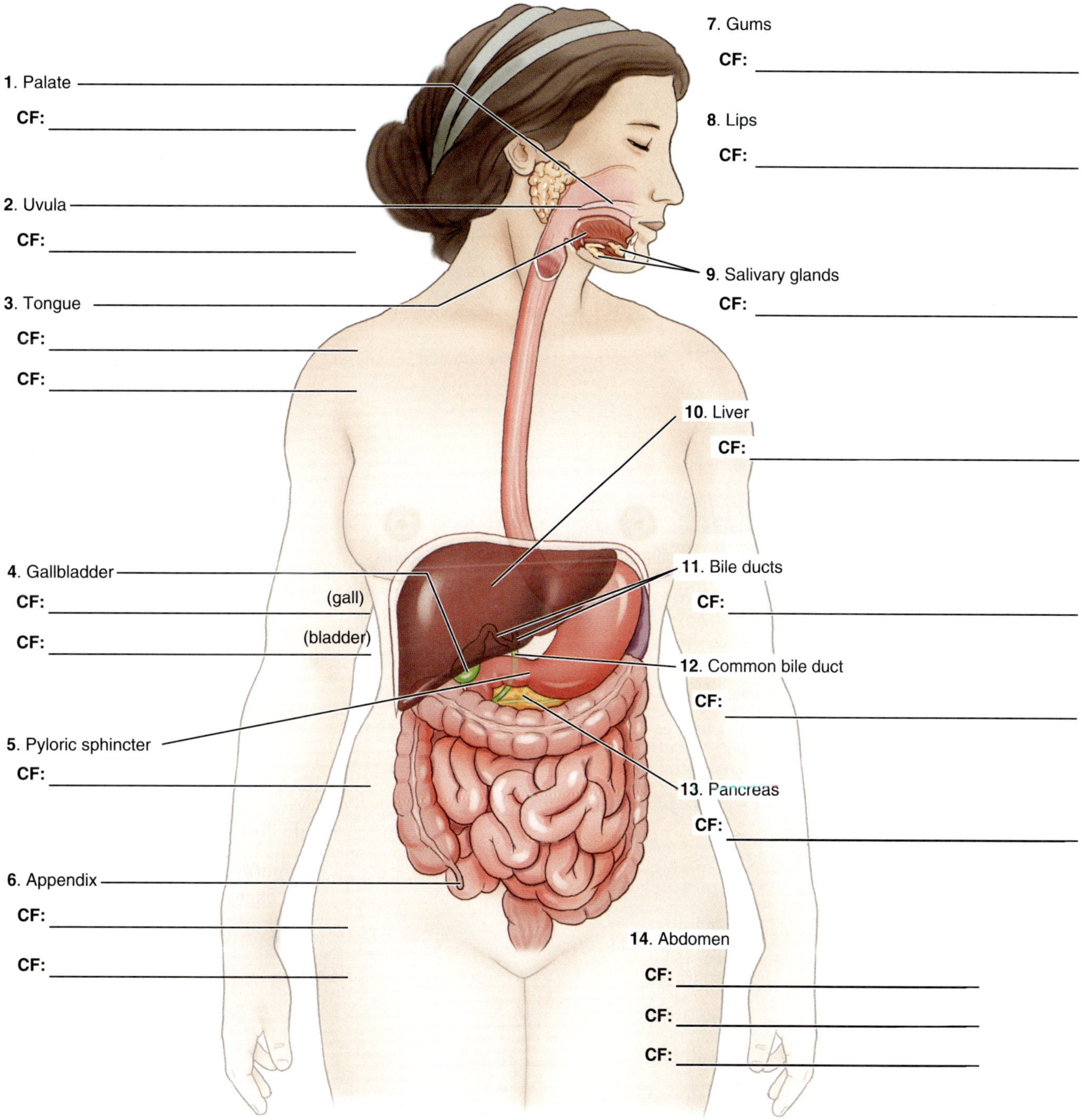

EXERCISE 5

Write the definitions of the following combining forms.

1. herni/o ____________
2. abdomin/o ____________
3. sial/o ____________
4. chol/e ____________
5. diverticul/o ____________
6. gingiv/o ____________
7. appendic/o ____________
8. gloss/o ____________
9. hepat/o ____________
10. cheil/o ____________
11. peritone/o ____________
12. palat/o ____________
13. pancreat/o ____________
14. lapar/o ____________
15. lingu/o ____________
16. choledoch/o ____________
17. pylor/o ____________
18. uvul/o ____________
19. cholangi/o ____________
20. polyp/o ____________
21. celi/o ____________
22. steat/o ____________
23. append/o ____________

EXERCISE 6

Write the combining form for each of the following.

1. palate ____________
2. saliva, salivary gland ____________
3. pancreas ____________
4. peritoneum ____________
5. tongue a. ____________ b. ____________
6. gum ____________
7. pylorus, pyloric sphincter ____________
8. liver ____________
9. gall, bile ____________
10. abdomen a. ____________ b. ____________ c. ____________
11. hernia ____________
12. diverticulum ____________
13. lip ____________
14. appendix a. ____________ b. ____________
15. uvula ____________
16. bile duct ____________
17. common bile duct ____________
18. small growth ____________
19. fat ____________

Prefix

Prefix	Definition
hemi-	half

Suffix

Suffix	Definition
-pepsia	digestion

Refer to **Appendix A** and **Appendix B** for a complete listing of word parts.

EXERCISE 7

Write the definition of the following prefix and suffix.

1. -pepsia ____________________
2. hemi- ____________________

EXERCISE 8

Write the prefix and suffix for the following definition.

1. digestion ____________________
2. half ____________________

EXERCISE FIGURE C

Fill in the blanks to complete labeling of the diagram.

1
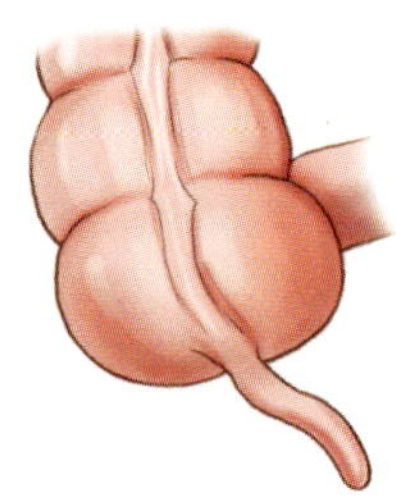

1. Normal appendix.

2
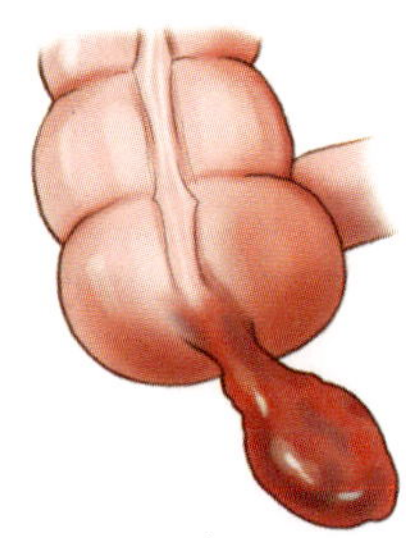

2. ______ / ______.
appendix / inflammation

MEDICAL TERMS

The terms you need to learn to complete this chapter are listed below. The exercises following each list will help you learn the definition and the spelling of each word.

For terms relating to nutrition, go to http://evolve.elsevier.com. Refer to p. 18 for your Evolve Access Information. Select **Appendices, Appendix J, Nutritional Terms**.

Disease and Disorder Terms

Built from Word Parts

The following terms are built from word parts you have already learned and can be translated literally to find their meanings. Further explanation of terms beyond the definition of their word parts, if needed, is included in parentheses.

Term	Definition
appendicitis (a-*pen*-di-SĪ-tis)	inflammation of the appendix (Exercise Figure C)
cholangioma (kō-LAN-jē-Ō-ma)	tumor of the bile duct

Disease and Disorder Terms—*cont'd*

Built from Word Parts

Term	Definition
cholecystitis (*kō*-lē-sis-TĪ-tis)	inflammation of the gallbladder
choledocholithiasis (kō-*led*-o-kō-li-THĪ-a-sis)	condition of stones in the common bile duct (Exercise Figure D)
cholelithiasis (*kō*-le-li-THĪ-a-sis)	condition of gallstones (Exercise Figure D)
diverticulitis (*dī*-ver-*tik*-ū-LĪ-tis)	inflammation of a diverticulum (see Figure 11-6)
diverticulosis (*dī*-ver-*tik*-ū-LŌ-sis)	abnormal condition of having diverticula (see Figures 11-6 and 11-17, *A*)
esophagitis (e-*sof*-a-JĪ-tis)	inflammation of the esophagus
gastritis (gas-TRĪ-tis)	inflammation of the stomach
gastroenteritis (*gas*-trō-*en*-te-RĪ-tis)	inflammation of the stomach and intestines

EXERCISE FIGURE D

Fill in the blanks to complete labeling of the diagram.

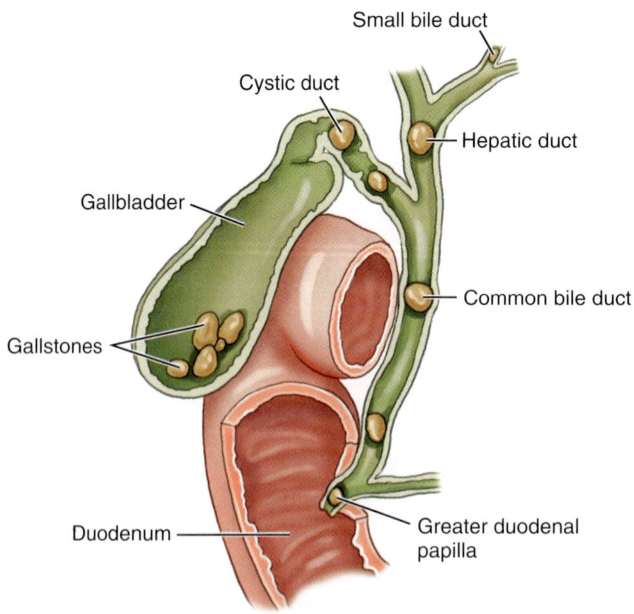

Common sites of

_____ / _____ / _____ / _____ and _____ / _____ / _____ / _____

gall / cv / stone / condition of   common bile duct / cv / stone / condition of

Term	Definition
gastroenterocolitis (*gas*-trō-*en*-ter-ō-kōl-Ī-tis)	inflammation of the stomach, intestines, and colon
gingivitis (*jin*-ji-VĪ-tis)	inflammation of the gums
hepatitis (*hep*-a-TĪ-tis)	inflammation of the liver
hepatoma (*hep*-a-TŌ-ma)	tumor of the liver
palatitis (*pal*-a-TĪ-tis)	inflammation of the palate
pancreatitis (*pan*-krē-a-TĪ-tis)	inflammation of the pancreas
peritonitis (*per*-i-tō-NĪ-tis) (NOTE: the *e* is dropped from the combining form peritone/o.)	inflammation of the peritoneum
polyposis (*pol*-i-PŌ-sis)	abnormal condition of (multiple) polyps (in the mucous membrane of the intestine, especially the colon; high potential for malignancy) (Figure 11-8)
proctoptosis (*prok*-top-TŌ-sis)	prolapse of the rectum
rectocele (REK-tō-sēl)	protrusion of the rectum
sialolith (sī-AL-ō-lith)	stone in the salivary gland
steatohepatitis (*stē*-a-tō-*hep*-a-TĪ-tis)	inflammation of the liver associated with (excess) fat; (often caused by alcohol abuse and obesity; over time may cause cirrhosis)
uvulitis (*ū*-vū-LĪ-tis)	inflammation of the uvula

NASH

or nonalcoholic **steatohepatitis** may occur in nonalcoholic patients who are obese and/or suffer from type 2 diabetes mellitus.

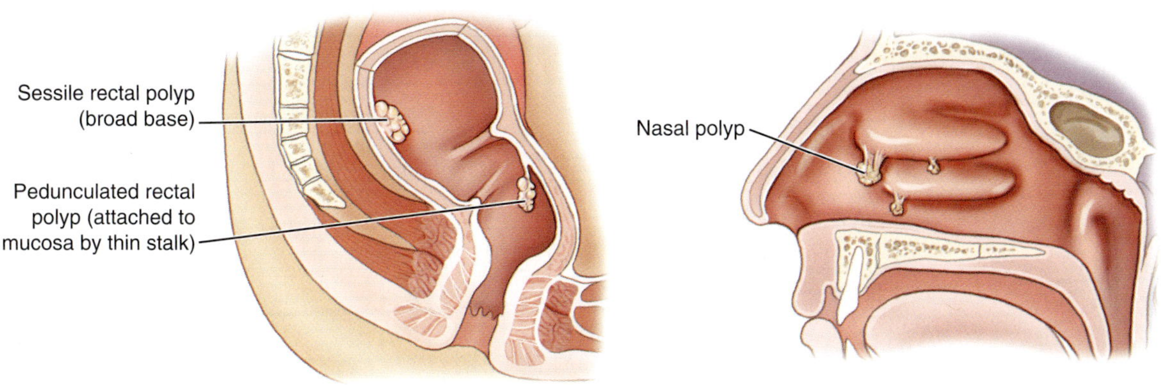

FIGURE 11-8
Polyp is a general term used to describe a protruding growth from a mucous membrane. Polyps are commonly found in the nose, uterus, intestines, and urinary bladder.

EXERCISE 9

Practice saying aloud each of the disease and disorder terms built from word parts on pp. 495-497.

To hear the terms, go to http://evolve.elsevier.com. Refer to p. 18 for your Evolve Access Information. Select Exercises & Review, Chapter 11, Chapter Exercises, Pronunciation.

☐ Place a check mark in the box when you have completed this exercise.

EXERCISE 10

Analyze and define the following terms.

1. cholelithiasis ____________________
2. diverticulosis ____________________
3. sialolith ____________________
4. hepatoma ____________________
5. uvulitis ____________________
6. pancreatitis ____________________
7. proctoptosis ____________________
8. gingivitis ____________________
9. gastritis ____________________
10. rectocele ____________________
11. palatitis ____________________
12. hepatitis ____________________
13. appendicitis ____________________
14. cholecystitis ____________________
15. diverticulitis ____________________
16. gastroenteritis ____________________
17. gastroenterocolitis ____________________
18. choledocholithiasis ____________________
19. cholangioma ____________________
20. polyposis ____________________
21. esophagitis ____________________
22. peritonitis ____________________
23. steatohepatitis ____________________

EXERCISE 11

Build disease and disorder terms for the following definitions by using the word parts you have learned.

1. tumor of the liver ________ / ________ (WR / S)
2. inflammation of the stomach ________ / ________ (WR / S)
3. stone in the salivary gland ________ / CV / ________ (WR / CV / WR)
4. inflammation of the appendix ________ / ________ (WR / S)
5. inflammation of a diverticulum ________ / ________ (WR / S)
6. inflammation of the gallbladder ________ / CV / ________ / ________ (WR / CV / WR / S)
7. abnormal condition of having diverticula ________ / ________ (WR / S)
8. inflammation of the stomach and intestines ________ / CV / ________ / ________ (WR / CV / WR / S)
9. prolapse of the rectum ________ / CV / ________ (WR / CV / S)
10. protrusion of the rectum ________ / CV / ________ (WR / CV / S)
11. inflammation of the uvula ________ / ________ (WR / S)
12. inflammation of the gums ________ / ________ (WR / S)
13. inflammation of the liver ________ / ________ (WR / S)
14. inflammation of the palate ________ / ________ (WR / S)
15. condition of gallstones ________ / CV / ________ / ________ (WR / CV / WR / S)
16. inflammation of the liver associated with (excess) fat ________ / CV / ________ / ________ (WR / CV / WR / S)
17. inflammation of the stomach, intestines, and colon ________ / CV / ________ / CV / ________ / ________ (WR / CV / WR / CV / WR / S)

18. inflammation of the pancreas ______ / ______
WR / S

19. tumor of the bile duct ______ / ______
WR / S

20. inflammation of the esophagus ______ / ______
WR / S

21. condition of stones in the common bile duct ______ / ______ / ______ / ______
WR / CV / WR / S

22. abnormal condition of (multiple) polyps ______ / ______
WR / S

23. inflammation of the peritoneum ______ / ______
WR / S

EXERCISE 12

Spell each of the disease and disorder terms built from word parts on pp. 495-497 by having someone dictate them to you.

To hear and spell the terms, go to http://evolve.elsevier.com. Refer to p. 18 for your Evolve Access Information. Select Exercises & Review, Chapter 11, Chapter Exercises, Spelling.

☐ Place a check mark in the box if you have completed this exercise online.

1. ______
2. ______
3. ______
4. ______
5. ______
6. ______
7. ______
8. ______
9. ______
10. ______
11. ______
12. ______
13. ______
14. ______
15. ______
16. ______
17. ______
18. ______
19. ______
20. ______
21. ______
22. ______
23. ______

Disease and Disorder Terms

Not Built from Word Parts

In some of the following terms, you may recognize word parts you have already learned; however, the full meaning of the terms cannot be discerned by the definition of their word parts.

Term	Definition
adhesion (ad-HĒ-zhun)	abnormal growing together of two surfaces that normally are separated. This may occur after abdominal surgery; surgical treatment is called **adhesiolysis** or **adhesiotomy** (Figure 11-9, *A*).
anorexia nervosa (*an*-ō-REK-sē-a) (ner-VŌ-sa)	eating disorder characterized by a prolonged refusal to eat, resulting in emaciation, amenorrhea in females, and abnormal fear of becoming obese. It occurs primarily in adolescents and young adults.
bulimia nervosa (bū-LĒ-mē-a) (ner-VŌ-sa)	an eating disorder involving gorging with food, followed by induced vomiting or laxative abuse (binging and purging)

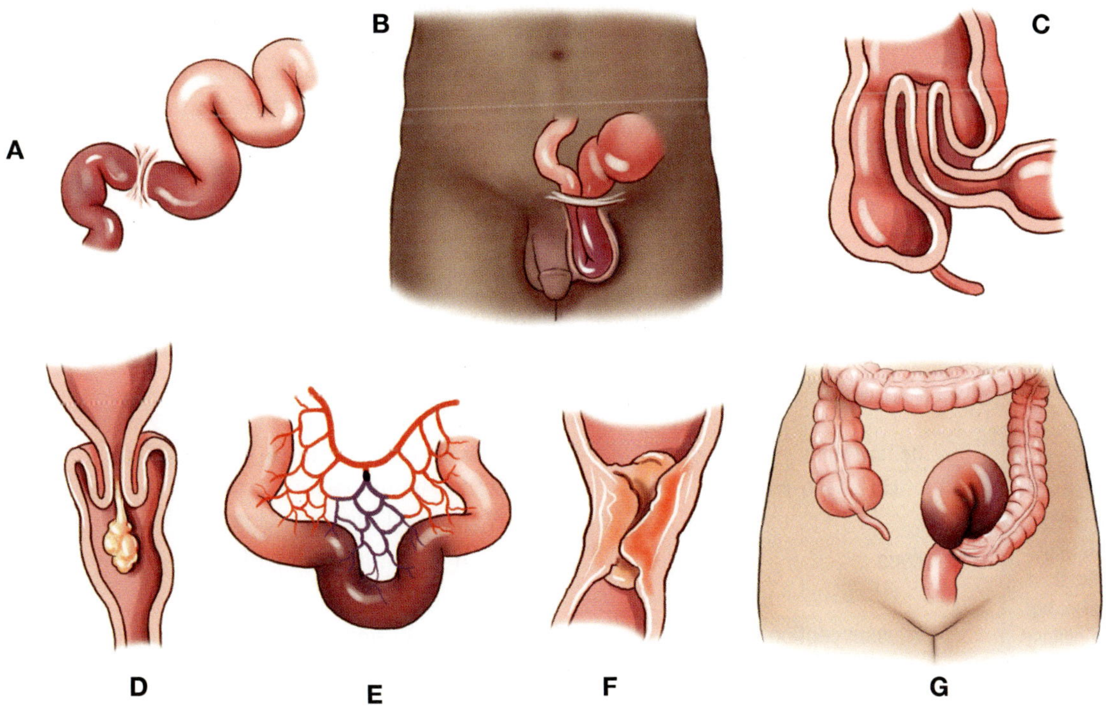

FIGURE 11-9
Causes of intestinal obstruction. **A**, Adhesions. **B**, Strangulated inguinal hernia. **C**, Ileocecal intussusception. **D**, Intussusception caused by polyps. **E**, Mesenteric vascular occlusion. **F**, Neoplasm. **G**, Volvulus of the sigmoid colon.

GASTROESOPHAGEAL REFLUX DISEASE (GERD)

is a common gastrointestinal disorder. The acidity of the regurgitated stomach contents causes irritation and inflammation of the esophagus (reflux esophagitis). **Barrett esophagus,** or cellular changes in the lower esophagus increasing the risk of cancer, may develop as a result of chronic GERD.

CAM TERM

Vitamin therapy is the use of nutrition, through diet and supplements, to decrease the incidence of disease and symptoms and to support wellness. Studies of probiotic therapies have shown promise in addressing a variety of gastrointestinal disturbances including **irritable bowel syndrome,** lactose intolerance, and alcohol-induced liver disease.

OBESITY

is when the BMI (body mass index) is greater than 30 kg/m^2. **Overweight** is defined as BMI between 25 and 29.9 kg/m^2. **Morbid obesity** is defined as BMI over 40 kg/m^2. BMI is calculated by dividing weight in kilograms by the square of height in meters (or by dividing weight in pounds by height in inches squared and then multiplying by 703).

Disease and Disorder Terms—*cont'd*

Not Built from Word Parts

Term	Definition
celiac disease (SĒ-lē-ak) (di-ZĒZ)	a malabsorption syndrome caused by an immune reaction to gluten (a protein in wheat, rye, and barley), which may damage the lining of the small intestine that is responsible for absorption of food into the bloodstream. Celiac disease is considered a multisystem disorder with varying symptoms, including abdominal bloating and pain, chronic diarrhea or constipation, steatorrhea, vomiting, weight loss, fatigue, iron deficiency anemia, and a pruritic skin rash known as dermatitis herpetiformis (also called **gluten enteropathy**).
cirrhosis (sir-RŌ-sis)	chronic disease of the liver with gradual destruction of cells and formation of scar tissue; commonly caused by alcoholism and certain types of viral hepatitis
Crohn disease (krōn) (di-ZĒZ)	chronic inflammation of the intestinal tract usually affecting the ileum and colon; characterized by cobblestone ulcerations and the formation of scar tissue that may lead to intestinal obstruction (also called **regional ileitis** or **regional enteritis.**)
gastroesophageal reflux disease (GERD) (gas-trō-e-sof-a-JĒ-al) (RĒ-fluks) (di-ZĒZ)	the abnormal backward flow of the gastrointestinal contents into the esophagus, causing heartburn and the gradual breakdown of the mucous barrier of the esophagus
hemochromatosis (hē-mō-krō-ma-TŌ-sis)	an iron metabolism disorder that occurs when too much iron is absorbed from food, resulting in excessive deposits of iron in the tissue; can cause congestive heart failure, diabetes, cirrhosis, or cancer of the liver
hemorrhoids (HEM-o-roydz)	swollen or distended veins in the rectal area, which may be internal or external, and can be a source of rectal bleeding (Figure 11-10)
ileus (IL-ē-us)	obstruction of the intestine, often caused by failure of peristalsis
intussusception (*in*-tu-sus-SEP-shun)	telescoping of a segment of the intestine (Figure 11-9, *C* and *D*)
irritable bowel syndrome (IBS) (IR-i-ta-bl) (BOW-el) (SIN-drōm)	periodic disturbances of bowel function, such as diarrhea and/or constipation, usually associated with abdominal pain
obesity (ō-BĒS-i-tē)	excess of body fat (not body weight)

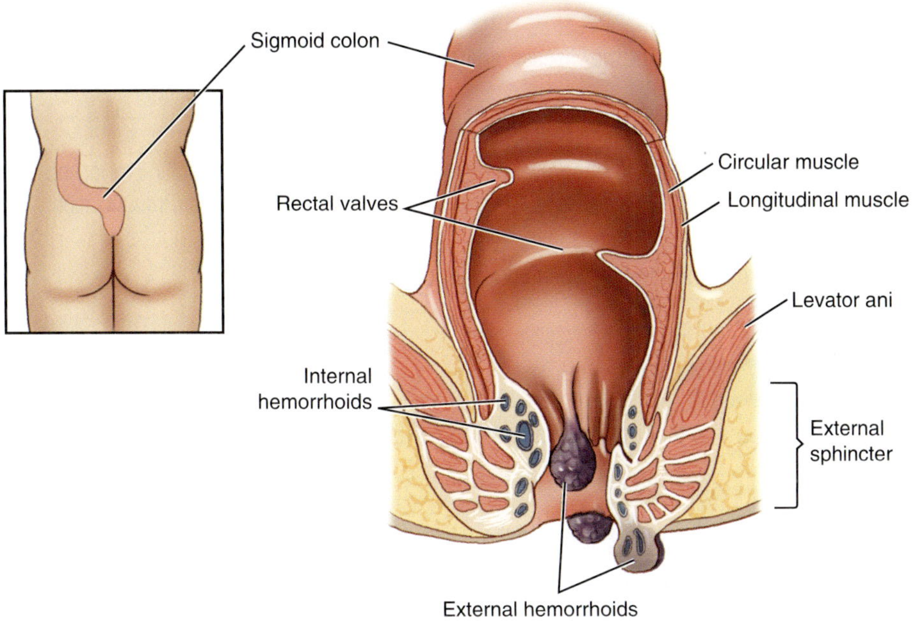

FIGURE 11-10
Hemorrhoids.

Term	Definition
peptic ulcer (PEP-tik) (UL-ser)	eroded area of the mucous membrane of the stomach or duodenum associated with increased secretion of acid from the stomach, bacterial infection (*H. pylori*), or nonsteroidal anti-inflammatory drugs (often referred to as **gastric** or **duodenal ulcer**, depending on its location)
polyp (POL-ip)	tumorlike growth extending outward from a mucous membrane; usually benign; common sites are in the nose, throat, and intestines (see Figures 11-8 and 11-14)
ulcerative colitis (UL-ser-a-tiv) (kō-LĪ-tis)	inflammation of the colon with the formation of ulcers. The main symptom is bloody diarrhea. An ileostomy may be performed to treat this condition.
volvulus (VOL-vū-lus)	twisting or kinking of the intestine, causing intestinal obstruction (see Figure 11-9, *G*)

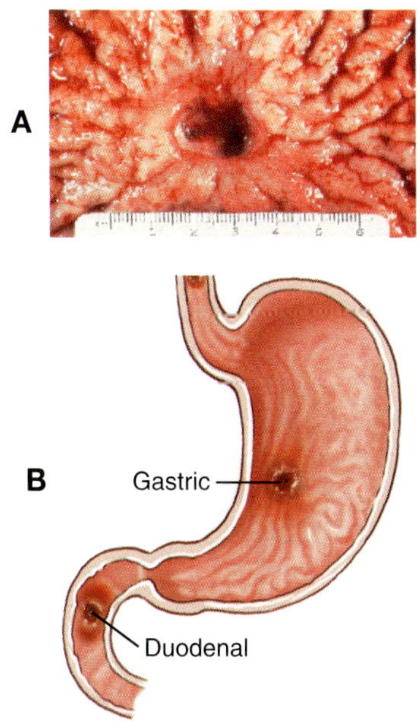

FIGURE 11-11
A. Peptic ulcer. B. Sites of peptic ulcers.

EXERCISE 13

Practice saying aloud each of the disease and disorder terms not built from word parts on pp. 501-503.

To hear the terms, go to http://evolve.elsevier.com. Refer to p. 18 for your Evolve Access Information. Select Exercises & Review, Chapter 11, Chapter Exercises, Pronunciation.

☐ Place a check mark in the box when you have completed this exercise.

EXERCISE 14

Match the definitions in the first column with the correct terms in the second column.

_____ 1. prolonged refusal to eat
_____ 2. chronic disease of the liver
_____ 3. chronic inflammation of the intestinal tract usually affecting the ileum and colon
_____ 4. abnormal growing together of two surfaces
_____ 5. twisted intestine
_____ 6. eroded area of the mucous membrane of the stomach or duodenum
_____ 7. telescoping of a segment of the intestine
_____ 8. tumorlike growth
_____ 9. formation of ulcers in the colon
_____ 10. eating disorder involving gorging food, followed by induced vomiting
_____ 11. obstruction of the intestine
_____ 12. periodic disturbance of bowel function
_____ 13. abnormal backward flow of the gastrointestinal contents into the esophagus
_____ 14. excess of body fat
_____ 15. malabsorption syndrome caused by an immune reaction to gluten
_____ 16. swollen or distended veins in the rectal area
_____ 17. an iron metabolism disorder

a. intussusception
b. cirrhosis
c. gastroesophageal reflux disease
d. volvulus
e. Crohn disease
f. anorexia nervosa
g. peptic ulcer
h. ulcerative colitis
i. irritable bowel syndrome
j. bulimia nervosa
k. polyp
l. obesity
m. ileus
n. adhesion
o. celiac disease
p. hemorrhoids
q. hemochromatosis

EXERCISE 15

Write the definitions of the following terms.

1. peptic ulcer ______
2. anorexia nervosa ______
3. Crohn disease ______
4. volvulus ______
5. adhesion ______
6. cirrhosis ______
7. intussusception ______
8. celiac disease ______
9. ulcerative colitis ______
10. bulimia nervosa ______
11. hemorrhoids ______
12. polyp ______
13. irritable bowel syndrome ______
14. ileus ______
15. gastroesophageal reflux disease ______
16. obesity ______
17. hemochromatosis ______

EXERCISE 16

Spell each of the disease and disorder terms not built from word parts on pp. 501-503 by having someone dictate them to you.

To hear and spell the terms, go to http://evolve.elsevier.com. Refer to p. 18 for your Evolve Access Information. Select Exercises & Review, Chapter 11, Chapter Exercises, Spelling.
☐ Place a check mark in the box if you have completed this exercise online.

1. ______
2. ______
3. ______
4. ______
5. ______
6. ______
7. ______
8. ______
9. ______
10. ______
11. ______
12. ______
13. ______
14. ______
15. ______
16. ______
17. ______

Surgical Terms

Built from Word Parts

The following terms are built from word parts you have already learned and can be translated literally to find their meanings. Further explanation of terms beyond the definition of their word parts, if needed, is included in parentheses.

CHOLECYSTECTOMY

was first performed in 1882 by a German surgeon. **Laparoscopic cholecystectomy** was first performed in 1987 in France.

Term	Definition
abdominocentesis (ab-*dom*-i-nō-sen-TĒ-sis)	surgical puncture to remove fluid from the abdominal cavity (also called **paracentesis**)
abdominoplasty (ab-DOM-i-nō-*plas*-tē)	surgical repair of the abdomen
anoplasty (Ā-nō-*plas*-tē)	surgical repair of the anus
antrectomy (an-TREK-to-mē)	excision of the antrum
appendectomy (*ap*-en-DEK-to-mē)	excision of the appendix
celiotomy (*sē*-lē-OT-o-mē)	incision into the abdominal cavity
cheilorrhaphy (kī-LOR-a-fē)	suture of the lip
cholecystectomy (*kō*-le-sis-TEK-to-mē)	excision of the gallbladder (Figure 11-12)
choledocholithotomy (kō-*led*-o-kō-li-THOT-o-mē)	incision into the common bile duct to remove a stone
colectomy (kō-LEK-to-mē)	excision of the colon
colostomy (ko-LOS-to-mē)	creation of an artificial opening into the colon (through the abdominal wall). (Used for the passage of stool. A colostomy, which creates a mouthlike opening on the abdominal wall called a **stoma**, may be permanent or temporary; performed as treatment for bowel obstruction, cancer, or diverticulitis.) (Exercise Figure E)
diverticulectomy (*dī*-ver-*tik*-ū-LEK-to-mē)	excision of a diverticulum
enterorrhaphy (*en*-ter-OR-a-fē)	suture of the intestine
esophagogastroplasty (e-*sof*-a-gō-GAS-trō-*plas*-tē)	surgical repair of the esophagus and the stomach

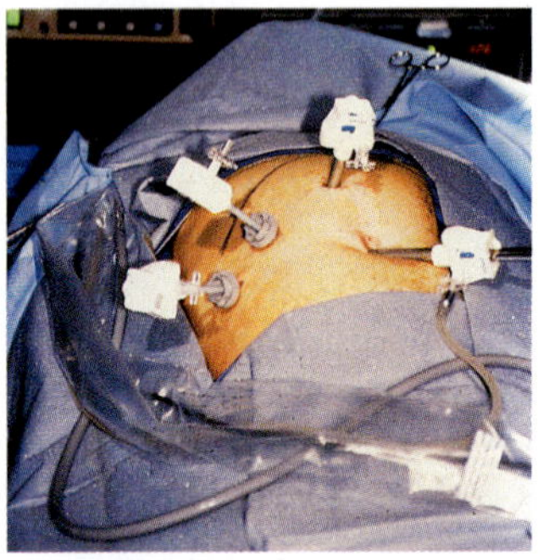

FIGURE 11-12
In laparoscopic cholecystectomy, a type of endoscopic surgery, CO_2 is used to insufflate the surgical area for better visualization. A small incision is made in the folds of the umbilicus for the insertion of the laparoscope. Three additional small incisions are made for the insertion of operative sheaths to accommodate accessory instrumentation. **Polypectomy, adhesiolysis, bariatric surgery, herniorrhaphy,** and **splenectomy** may also be performed using endoscopic surgery rather than large incision surgery.

EXERCISE FIGURE E

Fill in the blanks to complete labeling of the diagram.

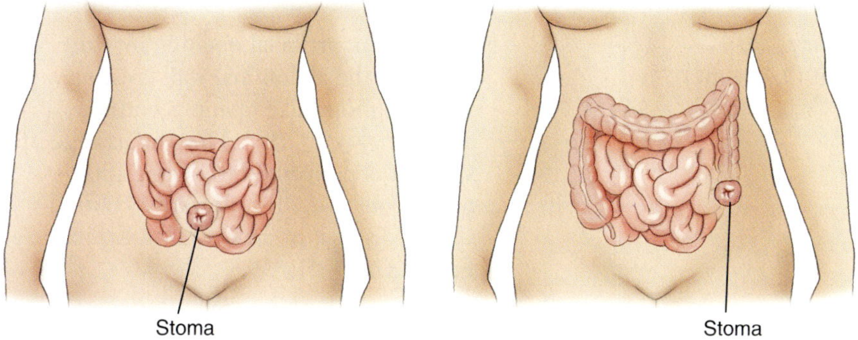

1. ______ / ______ / ______ after total colectomy.
   ileum / cv / creation of an artificial opening

2. ______ / ______ / ______ after abdominoperineal resection.
   colon / cv / creation of an artificial opening

EXERCISE FIGURE F

Fill in the blanks to label the diagram.

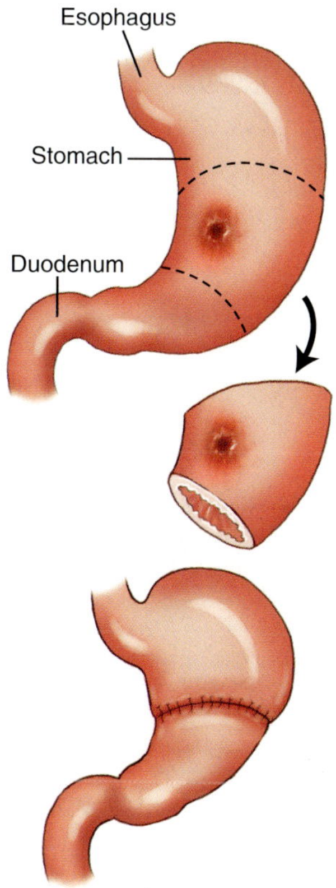

______ / ______
stomach / surgical removal

Term	Definition
gastrectomy (gas-TREK-to-mē)	excision of the stomach (or part of the stomach) (Exercise Figure F)
gastrojejunostomy (*gas*-trō-je-jū-NOS-to-mē)	creation of an artificial opening between the stomach and jejunum
gastroplasty (GAS-trō-*plas*-tē)	surgical repair of the stomach (see Table 11-1)
gastrostomy (gas-TROS-to-mē)	creation of an artificial opening into the stomach (through the abdominal wall). (A tube is inserted through the opening for administration of food when swallowing is impossible.) (Figure 11-13)
gingivectomy (*jin*-ji-VEK-to-mē)	surgical removal of gum (tissue)
glossorrhaphy (glo-SOR-a-fē)	suture of the tongue
hemicolectomy (*hem*-ē-kō-LEK-to-mē)	excision of half of the colon
herniorrhaphy (*her*-nē-OR-a-fē)	suturing of a hernia (for repair)

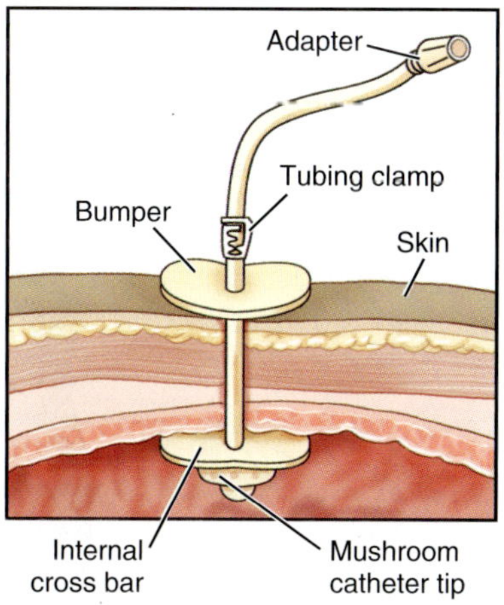

FIGURE 11-13
Percutaneous endoscopic gastrostomy (PEG) was first described in 1980. It is an alternative to **traditional gastrostomy**. An **endoscope** is used to place a tube in the stomach. Cost and discomfort to the patient are reduced when **PEG** is used instead of traditional gastrostomy.

Surgical Terms—*cont'd*

Built from Word Parts

Term	Definition
ileostomy (*il*-ē-OS-to-mē)	creation of an artificial opening into the ileum (through the abdominal wall creating a stoma, a mouthlike opening on the abdominal wall). (Used for the passage of stool. It is performed following total proctocolectomy for ulcerative colitis, Crohn disease, or cancer.) (see Exercise Figure E)
laparotomy (*lap*-a-ROT-o-mē)	incision into the abdominal cavity
palatoplasty (PAL-a-tō-*plas*-tē)	surgical repair of the palate
polypectomy (*pol*-i-PEK-to-mē)	excision of a polyp (Figure 11-14)
pyloromyotomy (pī-*lor*-ō-mī-OT-o-mē)	incision into the pyloric muscle
pyloroplasty (pī-LOR-ō-*plas*-tē)	surgical repair of the pylorus
uvulectomy (*ū*-vū-LEK-to-mē)	excision of the uvula
uvulopalatopharyngoplasty (UPPP) (*ū*-vū-lō-*pal*-a-*tō*-fa-RING-gō-*plas*-tē)	surgical repair of the uvula, palate, and pharynx (performed to correct obstructive sleep apnea) (see Figure 5-7)

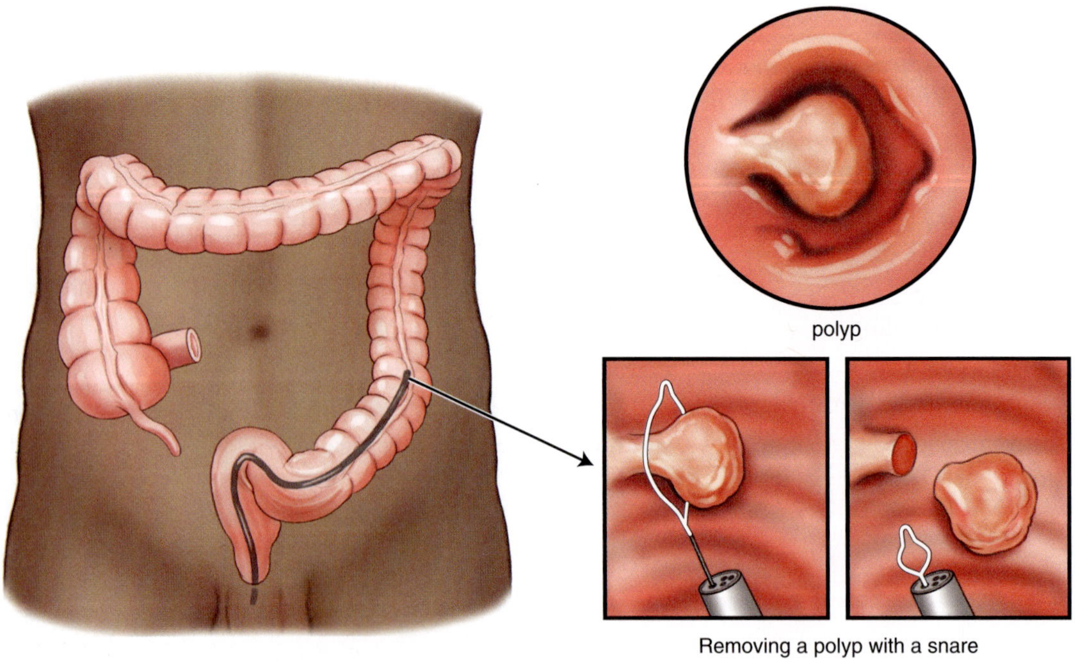

FIGURE 11-14
Polypectomy performed using a colonoscope.

EXERCISE 17

Practice saying aloud each of the surgical terms built from word parts on pp. 506-508.

To hear the terms, go to http://evolve.elsevier.com. Refer to p. 18 for your Evolve Access Information. Select Exercises & Review, Chapter 11, Chapter Exercises, Pronunciation.

☐ Place a check mark in the box when you have completed this exercise.

EXERCISE 18

Analyze and define the following surgical terms.

1. gastrectomy ______
2. esophagogastroplasty ______
3. diverticulectomy ______
4. antrectomy ______
5. palatoplasty ______
6. uvulectomy ______
7. gastrojejunostomy ______
8. cholecystectomy ______
9. colectomy ______
10. colostomy ______
11. pyloroplasty ______
12. anoplasty ______
13. appendectomy ______

14. cheilorrhaphy ______________________________
15. gingivectomy ______________________________
16. laparotomy ______________________________
17. ileostomy ______________________________
18. gastrostomy ______________________________
19. herniorrhaphy ______________________________
20. glossorrhaphy ______________________________
21. choledocholithotomy ______________________________
22. hemicolectomy ______________________________
23. polypectomy ______________________________
24. enterorrhaphy ______________________________
25. abdominoplasty ______________________________
26. pyloromyotomy ______________________________
27. uvulopalatopharyngoplasty ______________________________
28. celiotomy ______________________________
29. gastroplasty ______________________________
30. abdominocentesis ______________________________

EXERCISE 19

Build surgical terms for the following definitions by using the word parts you have learned.

1. excision of the appendix ________ / ________
   WR / S
2. suture of the tongue ________ /CV/ ________
   WR / CV / S
3. surgical repair of the esophagus and stomach ________ /CV/ ________ /CV/ ________
   WR / CV / WR / CV / S
4. excision of a diverticulum ________ / ________
   WR / S
5. artificial opening into the ileum ________ /CV/ ________
   WR / CV / S
6. surgical removal of gum tissue ________ / ________
   WR / S
7. incision into the abdominal cavity
   a. ________ /CV/ ________
   WR / CV / S
   b. ________ /CV/ ________
   WR / CV / S
8. surgical repair of the anus ________ /CV/ ________
   WR / CV / S
9. excision of the antrum ________ / ________
   WR / S
10. excision of the gallbladder ________ /CV/ ________ / ________
    WR / CV / WR / S
11. excision of the colon ________ / ________
    WR / S
12. creation of an artificial opening into the colon ________ /CV/ ________
    WR / CV / S
13. excision of the stomach ________ / ________
    WR / S
14. creation of an artificial opening into the stomach ________ /CV/ ________
    WR / CV / S
15. creation of an artificial opening between the stomach and jejunum ________ /CV/ ________ /CV/ ________
    WR / CV / WR / CV / S

16. excision of the uvula ______ / ______
WR / S

17. surgical repair of the palate ______ /CV/ ______
WR /CV/ S

18. surgical repair of the pylorus ______ /CV/ ______
WR /CV/ S

19. suture of a hernia ______ /CV/ ______
WR /CV/ S

20. suture of the lip ______ /CV/ ______
WR /CV/ S

21. excision of half of the colon ______ / ______ / ______
P / WR / S

22. incision into the common bile duct to remove a stone ______ /CV/ ______ /CV/ ______
WR /CV/ WR /CV/ S

23. excision of a polyp ______ / ______
WR / S

24. suture of the intestine ______ /CV/ ______
WR /CV/ S

25. surgical repair of the abdomen ______ /CV/ ______
WR /CV/ S

26. incision into the pylorus muscle ______ /CV/ ______ /CV/ ______
WR /CV/ WR /CV/ S

27. surgical repair of the uvula, palate, and pharynx ______ /CV/ ______ /CV/ ______ /CV/ ______
WR /CV/ WR /CV/ WR /CV/ S

28. surgical repair of the stomach ______ /CV/ ______
WR /CV/ S

29. surgical puncture to remove fluid from the abdominal cavity ______ /CV/ ______
WR /CV/ S

EXERCISE 20

Spell each of the surgical terms built from word parts on pp. 506-508 by having someone dictate them to you.

To hear and spell the terms, go to http://evolve.elsevier.com. Refer to p. 18 for your Evolve Access Information. Select Exercises & Review, Chapter 11, Chapter Exercises, Spelling.
☐ Place a check mark in the box if you have completed this exercise online.

1. ______________	16. ______________
2. ______________	17. ______________
3. ______________	18. ______________
4. ______________	19. ______________
5. ______________	20. ______________
6. ______________	21. ______________
7. ______________	22. ______________
8. ______________	23. ______________
9. ______________	24. ______________
10. ______________	25. ______________
11. ______________	26. ______________
12. ______________	27. ______________
13. ______________	28. ______________
14. ______________	29. ______________
15. ______________	30. ______________

Surgical Terms

Not Built from Word Parts

In some of the following terms, you may recognize word parts you have already learned; however, the full meaning of the terms cannot be discerned by the definition of their word parts.

Term	Definition
abdominoperineal resection (A&P resection) (ab-*dom*-i-nō-per-i-NĒ-el) (rē-SEK-shun)	removal of the distal colon and rectum through both abdominal and perineal approaches; performed to treat colorectal cancer and inflammatory diseases of the lower large intestine. The patient will have a colostomy. (see Exercise Figure E, *2*)

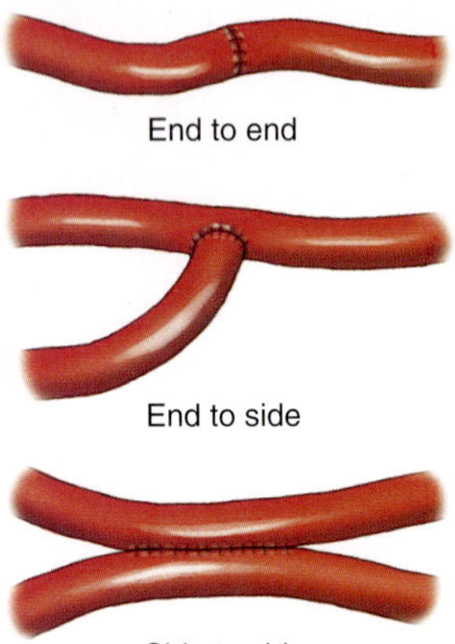

FIGURE 11-15
Types of anastomoses.

Surgical Terms—*cont'd*

Not Built from Word Parts

Term	Definition
anastomosis (*pl.* **anastomoses**) (a-*nas*-to-MŌ-sis) (a-*nas*-to-MŌ-sēz)	an opening created by surgically joining two structures, such as blood vessels or bowel segments (Figure 11-15)
bariatric surgery (*bar*-ē-AT-rik) (SUR-jer-ē)	surgical reduction of gastric capacity to treat morbid obesity causing serious illness (Table 11-1)
hemorrhoidectomy (*hem*-o-royd-EK-to-mē)	excision of hemorrhoids, the swollen or distended veins in the rectal region
vagotomy (vā-GOT-o-mē)	cutting of certain branches of the vagus nerve, performed with gastric surgery to reduce the amount of gastric acid produced and thus reduce the recurrence of ulcers

BARIATRIC

contains the word roots **bar**, meaning **weight**, and **iatr**, meaning **treatment**.

EXERCISE 21

Practice saying aloud each of the surgical terms not built from word parts on pp. 513-514.

To hear the terms, go to http://evolve.elsevier.com. Refer to p. 18 for your Evolve Access Information. Select Exercises & Review, Chapter 11, Chapter Exercises, Pronunciation.

☐ Place a check mark in the box when you have completed this exercise.

EXERCISE 22

Write the term for each of the following definitions.

1. cutting certain branches of the vagus nerve ______________________
2. opening created by surgically joining two structures ______________________
3. removal of the distal colon and rectum ______________________
4. surgical reduction of gastric capacity to treat morbid obesity ______________________
5. excision of the swollen or distended veins in the rectal region ______________________

TABLE 11-1
Bariatric Surgery

Bariatric surgery may be used to treat morbid obesity for patients with a BMI greater than 40 or those with a BMI greater than 35 associated with a serious medical condition. During surgery, a small stomach pouch is created for the purpose of restricting the amount of food an individual can eat. The following are three types of surgeries performed.

Roux-en-Y Gastric Bypass (RYGB)

Creation of a small gastric pouch with drainage of food to the rest of the gastrointestinal tract through a restricted stoma; the duodenum and part of the jejunum are bypassed. RYGB, the most common form of bariatric surgery performed in the United States, restricts food intake and calorie absorption rate.

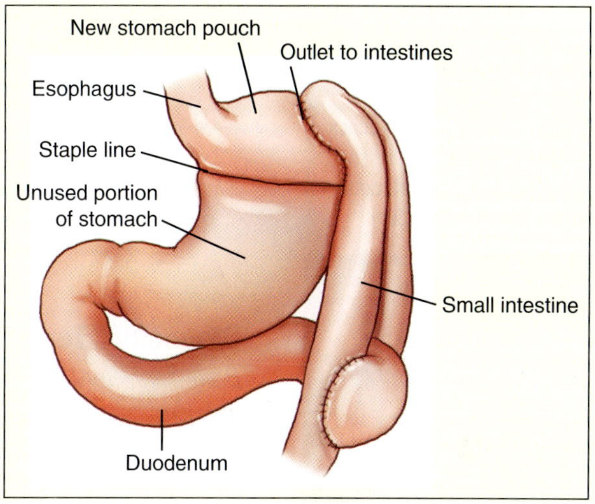

Vertical Banded Gastroplasty (VBG)

Creation of a small gastric pouch with a vertical line of staples and the connection of a band for the drainage of food into the small intestine; also called stomach stapling.

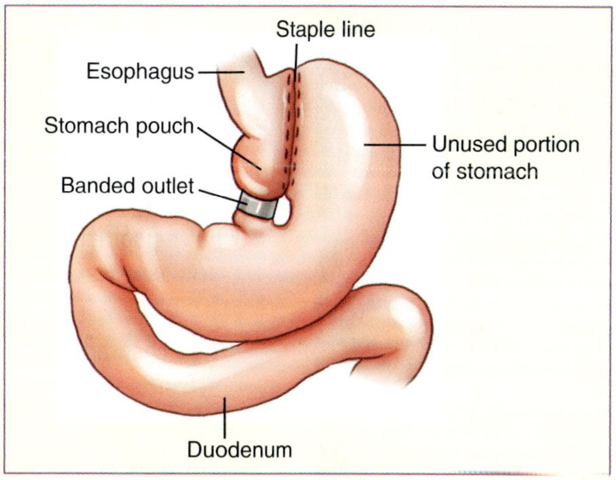

Laparoscopic Adjustable Gastric Banding (LAGB)

Creation of a small gastric pouch by the placement of a band around the upper portion of the stomach; the band can be adjusted to change the size of the stomach through a subcutaneous port.

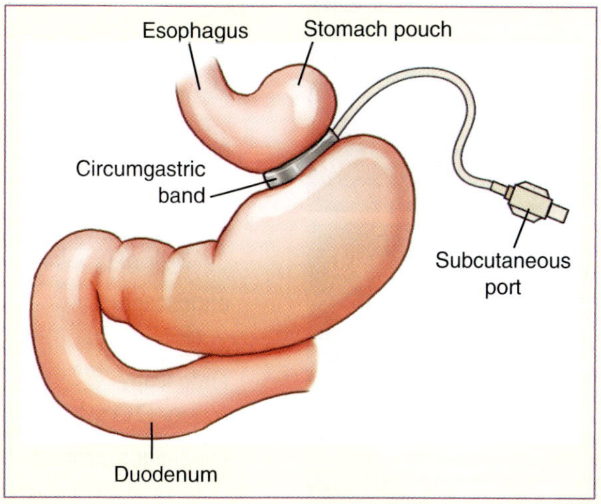

OPERATIVE CHOLANGIOGRAPHY

is performed during surgery to check for residual stones after the removal of the gallbladder. Postoperative cholangiography, also called T-tube cholangiography, is performed in the radiology department after a cholecystectomy, also to check for residual stones. Both use the injection of contrast media into the common bile duct.

A

B

C

D

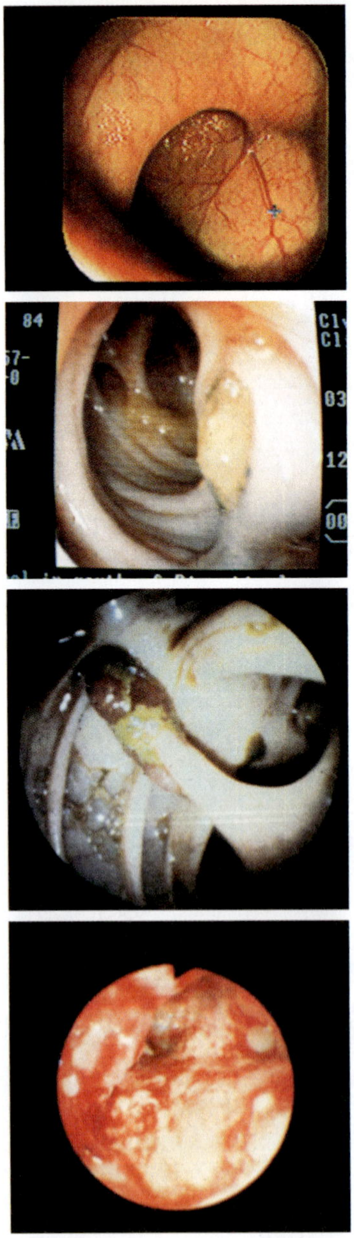

FIGURE 11-16
Images obtained during colonoscopy reveal normal colon **(A),** diverticulosis **(B),** colon polyp **(C),** and colon cancer **(D).**

EXERCISE 23

Spell each of the surgical terms not built from word parts on pp. 513-514 by having someone dictate them to you.

To hear and spell the terms, go to http://evolve.elsevier.com. Refer to p. 18 for your Evolve Access Information. Select Exercises & Review, Chapter 11, Chapter Exercises, Spelling.
☐ Place a check mark in the box if you have completed this exercise online.

1. ______________________
2. ______________________
3. ______________________
4. ______________________
5. ______________________

Diagnostic Terms

Built from Word Parts

The following terms are built from word parts you have already learned and can be translated literally to find their meanings. Further explanation of terms beyond the definition of their word parts, if needed, is included in parentheses.

Term	Definition
DIAGNOSTIC IMAGING	
cholangiogram (kō-LAN-jē-ō-gram)	radiographic image of bile ducts
cholangiography (kō-*lan*-jē-OG-ra-fē)	radiographic imaging of the bile ducts (after administration of contrast media to outline the ducts)
CT colonography (*kō*-lon-OG-ra-fē)	radiographic imaging of the colon (using a CT scanner and software)
esophagogram (e-SOF-a-gō-gram)	radiographic image of the esophagus. (Barium is used as contrast media; also called **esophagram** and **barium swallow**)
ENDOSCOPY	
colonoscope (kō-LON-ō-skōp)	instrument used for visual examination of the colon (see Figure 11-14)
colonoscopy (*kō*-lon-OS-ko-pē)	visual examination of the colon (see Figures 11-16 and 11-17)
endoscope (EN-dō-skōp)	instrument used for visual examination within a hollow organ
endoscopy (en-DOS-ko-pē)	visual examination within a hollow organ (Figure 11-18)
esophagogastroduodenoscopy (EGD) (*e-sof*-a-gō-*gas*-trō-*dū*-od-e-NOS-ko-pē)	visual examination of the esophagus, stomach, and duodenum
esophagoscopy (e-*sof*-a-GOS-ko-pē)	visual examination of the esophagus
gastroscope (GAS-trō-skōp)	instrument used for visual examination of the stomach (Exercise Figure G)

Term	Definition
gastroscopy (gas-TROS-ko-pē)	visual examination of the stomach (Exercise Figure G)
laparoscope (LAP-a-rō-skōp)	instrument used for visual examination of the abdominal cavity. (Also used to perform laparoscopic surgery, a method that sometimes replaces **laparotomy,** open abdominal incisional surgery.) (See Figure 11-12)
laparoscopy (*lap*-a-ROS-ko-pē)	visual examination of the abdominal cavity

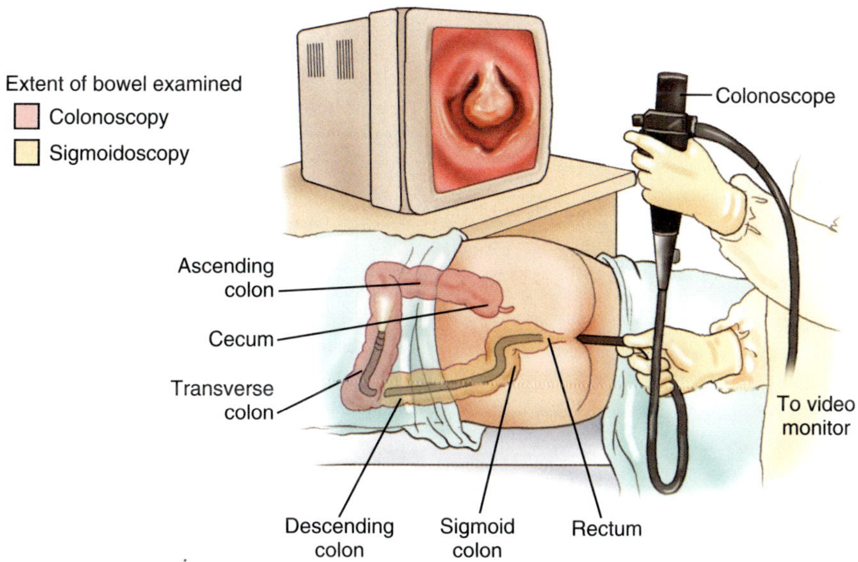

FIGURE 11-17
Sigmoidoscopy, colonoscopy.

COMPUTED TOMOGRAPHY (CT) COLONOGRAPHY

also called **virtual colonoscopy**, is a new method to test for colon polyps and colon cancer. It involves using a CT scanner and computer software that allows the physician to see the colon in multiple dimensions. It is less invasive than the conventional method of colonoscopy to screen for colon cancer.

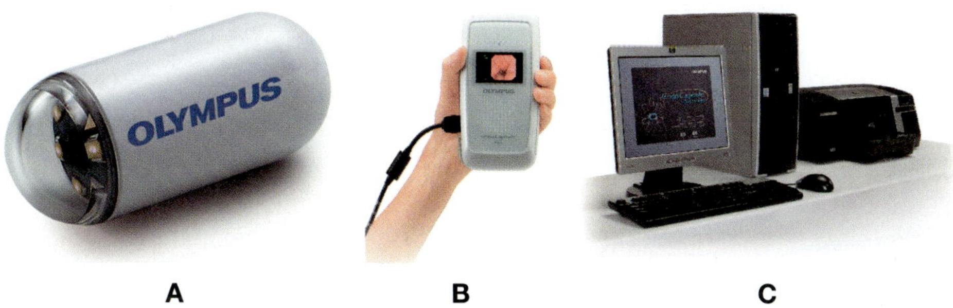

FIGURE 11-18
CAPSULE ENDOSCOPY, also known as **camera endoscopy**, was approved for use in 2001 by the Food and Drug Administration. **(A)** Patients swallow a capsule containing a camera, about the size of a large vitamin pill. Pictures are taken by the camera every second as it moves naturally through the digestive tract. **(B)** The images are recorded on a small device worn around the patient's waist. The recorded device is returned to the physician's office after 8 hours. **(C)** The images are transferred to a computer and examined. The video capsule is expelled in the bowel movement and not retrieved.

Capsule endoscopy replaces the standard endoscopy performed by pushing an endoscopic tube through the small intestine. It is especially helpful in identifying the cause of obscure intestinal bleeding, and diagnosing the causes of abdominal pain.

Diagnostic Terms—*cont'd*

Built from Word Parts

Term	Definition
proctoscope (PROK-tō-skōp)	instrument used for visual examination of the rectum
proctoscopy (prok-TOS-ko-pē)	visual examination of the rectum
sigmoidoscopy (*sig*-moy-DOS-ko-pē)	visual examination of the sigmoid colon (see Figure 11-17)

EXERCISE FIGURE G

Fill in the blanks to complete labeling of the diagram.

A

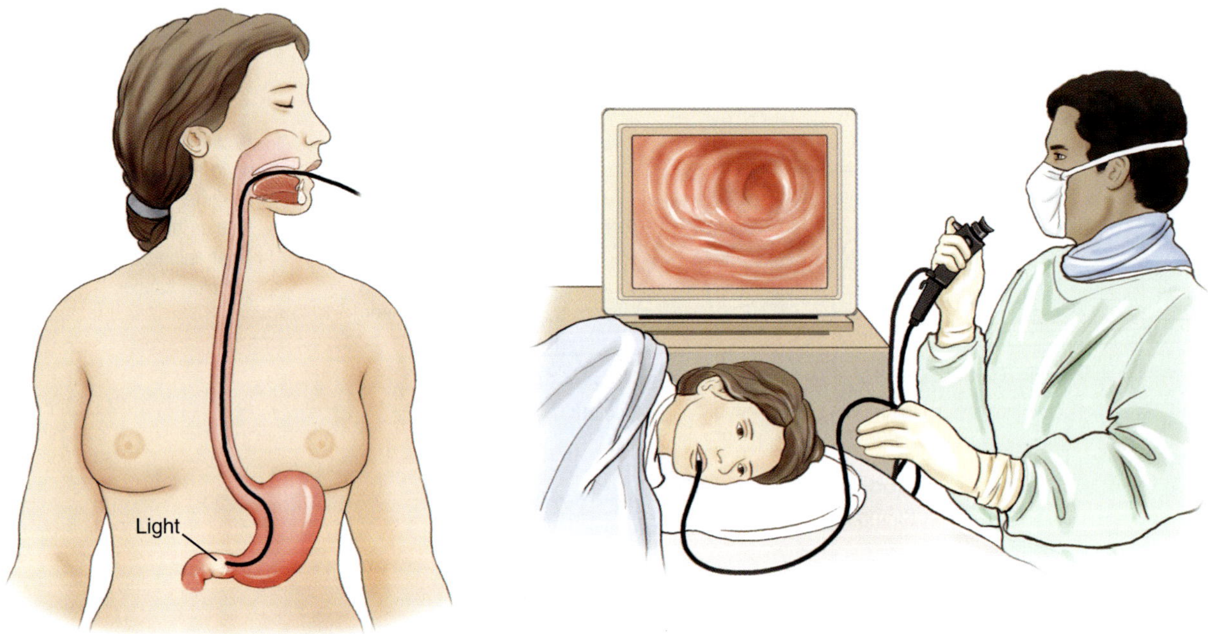

A, ______ / ______ / ______
stomach / cv / visual examination

B

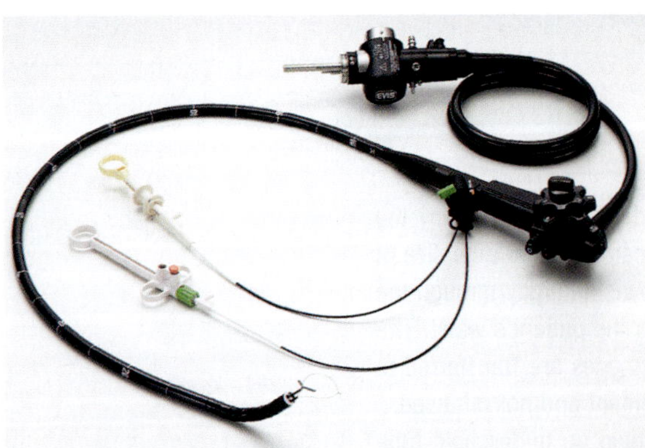

B, Fiberscope, a type of ______ / ______ / ______ that
stomach / cv / instrument used for visual examination
has glass fibers in a flexible tube, allows for light to be transmitted back to the examiner.

EXERCISE 24

Practice saying aloud each of the diagnostic terms built from word parts on pp. 516-518.

To hear the terms, go to http://evolve.elsevier.com. Refer to p. 18 for your Evolve Access Information. Select Exercises & Review, Chapter 11, Chapter Exercises, Pronunciation.

☐ Place a check mark in the box when you have completed this exercise.

EXERCISE 25

Analyze and define the following diagnostic terms.

1. esophagoscopy ______________________________
2. gastroscope ______________________________
3. gastroscopy ______________________________
4. proctoscope ______________________________
5. proctoscopy ______________________________
6. endoscope ______________________________
7. endoscopy ______________________________
8. sigmoidoscopy ______________________________
9. cholangiogram ______________________________
10. esophagogastroduodenoscopy ______________________________
11. colonoscope ______________________________
12. laparoscope ______________________________
13. colonoscopy ______________________________
14. laparoscopy ______________________________
15. CT colonography ______________________________
16. esophagogram ______________________________
17. cholangiography ______________________________

EXERCISE 26

Build diagnostic terms that correspond to the following definitions by using the word parts you have learned.

1. visual examination within a hollow organ
   ______ / ______
   P / S(WR)
2. instrument used for visual examination of the stomach
   ______ /CV/ ______
   WR /CV/ S
3. instrument used for visual examination of the rectum
   ______ /CV/ ______
   WR /CV/ S
4. instrument used for visual examination within a hollow organ
   ______ / ______
   P / S(WR)
5. visual examination of the rectum
   ______ /CV/ ______
   WR /CV/ S
6. visual examination of the esophagus
   ______ /CV/ ______
   WR /CV/ S
7. visual examination of the sigmoid colon
   ______ /CV/ ______
   WR /CV/ S
8. radiographic image of bile ducts
   ______ /CV/ ______
   WR /CV/ S
9. visual examination of the stomach
   ______ /CV/ ______
   WR /CV/ S
10. instrument used for visual examination of the abdominal cavity
    ______ /CV/ ______
    WR /CV/ S
11. visual examination of the esophagus, stomach, and duodenum
    ______ /CV/ ______ /CV/ ______ /CV/ ______
    WR /CV/ WR /CV/ WR /CV/ S
12. visual examination of the colon
    ______ /CV/ ______
    WR /CV/ S

13. visual examination of the abdominal cavity ______ WR / CV / ______ S

14. instrument used for visual examination of the colon ______ WR / CV / ______ S

15. radiographic imaging of the colon CT ______ WR / CV / ______ S

16. radiographic imaging of the bile ducts ______ WR / CV / ______ S

17. radiographic image of the esophagus ______ WR / CV / ______ S

EXERCISE 27

Spell each of the diagnostic terms built from word parts on pp. 516-518 by having someone dictate them to you.

To hear and spell the terms, go to http://evolve.elsevier.com. Refer to p. 18 for your Evolve Access Information. Select Exercises & Review, Chapter 11, Chapter Exercises, Spelling.
☐ Place a check mark in the box if you have completed this exercise online.

1. ______
2. ______
3. ______
4. ______
5. ______
6. ______
7. ______
8. ______
9. ______
10. ______
11. ______
12. ______
13. ______
14. ______
15. ______
16. ______
17. ______

Diagnostic Terms

Not Built from Word Parts

In some of the following terms, you may recognize word parts you have already learned; however, the full meaning of the terms cannot be discerned by the definition of their word parts.

Term	Definition
DIAGNOSTIC IMAGING	
abdominal ultrasonography (ab-DOM-i-nal) (*ul*-tra-so-NOG-ra-fē)	process of recording images of internal organs using high-frequency sound waves produced by a transducer placed directly on the skin covering the abdominal cavity. Images may be viewed on a monitor and/or recorded for later use. The size and structure of organs such as the aorta, liver, gallbladder, bile ducts, and pancreas can be visualized. Liver cysts, abscesses, tumors, cholelithiasis, pancreatitis, and pancreatic tumors may be detected. May also be used to evaluate the kidneys and the portion of the aorta extending through the abdominal cavity (Table 11-2).
barium enema (BE) (BAR-ē-um) (EN-e-ma)	series of radiographic images taken of the large intestine after the contrast agent barium has been administered rectally (also called **lower GI series**) (Figure 11-19)
endoscopic retrograde cholangiopancreatography (ERCP) (*en*-dō-SKOP-ic) (RET-rō-grād) (kō-*lan*-jē-ō-*pan*-krē-a-TOG-rah-fē)	radiographic examination of the biliary ducts and pancreatic ducts with contrast media, fluoroscopy, and endoscopy; used to evaluate and diagnose obstructions, strictures, stone diseases, pancreatitis, and pancreatic cancer. (Figure 11-20)
upper GI (gastrointestinal) series	series of radiographic images taken of the stomach and duodenum after the contrast agent barium has been swallowed
ENDOSCOPY	
endoscopic ultrasound (EUS) (*en*-dō-SKOP-ic) (UL-tra-sound)	a procedure using an endoscope fitted with an ultrasound probe that provides images of layers of the intestinal wall; used to detect tumors and cystic growths and for staging of malignant tumors (Figure 11-20)
LABORATORY	
fecal occult blood test (FOBT) (FĒ-kl) (o-KULT) (blud)	a test to detect occult blood in feces. It is used to screen for colon cancer or polyps. Occult blood refers to blood that is present but can only be detected by chemical testing (also called **guaiac test**).
***Helicobacter pylori (H. pylori)* antibodies test** (*hel*-i-kō-BAK-ter) (pī-LŌ-rē) (AN-ti-bod-ēs)	a blood test to determine the presence of *H. pylori* bacteria. The bacteria can be found in the lining of the stomach and can cause peptic ulcers. Tests for *H. pylori* are also performed on biopsy specimens and by breath test.

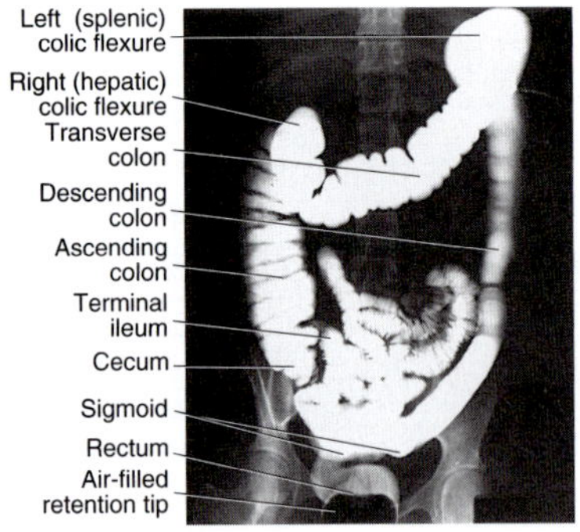

FIGURE 11-19
Barium enema, also called **lower GI** series.

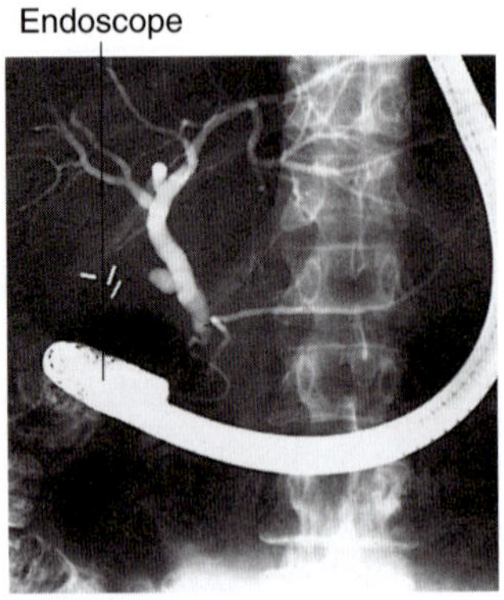

FIGURE 11-20
Endoscopic retrograde cholangiopancreatography (ERCP) is used to diagnose biliary and pancreatic pathologic conditions.

TABLE 11-2
Abdominal Ultrasonography

AREAS VISUALIZED AND POSSIBLE FINDINGS

- **Liver**—cysts, abscess, tumors
- **Gallbladder and Bile Ducts**—cholelithiasis, polyps, tumors
- **Pancreas**—inflammation, tumors, abscess, pseudocysts
- **Kidney**—calculi, cysts, tumors, hydronephrosis, malformations, abscess
- **Aorta**—aneurysm

IMAGE
Abdominal ultrasound showing cholelithiasis.
GB = gallbladder
St = Stone

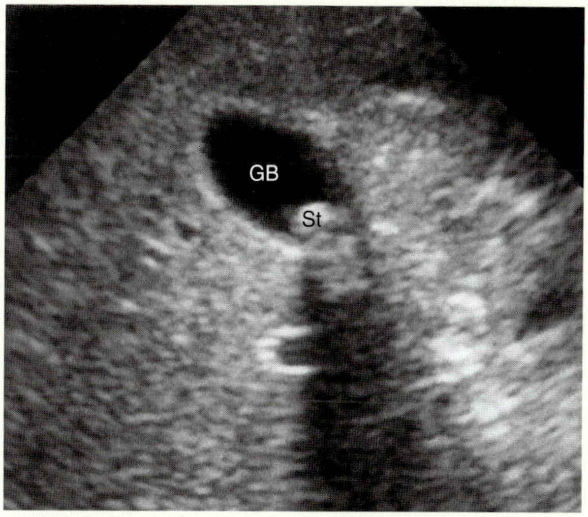

EXERCISE 28

Practice saying aloud each of the diagnostic terms not built from word parts on p. 522.

To hear the terms, go to http://evolve.elsevier.com. Refer to p. 18 for your Evolve Access Information. Select Exercises & Review, Chapter 11, Chapter Exercises, Pronunciation.

☐ Place a check mark in the box when you have completed this exercise.

EXERCISE 29

Write definitions for the following terms.

1. upper GI series ______
2. barium enema ______
3. endoscopic retrograde cholangiopancreatography ______
4. endoscopic ultrasound ______
5. *Helicobacter pylori* antibodies test ______
6. fecal occult blood test ______
7. abdominal ultrasonography ______

EXERCISE 30

Match the procedures in the first column with their correct definitions in the second column.

_____ 1. fecal occult blood test
_____ 2. barium enema
_____ 3. *Helicobacter pylori* antibodies test
_____ 4. upper GI series
_____ 5. endoscopic retrograde cholangiopancreatography
_____ 6. abdominal ultrasonography
_____ 7. endoscopic ultrasound

a. used to diagnose peptic ulcers
b. radiographic image of the stomach and duodenum
c. provides images of layers of the intestinal wall
d. detects blood in feces
e. radiographic image of the esophagus
f. radiographic image of the large intestine
g. process of recording images of internal organs by using sound waves
h. examination of biliary ducts and pancreatic ducts

EXERCISE 31

Spell each of the diagnostic terms not built from word parts on p. 522 by having someone dictate them to you.

To hear and spell the terms, go to http://evolve.elsevier.com. Refer to p. 18 for your Evolve Access Information. Select Exercises & Review, Chapter 11, Chapter Exercises, Spelling.
☐ Place a check mark in the box if you have completed this exercise online.

1. ______________________
2. ______________________
3. ______________________
4. ______________________
5. ______________________
6. ______________________
7. ______________________

Complementary Terms

Built from Word Parts

The following terms are built from word parts you have already learned and can be translated literally to find their meanings. Further explanation of terms beyond the definition of their word parts, if needed, is included in parentheses.

Term	Definition
abdominal (ab-DOM-i-nal)	pertaining to the abdomen
anal (Ā-nal)	pertaining to the anus
aphagia (a-FĀ-ja)	without swallowing (the inability to)
celiac (SĒ-lē-ak)	pertaining to the abdomen
colorectal (*kō*-lō-REK-tal)	pertaining to the colon and rectum
duodenal (dū-OD-e-nal)	pertaining to the duodenum
dyspepsia (dis-PEP-sē-a)	difficult digestion (often used to describe GI symptoms, such as abdominal pain and bloating)
dysphagia (dis-FĀ-ja)	difficult swallowing
enteropathy (*en*-ter-OP-a-thē)	disease of the intestine
esophageal (e-*sof*-a-JĒ-al)	pertaining to the esophagus
gastric (GAS-trik)	pertaining to the stomach
gastroenterologist (*gas*-trō-*en*-ter-OL-o-jist)	a physician who studies and treats diseases of the stomach and intestines (GI tract and accessory organs)
gastroenterology (*gas*-trō-*en*-ter-OL-o-jē)	study of the stomach and intestines (a branch of medicine that deals with treating diseases of the GI tract and accessory organs)
gastromalacia (*gas*-trō-ma-LĀ-sha)	softening of the stomach
glossopathy (glos-OP-a-thē)	disease of the tongue
ileocecal (*il*-ē-ō-SĒ-kal)	pertaining to the ileum and cecum
nasogastric (*nā*-zō-GAS-trik)	pertaining to the nose and stomach

Term	Definition
oral (OR-al)	pertaining to the mouth
pancreatic (*pan*-krē-AT-ik)	pertaining to the pancreas
peritoneal (*per*-i-tō-NĒ-al)	pertaining to the peritoneum
proctologist (prok-TOL-o-jist)	physician who studies and treats diseases of the rectum
proctology (prok-TOL-o-jē)	study of the rectum (a branch of medicine that deals with disorders of the rectum and anus)
rectal (REK-tal)	pertaining to the rectum
steatorrhea (*stē*-a-tō-RĒ-a)	discharge of fat (excessive amount of fat in the stool, causing frothy, foul-smelling fecal matter usually associated with the malabsorption of fat in conditions such as chronic pancreatitis and celiac disease)
steatosis (*stē*-a-tō-sis)	abnormal condition of fat (increased fat at the cellular level often affecting the liver)
stomatitis (*stō*-ma-TĪ-tis)	inflammation of the mouth (mucous membrane)
stomatogastric (*stō*-ma-tō-GAS-trik)	pertaining to the mouth and stomach
sublingual (sub-LING-gwal)	pertaining to under the tongue

EXERCISE 32

Practice saying aloud each of the complementary terms built from word parts on pp. 525-526.

To hear the terms, go to http://evolve.elsevier.com. Refer to p. 18 for your Evolve Access Information. Select Exercises & Review, Chapter 11, Chapter Exercises, Pronunciation.

☐ Place a check mark in the box when you have completed this exercise.

EXERCISE 33

Analyze and define the following complementary terms.

1. aphagia ______
2. dyspepsia ______
3. anal ______
4. dysphagia ______
5. glossopathy ______
6. ileocecal ______
7. oral ______
8. stomatogastric ______
9. gastromalacia ______
10. pancreatic ______
11. peritoneal ______
12. steatosis ______
13. sublingual ______
14. proctology ______
15. nasogastric ______
16. abdominal ______
17. proctologist ______
18. gastroenterology ______
19. gastroenterologist ______
20. colorectal ______
21. rectal ______
22. steatorrhea ______
23. stomatitis ______
24. enteropathy ______
25. gastric ______
26. duodenal ______
27. esophageal ______
28. celiac ______

EXERCISE 34

Build the complementary terms for the following definitions by using the word parts you have learned.

1. disease of the tongue ______ / ______ / ______
   WR / CV / S
2. without swallowing (the inability to) ______ / ______
   P / S(WR)
3. pertaining to under the tongue ______ / ______ / ______
   P / WR / S
4. pertaining to the nose and the stomach ______ / ______ / ______ / ______
   WR / CV / WR / S
5. pertaining to the mouth and the stomach ______ / ______ / ______ / ______
   WR / CV / WR / S
6. pertaining to the anus ______ / ______
   WR / S
7. pertaining to the peritoneum ______ / ______
   WR / S
8. pertaining to the abdomen a. ______ / ______
   WR / S

   b. ______ / ______
   WR / S
9. difficult swallowing ______ / ______
   P / S(WR)
10. pertaining to the ileum and cecum ______ / ______ / ______ / ______
    WR / CV / WR / S
11. softening of the stomach ______ / ______ / ______
    WR / CV / S
12. physician who studies and treats diseases of the rectum ______ / ______ / ______
    WR / CV / S
13. difficult digestion ______ / ______
    P / S(WR)
14. pertaining to the pancreas ______ / ______
    WR / S

15. study of the rectum ______ / ______ / ______
WR / CV / S

16. discharge of fat ______ / ______ / ______
WR / CV / S

17. pertaining to the mouth ______ / ______
WR / S

18. physician who studies and treats diseases of the stomach and intestines ______ / ______ / ______ / ______ / ______
WR / CV / WR / CV / S

19. study of the stomach and intestines ______ / ______ / ______ / ______ / ______
WR / CV / WR / CV / S

20. pertaining to the colon and rectum ______ / ______ / ______ / ______
WR / CV / WR / S

21. pertaining to the rectum ______ / ______
WR / S

22. abnormal condition of fat ______ / ______
WR / S

23. pertaining to the esophagus ______ / ______
WR / S

24. pertaining to the stomach ______ / ______
WR / S

25. pertaining to the duodenum ______ / ______
WR / S

26. disease of the intestine ______ / ______ / ______
WR / CV / S

27. inflammation of the mouth (mucous membrane) ______ / ______
WR / S

EXERCISE 35

Spell each of the complementary terms built from word parts on pp. 525-526 by having someone dictate them to you.

To hear and spell the terms, go to http://evolve.elsevier.com. Refer to p. 18 for your Evolve Access Information. Select Exercises & Review, Chapter 11, Chapter Exercises, Spelling.
☐ Place a check mark in the box if you have completed this exercise online.

1. ______________	15. ______________
2. ______________	16. ______________
3. ______________	17. ______________
4. ______________	18. ______________
5. ______________	19. ______________
6. ______________	20. ______________
7. ______________	21. ______________
8. ______________	22. ______________
9. ______________	23. ______________
10. ______________	24. ______________
11. ______________	25. ______________
12. ______________	26. ______________
13. ______________	27. ______________
14. ______________	28. ______________

Complementary Terms

Not Built from Word Parts

In some of the following terms, you may recognize word parts you have already learned; however, the full meaning of the terms cannot be discerned by the definition of their word parts.

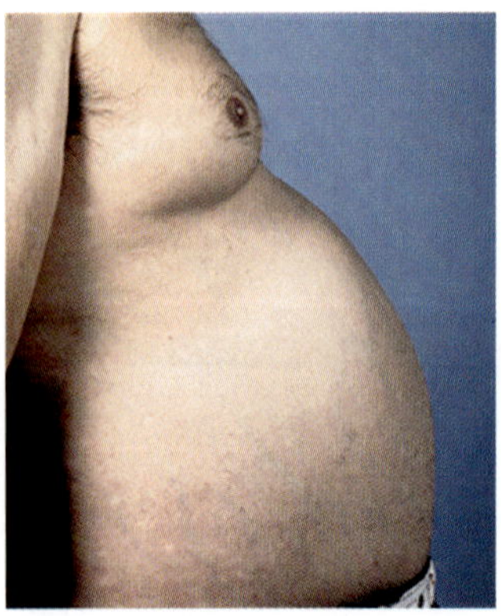

FIGURE 11-21
Ascites.

Term	Definition
ascites (a-SĪ-tēz)	abnormal collection of fluid in the peritoneal cavity (Figure 11-21)
diarrhea (dī-a-RĒ-a) (NOTE: diarrhea is composed of *dia-*, meaning through, and *-rrhea*, meaning flow.)	frequent discharge of liquid stool
dysentery (DIS-en-*ter*-ē)	disorder that involves inflammation of the intestine (usually the large intestine) associated with diarrhea and abdominal pain

Complementary Terms—*cont'd*

Not Built from Word Parts

Term	Definition
emesis (EM-e-sis)	expelling matter from the stomach through the mouth (also called **vomiting**)
feces (FĒ-sēz)	waste from the digestive tract expelled through the rectum (also called **stool** or **fecal matter**)
flatus (FLĀ-tus)	gas in the digestive tract or expelled through the anus
gastric lavage (GAS-trik) (la-VOZH)	washing out of the stomach
gavage (ga-VOZH)	process of feeding a person through a nasogastric tube
hematemesis (*hē*-ma-TEM-e-sis)	vomiting of blood
hematochezia (*hē*-ma-to-KĒ-zha)	passage of bloody feces
malabsorption (*mal*-ab-SORP-shun)	impaired digestion or intestinal absorption of nutrients
melena (me-LĒ-na)	black, tarry stool that contains digested blood; usually a result of bleeding in the upper GI tract
nausea (NAW-zē-a)	urge to vomit
peristalsis (*per*-i-STAL-sis)	involuntary wavelike contractions that propel food along the digestive tract
reflux (RĒ fluks)	abnormal backward flow. In esophageal reflux, the stomach contents flow back into the esophagus.
stoma (STŌ-ma)	surgical opening between an organ and the surface of the body, such as the opening established in the abdominal wall by colostomy, ileostomy, or a similar operation. Stoma may also refer to an opening created between body structures or between portions of the intestines. (see Exercise Figure E)
vomiting (VOM-it-ing)	expelling matter from the stomach through the mouth (also called **emesis**)

Refer to **Appendix D** for pharmacology terms related to the digestive system.

For a list of nutritional terms, go to http://evolve.elsevier.com. Refer to p. 18 for your Evolve Access Information. Select **Appendices, Appendix J, Nutritional Terms**.

EXERCISE 36

Practice saying aloud each of the complementary terms not built from word parts on pp. 530-531.

To hear the terms, go to http://evolve.elsevier.com. Refer to p. 18 for your Evolve Access Information. Select Exercises & Review, Chapter 11, Chapter Exercises, Pronunciation.

☐ Place a check mark in the box when you have completed this exercise.

EXERCISE 37

Match the definitions in the first column with the correct terms in the second column.

_____	1. abnormal collection of fluid	a.	hematemesis
_____	2. expelling matter from the stomach	b.	flatus
_____	3. feeding a person through a tube	c.	gastric lavage
_____	4. washing out of the stomach	d.	reflux
_____	5. urge to vomit	e.	vomiting, emesis
_____	6. frequent discharge of liquid stool	f.	gavage
_____	7. waste expelled from the rectum	g.	melena
_____	8. vomiting of blood	h.	dysentery
_____	9. abnormal backward flow	i.	diarrhea
_____	10. inflammation of the intestine associated with diarrhea and abdominal pain	j.	peristalsis
_____	11. gas expelled through the anus	k.	feces
_____	12. involuntary wavelike contractions	l.	nausea
_____	13. black, tarry stools	m.	ascites
_____	14. surgical opening between an organ and the surface of the body	n.	hematochezia
_____	15. passage of bloody feces	o.	stoma
_____	16. impaired digestion or intestinal absorption	p.	malabsorption

EXERCISE 38

Write definitions for each of the following terms.

1. ascites _______________
2. gavage _______________
3. gastric lavage _______________
4. feces _______________
5. nausea _______________

6. vomiting ______
7. dysentery ______
8. diarrhea ______
9. flatus ______
10. reflux ______
11. hematemesis ______
12. peristalsis ______
13. melena ______
14. stoma ______
15. hematochezia ______
16. emesis ______
17. malabsorption ______

EXERCISE 39

Spell each of the complementary terms not built from word parts on pp. 530-531 by having someone dictate them to you.

To hear and spell the terms, go to http://evolve.elsevier.com. Refer to p. 18 for your Evolve Access Information. Select Exercises & Review, Chapter 11, Chapter Exercises, Spelling.
☐ Place a check mark in the box if you have completed this exercise online.

1. ______
2. ______
3. ______
4. ______
5. ______
6. ______
7. ______
8. ______
9. ______
10. ______
11. ______
12. ______
13. ______
14. ______
15. ______
16. ______
17. ______

Abbreviations

A&P resection	abdominoperineal resection
BE	barium enema
EGD	esophagogastroduodenoscopy
ERCP	endoscopic retrograde cholangiopancreatography
EUS	endoscopic ultrasound
FOBT	fecal occult blood test
GERD	gastroesophageal reflux disease
GI	gastrointestinal
H. pylori	*Helicobacter pylori*
IBS	irritable bowel syndrome
N&V	nausea and vomiting
PEG	percutaneous endoscopic gastrostomy
UGI	upper gastrointestinal
UPPP	uvulopalatopharyngoplasty

Refer to **Appendix C** for a complete list of abbreviations.

EXERCISE 40

Write the meaning of the following abbreviations.

1. ERCP ______________ ______________ ______________
2. EUS ______________ ______________
3. N&V ______________ ______________ ______________
4. IBS ______________ ______________ ______________
5. PEG ______________ ______________ ______________
6. UGI ______________ ______________
7. UPPP ______________
8. GERD ______________ ______________ ______________
9. GI ______________
10. *H. pylori* ______________ ______________
11. BE ______________ ______________
12. EGD ______________
13. A&P resection ______________ ______________
14. FOBT ______________ ______________ ______________ ______________

PRACTICAL APPLICATION

EXERCISE 41 *Interact with Medical Documents*

Complete any two of the following:

A. Complete the endoscopy report by writing the medical terms in the blanks. Use the list of definitions with the corresponding numbers.

University Hospital and Medical Center
4700 North Main Street • Wellness, Arizona 54321 • (987) 555-3210

PATIENT NAME: Ruth Clifton **CASE NUMBER:** 77721-DIG
DATE OF BIRTH: 09/15/19XX **DATE:** 12/27/20XX

ENDOSCOPY REPORT

CASE HISTORY: This is a 40-year-old African American woman who was referred to the 1. ________________ clinic for evaluation. Patient reports 2. ________________ and vomiting with upper abdominal pain. She has also had a problem with 3. ________________ but denies any 4. ________________ or 5. ________________. She has not used any alcohol or salicylates. She is currently taking several medications but they are not known for ulcerogenic side effects.

PROCEDURE: 6. ____________________________________: The patient was given 2 mg of intravenous Versed along with lidocaine spray to the pharynx. After the patient was placed in the left lateral decubitus position, the Olympus 7. ________________ was passed into the esophagus without difficulty. The esophagus in its entirety was essentially free of mucosal abnormalities. No evidence of 8. ________________. The stomach was entered and some gastric juices were aspirated. The esophagus, cardia, and body of the stomach were free of abnormalities. A biopsy of the gastric mucosa was taken for 9. ________________. In the distal antral area some mild erythematous changes were noted. The pylorus had normal peristaltic activity. The first part of the duodenum, however, revealed evidence of ulcerations, both anterosuperiorly as well as posteroinferiorly, with surrounding erythema. These 10. ________________ were less than 1 cm in size. The second part of the duodenum was free of mucosal abnormalities. Withdrawing the scope confirmed the findings upon entry. The patient tolerated the procedure quite well and recovered uneventfully.

Vital signs will be taken every half hour for the next 2 hours.

POSTPROCEDURAL DIAGNOSIS:
11. ________________
12. ________________ uclers

____
Jesus Garcia, MD

JG/mcm

1. visual examination within a hollow organ
2. urge to vomit
3. difficult digestion
4. vomiting of blood
5. black, tarry stool that contains digested blood
6. visual examination of the esophagus, stomach, and duodenum
7. instrument used for visual examination of the stomach
8. abnormal backward flow
9. abbreviation for *Helicobacter pylori*
10. eroded areas
11. inflammation of the stomach
12. pertaining to the duodenum

EXERCISE 41 *Interact with Medical Documents—cont'd*

B. Read the radiology report and answer the questions following it.

028200 CARBIA, WANDA

File Patient Navigate Custom Fields Help

Patient Chart | Lab | Rad | Notes | Documents | Rx | Scheduling | Images | Billing

Name: **CARBIA, WANDA** MR#: **028200** DOB: **10/13/19XX** Sex: **Female**

RADIOLOGY REPORT

ENCOUNTER DATE: 2/17/20XX

EXAMINATION: Abdominal Ultrasound

HISTORY: Nausea, fatigue, and jaundice.

FINDINGS: Multiple scans of the upper abdomen show no focal hepatic lesions. There are numerous small shadowing calculi within the gallbladder. The gallbladder wall is not thickened, there is no pericholecystic fluid collection. The common bile duct is normal in caliber, measuring 4 mm in maximum diameter. No calculi are seen within the common bile duct.
The spleen is not enlarged. No focal abnormality is identified within the pancreas.

IMPRESSION: Cholelithiasis. No associated biliary dilation. The upper abdominal sonogram is otherwise normal.

Electronically signed by: Jose Garza, MD 2/17/20XX 11:24 AM

JG/bab

Start | Log On/Off | Print | Edit

1. The exam included which diagnostic procedure:
   a. radiographic imaging of the colon with computerized tomography
   b. radiographic imaging of the bile ducts after administration of contrast media
   c. use of an endoscope fitted with an ultrasound probe to obtain images of layers of the intestinal wall
   d. recording images of organs with sound waves produced by a transducer placed directly on the skin

2. The patient's symptoms included:
   a. expelling matter from the stomach through the mouth
   b. condition characterized by a yellow tinge to the skin
   c. bluish discoloration of the skin
   d. erythroderma

3. The examination revealed the presence of:
   a. stones within the gallbladder
   b. stones within the common bile duct
   c. lesions in the liver
   d. inflammation of the pancreas

4. "Biliary dilation" would most likely refer to:
   a. inflammation of the pancreas
   b. the presence of fluid in the upper abdomen
   c. choledocholithiasis
   d. widening of the bile ducts or gallbladder

EXERCISE 41 *Interact with Medical Documents—cont'd*

C. Read the radiology report and answer the questions following it.

028200 CARBIA, WANDA

File Patient Navigate Custom Fields Help

Patient Chart | Lab | Rad | Notes | Documents | Rx | Scheduling | Images | Billing

Name: **CARBIA, WANDA** MR#: **028200** DOB: **10/13/19XX** Sex: **Female**

RADIOLOGY REPORT

ENCOUNTER DATE: 11/19/20XX

EXAMINATION: CT Colonography

HISTORY: Intestinal obstruction

FINDINGS: The colon is moderately well distended. There is a moderate amount of residual fluid within the sigmoid, ascending, and descending colons. Mild to moderate amount of barium-tagged stool within the left colon. There are a few scattered adherent, homogeneous filling defects that may relate to adherent, nontagged stool. No definite polyp or mass greater than 7 mm identified. No annular constricting masses. No abnormal bowel dilation to suggest small bowel obstruction currently. No ascites or enlarged lymph nodes within the abdomen. Status post cholecystectomy. A uterus is not visualized. There is streak artifact from several surgical clips within the retroperitoneum and pelvis.

IMPRESSION: CT colonography with above described limitations. However, no specific evidence for polyp or mass greater than 7 mm.

Electronically signed by: Elousie Klint, MD 11/19/20XX 7:37 PM

EK/bab

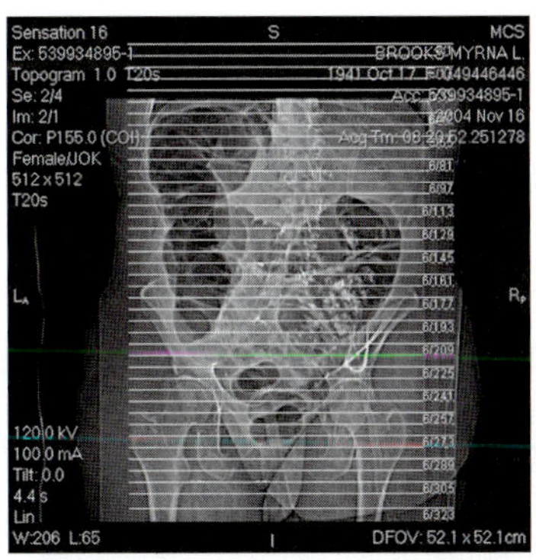

Start | Log On/Off | Print | Edit

1. No ascites indicates:
   a. no fluid accumulation in the peritoneal cavity
   b. no inflammation of the intestine associated with diarrhea and abdominal pain
   c. no residual fluid within the sigmoid colon
   d. no kinking of the intestine

2. The CT colonography was performed:
   a. before excision of the colon
   b. after excision of the appendix
   c. before creation of an artificial opening into the colon
   d. after excision of the gallbladder

3. The report most clearly suggests that the intestinal obstruction was probably *not* caused by a(n):
   a. adhesion
   b. volvulus
   c. intussusception
   d. polyp or mass

EXERCISE 41 *Interact with Medical Documents—cont'd*

D. Read the history and physical report and answer the questions following it.

University Hospital and Medical Center
4700 North Main Street • Wellness, Arizona 54321 • (987) 555-3210

PATIENT NAME: Riffle, Dorothy **MR #:** 041107
DATE OF BIRTH: 10/16/19XX **ADMIT DATE:** 07/27/20XX
SIGNED BY: SULIMAN MD, MADHAVAN **SIGNED DATE/TIME:** 07/27/20XX 12:36

HISTORY AND PHYSICAL REPORT

CHIEF COMPLAINT: Abdominal pain times 1 day.

HISTORY OF PRESENT ILLNESS: This is a 67-year-old female with a past medical history of recurrent bowel obstruction and previous history of **ovarian cancer** which was resected in 1992. At that time also a tumor was found with **adhesions** to the ileum, and she had a small bowel resection at the time of surgery. Since then the patient has had a recurrent history of small-bowel obstruction treated conservatively. Her last attack was 8 years ago, but throughout this time the patient has had more than 20 attacks of small-bowel obstruction. She is also known to have a history of **coronary artery disease** when she presented with **anginal** pain. She had an abnormal **exercise stress test,** and she had **coronary stent** placement in January of this year.

She presented yesterday to the emergency department complaining of **abdominal** pain, **nausea,** and **vomiting.** She had no fever, no chills, and no rigors. She had mild abdominal distention. She had a bowel movement yesterday. She had no loss of consciousness in the ED. She had an abdominal **CT scan,** which showed small bowel dilatation. There was no mass seen on the CT scan. The patient was started on **nasogastric** tube suction. She was also noted to have a high **leukocyte** count, and she was started on **IV** antibiotics.

PAST MEDICAL HISTORY:

1 Coronary artery disease status post coronary stent placement in January.
2 **Hypertension.**
3 **Chronic obstructive pulmonary disease** (COPD).
4 Osteoarthritis.
5 History of ovarian cancer, as above.
6 Status post **appendectomy.**
7 Status post **cholecystectomy.**
8 Status post **hysterectomy.**

ALLERGIES: She has no known drug allergies, but she received ciprofloxacin for a **urinary tract infection** and she developed severe nausea with that. She had no itching or rash with ciprofloxacin.

SOCIAL HISTORY: The patient is married. Her husband is a retired **cardiologist.** She does not smoke, and she does not drink alcohol or use illicit drugs.

FAMILY HISTORY: Reviewed and not significant.

REVIEW OF SYSTEMS: As per history of present illness. All other systems are negative.

PHYSICAL EXAMINATION:

General: The patient is alert and oriented. She is comfortable in bed. She is in no **acute** distress. She has an NG tube in place.

Vital signs: Temperature 97.8. **Pulse** rate 78. Respiratory rate 16. **Blood pressure** 122/76 mm Hg. Oxygen saturation 98% on room air.

HEENT: Her pupils are reactive to light and accommodation. She has no scleral icterus. Her ears, nose, and throat are clear. Her mouth is clear.

Neck: Supple. She has no raised JVD. She has no cervical **lymphadenopathy.**

Chest: Clear to **auscultation** bilaterally.

Cardiovascular: Regular rate and rhythm without a gallop or a murmur.

Abdomen: Soft. Nontender. She has positive bowel sounds in all 4 quadrants. There is no mass felt.

Extremities: Lower limbs have no **edema.**

Neurologic: There are no focal neurologic signs observed.

LABORATORY DATA: Her initial lab evaluation showed white blood cell count 16.5, **hemoglobin** 13.8, **hematocrit** 41.7, and platelet 325. INR 0.9, PTT 17. Glucose 153, calcium 9.5, BUN 15, creatinine 0.75, sodium 135, potassium 3.5, chloride 99, bicarbonate 126, alkaline phosphatase 53, ALT 36, AST 46, amylase 68, lipase 20, and total bilirubin 0.8.
She had a CT scan that showed small bowel dilatation and bilateral lower lobe **atelectasis.**
ASSESSMENT: This is a 67-year-old female with a previous history of recurrent intestinal obstructions secondary to adhesions, history of ovarian cancer, resected in 1992, and history of coronary artery disease and hypertension.
PLAN:
1. We will admit the patient to the medical floor.
2. We will keep the patient n.p.o. and we will continue NG tube suction.
3. We will replete her potassium.
4. We will start the patient on Levaquin and Flagyl for **leukocytosis.**
5. A blood culture was drawn in the ED.
6. We will continue to follow the patient conservatively.
7. We will obtain a surgical consult.
8. Further treatment recommendations will depend on the patient's progress.

____

MADHAVAN SULIMAN, MD
D: 07/27/20XX 07:04:41
T: 07/27/20XX 07:12:04
#: 1274211 Doc ID: 1724156
Author: SULIMAN MD, MADHAVAN Signed on: 07.27.20XX.12:36 PM

1. Read the report on pp. 538-539 aloud taking special effort to pronounce the terms in bold. These are terms you have already learned in this and previous chapters. Evaluate your comprehension of these terms. This is a good example of the number of medical terms that can appear in one document, and it highlights the importance of the language.

2. Under the heading PLAN, the doctor ordered two medications, Flagyl and Levaquin, because of:
   a. increased number of white blood cells
   b. decreased number of white blood cells
   c. enlarged white blood cells

3. List three symptoms relating to the digestive system that the patient was experiencing upon entering the emergency department.
   a. ______________________________
   b. ______________________________
   c. ______________________________

4. Write the body system affected by the disease or surgery listed under the heading PAST MEDICAL HISTORY.

Condition/Surgery	Body System
a. hysterectomy	______________
b. hypertension	______________
c. cholecystectomy	______________
d. COPD	______________
e. ovarian cancer	______________
f. appendectomy	______________
g. coronary stent placement	______________

EXERCISE 42 *Interpret Medical Terms*

To test your understanding of the terms introduced in this chapter, circle the words that correctly complete the sentences. The italicized words refer to the correct answer.

1. Mr. Gomez was tentatively diagnosed with *gallstones*, or (**cholelithiasis, cholecystitis, sialolithiasis**).
2. An abdominal ultrasound confirmed the diagnosis, and Mr. Gomez is now scheduled for a laparoscopic *excision of the gallbladder*, or (**cholecystostomy, cholecystectomy, colectomy**).
3. The plural spelling of the term meaning *opening created by surgically joining two structures* is (**anastomoses, anastomosis, anastomosices**).
4. The patient was diagnosed with a condition of *inflammation of the colon and formation of ulcers*, called (**cirrhosis, ulcerative colitis, peptic ulcer**).
5. A *prolapse of the rectum* is (**rectocele, intussusception, proctoptosis**).
6. An *abnormal growing together of two surfaces* is (**anastomosis, adhesion, amniocentesis**).
7. Named for their location, gastric ulcers and duodenal ulcers are forms of *eroded areas of the mucous membrane of the stomach* and *duodenum* (**irritable bowel syndrome, peptic ulcers, ulcerative colitis**).
8. Tests used to diagnosis peptic ulcers include *Helicobacter pylori* antibodies test, *series of radiographic images taken of the stomach and duodenum after the contrast agent barium has been swallowed* (**barium enema, upper GI series, endoscopic ultrasound**), and *visual examination of the esophagus, stomach and duodenum* (**esophagogastroduodenoscopy, endoscopic ultrasound, laparoscopy**).
9. Three surgical procedures that may be performed on a patient with peptic ulcers are (1) *excision of the stomach*, or (**gastrotomy, gastrostomy, gastrectomy**); (2) *surgical repair of the pylorus*, or (**pyloroplasty, cheilorrhaphy, gastrojejunostomy**); and (3) *cutting of certain branches of the vagus nerve*, or (**colostomy, vagotomy, gingivectomy**).
10. *Difficult digestion* is (**dyspepsia, dysphagia, aphagia**).
11. *Feeding* a person *through a gastric tube* is called (**lavage, gavage, gastrostomy**).
12. The *surgical procedure to remove the colon and rectum and create an artificial opening into the colon* are (**colectomy and colostomy, abdominoperineal resection and colostomy, abdominoperineal resection and ileostomy**).
13. To rule out cancer of the colon, the doctor performed a diagnostic procedure to *visually examine the colon* or (**colonoscopy, colonoscope, colostomy**).
14. The doctor diagnosed the patient as having *an obstruction of the intestine* or (**polyp, irritable bowel syndrome, ileus**).
15. The following test is used to screen for colon cancer (**fecal occult blood test, *Helicobacter pylori* antibodies test, upper GI series**).
16. (**Stoma, Stomata, Stomaes**) is the plural spelling of the term meaning *surgical opening between an organ and the surface of the body.*

WEB LINK

For more information about diseases and disorders of the digestive system and the latest treatments available, please visit the National Digestive Diseases Information Clearing House at ***http://digestive.niddk.nih.gov.***

EXERCISE 43 *Read Medical Terms in Use*

Practice pronunciation of terms by reading the following discussion. Use the pronunciation key following the medical term to assist you in saying the word.

To hear these terms, go to http://evolve.elsevier.com. Refer to p. 18 for your Evolve Access Information. Select Exercises & Review, Chapter 11, Chapter Exercises, Read Medical Terms in Use.

COLORECTAL CANCER

Colorectal (kō-lō-REK-tal) cancer begins in the colon or rectum and is the second leading cause of cancer deaths in the United States. Most are adenocarcinomas that originate as a benign, adenomatous **polyp** (POL-ip).

Many people have no symptoms until the tumor is quite advanced, and symptoms vary depending on the location of the tumor. Warning signs are altered bowel habits, **rectal** (REK-tal) bleeding, **abdominal** (ab-DOM-i-nal) cramps, **flatus** (FLĀ-tus) and bloating, iron deficiency anemia, and weight loss.

Screening and diagnostic tests for colorectal cancer include digital rectal examination, **fecal** (FĒ-kl) **occult** (o-KULT) blood test, **sigmoidoscopy** (*sig*-moy-DOS-ko-pē), **colonoscopy** (kō-lon-OS-ko-pē), and **barium** (BAR-ē-um) **enema** (EN-e-ma). As well as being an important diagnostic tool, colonoscopy may be used for biopsy and for the removal of **polyps.** To perform a **polypectomy** (pol-i-PEK-to-mē), a braided wire snare is inserted into the **colonoscope** (kō-LON-ō-skōp). A snare loop, like a noose, is placed around the stem of the polyp. With electrosurgical power attached to the snare, the polyp is detached. The polyp is removed from the colon for histologic examination.

For cancer beyond the early stage, conventional surgery is the main treatment. The type of surgery depends on the location and stage of the tumor. Types of surgeries performed are left or right-sided **hemicolectomy** (*hem*-ē-kō-LEK-to-mē) with **anastomosis** (a-*nas*-to-MŌ-sis), sigmoid **colectomy** (kō-LEK-to-mē), and **abdominoperineal** (ab-*dom*-i-nō-*per*-i-NĒ-el) **resection** with **colostomy** (ko-LOS-to-mē).

EXERCISE 44 *Comprehend Medical Terms in Use*

Test your comprehension of terms in the previous medical discussion by circling the correct answer.

1. Which of the following is used for diagnosing colorectal cancer?
   a. visual exam of the stomach
   b. series of radiographic images of the small intestine
   c. visual exam of the colon
   d. radiographic image of the esophagus
2. T F A polypectomy may be performed during a colonoscopy.
3. T F Depending on the location of the tumor, a surgical treatment for colorectal cancer may be performed that creates an opening between the colon and abdominal wall for the passage of stool.
4. T F Vomiting blood is a warning sign for colorectal cancer.

CHAPTER REVIEW

ONLINE CHAPTER REVIEW

To access the Evolve website, go to http://evolve.elsevier.com. Refer to p. 18 for your Evolve Access Information. Select Exercises & Review, Chapter 11, then select Chapter Exercises, Practice Activities, Animations, or Games. Place a check mark in the box when you have completed an exercise or activity, watched an animation, or played a game. Have fun!

Chapter Exercises

Exercises in this section of your Evolve resources correlate to exercises in your textbook. You may have completed them as you worked through the chapter.

- ☐ Pronunciation
- ☐ Spelling
- ☐ Read Medical Terms in Use

Practice Activities

Practice in study mode, then test your learning in assessment mode. Keep track of your scores from assessment mode if you wish.

	SCORE
☐ Picture It	______
☐ Define Word Parts	______
☐ Build Medical Terms	______
☐ Word Shop	______
☐ Define Medical Terms	______
☐ Use It	______
☐ Hear It and Type It: Clinical Vignettes	______

Animations

- ☐ Adhesion–Bowel Obstruction
- ☐ Appendicitis
- ☐ Bariatric Surgery: Roux-en-Y Gastric Bypass
- ☐ Cirrhosis
- ☐ Colonoscopy with Polypectomy
- ☐ Diverticulitis
- ☐ Endoscopy
- ☐ ERCP
- ☐ Ileus
- ☐ Irritable Bowel Syndrome
- ☐ Nasogastric Tube Placement
- ☐ Peritonitis

Games

- ☐ Name that Word Part
- ☐ Term Storm
- ☐ Term Explorer
- ☐ Termbusters
- ☐ Medical Millionaire
- ☐ Crossword Puzzle

REVIEW OF WORD PARTS

Can you define and spell the following word parts?

Combining Forms

abdomin/o
an/o
antr/o
append/o
appendic/o
cec/o
celi/o
cheil/o
cholangi/o
chol/e
choledoch/o
col/o
colon/o
diverticul/o
duoden/o
enter/o
esophag/o
gastr/o
gingiv/o
gloss/o
hepat/o
herni/o
ile/o
jejun/o
lapar/o
lingu/o
or/o
palat/o
pancreat/o
peritone/o
polyp/o
proct/o
pylor/o
rect/o
sial/o
sigmoid/o
steat/o
stomat/o
uvul/o

Prefix

hemi-

Suffix

-pepsia

REVIEW OF TERMS

Can you define, pronounce, and spell the following terms *built from word parts*?

Diseases and Disorders

appendicitis
cholangioma
cholecystitis
choledocholithiasis
cholelithiasis
diverticulitis
diverticulosis
esophagitis
gastritis
gastroenteritis
gastroenterocolitis
gingivitis
hepatitis
hepatoma
palatitis
pancreatitis
peritonitis
polyposis
proctoptosis
rectocele
sialolith
steatohepatitis
uvulitis

Surgical

abdominocentesis
abdominoplasty
anoplasty
antrectomy
appendectomy
celiotomy
cheilorrhaphy
cholecystectomy
choledocholithotomy
colectomy
colostomy
diverticulectomy
enterorrhaphy
esophagogastroplasty
gastrectomy
gastrojejunostomy
gastroplasty
gastrostomy
gingivectomy
glossorrhaphy
hemicolectomy
herniorrhaphy
ileostomy
laparotomy
palatoplasty
polypectomy
pyloromyotomy
pyloroplasty
uvulectomy
uvulopalatopharyngoplasty (UPPP)

Diagnostic

cholangiogram
cholangiography
colonoscope
colonoscopy
CT colonography
endoscope
endoscopy
esophagogastroduodenoscopy (EGD)
esophagogram
esophagoscopy
gastroscope
gastroscopy
laparoscope
laparoscopy
proctoscope
proctoscopy
sigmoidoscopy

Complementary

abdominal
anal
aphagia
celiac
colorectal
duodenal
dyspepsia
dysphagia
enteropathy
esophageal
gastric
gastroenterologist
gastroenterology
gastromalacia
glossopathy
ileocecal
nasogastric
oral
pancreatic
peritoneal
proctologist
proctology
rectal
steatorrhea
steatosis
stomatitis
stomatogastric
sublingual

Can you build, analyze, define, pronounce, and spell the following terms *not built from word parts?*

Diseases and Disorders

adhesion
anorexia nervosa
bulimia nervosa
celiac disease
cirrhosis
Crohn disease
gastroesophageal reflux disease (GERD)
hemochromatosis
hemorrhoids
ileus
intussusception
irritable bowel syndrome (IBS)
obesity
peptic ulcer
polyp
ulcerative colitis
volvulus

Surgical

abdominoperineal resection (A&P resection)
anastomosis (*pl.* anastomoses)
bariatric surgery
hemorrhoidectomy
vagotomy

Diagnostic

abdominal ultrasonography
barium enema (BE)
endoscopic retrograde cholangiopancreatography (ERCP)
endoscopic ultrasound (EUS)
fecal occult blood test (FOBT)
Helicobacter pylori antibodies test
upper GI (gastrointestinal) series

Complementary

ascites
diarrhea
dysentery
emesis
feces
flatus
gastric lavage
gavage
hematemesis
hematochezia
malabsorption
melena
nausea
peristalsis
reflux
stoma
vomiting

ANSWERS

Exercise Figures

Exercise Figure

A. 1. mouth: or/o, stomat/o
2. esophagus: esophag/o
3. duodenum: duoden/o
4. colon: col/o, colon/o
5. cecum: cec/o
6. anus: an/o
7. stomach: gastr/o
8. antrum: antr/o
9. jejunum: jejun/o
10. ileum: ile/o
11. sigmoid colon: sigmoid/o
12. rectum: proct/o, rect/o

Exercise Figure

B. 1. palate: palat/o
2. uvula: uvul/o
3. tongue: gloss/o, lingu/o
4. gallbladder: chol/e (gall), cyst/o (bladder)
5. pyloric sphincter: pylor/o
6. appendix: append/o, appendic/o
7. gum: gingiv/o
8. lip: cheil/o
9. salivary glands: sial/o
10. liver: hepat/o
11. bile duct: cholangi/o
12. common bile duct: choledoch/o
13. pancreas: pancreat/o
14. abdomen: abdomin/o, celi/o, lapar/o

Exercise Figure

C. 2. appendic/itis

Exercise Figure

D. chol/e/lith/iasis, choledoch/o/lith/iasis

Exercise Figure

E. 1. ile/o/stomy
2. col/o/stomy

Exercise Figure

F. gastr/ectomy

Exercise Figure

G. A. gastr/o/scopy
B. gastr/o/scope

Exercise 1

1. alimentary canal
2. gastrointestinal tract
3. pharynx
4. esophagus
5. stomach
6. duodenum
7. jejunum
8. ileum
9. cecum
10. ascending colon
11. transverse colon
12. descending colon
13. sigmoid colon
14. rectum
15. anus

Exercise 2

1. l
2. d
3. a
4. h
5. m
6. j
7. b
8. i
9. c
10. g
11. e
12. k
13. f

Exercise 3

1. rectum
2. stomach
3. anus
4. cecum
5. ileum
6. mouth
7. duodenum
8. colon
9. mouth
10. intestine
11. rectum
12. antrum
13. esophagus
14. jejunum
15. sigmoid colon
16. colon

Exercise 4

1. cec/o
2. gastr/o
3. ile/o
4. jejun/o
5. sigmoid/o
6. esophag/o
7. a. rect/o
   b. proct/o
8. enter/o
9. duoden/o
10. a. col/o
    b. colon/o
11. a. or/o
    b. stomat/o
12. an/o
13. antr/o

Exercise 5

1. hernia
2. abdomen
3. saliva, salivary gland
4. gall, bile
5. diverticulum
6. gum
7. appendix
8. tongue
9. liver
10. lip
11. peritoneum
12. palate
13. pancreas
14. abdomen
15. tongue
16. common bile duct
17. pylorus, pyloric sphincter
18. uvula
19. bile duct
20. polyp, small growth
21. abdomen
22. fat
23. appendix

Exercise 6

1. palat/o
2. sial/o
3. pancreat/o
4. peritone/o
5. a. gloss/o
   b. lingu/o
6. gingiv/o
7. pylor/o
8. hepat/o
9. chol/e
10. a. abdomin/o
    b. celi/o
    c. lapar/o
11. herni/o
12. diverticul/o
13. cheil/o
14. a. append/o
    b. appendic/o
15. uvul/o
16. cholangi/o
17. choledoch/o
18. polyp/o
19. steat/o

Exercise 7

1. digestion
2. half

Exercise 8

1. -pepsia
2. hemi-

Exercise 9

Pronunciation Exercise

Exercise 10

1. WR CV WR S
chol/e/lith/iasis
CF
condition of gallstones
2. WR S
diverticul/osis
abnormal condition of having diverticula
3. WR CV WR
sial/o/lith
CF
stone in the salivary gland
4. WR S
hepat/oma
tumor of the liver
5. WR S
uvul/itis
inflammation of the uvula
6. WR S
pancreat/itis
inflammation of the pancreas
7. WR CV S
proct/o/ptosis
CF
prolapse of the rectum
8. WR S
gingiv/itis
inflammation of the gums
9. WR S
gastr/itis
inflammation of the stomach
10. WR CV S
rect/o/cele
CF
protrusion of the rectum
11. WR S
palat/itis
inflammation of the palate
12. WR S
hepat/itis
inflammation of the liver
13. WR S
appendic/itis
inflammation of the appendix
14. WR CV WR S
chol/e/cyst/itis
CF
inflammation of the gallbladder
15. WR S
diverticul/itis
inflammation of a diverticulum
16. WR CV WR S
gastr/o/enter/itis
CF
inflammation of the stomach and intestines
17. WR CV WR CV WR S
gastr/o/enter/o/col/itis
CF CF
inflammation of the stomach, intestines, and colon
18. WR CV WR S
choledoch/o/lith/iasis
CF
condition of stones in the common bile duct
19. WR S
cholangi/oma
tumor of the bile duct
20. WR S
polyp/osis
abnormal condition of (multiple) polyps
21. WR S
esophag/itis
inflammation of the esophagus
22. WR S
periton/itis
inflammation of the peritoneum
23. WR CV WR S
steat/o/hepat/itis
CF
inflammation of the liver associated with (excess) fat

Exercise 11

1. hepat/oma
2. gastr/itis
3. sial/o/lith
4. appendic/itis
5. diverticul/itis
6. chol/e/cyst/itis
7. diverticul/osis
8. gastr/o/enter/itis
9. proct/o/ptosis
10. rect/o/cele
11. uvul/itis
12. gingiv/itis
13. hepat/itis
14. palat/itis
15. chol/e/lith/iasis
16. steat/o/hepat/itis
17. gastr/o/enter/o/col/itis
18. pancreat/itis
19. cholangi/oma
20. esophag/itis
21. choledoch/o/lith/iasis
22. polyp/osis
23. periton/itis

Exercise 12

Spelling Exercise; see text pp. 495-497.

Exercise 13

Pronunciation Exercise

Exercise 14

1. f	10. j
2. b	11. m
3. e	12. i
4. n	13. c
5. d	14. l
6. g	15. o
7. a	16. p
8. k	17. q
9. h	

Exercise 15

1. eroded area of the mucous membrane of the stomach or duodenum
2. eating disorder characterized by a prolonged refusal to eat
3. chronic inflammation of the intestinal tract usually affecting the ileum and colon
4. twisting or kinking of the intestine
5. abnormal growing together of two surfaces that normally are separated
6. chronic disease of the liver with gradual destruction of cells
7. telescoping of segment of the intestine
8. malabsorption syndrome caused by an immune reaction to gluten
9. inflammation of the colon with the formation of ulcers
10. eating disorder involving gorging food followed by induced vomiting
11. swollen or distended veins in the rectal area
12. tumorlike growth extending out from a mucous membrane
13. disturbance of bowel function
14. obstruction of the intestine, often caused by failure of peristalsis
15. abnormal backward flow of the gastrointestinal contents into the esophagus
16. excess body fat
17. an iron metabolism disorder

Exercise 16

Spelling Exercise; see text pp. 501-503.

Exercise 17

Pronunciation Exercise

Exercise 18

1. WR S
gastr/ectomy
excision of the stomach
2. WR CV WR CV S
esophag/o/gastr/o/plasty
CF CF
surgical repair of the esophagus and the stomach

3. WR S
diverticul/ectomy
excision of a diverticulum

4. WR S
antr/ectomy
excision of the antrum

5. WR CV S
palat/o/plasty
CF
surgical repair of the palate

6. WR S
uvul/ectomy
excision of the uvula

7. WR CV WR CV S
gastr/o/jejun/o/stomy
CF CF
creation of an artificial opening between the stomach and the jejunum

8. WR CV WR S
chol/e/cyst/ectomy
CF
excision of the gallbladder

9. WR S
col/ectomy
excision of the colon

10. WR CV S
col/o/stomy
CF
creation of an artificial opening into the colon

11. WR CV S
pylor/o/plasty
CF
surgical repair of the pylorus

12. WR CV S
an/o/plasty
CF
surgical repair of the anus

13. WR S
append/ectomy
excision of the appendix

14. WR CV S
cheil/o/rrhaphy
CF
suture of the lip

15. WR S
gingiv/ectomy
surgical removal of gum (tissue)

16. WR CV S
lapar/o/tomy
CF
incision into the abdominal cavity

17. WRCV S
ile/o/stomy
CF
creation of an artificial opening into the ileum

18. WR CV S
gastr/o/stomy
CF
creation of an artificial opening into the stomach

19. WR CV S
herni/o/rrhaphy
CF
suturing of a hernia

20. WR CV S
gloss/o/rrhaphy
CF
suture of the tongue

21. WR CVWR CV S
choledoch/o/lith/o/tomy
CF CF
incision into the common bile duct to remove a stone

22. P WR S
hemi/col/ectomy
excision of half of the colon

23. WR S
polyp/ectomy
excision of a polyp

24. WR CV S
enter/o/rrhaphy
CF
suture of the intestine

25. WR CV S
abdomin/o/plasty
CF
surgical repair of the abdomen

26. WR CV WR CV S
pylor/o/my/o/tomy
CF CF
incision into the pylorus muscle

27. WR CV WR CV WR CV S
uvul/o/palat/o/pharyng/o/plasty
CF CF CF
surgical repair of the uvula, palate, and pharynx

28. WR CV S
celi/o/tomy
CF
incision into the abdominal cavity

29. WR CV S
gastr/o/plasty
CF
surgical repair of the stomach

30. WR CV S
abdomin/o/centesis
CF
surgical puncture to remove fluid from the abdominal cavity

Exercise 19

1. append/ectomy
2. gloss/o/rrhaphy
3. esophag/o/gastr/o/plasty
4. diverticul/ectomy
5. ile/o/stomy
6. gingiv/ectomy
7. a. lapar/o/tomy
   b. celi/o/tomy
8. an/o/plasty
9. antr/ectomy
10. chol/e/cyst/ectomy
11. col/ectomy
12. col/o/stomy
13. gastr/ectomy
14. gastr/o/stomy
15. gastr/o/jejun/o/stomy
16. uvul/ectomy
17. palat/o/plasty
18. pylor/o/plasty
19. herni/o/rrhaphy
20. cheil/o/rrhaphy
21. hemi/col/ectomy
22. choledoch/o/lith/o/tomy
23. polyp/ectomy
24. enter/o/rrhaphy
25. abdomin/o/plasty
26. pylor/o/my/o/tomy
27. uvul/o/palat/o/pharyng/o/plasty
28. gastr/o/plasty
29. abdomin/o/centesis

Exercise 20

Spelling Exercise; see text pp. 506-508.

Exercise 21

Pronunciation Exercise

Exercise 22

1. vagotomy
2. anastomosis
3. abdominoperineal resection
4. bariatric surgery
5. hemorrhoidectomy

Exercise 23

Spelling Exercise; see text pp. 513-514.

Exercise 24

Pronunciation Exercise

Exercise 25

1. WR CV S
esophag/o/scopy
CF
visual examination of the esophagus

2. WR CV S
gastr/o/scope
CF
instrument used for visual examination of the stomach

3. WR CV S
gastr/o/scopy
CF
visual examination of the stomach
4. WR CV S
proct/o/scope
CF
instrument used for visual examination of the rectum
5. WR CV S
proct/o/scopy
CF
visual examination of the rectum
6. P S(WR)
endo/scope
instrument used for visual examination within a hollow organ
7. P S(WR)
endo/scopy
visual examination within a hollow organ
8. WR CV S
sigmoid/o/scopy
CF
visual examination of the sigmoid colon
9. WR CV S
cholangi/o/gram
CF
radiographic image of bile ducts
10. WR CV WR CV WR CV S
esophag/o/gastr/o/duoden/o/scopy
CF CF CF
visual examination of the esophagus, stomach, and duodenum
11. WR CV S
colon/o/scope
CF
instrument used for visual examination of the colon
12. WR CV S
lapar/o/scope
CF
instrument used for visual examination of the abdominal cavity
13. WR CV S
colon/o/scopy
CF
visual examination of the colon
14. WR CV S
lapar/o/scopy
CF
visual examination of the abdominal cavity
15. WR CV S
CT colon/o/graphy
CF
radiographic imaging of the colon
16. WR CV S
esophag/o/gram
CF
radiographic image of the esophagus
17. WR CV S
cholangi/o/graphy
CF
radiographic imaging of the bile ducts

Exercise 26

1. endo/scopy
2. gastr/o/scope
3. proct/o/scope
4. endo/scope
5. proct/o/scopy
6. esophag/o/scopy
7. sigmoid/o/scopy
8. cholangi/o/gram
9. gastr/o/scopy
10. lapar/o/scope
11. esophag/o/gastr/o/duoden/o/scopy
12. colon/o/scopy
13. lapar/o/scopy
14. colon/o/scope
15. CT colon/o/graphy
16. cholangi/o/graphy
17. esophag/o/gram

Exercise 27

Spelling Exercise; see text pp. 516-518.

Exercise 28

Pronunciation Exercise

Exercise 29

1. series of radiographic images taken of the stomach and duodenum after the contrast agent barium has been swallowed
2. series of radiographic images taken of the large intestine after the contrast agent barium has been administered rectally
3. radiographic examination of the biliary tract and pancreatic ducts
4. an endoscope fitted with an ultrasound probe providing images of layers of the intestinal wall
5. a blood test to determine the presence of *Helicobacter pylori* bacteria, a cause of peptic ulcers
6. a test to detect fecal occult blood
7. process of recording images of internal organs using sound waves

Exercise 30

1. d
2. f
3. a
4. b
5. h
6. g
7. c

Exercise 31

Spelling Exercise; see text p. 522.

Exercise 32

Pronunciation Exercise

Exercise 33

1. P S(WR)
a/phagia
without swallowing (inability to)
2. P S(WR)
dys/pepsia
difficult digestion
3. WR S
an/al
pertaining to the anus
4. P S(WR)
dys/phagia
difficult swallowing
5. WR CV S
gloss/o/pathy
CF
disease of the tongue
6. WR CV WR S
ile/o/cec/al
CF
pertaining to the ileum and cecum

7. WR S
or/al
pertaining to the mouth
8. WR CV WR S
stomat/o/gastr/ic
CF
pertaining to the mouth and stomach
9. WR CV S
gastr/o/malacia
CF
softening of the stomach
10. WR S
pancreat/ic
pertaining to the pancreas
11. WR S
peritone/al
pertaining to the peritoneum
12. WR S
steat/osis
abnormal condition of fat
13. P WR S
sub/lingu/al
pertaining to under the tongue
14. WR CV S
proct/o/logy
CF
study of the rectum
15. WR CV WR S
nas/o/gastr/ic
CF
pertaining to the nose and stomach
16. WR S
abdomin/al
pertaining to the abdomen
17. WR CV S
proct/o/logist
CF
physician who studies and treats diseases of the rectum
18. WR CV WR CV S
gastr/o/enter/o/logy
CF CF
study of the stomach and intestines
19. WR CV WR CV S
gastr/o/enter/o/logist
CF CF
physician who studies and treats diseases of the stomach and intestines
20. WR CV WR S
col/o/rect/al
CF
pertaining to the colon and rectum
21. WR S
rect/al
pertaining to the rectum
22. WR CV S
steat/o/rrhea
CF
discharge of fat
23. WR S
stomat/itis
inflammation of the mouth (mucous membrane)
24. WR CV S
enter/o/pathy
CF
disease of the intestine
25. WR S
gastr/ic
pertaining to the stomach
26. WR S
duoden/al
pertaining to the duodenum
27. WR S
esophag/eal
pertaining to the esophagus
28. celi/ac
pertaining to the abdomen

Exercise 34

1. gloss/o/pathy
2. a/phagia
3. sub/lingu/al
4. nas/o/gastr/ic
5. stomat/o/gastr/ic
6. an/al
7. peritone/al
8. abdomin/al, celi/ac
9. dys/phagia
10. ile/o/cec/al
11. gastr/o/malacia
12. proct/o/logist
13. dys/pepsia
14. pancreat/ic
15. proct/o/logy
16. steat/o/rrhea
17. or/al
18. gastr/o/enter/o/logist
19. gastr/o/enter/o/logy
20. col/o/rect/al
21. rect/al
22. steat/osis
23. esophag/eal
24. gastr/ic
25. duoden/al
26. enter/o/pathy
27. stomat/itis

Exercise 35

Spelling Exercise; see text pp. 525-526.

Exercise 36

Pronunciation Exercise

Exercise 37

1.	m	9.	d
2.	e	10.	h
3.	f	11.	b
4.	c	12.	j
5.	l	13.	g
6.	i	14.	o
7.	k	15.	n
8.	a	16.	p

Exercise 38

1. abnormal collection of fluid in the peritoneal cavity
2. process of feeding a person through a nasogastric tube
3. washing out of the stomach
4. waste from the digestive tract expelled through the rectum
5. urge to vomit
6. expelling matter from the stomach through the mouth
7. disorder that involves inflammation of the intestine
8. frequent discharge of liquid stool
9. gas expelled through the anus
10. abnormal backward flow
11. vomiting of blood
12. involuntary wavelike contractions that propel food along the digestive tract
13. black, tarry stools that contain digested blood
14. surgical opening between an organ and the surface of the body
15. passage of bloody feces
16. expelling matter from the stomach through the mouth
17. impaired digestion or intestinal absorption

Exercise 39

Spelling Exercise; see text pp. 530-531.

Exercise 40

1. endoscopic retrograde cholangiopancreatography
2. endoscopic ultrasound
3. nausea and vomiting
4. irritable bowel syndrome
5. percutaneous endoscopic gastrostomy
6. upper gastrointestinal
7. uvulopalatopharyngoplasty
8. gastroesophageal reflux disease
9. gastrointestinal
10. *Helicobacter pylori*
11. barium enema
12. esophagogastroduodenoscopy
13. abdominoperineal resection
14. fecal occult blood test

Exercise 41

A.
1. endoscopy
2. nausea
3. dyspepsia
4. hematemesis
5. melena
6. esophagogastroduodenoscopy
7. gastroscope
8. reflux
9. *H. pylori*
10. ulcers
11. gastritis
12. duodenal

B.
1. d
2. b
3. a
4. d

C.
1. a
2. d
3. d

D.
1. Pronunciation Exercise
2. a
3. a. abdominal pain
   b. nausea
   c. vomiting
4. a. female reproductive system
   b. cardiovascular system
   c. digestive system
   d. respiratory system
   e. female reproductive system
   f. digestive system
   g. cardiovascular system

Exercise 42

1. cholelithiasis
2. cholecystectomy
3. anastomoses
4. ulcerative colitis
5. proctoptosis
6. adhesion
7. peptic ulcers
8. upper GI series, esophagogastroduodenoscopy
9. gastrectomy, pyloroplasty, vagotomy
10. dyspepsia
11. gavage
12. abdominoperineal resection and colostomy
13. colonoscopy
14. ileus
15. fecal occult blood test
16. stomata

Exercise 43

Reading Exercise

Exercise 44

1. c
2. *T*
3. *T*
4. *F*, vomiting blood is not a warning sign of colorectal cancer.

NOTES

NOTES

Chapter 12

Eye

OUTLINE

OBJECTIVES

Upon completion of this chapter you will be able to:

1. Identify organs and structures of the eye.
2. Define and spell word parts related to the eye.
3. Define, pronounce, and spell disease and disorder terms related to the eye.
4. Define, pronounce, and spell surgical terms related to the eye.
5. Define, pronounce, and spell diagnostic terms related to the eye.
6. Define, pronounce, and spell complementary terms related to the eye.
7. Interpret the meaning of abbreviations related to the eye.
8. Interpret, read, and comprehend medical language in simulated medical statements and documents.

ANATOMY

Function

The eyes are organs of vision and are located in a bony protective cavity of the skull called the **orbit.** Only a small portion of the eye is visible from the exterior (Figures 12-1 and 12-2).

Structures of the Eye

Term	Definition
sclera	outer protective layer of the eye; the portion seen on the anterior portion of the eyeball is referred to as the **white of the eye**
cornea	transparent anterior part of the sclera, which is anterior to the aqueous humor and lies over the iris. It allows the light rays to enter the eye.
choroid	middle layer of the eye, which is interlaced with many blood vessels that supply nutrients to the eye
iris	the pigmented muscular structure that regulates the amount of light entering the eye by controlling the size of the pupil
pupil	opening in the center of the iris
lens	lies directly behind the pupil; its function is to focus and bend light
retina	innermost layer of the eye, which contains the vision receptors (see Figure 12-3)
aqueous humor	watery liquid found in the anterior cavity of the eye. It provides nourishment to nearby structures and maintains shape in the anterior part of the eye
vitreous humor	jellylike substance found behind the lens in the posterior cavity of the eye that maintains its shape
meibomian glands	oil glands found in the upper and lower edges of the eyelids that help lubricate the eye
lacrimal glands and ducts	produce and drain tears
optic nerve	carries visual impulses from the retina to the brain
conjunctiva	mucous membrane lining the eyelids and covering the anterior portion of the sclera

IRIS

was the special messenger of the Queen of Heaven according to Greek mythology. In this role she passed from heaven to earth over the rainbow while dressed in rainbow hues. Her name was applied to the ***circular eye muscle*** because of its varied colors.

A & P Booster
For students desiring more anatomy and physiology, go to http://evolve.elsevier.com. Refer to p. 18 for your Evolve Access Information. Select A & P Booster, Chapter 12.

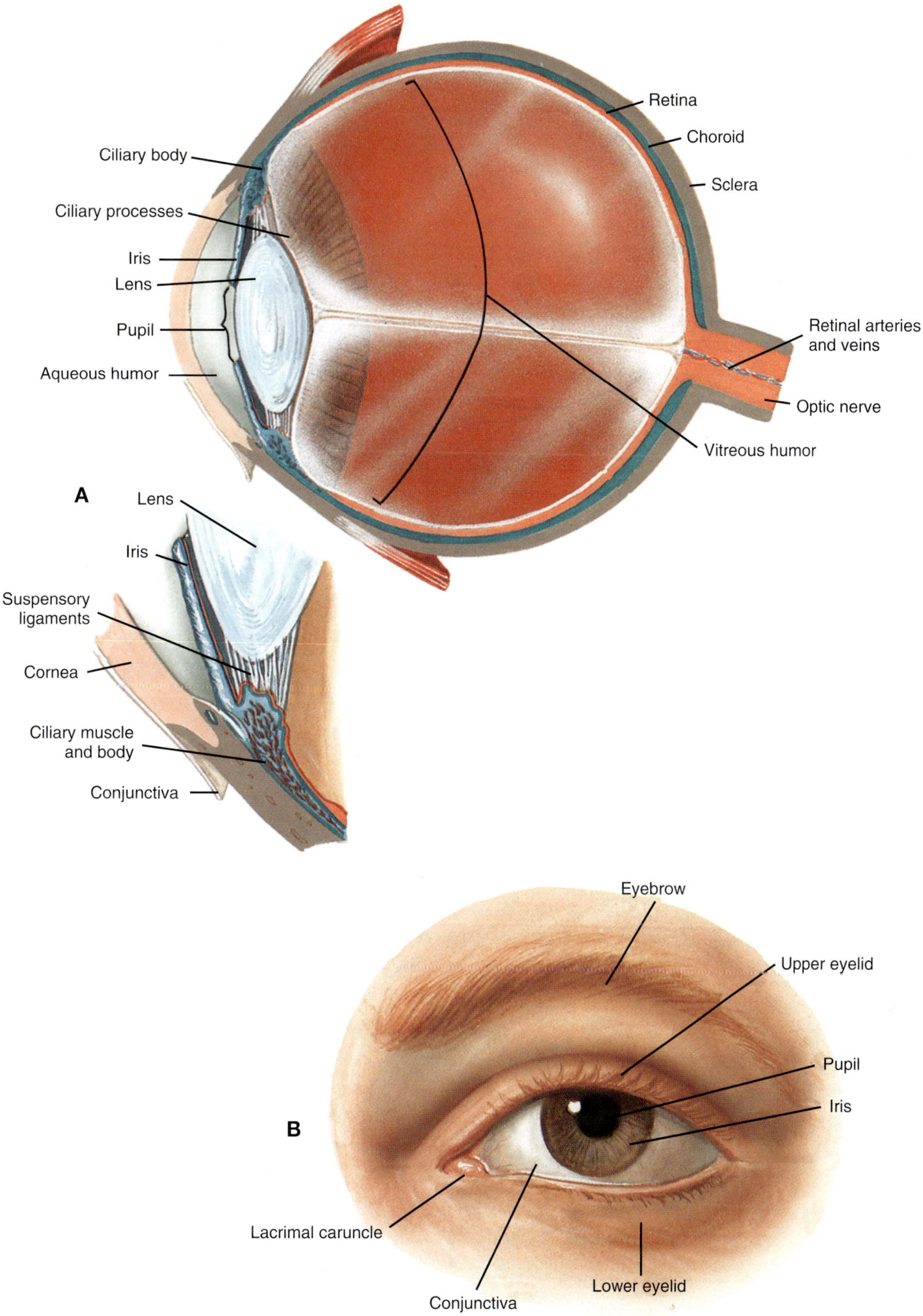

FIGURE 12-1
A, Anatomy of the eye. **B,** Visible surface of the eye.

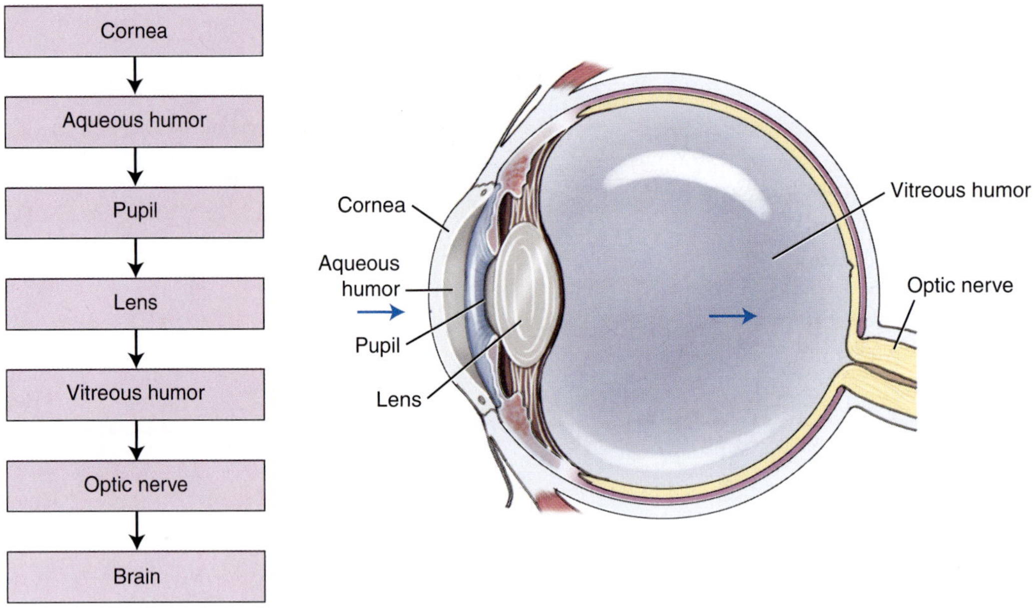

FIGURE 12-2
Pathway of light.

EXERCISE 1

Match the anatomic terms in the first column with the correct definitions in the second column. *To check your answers to the exercises in this chapter, go to Answers, p. 590, at the end of the chapter.*

_____ 1. aqueous humor
_____ 2. choroid
_____ 3. conjunctiva
_____ 4. cornea
_____ 5. iris
_____ 6. lacrimal glands
_____ 7. lens

a. lies directly behind the pupil
b. the pigmented muscular structure
c. middle layer of the eye
d. watery liquid found in the anterior cavity of the eye
e. produce tears
f. mucous membrane lining the eyelids
g. jellylike substance behind the lens and in the posterior cavity
h. transparent anterior part of the sclera

EXERCISE 2

Match the anatomic terms in the first column with the correct definitions in the second column.

_____ 1. meibomian glands
_____ 2. optic nerve
_____ 3. pupil
_____ 4. retina
_____ 5. sclera
_____ 6. vitreous humor

a. outer protective layer of the eye
b. innermost layer of the eye
c. jellylike substance found behind the lens and in the posterior cavity of the eye
d. oil glands in eyelids that help lubricate the eye
e. opening in the center of the iris
f. carries visual impulses from the retina to the brain
g. middle layer of the eye

WORD PARTS

Combining Forms of the Eye

Word parts you need to learn to complete this chapter are listed on the following pages. The exercises at the end of each list will help you learn their definitions and spellings.

Use the flashcards accompanying this text or electronic flashcards to assist you in memorizing the word parts for this chapter.

To use electronic flashcards, go to http://evolve.elsevier.com. Refer to p. 18 for your Evolve Access Information. Select Flashcards, Chapter 12.

Combining Form	Definition
blephar/o	eyelid
conjunctiv/o	conjunctiva
cor/o, core/o, pupill/o (NOTE: pupil has one *l*; the combining form has two *l*s.)	pupil
corne/o, kerat/o (NOTE: *kerat/o* also means *hard* or *horny tissue;* see Chapter 4.)	cornea
dacry/o, lacrim/o	tear, tear duct
ir/o, irid/o	iris
ocul/o, ophthalm/o	eye
opt/o	vision
phac/o, phak/o	lens
retin/o	retina (Figure 12-3)
scler/o	sclera

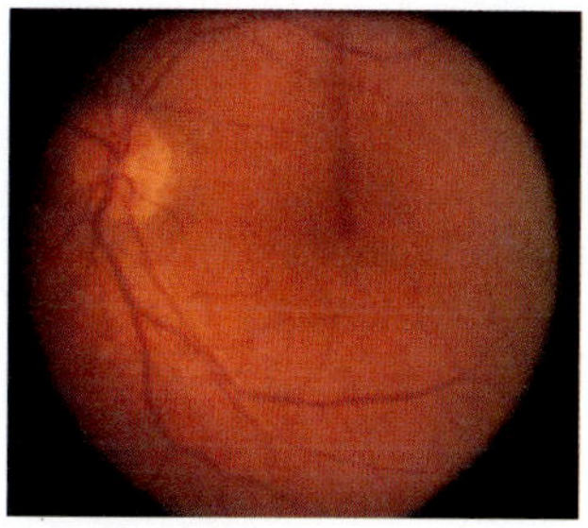

FIGURE 12-3
Ophthalmoscopic view of the retina.

Spelling Ophthalm
Look closely at the spelling of the word root **ophthalm.** Medical terms containing **ophthalm** are often misspelled by omitting the first h; **ph** gives the **f** sound followed by the sound of **thal.** Think pronunciation when spelling terms that contain **ophthalm,** as in ophthalmology (of[ph]-thal-MOL-o-jē).

EXERCISE 3

Write the definitions of the following combining forms.

1. ocul/o ____________________
2. blephar/o____________________
3. corne/o ____________________
4. lacrim/o____________________
5. retin/o ____________________
6. pupill/o ____________________
7. scler/o ____________________
8. irid/o ____________________
9. conjunctiv/o ________________
10. cor/o ____________________
11. ophthalm/o________________
12. kerat/o____________________
13. ir/o____________________
14. core/o ____________________
15. opt/o ____________________
16. dacry/o ____________________
17. phac/o, phak/o ______________

EXERCISE FIGURE A

Diagrams of the eye. Fill in the blanks with combining forms. *To check your answers, go to p. 590.*

1. Eye

   CF: ______________________________

   CF: ______________________________

2. Eyelid

   CF: ______________________________

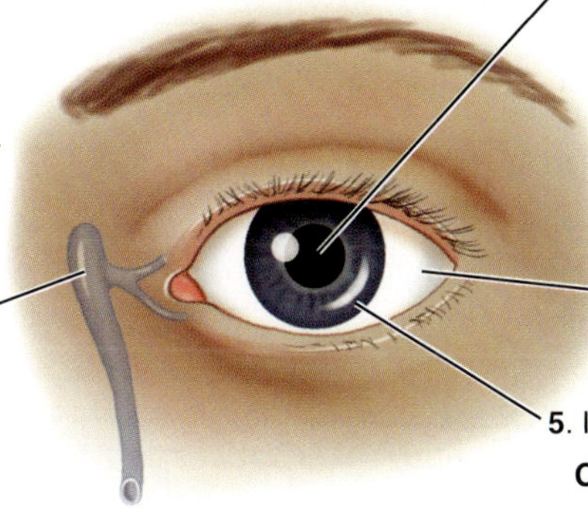

3. Pupil

   CF: ______________________________

   CF: ______________________________

   CF: ______________________________

4. Sclera

   CF: ______________________________

5. Iris

   CF: ______________________________

   CF: ______________________________

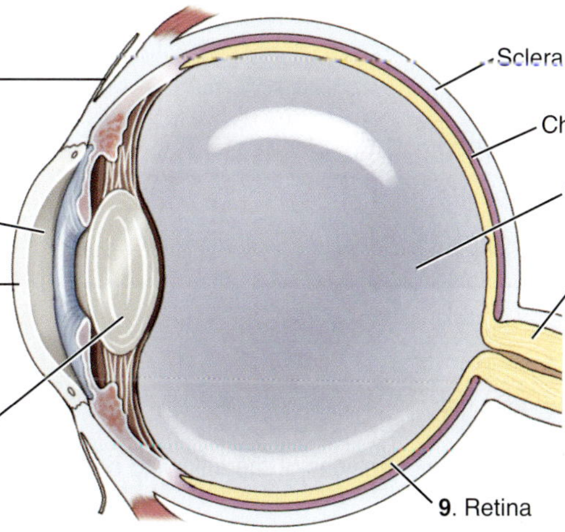

6. Conjunctiva

   CF: ______________________________

7. Cornea

   CF: ______________________________

   CF: ______________________________

8. Lens

   CF: ______________________________

   CF: ______________________________

9. Retina

   CF: ______________________________

EXERCISE 4

Write the combining form for each of the following terms.

1. eye a. ____________ b. ____________
2. cornea a. ____________ b. ____________
3. conjunctiva ____________
4. tear, tear duct a. ____________ b. ____________
5. eyelid ____________
6. pupil a. ____________ b. ____________ c. ____________
7. sclera ____________
8. retina ____________
9. iris a. ____________ b. ____________
10. vision ____________
11. lens a. ____________ b. ____________

Combining Forms Commonly Used with the Eye

Combining Form	Definition
cry/o	cold
dipl/o	two, double
is/o	equal
phot/o	light
ton/o	tension, pressure

EXERCISE 5

Write the definitions of the following combining forms.

1. ton/o ____________________
2. phot/o ____________________
3. cry/o ____________________
4. dipl/o ____________________
5. is/o ____________________

EXERCISE 6

Write the combining form for each of the following.

1. cold ____________________
2. tension, pressure ____________
3. two, double ____________
4. light ____________________
5. equal ____________________

Prefixes and Suffixes

Prefixes	Definition
bi-, bin-	two

Suffixes	Definitions
-opia	vision (condition)
-phobia	abnormal fear of or aversion to specific things
-plegia	paralysis

Refer to **Appendix A** and **Appendix B** for a complete listing of word parts.

EXERCISE 7

Write the definition of the following prefixes and suffixes.

1. -opia ____________________
2. bi- ____________________
3. -plegia ____________________
4. -phobia ____________________
5. bin- ____________________

EXERCISE 8

Write the prefixes or suffixes for each of the following definitions.

1. paralysis ____________________
2. two a. ____________________
   b. ____________________
3. abnormal fear of or aversion to specific things ____________________
4. vision (condition) ____________________

EXERCISE FIGURE B

Fill in the blanks to label the diagram.

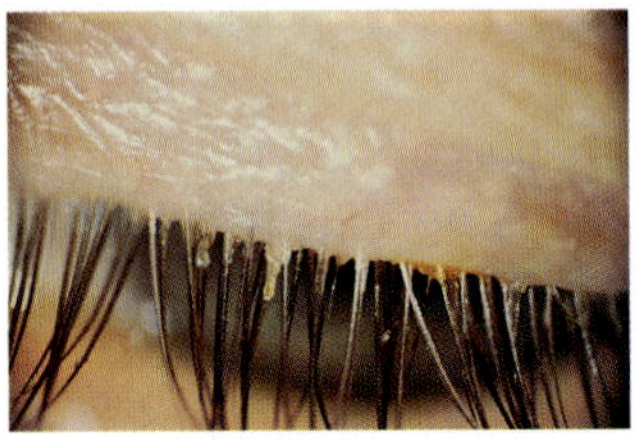

_____ / _____
eyelid / inflammation
with thickened lids and crusts around the lashes.

EXERCISE FIGURE C

Fill in the blanks to label the diagram.

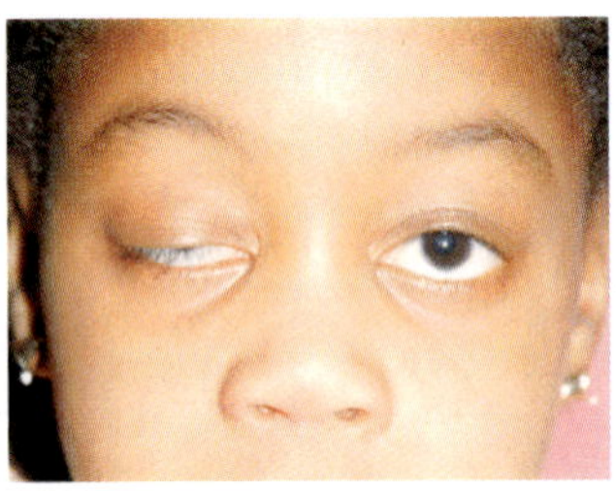

_____ / _____ / _____
eyelid / cv / drooping

EXERCISE FIGURE D

Fill in the blanks to label the diagram.

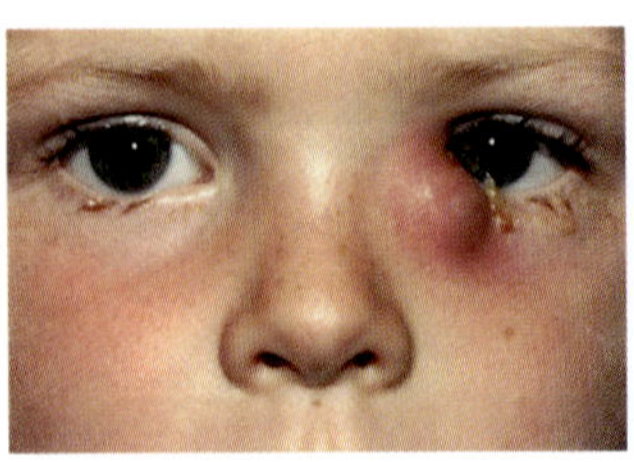

_____ / _____ / _____ / _____
tear / cv / sac / inflammation

MEDICAL TERMS

The terms you need to learn to complete this chapter are listed on the following pages. The exercises following each list will help you learn the definition and the spelling of each word.

Disease and Disorder Terms

Built from Word Parts

The following terms are built from word parts you have already learned and can be translated literally to find their meanings. Further explanation of terms beyond the definition of their word parts, if needed, is included in parentheses.

Term	Definition
aphakia (a-FĀ-kē-a)	condition of without a lens (may be congenital, though often is the result of extraction of a cataract without the placement of an intraocular lens)
blepharitis (*blef*-a-RĪ-tis)	inflammation of the eyelid (Exercise Figure B)
blepharoptosis (*blef*-ar-op-TŌ-sis)	drooping of the eyelid (Exercise Figure C) (commonly called **ptosis**)
conjunctivitis (kon-*junk*-ti-VĪ-tis)	inflammation of the conjunctiva (commonly called **pinkeye**)
dacryocystitis (*dak*-rē-ō-sis-TĪ-tis)	inflammation of the tear (lacrimal) sac (Exercise Figure D)
diplopia (di-PLŌ-pē-a)	double vision
endophthalmitis (*en*-dof-thal-MĪ-tis) (NOTE: the *o* in *endo* is dropped.)	inflammation within the eye
iridoplegia (*īr*-i-dō-PLĒ-ja)	paralysis of the iris
iritis (*ī*-RĪ-tis)	inflammation of the iris
keratitis (*ker*-a-TĪ-tis)	inflammation of the cornea
keratomalacia (*ker*-a-tō-ma-LĀ-sha)	softening of the cornea (usually a bilateral condition associated with vitamin A deficiency)
leukocoria (*lū*-kō-KŌ-rē-a)	condition of white pupil
oculomycosis (*ok*-ū-lō-mī-KŌ-sis)	abnormal condition of the eye caused by a fungus
ophthalmalgia (*of-thal*-MAL-ja)	pain in the eye
ophthalmoplegia (of-thal-mō-PLĒ-ja)	paralysis of the eye (muscle)
phacomalacia (*fāk*-ō-ma-LĀ-sha)	softening of the lens

Term	Definition
photophobia (*fō*-tō-FŌ-bē-a)	abnormal fear of (sensitivity to) light
retinoblastoma (*ret*-i-nō-blas-TŌ-ma)	tumor arising from a developing retinal cell (a congenital, malignant tumor)
retinopathy (*ret*-i-NOP-a-thē)	(any noninflammatory) disease of the retina (such as diabetic retinopathy)
sclerokeratitis (*sklĕr*-ō-*ker*-a-TĪ-tis)	inflammation of the sclera and the cornea
scleromalacia (*sklĕr*-ō-ma-LĀ-sha)	softening of the sclera
xerophthalmia (*zēr*-of-THAL-mē-a)	condition of dry eye (conjunctiva and cornea) (caused by vitamin A deficiency)

CAM TERM

Yoga is the practice of physical postures, conscious breathing, and meditation. Regular practice of yoga has demonstrated efficacy in relieving dry eye and other uncomfortable symptoms of computer vision syndrome.

EXERCISE 9

Practice saying aloud each of the disease and disorder terms built from word parts on these two pages.

To hear the terms, go to http://evolve.elsevier.com. Refer to p. 18 for your Evolve Access Information. Select Exercises & Review, Chapter 12, Chapter Exercises, Pronunciation.

☐ Place a check mark in the box when you have completed this exercise.

EXERCISE 10

Analyze and define the following terms.

1. sclerokeratitis ____________________
2. ophthalmalgia ____________________
3. blepharoptosis ____________________
4. diplopia ____________________
5. conjunctivitis ____________________
6. leukocoria ____________________
7. iridoplegia ____________________
8. scleromalacia ____________________
9. photophobia ____________________
10. blepharitis ____________________
11. oculomycosis ____________________
12. dacryocystitis ____________________

13. endophthalmitis ______________________
14. iritis ______________________
15. retinoblastoma ______________________
16. keratitis ______________________
17. ophthalmoplegia ______________________
18. retinopathy ______________________
19. xerophthalmia ______________________
20. keratomalacia ______________________
21. phacomalacia ______________________
22. aphakia ______________________

EXERCISE 11

Build disease and disorder terms for the following definitions by using the word parts you have learned.

1. inflammation of the conjunctiva ______ / ______
   WR / S
2. abnormal eye condition caused by a fungus ______ / / ______ / ______
   WR / CV / WR / S
3. pain in the eye ______ / ______
   WR / S
4. double vision ______ / ______
   WR / S
5. inflammation of the eyelid ______ / ______
   WR / S
6. condition of white pupil ______ / / ______ / ______
   WR / CV / WR / S
7. paralysis of the iris ______ / / ______
   WR / CV / S
8. drooping of the eyelid ______ / / ______
   WR / CV / S
9. inflammation of the iris ______ / ______
   WR / S
10. tumor arising from a developing retinal cell ______ / / ______ / ______
    WR / CV / WR / S
11. softening of the sclera ______ / / ______
    WR / CV / S
12. inflammation of a tear (lacrimal) sac ______ / / ______ / ______
    WR / CV / WR / S

13. inflammation of the sclera and cornea ______ / ______ / ______ / ______
WR / CV / WR / S

14. abnormal fear of (sensitivity to) light ______ / ______ / ______
WR / CV / S

15. inflammation of the cornea ______ / ______
WR / S

16. disease of the retina ______ / ______ / ______
WR / CV / S

17. inflammation within the eye ______ / ______ / ______
P / WR / S

18. paralysis of the eye (muscle) ______ / ______ / ______
WR / CV / S

19. condition of dry eye ______ / ______ / ______
WR / WR / S

20. softening of the cornea ______ / ______ / ______
WR / CV / S

21. condition of without a lens ______ / ______ / ______
P / WR / S

22. softening of the lens ______ / ______ / ______
WR / CV / S

EXERCISE 12

Spell each of the disease and disorder terms built from word parts on pp. 562-563 by having someone dictate them to you.

To hear and spell the terms, go to http://evolve.elsevier.com. Refer to p. 18 for your Evolve Access Information. Select Exercises & Review, Chapter 12, Chapter Exercises, Spelling.
☐ Place a check mark in the box if you have completed this exercise online.

1. ______
2. ______
3. ______
4. ______
5. ______
6. ______
7. ______
8. ______
9. ______
10. ______
11. ______
12. ______
13. ______
14. ______
15. ______
16. ______
17. ______
18. ______
19. ______
20. ______
21. ______
22. ______

CATARACT

is derived from the Greek **kato,** meaning **down,** and **raktos,** meaning **precipice.** Together, the words were interpreted as **waterfall.** The cataract sufferer sees things as through a watery veil of mist, or waterfall.

Disease and Disorder Terms

Not Built from Word Parts

In some of the following terms, you may recognize word parts you have already learned; however, the full meaning of the terms cannot be discerned by the definition of their word parts.

Term	Definition
amblyopia (*am*-ble-Ō-pē-a)	reduced vision in one eye caused by disuse or misuse associated with strabismus, unequal refractive errors, or otherwise impaired vision. The brain suppresses images from the impaired eye to avoid double vision (also called **lazy eye**).
astigmatism (Ast) (a-STIG-ma-tizm)	defective curvature of the refractive surfaces (cornea or lens) of the eye (Figure 12-4, *C*)
cataract (KAT-a-rakt)	clouding of the lens of the eye (Figure 12-5)
chalazion (ka-LĀ-zē-on)	obstruction of an oil gland of the eyelid (also called **meibomian cyst**) (Figure 12-6)
detached retina (RET-in-a)	separation of the retina from the choroid in back of the eye (Figure 12-7)

A
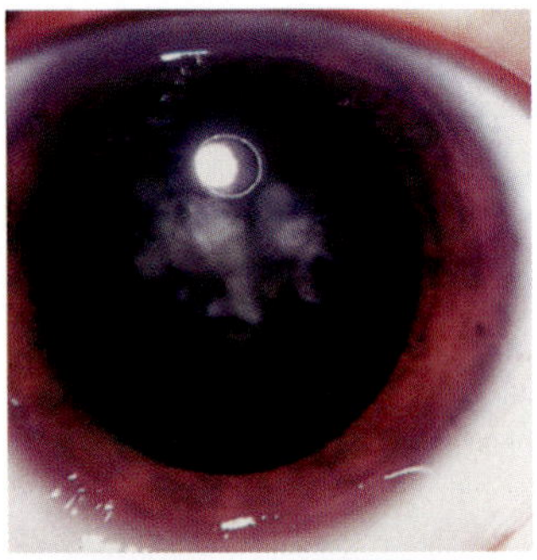

B
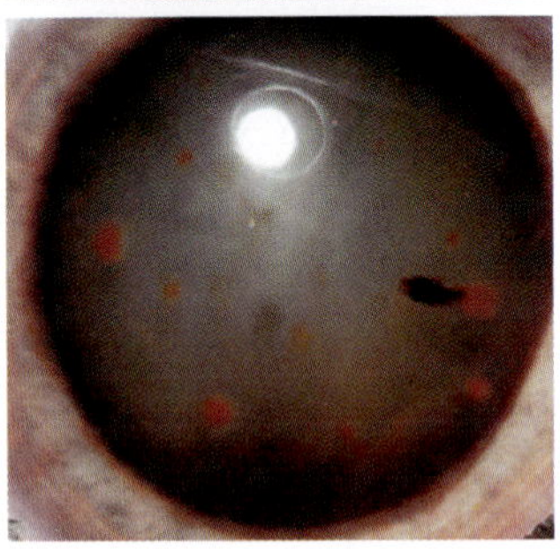

FIGURE 12-5
A, Snowflake cataract. **B,** Senile cataract.

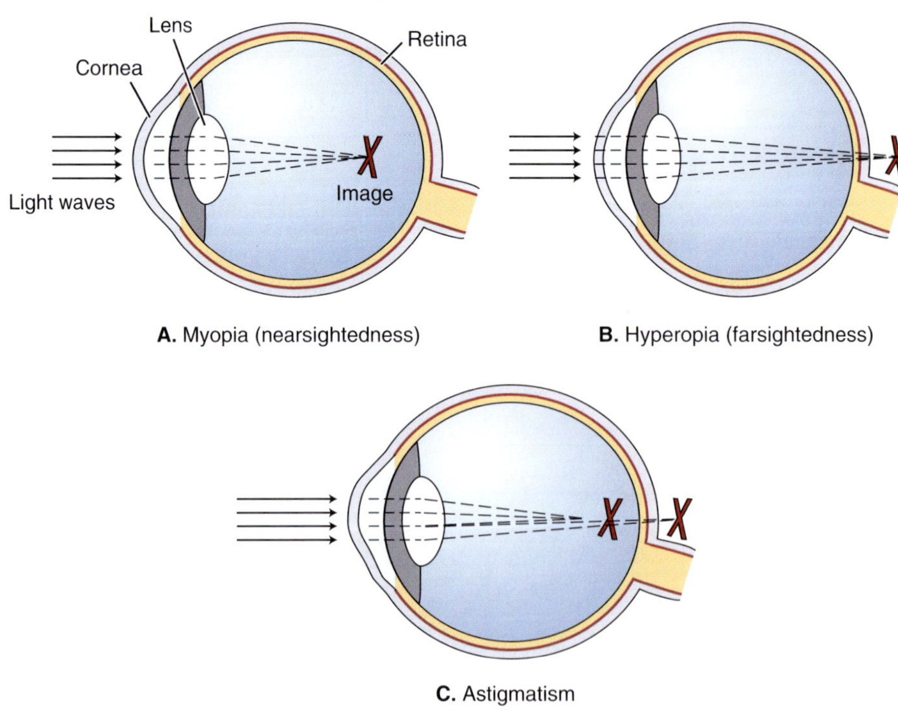

FIGURE 12-4
Refraction errors. **A,** Myopia, nearsightedness. **B,** Hyperopia, farsightedness. **C,** Astigmatism.

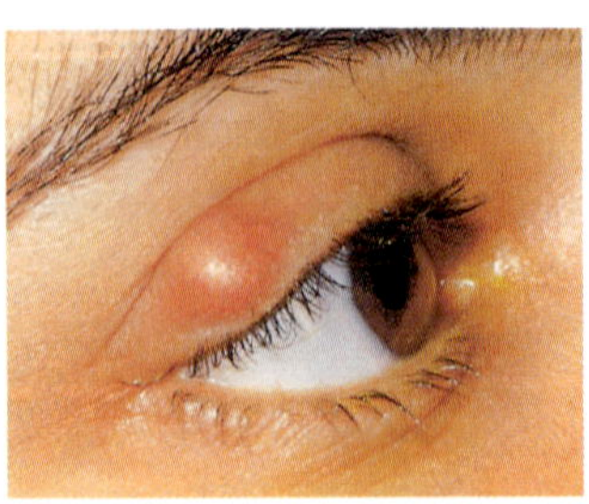

FIGURE 12-6
Chalazion (right upper eyelid).

Term	Definition
glaucoma (glaw-KŌ-ma)	eye disorder characterized by optic nerve damage usually caused by the abnormal increase of intraocular pressure (IOP). If not treated it will lead to blindness.
hyperopia (*hī*-per-Ō-pē-a)	farsightedness (Figure 12-4, *B*)
macular degeneration (MAC-ū-lar) (dē-*gen*-e-RĀ-shun)	a progressive deterioration of the portion of the retina called the **macula lutea**, resulting in loss of central vision (Figure 12-8)
myopia (mī-Ō-pē-a)	nearsightedness (see Figure 12-4, *A*)
nyctalopia (*nik*-ta-LŌ-pē-a)	poor vision at night or in faint light (also called **night blindness**)
nystagmus (nis-TAG-mus)	involuntary, jerking movements of the eyes
pinguecula (ping-GWEH-kū-la)	yellowish mass on the conjunctiva that may be related to exposure to ultraviolet light, dry climates, and dust. A pinguecula that spreads onto the cornea becomes a **pterygium.**

GLAUCOMA

is composed of the Greek **glaukos**, meaning **blue-gray** or **sea green**, and **oma**, meaning a morbid condition. The term was given to any condition in which gray or green replaced the black in the pupil.

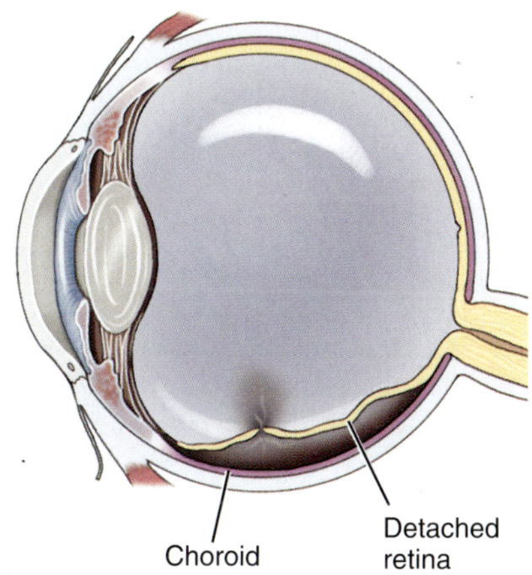

FIGURE 12-7

Detached retina. Vitreous fluid has seeped through a tear in the retina, causing the choroid coat and retina to separate.

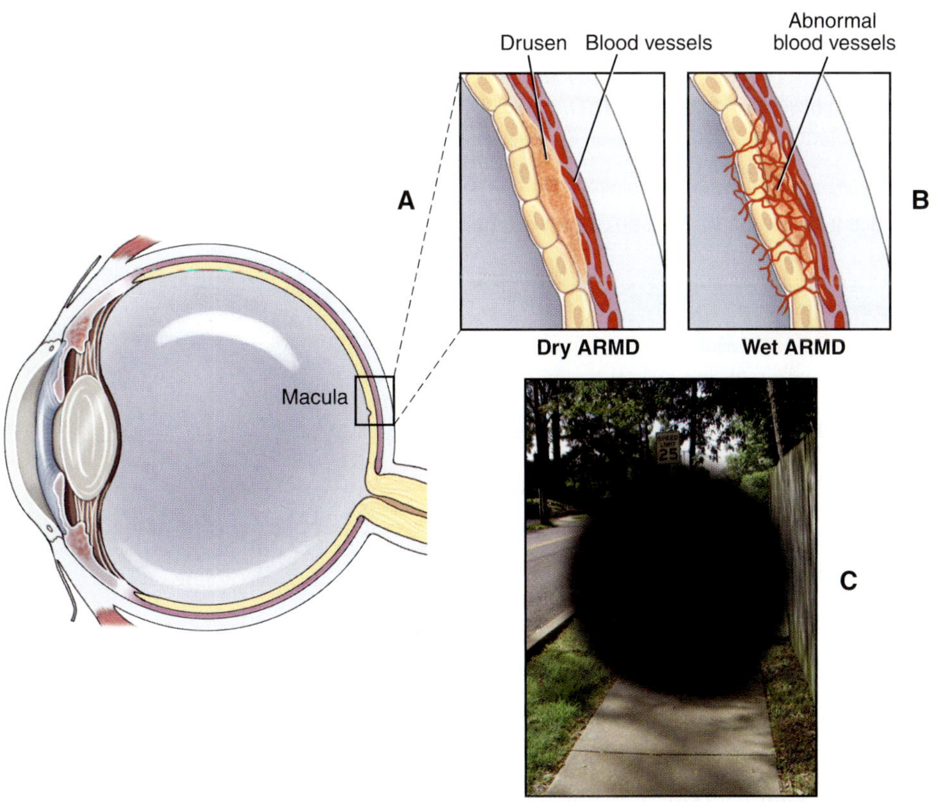

FIGURE 12-8

Macular degeneration. **A, Dry macular degeneration**, where blood vessels under the macula become brittle and yellow deposits called drusen form, is the most common form of age-related macular degeneration (ARMD). **B, Wet macular degeneration**, where new abnormal blood vessels form under the macula, is less common though more likely to cause legal blindness. **C,** Central vision loss as may be experienced in ARMD.

AGE-RELATED MACULAR DEGENERATION (ARMD)

is the leading cause of legal blindness in persons older than 65 years. Onset occurs between the ages of 50 and 60 (see Figure 12-8).

Disease and Disorder Terms—*cont'd*

Not Built from Word Parts

Term	Definition
presbyopia (*pres*-bē-Ō-pē-a)	impaired vision as a result of aging
pterygium (te-RIJ-ē-um)	thin tissue growing into the cornea from the conjunctiva, usually caused from sun exposure
retinitis pigmentosa (*ret*-i-NĪ-tis) (*pig*-men-TŌ-sa)	hereditary, progressive disease marked by night blindness with atrophy and retinal pigment changes
strabismus (stra-BIZ-mus)	abnormal condition of squint or crossed eyes caused by the visual axes not meeting at the same point
sty (stī)	infection of an oil gland of the eyelid (Figure 12-9) (also spelled **stye** and also called **hordeolum**)

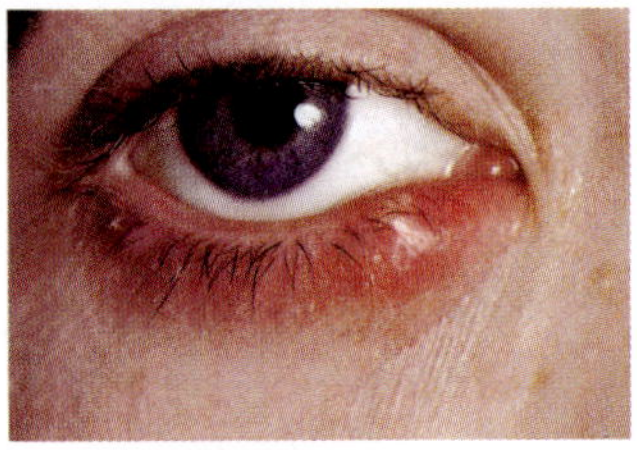

FIGURE 12-9
Sty, stye, or hordeolum.

EXERCISE 13

Practice saying aloud each of the disease and disorder terms not built from word parts on pp. 566-568.

To hear the terms, go to http://evolve.elsevier.com. Refer to p. 18 for your Evolve Access Information. Select Exercises & Review, Chapter 12, Chapter Exercises, Pronunciation.

☐ Place a check mark in the box when you have completed this exercise.

EXERCISE 14

Fill in the blanks with the correct terms.

1. Another name for nearsightedness is ______________________.
2. Impaired vision as a result of aging is ______________________.
3. The abnormal condition of squinted or crossed eyes caused by visual axes not meeting at the same point is called ______________________.
4. An obstruction of an oil gland of the eyelid is called a(n) ______________.
5. A defective curvature of the refractive surfaces of the eye causes a condition known as ______________________.
6. ______________________ is the name given to involuntary, jerking movements of the eye.
7. A clouding of the lens of the eye is called a(n) ______________________.
8. ______________________ is the name given to an infection of an oil gland of the eyelids.

9. A disorder usually caused by the abnormal increase of intraocular pressure is ______________________________.

10. A(n) ______________________________ ______________________________ is a separation of the retina from the choroid in the back of the eye.

11. Another name for farsightedness is ______________________________.

12. ______________________________ ______________________________ is a hereditary, progressive disease causing night blindness with retinal pigment changes and atrophy.

13. Another name for night blindness is ______________________________.

14. A thin tissue growing into the cornea from the conjunctiva is called a(n) ______________________________.

15. ______________________________ ______________________________ is the progressive deterioration of the macula lutea.

16. Another name for lazy eye is ______________________________.

17. ______________________________ may be related to exposure to ultraviolet light, dry climates, and dust and may spread onto the cornea to become a pterygium.

EXERCISE 15

Match the terms in the first column with the correct definitions in the second column.

	Term		Definition
______	1. astigmatism	a.	infection of an oil gland of the eyelid
______	2. cataract	b.	deterioration of the macula lutea
______	3. chalazion	c.	crossed eyes or squinting caused by visual axes not meeting at the same point
______	4. detached retina	d.	involuntary, jerking movements of the eye
______	5. glaucoma	e.	impaired vision caused by aging
______	6. myopia	f.	defective curvature of the refractive surfaces of the eye
______	7. nystagmus	g.	clouding of a lens of the eye
______	8. hyperopia	h.	hereditary, progressive disease marked by night blindness
______	9. presbyopia	i.	nearsightedness
______	10. strabismus	j.	obstruction of an oil gland of the eye
______	11. sty	k.	usually caused from sun exposure
______	12. pterygium	l.	eye disorder characterized by optic nerve damage
______	13. retinitis pigmentosa	m.	separation of the retina from the choroid in the back of the eye
______	14. nyctalopia	n.	poor vision at night or in faint light
______	15. macular degeneration	o.	farsightedness
______	16. pinguecula	p.	double vision
______	17. amblyopia	q.	yellow mass on the conjunctiva
		r.	reduced vision in one eye caused by disuse or misuse

EXERCISE 16

Spell each of the disease and disorder terms not built from word parts on pp. 566-568 by having someone dictate them to you.

To hear and spell the terms, go to http://evolve.elsevier.com. Refer to p. 18 for your Evolve Access Information. Select Exercises & Review, Chapter 12, Chapter Exercises, Spelling.
☐ Place a check mark in the box if you have completed this exercise online.

1. ______________________
2. ______________________
3. ______________________
4. ______________________
5. ______________________
6. ______________________
7. ______________________
8. ______________________
9. ______________________
10. ______________________
11. ______________________
12. ______________________
13. ______________________
14. ______________________
15. ______________________
16. ______________________
17. ______________________

Surgical Terms

Built from Word Parts

The following terms are built from word parts you have already learned and can be translated literally to find their meanings. Further explanation of terms beyond the definition of their word parts, if needed, is included in parentheses.

Term	Definition
blepharoplasty (BLEF-a-rō-*plas*-tē)	surgical repair of the eyelid
cryoretinopexy (*krī*-ō-RE-tin-ō-*pek*-sē)	surgical fixation of the retina by using extreme cold (carbon dioxide)
dacryocystorhinostomy (*dak*-rē-ō-*sis*-tō-rī-NOS-to-mē)	creation of an artificial opening between the tear (lacrimal) sac and the nose (to restore drainage into the nose when the nasolacrimal duct is obstructed or obliterated)
dacryocystotomy (*dak*-rē-ō-sis-TOT-o-mē)	incision of the tear (lacrimal) sac
iridectomy (*ir*-i-DEK-to-mē)	excision (of part) of the iris
iridotomy (*ir*-i-DOT-o-mē)	incision of the iris

Term	Definition
keratoplasty (KER-a-tō-*plas*-tē)	surgical repair of the cornea (corneal transplant) (Figure 12-10)
sclerotomy (skle-ROT-o-mē)	incision of the sclera

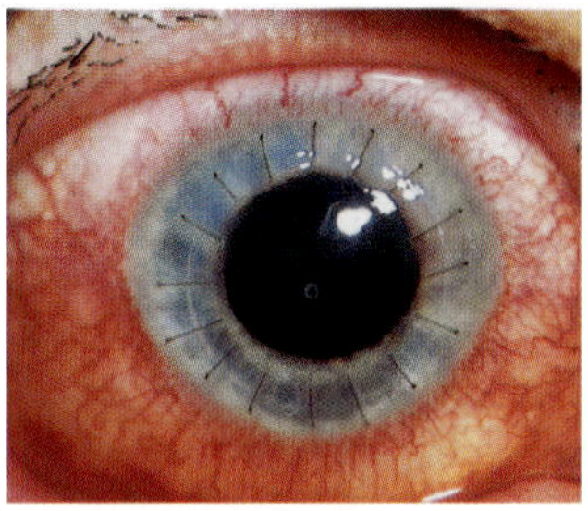

FIGURE 12-10
Appearance of eye after keratoplasty.

EXERCISE 17

Practice saying aloud each of the surgical terms built from word parts on these two pages.

To hear the terms, go to http://evolve.elsevier.com. Refer to p. 18 for your Evolve Access Information. Select Exercises & Review, Chapter 12, Chapter Exercises, Pronunciation.

☐ Place a check mark in the box when you have completed this exercise.

EXERCISE 18

Analyze and define the following surgical terms.

1. keratoplasty ______________________________
2. sclerotomy ______________________________
3. dacryocystotomy ______________________________
4. cryoretinopexy ______________________________
5. blepharoplasty ______________________________
6. iridectomy ______________________________
7. dacryocystorhinostomy ______________________________
____
8. iridotomy ______________________________

EXERCISE 19

Build surgical terms for the following definitions by using the word parts you have learned.

1. creation of an artificial opening between the tear (lacrimal) sac and the nose
   ______ / ______ / ______ / ______ / ______ / ______ / ______
   WR / CV / WR / CV / WR / CV / S
2. excision of the iris
   ______ / ______
   WR / S
3. surgical repair of the cornea
   ______ / ______ / ______
   WR / CV / S
4. incision of the sclera
   ______ / ______ / ______
   WR / CV / S
5. incision of the iris
   ______ / ______ / ______
   WR / CV / S
6. surgical repair of the eyelid
   ______ / ______ / ______
   WR / CV / S
7. surgical fixation of the retina using extreme cold
   ______ / ______ / ______ / ______ / ______
   WR / CV / WR / CV / S
8. incision of the (lacrimal) tear sac
   ______ / ______ / ______ / ______ / ______
   WR / CV / WR / CV / S

EXERCISE 20

Spell each of the surgical terms built from word parts on pp. 570-571 by having someone dictate them to you.

To hear and spell the terms, go to http://evolve.elsevier.com. Refer to p. 18 for your Evolve Access Information. Select Exercises & Review, Chapter 12, Chapter Exercises, Spelling.
☐ Place a check mark in the box if you have completed this exercise online.

1. ______________________
2. ______________________
3. ______________________
4. ______________________
5. ______________________
6. ______________________
7. ______________________
8. ______________________

Surgical Terms

Not Built from Word Parts

In some of the following terms, you may recognize word parts you have already learned; however, the full meaning of the terms cannot be discerned by the definition of their word parts.

Term	Definition
enucleation (ē-*nū*-klē-Ā-shun)	surgical removal of the eyeball (also, the removal of any organ that comes out clean and whole)
LASIK (laser-assisted in situ keratomileusis) (LĀ-sik)	a laser procedure that reshapes the corneal tissue beneath the surface of the cornea to correct astigmatism, hyperopia, and myopia. LASIK is a combination of Excimer laser and lamellar keratoplasty. It differs from PRK in that it reshapes corneal tissue beneath the surface rather than on the surface (Figure 12-11, *B*).
phacoemulsification (PHACO) (*fa*-kō-ē-*mul*-si-fi-KĀ-shun)	method to remove cataracts in which an ultrasonic needle probe breaks up the lens, which is then aspirated
PRK (photorefractive keratectomy) (*fō*-tō-rē-FRAK-tiv) (*ker*-a-TEK-to-mē)	a procedure for the treatment of nearsightedness in which an Excimer laser is used to reshape (flatten) the corneal surface by removing a portion of the cornea (Figure 12-11, *A*)
retinal photocoagulation (RET-in-al) (*fō*-tō-kō-*ag*-ū-LĀ-shun)	an intense beam of light from a laser condenses retinal tissue to seal leaking blood vessels, to destroy abnormal tissue or lesions, or to bond the retina to the back of the eye. Used to treat retinal tears and detachment, diabetic retinopathy, wet macular degeneration, glaucoma, and intraocular tumors.
scleral buckling (SKLER-al) (BUK-ling)	a procedure to repair a detached retina. A strip of sclera is resected, or a fold is made in the sclera. An exoplant is used to hold and buckle the sclera (Figure 12-12).
trabeculectomy (tra-*bek*-ū-LEK-to-mē)	surgical creation of a drain to reduce intraocular pressure (used to treat glaucoma)
vitrectomy (vi-TREK-to-mē)	surgical removal of all or part of the vitreous humor (used to treat diabetic retinopathy)

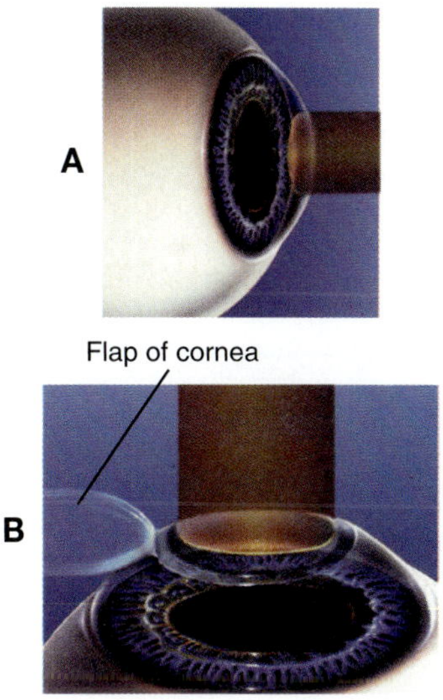

FIGURE 12-11
Excimer laser treatments for nearsightedness. **A, PRK** (photorefractive keratectomy): removes tissue from the surface of the cornea. **B, LASIK** (laser-assisted in situ keratomileusis): reshapes corneal tissue below the surface of the cornea. The Excimer laser was invented in the early 1980s. It is a computer-controlled ultraviolet beam of light that reshapes the cornea. It has replaced **RK** (radial keratotomy), a surgery in which spokelike incisions are made to reshape the cornea.

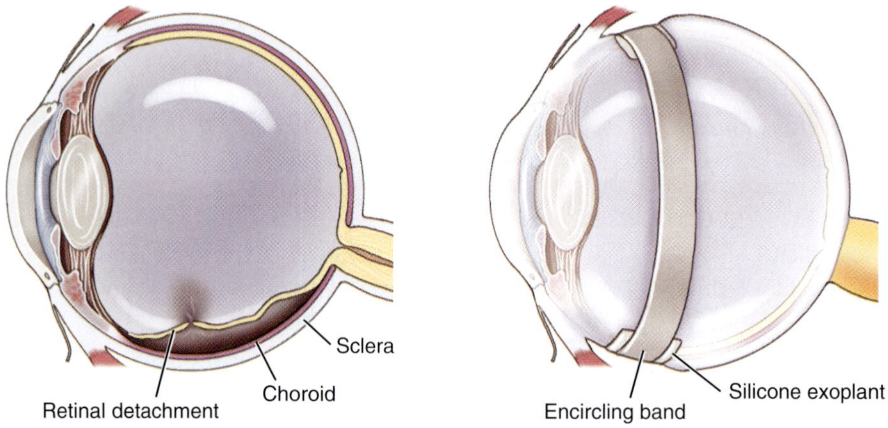

FIGURE 12-12
Scleral buckling. A surgical procedure to repair a detached retina.

EXERCISE 21

Practice saying aloud each of the surgical terms not built from word parts on p. 573.

To hear the terms, go to http://evolve.elsevier.com. Refer to p. 18 for your Evolve Access Information. Select Exercises & Review, Chapter 12, Chapter Exercises, Pronunciation.

☐ Place a check mark in the box when you have completed this exercise.

EXERCISE 22

Fill in the blank with the correct terms.

1. ______________ ____________________________ is the use of a laser beam to condense retinal tissue to seal leaking blood vessels, destroy abnormal tissue, or bond the retina to the back of the eye.
2. Surgical removal of an eyeball is called a(n) ____________________________.
3. ____________________________ is the name given to the procedure that breaks up the lens with ultrasound and then aspirates it.
4. A procedure using the Excimer laser and lamellar keratoplasty to correct hyperopia, myopia, and astigmatism is called ______________.
5. ______________________ is the surgical creation of a drain to reduce intraocular pressure.
6. An operation to repair a detached retina in which the sclera is folded or resected and an exoplant is used to buckle and hold the sclera is called ______________ ______________.
7. Surgery to remove vitreous humor from the eye is called ______________.
8. ______________ is a procedure for the treatment of nearsightedness in which an Excimer laser is used to reshape the corneal surface.

EXERCISE 23

Match the terms in the first column with their correct definitions in the second column.

_____ 1. LASIK
_____ 2. enucleation
_____ 3. trabeculectomy
_____ 4. retinal photocoagulation
_____ 5. phacoemulsification
_____ 6. scleral buckling
_____ 7. vitrectomy
_____ 8. PRK

a. use of a laser beam to repair retinal tears and detachment, as well as other retinopathies
b. surgical creation of a permanent drain to reduce intraocular pressure
c. procedure for the treatment of nearsightedness in which an Excimer laser is used to reshape the corneal surface
d. procedure in which the lens is broken up by ultrasound and aspirated
e. procedure used to correct astigmatism, nearsightedness, and farsightedness by reshaping tissue beneath the corneal surface
f. surgical removal of an eyeball
g. surgical removal of vitreous humor
h. operation in which a cataract is lifted from the eye with an extremely cold probe
i. detached retina surgery in which the sclera is folded and an exoplant is used to buckle and hold the sclera
j. surgical incision of the sclera

EXERCISE 24

Spell each of the surgical terms not built from word parts on p. 573 by having someone dictate them to you.

To hear and spell the terms, go to http://evolve.elsevier.com. Refer to p. 18 for your Evolve Access Information. Select Exercises & Review, Chapter 12, Chapter Exercises, Spelling.
☐ Place a check mark in the box if you have completed this exercise online.

1. ____________________ 5. ____________________
2. ____________________ 6. ____________________
3. ____________________ 7. ____________________
4. ____________________ 8. ____________________

Diagnostic Terms

Built from Word Parts

The following terms are built from word parts you have already learned and can be translated literally to find their meanings. Further explanation of terms beyond the definition of their word parts, if needed, is included in parentheses.

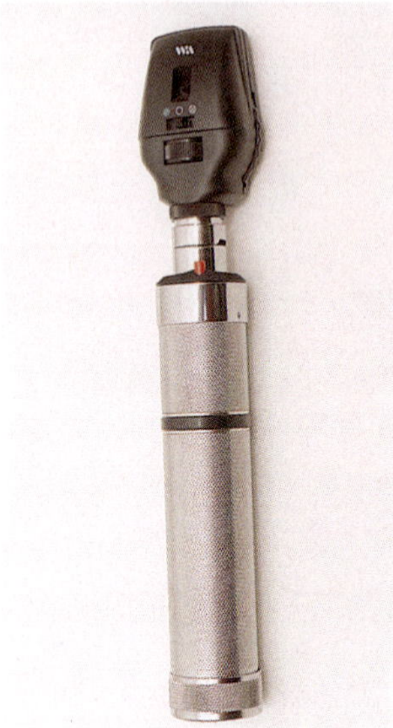

FIGURE 12-13 Ophthalmoscope.

Term	Definition
DIAGNOSTIC IMAGING	
fluorescein angiography (flō-RES-ēn) (*an*-jē-OG-ra-fē)	(digital) process of recording blood vessels (of the eye with fluorescing dye)
OPHTHALMIC EVALUATION	
keratometer (*ker*-a-TOM-e-ter)	instrument used to measure (the curvature of) the cornea (used for fitting contact lenses)
ophthalmoscope (of-THAL-mō-skōp)	instrument used for visual examination (the interior) of the eye (Figure 12-13)
ophthalmoscopy (*of*-thal-MOS-ko-pē)	visual examination of the eye
optometry (op-TOM-e-trē)	measurement of vision (visual acuity and the prescribing of corrective lenses)
pupillometer (*pū*-pil-OM-e-ter)	instrument used to measure (the diameter of) the pupil
pupilloscope (pū-PIL-ō-skōp)	instrument used for visual examination of the pupil
retinoscopy (*ret*-i-NOS-ko-pē)	visual examination of the retina (to determine refractive error)
tonometer (tō-NOM-e-ter)	instrument used to measure pressure (within the eye, used to diagnose glaucoma)
tonometry (tō-NOM-e-trē)	measurement of pressure (within the eye)

EXERCISE 25

Practice saying aloud each of the diagnostic terms built from word parts above.

To hear the terms, go to http://evolve.elsevier.com. Refer to p. 18 for your Evolve Access Information. Select Exercises & Review, Chapter 12, Chapter Exercises, Pronunciation.

☐ Place a check mark in the box when you have completed this exercise.

EXERCISE 26

Analyze and define the following diagnostic terms.

1. pupilloscope ______________________
2. optometry ______________________
3. ophthalmoscope ______________________
4. tonometry ______________________
5. pupillometer ______________________
6. tonometer ______________________
7. keratometer ______________________
8. ophthalmoscopy ______________________
9. (fluorescein) angiography ______________________
10. retinoscopy ______________________

EXERCISE 27

Build diagnostic terms that correspond to the following definitions by using the word parts you have learned.

1. measurement of pressure (within the eye) ______ / ______ / ______ (WR / CV / S)
2. instrument used to measure (the diameter of) the pupil ______ / ______ / ______ (WR / CV / S)
3. instrument used to measure (the curvature of) the cornea ______ / ______ / ______ (WR / CV / S)
4. measurement of vision ______ / ______ / ______ (WR / CV / S)
5. instrument used for visual examination of the eye ______ / ______ / ______ (WR / CV / S)
6. instrument used to measure pressure (within the eye) ______ / ______ / ______ (WR / CV / S)
7. instrument used for visual examination of the pupil ______ / ______ / ______ (WR / CV / S)

8. visual examination of the eye ______ WR / CV / ______ S

9. process of recording blood vessels (of the eye with fluorescing dye) fluorescein ______ WR / CV / ______ S

10. visual examination of the retina ______ WR / CV / ______ S

EXERCISE 28

Spell each of the diagnostic terms built from word parts on p. 576 by having someone dictate them to you.

To hear and spell the terms, go to http://evolve.elsevier.com. Refer to p. 18 for your Evolve Access Information. Select Exercises & Review, Chapter 12, Chapter Exercises, Spelling.
☐ Place a check mark in the box if you have completed this exercise online.

1. ______
2. ______
3. ______
4. ______
5. ______
6. ______
7. ______
8. ______
9. ______
10. ______

Complementary Terms

Built from Word Parts

The following terms are built from word parts you have already learned and can be translated literally to find their meanings. Further explanation of terms beyond the definition of their word parts, if needed, is included in parentheses.

Term	Definition
anisocoria (an-ī-sō-KŌR-ē-a)	condition of absence of equal pupil (size) (unequal size of pupils)
binocular (bin-OK-ū-lar)	pertaining to two or both eyes
corneal (KOR-nē-al)	pertaining to the cornea
intraocular (*in*-tra-OK-ū-lar)	pertaining to within the eye
isocoria (ī-sō-KŌR-ē-a)	condition of equal pupil (size)
lacrimal (LAK-ri-mal)	pertaining to tears

Term	Definition
nasolacrimal (*nā*-zō-LAK-ri-mal)	pertaining to the nose and tear ducts
ophthalmic (of-THAL-mik)	pertaining to the eye
ophthalmologist (*of*-thal-MOL-o-jist)	physician who studies and treats diseases of the eye
ophthalmology (Ophth) (*of*-thal-MOL-o-jē)	study of the eye (a branch of medicine that deals with treating diseases of the eye)
ophthalmopathy (*of*-thal-MOP-a-thē)	(any) disease of the eye
optic (OP-tik)	pertaining to vision
pseudophakia (*soo*-dō-FĀ-ke-a)	condition of false lens (placement of an intraocular lens during surgery to treat cataracts)
pupillary (PŪ-pi-lar-ē)	pertaining to the pupil
retinal (RET-i-nal)	pertaining to the retina

EXERCISE 29

Practice saying aloud each of the complementary terms built from word parts on these two pages.

To hear the terms, go to http://evolve.elsevier.com. Refer to p. 18 for your Evolve Access Information. Select Exercises & Review, Chapter 12, Chapter Exercises, Pronunciation.

☐ Place a check mark in the box when you have completed this exercise.

EXERCISE 30

Analyze and define the following complementary terms.

1. ophthalmology ________________
2. binocular ________________
3. lacrimal ________________
4. pupillary ________________
5. ophthalmologist ________________
6. corneal ________________
7. ophthalmic ________________
8. nasolacrimal ________________
9. optic ________________

10. intraocular ______________________
11. retinal ______________________
12. ophthalmopathy ______________________
13. isocoria ______________________
14. anisocoria ______________________
15. pseudophakia ______________________

EXERCISE 31

Build the complementary terms for the following definitions by using the word parts you have learned.

1. study of the eye ______ / ______ / ______ (WR / CV / S)
2. pertaining to two or both eyes ______ / ______ / ______ (P / WR / S)
3. pertaining to the retina ______ / ______ (WR / S)
4. pertaining to within the eye ______ / ______ / ______ (P / WR / S)
5. physician who studies and treats diseases of the eye ______ / ______ / ______ (WR / CV / S)
6. pertaining to tears ______ / ______ (WR / S)
7. pertaining to vision ______ / ______ (WR / S)
8. pertaining to the eye ______ / ______ (WR / S)
9. pertaining to the cornea ______ / ______ (WR / S)
10. pertaining to the nose and tear ducts ______ / ______ / ______ / ______ (WR / CV / WR / S)
11. disease of the eye ______ / ______ / ______ (WR / CV / S)
12. pertaining to the pupil ______ / ______ (WR / S)
13. condition of false lens ______ / ______ / ______ / ______ (WR / CV / WR / S)
14. condition of equal pupil (size) ______ / ______ / ______ / ______ (WR / CV / WR / S)
15. condition of absence of equal pupil (size) ______ / ______ / ______ / ______ / ______ (P / WR / CV / WR / S)

EXERCISE 32

Spell each of the complementary terms built from word parts on pp. 578-579 by having someone dictate them to you.

To hear and spell the terms, go to http://evolve.elsevier.com. Refer to p. 18 for your Evolve Access Information. Select Exercises & Review, Chapter 12, Chapter Exercises, Spelling.
☐ Place a check mark in the box if you have completed this exercise online.

1. ______________________
2. ______________________
3. ______________________
4. ______________________
5. ______________________
6. ______________________
7. ______________________
8. ______________________
9. ______________________
10. ______________________
11. ______________________
12. ______________________
13. ______________________
14. ______________________
15. ______________________

Complementary Terms

Not Built from Word Parts

In some of the following terms, you may recognize word parts you have already learned; however, the full meaning of the terms cannot be discerned by the definition of their word parts.

Term	Definition
emmetropia (*em*-e-TRŌ-pē-a)	normal refractive condition of the eye
intraocular lens (IOL) (*in*-tra-OK-ū-lar) (lenz)	an artificial lens implanted within the eye during cataract surgery
miotic (mī-OT-ik)	agent that constricts the pupil
mydriatic (*mid*-rē-AT-ik)	agent that dilates the pupil
optician (op-TISH-in)	a specialist who fills prescriptions for lenses (cannot prescribe lenses)
optometrist (op-TOM-e-trist)	a health professional who prescribes corrective lenses and/or eye exercises
visual acuity (VA) (VIZH-ū-al) (a-KŪ-i-tē)	sharpness of vision for either distance or near

OPTOMETRIST

is derived from the Greek **optikos**, meaning **sight**, and **metron**, meaning **measure.** Literally, an optometrist is a person who measures sight.

Refer to **Appendix D** for pharmacology terms related to the eye.

EXERCISE 33

Practice saying aloud each of the complementary terms not built from word parts on p. 581.

To hear the terms, go to http://evolve.elsevier.com. Refer to p. 18 for your Evolve Access Information. Select Exercises & Review, Chapter 12, Chapter Exercises, Pronunciation.

☐ Place a check mark in the box when you have completed this exercise.

EXERCISE 34

Write the definitions for the following complementary terms.

1. optometrist ______________________________
2. mydriatic ______________________________
3. visual acuity ______________________________
4. miotic ______________________________
5. optician ______________________________
6. emmetropia ______________________________
7. intraocular lens ______________________________

EXERCISE 35

Fill in the blanks with the correct terms.

1. An agent that dilates a pupil is a(n) ______________.
2. An agent that constricts a pupil is a(n) ______________.
3. A health professional who prescribes corrective lenses and/or eye exercises is a(n) ______________________________.
4. Another term for sharpness of vision is ______________ ______________.
5. A specialist who fills prescriptions for lenses but who cannot prescribe lenses is a(n) ______________.
6. Normal refractive condition of the eye is called ______________________.
7. After the removal of the lens by phacoemulsification to treat cataracts, often an artificial lens, or ______________ ______________, is implanted within the eye.

EXERCISE 36

Spell each of the complementary terms not built from word parts on p. 581 by having someone dictate them to you.

To hear and spell the terms, go to http://evolve.elsevier.com. Refer to p. 18 for your Evolve Access Information. Select Exercises & Review, Chapter 12, Chapter Exercises, Spelling.
☐ Place a check mark in the box if you have completed this exercise online.

1. ______________________
2. ______________________
3. ______________________
4. ______________________
5. ______________________
6. ______________________
7. ______________________

Abbreviations

ARMD	age-related macular degeneration
Ast	astigmatism
Em	emmetropia
IOL	intraocular lens
IOP	intraocular pressure
Ophth	ophthalmology
PHACO	phacoemulsification
VA	visual acuity

EXERCISE 37

Write the meaning of the following abbreviations in the spaces provided.

1. VA ______________________ ______________________
2. Ast ______________________
3. IOP ______________________ ______________________
4. Em ______________________
5. Ophth ______________________
6. ARMD ______________________ ______________________ ______________________
7. PHACO ______________________
8. IOL ______________________ ______________________

PRACTICAL APPLICATION

EXERCISE 38 *Interact with Medical Documents*

A. Complete the progress note by writing the medical terms in the blanks. Use the list of definitions with the corresponding numbers.

University Hospital and Medical Center
4700 North Main Street • Wellness, Arizona 54321 • (987) 555-3210

PATIENT NAME: William Graves **CASE NUMBER:** 20066-OPH
DATE OF BIRTH: 06/27/19XX **DATE:** 04/05/20XX

PROGRESS NOTE

SUBJECTIVE: Mr. Graves is a 66-year-old white male here today for his annual 1. _________________exam. He has no current complaints. He has a family history of 2. _________________ in his brother. He has a history of hypertension and type 2 diabetes mellitus. A 3._________________ was removed from his right eye 5 years ago.

Current Medications: Glyburide 5 mg bid and Lopressor 50 mg bid.

Allergies: None.

OBJECTIVE:
Visual Acuities: Aided: right eye 20/25 left eye 20/30-1 both eyes 20/25
Unaided: right eye 20/100 left eye 20/80-1 both eyes 20/80

Externals: 2 mm 4. _________________ right eye. PERLA (pupils equal and reactive to light and accommodation). EOMI (extraocular movements intact).

Ophthalmoscopic: Lens: left eye showed early cortical spokes
Disk: margins normal
Cup-to-disk ratio: 0.2 both eyes
Fundus: Within normal limits, including DVM
Refraction: right eye-1.00-0.50 × 90 20/20, left eye-1.25-0.25 × 90 20/20
Tonometry: 14 mm Hg/right eye, 13 mm Hg/left eye

Visual Field: Full

ASSESSMENT: Patient has compound myopic 5. _________________ and 6. _________________ with diabetic 7. _________________ and grade II hypertension. He also shows an immature 8. _________________ in the left eye.

PLAN: Provide prescription for corrective lenses. See patient for follow-up visit in 6 months to reevaluate diabetic retinopathy and cataract. Counseled patient to report any sudden changes in vision.

____

Milli Bentley, MD

MB/mcm

1. study of the eye
2. eye disorder characterized by optic nerve damage usually caused by the abnormal increase of intraocular pressure
3. thin tissue growing into the cornea from the conjunctiva
4. drooping of eyelid
5. defective curvature of the refractive surface of the eye
6. impaired vision as a result of aging
7. (any noninflammatory) disease of the retina
8. clouding of the lens of the eye

EXERCISE 38 *Interact with Medical Documents—cont'd*

B. Read the following case study and answer the questions that follow.

Case Study

Patient Profile: This 70-year-old woman was admitted for surgical treatment of chronic, poorly controlled **glaucoma** and for **cataract** extraction.

Subjective: The patient reported a progressive loss of **visual acuity** in her right eye; she complained of headaches and problems with glare (particularly at night) and said she perceives halos around lights.

Objective: Vision testing and physical examination (i.e., **ophthalmoscopy,** slit lamp microscopy, and **tonometry**) revealed acuity (unaided) of 10/100 for the right eye and 20/60 for the left eye. Opacification of right lens was evident, as was moderate **corneal** edema.

Therapeutic Management: After a **mydriatic** agent was applied to the right pupil, a combined procedure **phacoemulsification** of the cataract and **trabeculectomy** with releasable sutures (to minimize **IOP**) was performed with the patient under local anesthesia. The patient tolerated the procedure well and returned to her room wearing a 12-hour collagen shield on the treated eye.

1. Vision testing and physical examination of the patient revealed opacification of the right lens, confirming the need for:
   a. PRK
   b. phacoemulsification
   c. scleral buckling
   d. enucleation

2. Application of a mydriatic agent would:
   a. reduce tears
   b. produce tears
   c. constrict the pupil
   d. dilate the pupil

3. A trabeculectomy was performed because the patient had a history of:
   a. abnormal condition of crossed eyes
   b. disorder characterized by optic nerve damage, usually caused by abnormal increased intraocular pressure
   c. nearsightedness
   d. a progressive deterioration of a portion of the retina

4. The abbreviation IOP stands for:
   a. both eyes
   b. normal vision
   c. intraocular pressure
   d. iris outer pupil

EXERCISE 39 *Interpret Medical Terms*

To test your understanding of the terms introduced in this chapter, circle the words that correctly complete the sentences. The italicized words refer to the correct answer.

1. The patient's *pupils* needed to be *dilated*; therefore, the doctor requested that a (**miotic, mydriatic, myopia**) medication be placed in each eye.
2. A person with a *defective curvature of the refractive surfaces* of the eye has a(n) (**astigmatism, glaucoma, strabismus**).
3. The doctor diagnosed the patient with the *clouded lens* of the eye as having a(n) (**nystagmus, astigmatism, cataract**).
4. To *measure the pressure within the patient's eye*, the physician used a(n) (**pupillometer, tonometer, keratometer**).
5. A person who is *farsighted* has (**hyperopia, myopia, diplopia**).
6. An *obstruction of an oil gland of the eyelid* is called a (**sty, chalazion, conjunctivitis**).
7. A patient with an *involuntary jerking movement of the eyes* has a condition known as (**astigmatism, strabismus, nystagmus**).
8. The name of the *surgery performed to create a permanent drain to reduce intraocular pressure* is (**trabeculectomy, iridectomy, phacoemulsification**).
9. The doctor ordered a *digital imaging of the blood vessels of the eye* or a(n) (**ophthalmoscopy, fluorescein angiography, optometer**).
10. *Condition of dry eye* (**oculomycosis, ophthalmoplegia, xerophthalmia**) begins with *night blindness* (**nyctalopia, photophobia, diplopia**) and may progress to *softening of the cornea* (**iridoplegia, keratomalacia, sclerokeratitis**).
11. The surgery schedule indicated the patient being treated for cataracts would undergo right eye *PHACO* (**photorefractive keratectomy, retinal photocoagulation, phacoemulsification**) with *IOL* (**intraocular pressure, intraocular lens**).
12. *Progressive deterioration of the retina, resulting in loss of central vision* (**retinitis pigmentosa, presbyopia, macular degeneration**) may be described as *dry*, where the blood vessels become thin and brittle, or *wet*, where new abnormal vessels develop under the macula lutea.
13. Diabetic *disease of the retina* (**blepharoptosis, retinopathy, ophthalmagia**), which may involve swelling and leaking of blood vessels or development of new abnormal blood vessels on the surface of the retina, may be surgically treated by *removal of all or part of the vitreous humor* (**trabeculectomy, vitrectomy, iridectomy**) and *intense beam of light from a laser to condense, destroy, or bond tissue* (**retinal photocoagulation, photorefractive keratectomy, phacoemulsification**).

WEB LINK

To learn more about conditions of the eye and vision, visit the **American Optometric Association's** website at ***www.aoa.org.***

EXERCISE 40 *Read Medical Terms in Use*

Practice pronunciation of terms by reading the following medical document. Use the pronunciation key following the medical terms to help you say the word.

To hear these terms, go to http://evolve.elsevier.com. Refer to p. 18 for your Evolve Access Information. Select Exercises & Review, Chapter 12, Chapter Exercises, Read Medical Terms in Use.

An elderly gentleman visited his **ophthalmologist** (*of*-thal-MOL-o-jist) because of decreased vision. A **tonometry** (ton-OM-e-trē) examination showed borderline readings. **Visual acuity** (VIZH-ū-al) (a-KŪ-i-tē) measurement indicated a mild degree of **myopia** (mī-Ō-pē–a) and **presbyopia** (*pres*-bē-Ō-pē-a). A diagnosis of **glaucoma** (glaw-KŌ-ma) is suspect in this case and Timoptic eye drops were prescribed, one drop daily.

A **cataract** (KAT-a-rakt) of the right eye was found. Lens implant surgery, which places an **intraocular lens** (in-tra-OK-ū-lar) (lenz), will be performed when the cataract matures sufficiently. Approximately 5 years ago the patient had a **detached retina** (RET-i-na) of the left eye. A **scleral buckling** (SKLER-al) (BUK-ling) procedure was performed and was successful in halting the process of retinal detachment.

EXERCISE 41 *Comprehend Medical Terms in Use*

Test your comprehension of terms in the previous medical document by circling the correct answer.

1. T F The ophthalmologist used an instrument to measure pressure within the patient's eyes to assist in the diagnosis of abnormally increased intraocular pressure.
2. Visual acuity measurement indicated:
   a. farsightedness and impaired vision as a result of aging
   b. nearsightedness and impaired vision as a result of aging
   c. poor night vision and farsightedness
   d. poor night vision and impaired vision because of aging
3. Timoptic eye drops were prescribed to address symptoms most likely caused by:
   a. inflammation of the cornea
   b. optic nerve damage caused by abnormally increased IOP
   c. separation of the retina from the choroid
   d. clouding of the lens of the eye
4. T F A scleral buckling procedure was used to correct clouding of the lens in the right eye.

CHAPTER REVIEW

ONLINE CHAPTER REVIEW

To access the Evolve website, go to http://evolve.elsevier.com. Refer to p. 18 for your Evolve Access Information. Select Exercises & Review, Chapter 12, then select Chapter Exercises, Practice Activities, Animations, or Games. Place a check mark in the box when you have completed an exercise or activity, watched an animation, or played a game. Have fun!

Chapter Exercises

Exercises in this section of your Evolve resources correlate to exercises in your textbook. You may have completed them as you worked through the chapter.

- ☐ Pronunciation
- ☐ Spelling
- ☐ Read Medical Terms in Use

Practice Activities

Practice in study mode, then test your learning in assessment mode. Keep track of your scores from assessment mode if you wish.

	SCORE
☐ Picture It	_____
☐ Define Word Parts	_____
☐ Build Medical Terms	_____
☐ Word Shop	_____
☐ Define Medical Terms	_____
☐ Use It	_____
☐ Hear It and Type It: Clinical Vignettes	_____

Animations

- ☐ Retinal Detachment

Games

- ☐ Name that Word Part
- ☐ Term Storm
- ☐ Term Explorer
- ☐ Termbusters
- ☐ Medical Millionaire
- ☐ Crossword Puzzle

REVIEW OF WORD PARTS

Can you define and spell the following word parts?

Combining Forms

blephar/o
conjunctiv/o
cor/o
core/o
corne/o
cry/o
dacry/o
dipl/o
ir/o
irid/o
is/o
kerat/o
lacrim/o
ocul/o
ophthalm/o
opt/o
phac/o
phak/o
phot/o
pupill/o
retin/o
scler/o
ton/o

Prefixes

bi-
bin-

Suffixes

-opia
-phobia
-plegia

REVIEW OF TERMS

Can you define, pronounce, and spell the following terms *built from word parts?*

Diseases and Disorders	Surgical	Diagnostic	Complementary
aphakia	blepharoplasty	fluorescein angiography	anisocoria
blepharitis	cryoretinopexy	keratometer	binocular
blepharoptosis	dacryocystorhinostomy	ophthalmoscope	corneal
conjunctivitis	dacryocystotomy	ophthalmoscopy	intraocular
dacryocystitis	iridectomy	optometry	isocoria
diplopia	iridotomy	pupillometer	lacrimal
endophthalmitis	keratoplasty	pupilloscope	nasolacrimal
iridoplegia	sclerotomy	retinoscopy	ophthalmic
iritis		tonometer	ophthalmologist
keratitis		tonometry	ophthalmology (Ophth)
keratomalacia			ophthalmopathy
leukocoria			optic
oculomycosis			pseudophakia
ophthalmalgia			pupillary
ophthalmoplegia			retinal
phacomalacia			
photophobia			
retinoblastoma			
retinopathy			
sclerokeratitis			
scleromalacia			
xerophthalmia			

Can you define, pronounce, and spell the following terms not *built from word parts?*

Diseases and Disorders		Surgical	Complementary
amblyopia	myopia	enucleation	emmetropia (Em)
astigmatism (Ast)	nyctalopia	LASIK (laser-assisted in situ keratomileusis)	intraocular lens (IOL)
cataract	nystagmus	phacoemulsification (PHACO)	miotic
chalazion	pinguecula	PRK (photorefractive keratectomy)	mydriatic
detached retina	presbyopia	retinal photocoagulation	optician
glaucoma	pterygium	scleral buckling	optometrist
hyperopia	retinitis pigmentosa	trabeculectomy	visual acuity (VA)
macular degeneration	strabismus	vitrectomy	
	sty (hordeolum)		

ANSWERS

Exercise Figures

Exercise Figure

A. 1. eye: ocul/o, ophthalm/o
2. eyelid: blephar/o
3. pupil: cor/o, core/o, pupill/o
4. sclera: scler/o
5. iris: irid/o, ir/o
6. conjunctiva: conjunctiv/o
7. cornea: corne/o, kerat/o
8. lens: phac/o, phak/o
9. retina: retin/o

Exercise Figure

B. blephar/itis

Exercise Figure

C. blephar/o/ptosis

Exercise Figure

D. dacry/o/cyst/itis

Exercise 1

1. d
2. c
3. f
4. h
5. b
6. e
7. a

Exercise 2

1. d
2. f
3. e
4. b
5. a
6. c

Exercise 3

1. eye
2. eyelid
3. cornea
4. tear, tear duct
5. retina
6. pupil
7. sclera
8. iris
9. conjunctiva
10. pupil
11. eye
12. cornea
13. iris
14. pupil
15. vision
16. tear, tear duct
17. lens

Exercise 4

1. a. ocul/o
   b. ophthalm/o
2. a. corne/o
   b. kerat/o
3. conjunctiv/o
4. a. dacry/o
   b. lacrim/o
5. blephar/o
6. a. cor/o
   b. core/o
   c. pupill/o
7. scler/o
8. retin/o
9. a. irid/o
   b. ir/o
10. opt/o
11. a. phac/o
    b. phak/o

Exercise 5

1. tension, pressure
2. light
3. cold
4. two, double
5. equal

Exercise 6

1. cry/o
2. ton/o
3. dipl/o
4. phot/o
5. is/o

Exercise 7

1. vision (condition)
2. two
3. paralysis
4. abnormal fear of or aversion to specific things
5. two

Exercise 8

1. -plegia
2. a. bi-
   b. bin-
3. -phobia
4. -opia

Exercise 9

Pronunciation Exercise

Exercise 10

1. WR CV WR S
   scler/o/kerat/itis
   CF
   inflammation of the sclera and the cornea
2. WR S
   ophthalm/algia
   pain in the eye
3. WR CV S
   blephar/o/ptosis
   CF
   drooping of the eyelid
4. WR S
   dipl/opia
   double vision
5. WR S
   conjunctiv/itis
   inflammation of the conjunctiva
6. WR CV WR S
   leuk/o/cor/ia
   CF
   condition of white pupil
7. WR CV S
   irid/o/plegia
   CF
   paralysis of the iris
8. WR CV S
   scler/o/malacia
   CF
   softening of the sclera
9. WR CV S
   phot/o/phobia
   CF
   abnormal fear of (sensitivity to) light
10. WR S
    blephar/itis
    inflammation of the eyelid
11. WR CV WR S
    ocul/o/myc/osis
    CF
    abnormal condition of the eye caused by a fungus
12. WR CV WR S
    dacry/o/cyst/itis
    CF
    inflammation of the tear (lacrimal) sac
13. P WR S
    end/ophthalm/itis
    inflammation within the eye
14. WR S
    ir/itis
    inflammation of the iris
15. WR CV WR S
    retin/o/blast/oma
    CF
    tumor arising from a developing retinal cell
16. WR S
    kerat/itis
    inflammation of the cornea
17. WR CV S
    ophthalm/o/plegia
    CF
    paralysis of the eye (muscles)
18. WR CV S
    retin/o/pathy
    CF
    disease of the retina
19. WR WR S
    xer/ophthalm/ia
    condition of dry eye
20. WR CV S
    kerat/o/malacia
    CF
    softening of the cornea

21. WR CV S
phac/o/malacia
CF
softening of the lens
22. P WR S
a/phak/ia
condition of without a lens

Exercise 11
1. conjunctiv/itis
2. ocul/o/myc/osis
3. ophthalm/algia
4. dipl/opia
5. blephar/itis
6. leuk/o/cor/ia
7. irid/o/plegia
8. blephar/o/ptosis
9. ir/itis
10. retin/o/blast/oma
11. scler/o/malacia
12. dacry/o/cyst/itis
13. scler/o/kerat/itis
14. phot/o/phobia
15. kerat/itis
16. retin/o/pathy
17. end/ophthalm/itis
18. ophthalm/o/plegia
19. xer/ophthalm/ia
20. kerat/o/malacia
21. a/phak/ia
22. phac/o/malacia

Exercise 12
Spelling Exercise; see text pp. 562-563.

Exercise 13
Pronunciation Exercise

Exercise 14
1. myopia
2. presbyopia
3. strabismus
4. chalazion
5. astigmatism
6. nystagmus
7. cataract
8. sty
9. glaucoma
10. detached retina
11. hyperopia
12. retinitis pigmentosa
13. nyctalopia
14. pterygium
15. macular degeneration
16. amblyopia
17. pinguecula

Exercise 15
1. f
2. g
3. j
4. m
5. l
6. i
7. d
8. o
9. e
10. c
11. a
12. k
13. h
14. n
15. b
16. q
17. r

Exercise 16
Spelling Exercise; see text pp. 566-568.

Exercise 17
Pronunciation Exercise

Exercise 18
1. WR CV S
kerat/o/plasty
CF
surgical repair of the cornea
2. WR CV S
scler/o/tomy
CF
incision of the sclera
3. WR CV WR CV S
dacry/o/cyst/o/tomy
CF CF
incision of the tear (lacrimal) sac
4. WR CV WR CV S
cry/o/retin/o/pexy
CF CF
surgical fixation of the retina by using extreme cold
5. WR CV S
blephar/o/plasty
CF
surgical repair of the eyelid
6. WR S
irid/ectomy
excision of the iris
7. WR CV WR CV WR CV S
dacry/o/cyst/o/rhin/o/stomy
CF CF CF
creation of an artificial opening between the tear (lacrimal) sac and the nose
8. WR CV S
irid/o/tomy
CF
incision of the iris

Exercise 19
1. dacry/o/cyst/o/rhin/o/stomy
2. irid/ectomy
3. kerat/o/plasty
4. scler/o/tomy
5. irid/o/tomy
6. blephar/o/plasty
7. cry/o/retin/o/pexy
8. dacry/o/cyst/o/tomy

Exercise 20
Spelling Exercise; see text pp. 570-571.

Exercise 21
Pronunciation Exercise

Exercise 22
1. retinal photocoagulation
2. enucleation
3. phacoemulsification
4. LASIK
5. trabeculectomy
6. scleral buckling
7. vitrectomy
8. PRK

Exercise 23
1. e
2. f
3. b
4. a
5. d
6. i
7. g
8. c

Exercise 24
Spelling Exercise; see text p. 573.

Exercise 25
Pronunciation Exercise

Exercise 26
1. WR CV S
pupill/o/scope
CF
instrument used for visual examination of the pupil
2. WR CV S
opt/o/metry
CF
measurement of vision
3. WR CV S
ophthalm/o/scope
CF
instrument used for visual examination of the eye
4. WR CV S
ton/o/metry
CF
measurement of pressure (within the eye)

5. WR CV S
pupill/o/meter
CF
instrument used to measure the pupil (diameter)
6. WR CV S
ton/o/meter
CF
instrument used to measure pressure (within the eye)
7. WR CV S
kerat/o/meter
CF
instrument used to measure (the curvature of) the cornea
8. WR CV S
ophthalm/o/scopy
CF
visual examination of the eye
9. WR CV S
(fluorescein) angi/o/graphy
CF
process of recording blood vessels (of the eye with fluorescing dye)
10. WR CV S
retin/o/scopy
CF
visual examination of the retina

Exercise 27
1. ton/o/metry
2. pupill/o/meter
3. kerat/o/meter
4. opt/o/metry
5. ophthalm/o/scope
6. ton/o/meter
7. pupill/o/scope
8. ophthalm/o/scopy
9. fluorescein angi/o/graphy
10. retin/o/scopy

Exercise 28
Spelling Exercise; see text p. 576.

Exercise 29
Pronunciation Exercise

Exercise 30
1. WR CV S
ophthalm/o/logy
CF
study of the eye
2. P WR S
bin/ocul/ar
pertaining to two or both eyes
3. WR S
lacrim/al
pertaining to tears
4. WR S
pupill/ary
pertaining to the pupil
5. WR CV S
ophthalm/o/logist
CF
physician who studies and treats diseases of the eye
6. WR S
corne/al
pertaining to the cornea
7. WR S
ophthalm/ic
pertaining to the eye
8. WR CV WR S
nas/o/lacrim/al
CF
pertaining to the nose and tear ducts
9. WR S
opt/ic
pertaining to vision
10. P WR S
intra/ocul/ar
pertaining to within the eye
11. WR S
retin/al
pertaining to the retina
12. WR CV S
ophthalm/o/pathy
CF
disease of the eye
13. WR CV WR S
is/o/cor/ia
CF
condition of equal pupil (size)
14. P WR CV WR S
an/is/o/cor/ia
CF
condition of absence of equal pupil (size)
15. WR CV WR S
pseud/o/phak/ia
CF
condition of false lens

Exercise 31
1. ophthalm/o/logy
2. bin/ocul/ar
3. retin/al
4. intra/ocul/ar
5. ophthalm/o/logist
6. lacrim/al
7. opt/ic
8. ophthalm/ic
9. corne/al
10. nas/o/lacrim/al
11. ophthalm/o/pathy
12. pupill/ary
13. pseud/o/phak/ia
14. is/o/cor/ia
15. an/is/o/cor/ia

Exercise 32
Spelling Exercise; see text pp. 578-579.

Exercise 33
Pronunciation Exercise

Exercise 34
1. a health professional who prescribes corrective lenses and/or eye exercises
2. agent that dilates the pupil
3. sharpness of vision
4. agent that constricts the pupil
5. a specialist who fills prescriptions for lenses
6. normal refractive condition of the eye
7. an artificial lens implanted within the eye

Exercise 35
1. mydriatic
2. miotic
3. optometrist
4. visual acuity
5. optician
6. emmetropia
7. intraocular lens

Exercise 36
Spelling Exercise; see text p. 581.

Exercise 37
1. visual acuity
2. astigmatism
3. intraocular pressure
4. emmetropia
5. ophthalmology
6. age-related macular degeneration
7. phacoemulsification
8. intraocular lens

Exercise 38
A. 1. ophthalmology
2. glaucoma
3. pterygium
4. blepharoptosis
5. astigmatism
6. presbyopia
7. retinopathy
8. cataract

B. 1. b
2. d
3. b
4. c

Exercise 39

1. mydriatic
2. astigmatism
3. cataract
4. tonometer
5. hyperopia
6. chalazion
7. nystagmus
8. trabeculectomy
9. fluorescein angiography
10. xerophthalmia, nyctalopia, keratomalacia
11. phacoemulsification, intraocular lens
12. macular degeneration
13. retinopathy, vitrectomy, retinal photocoagulation

Exercise 40

Reading Exercise

Exercise 41

1. *T*
2. b
3. b
4. *F*, scleral buckling was used to correct a detached retina and not a cataract.

Chapter 13

Ear

OUTLINE

OBJECTIVES

Upon completion of this chapter you will be able to:

1. Identify organs and structures of the ear.
2. Define and spell word parts related to the ear.
3. Define, pronounce, and spell disease and disorder terms related to the ear.
4. Define, pronounce, and spell surgical terms related to the ear.
5. Define, pronounce, and spell diagnostic terms related to the ear.
6. Define, pronounce, and spell complementary terms related to the ear.
7. Interpret the meaning of abbreviations related to the ear.
8. Interpret, read, and comprehend medical language in simulated medical statements and documents.

ANATOMY

Function

The two functions of the ear are to hear and to provide the sense of balance. The ear is made up of three parts: the *external* ear, the *middle* ear, and the *inner* ear, also called the *labyrinth* (Figure 13-1). We hear because sound waves vibrate through the ear (Figure 13-2) where they are transformed into nerve impulses that are then carried to the brain.

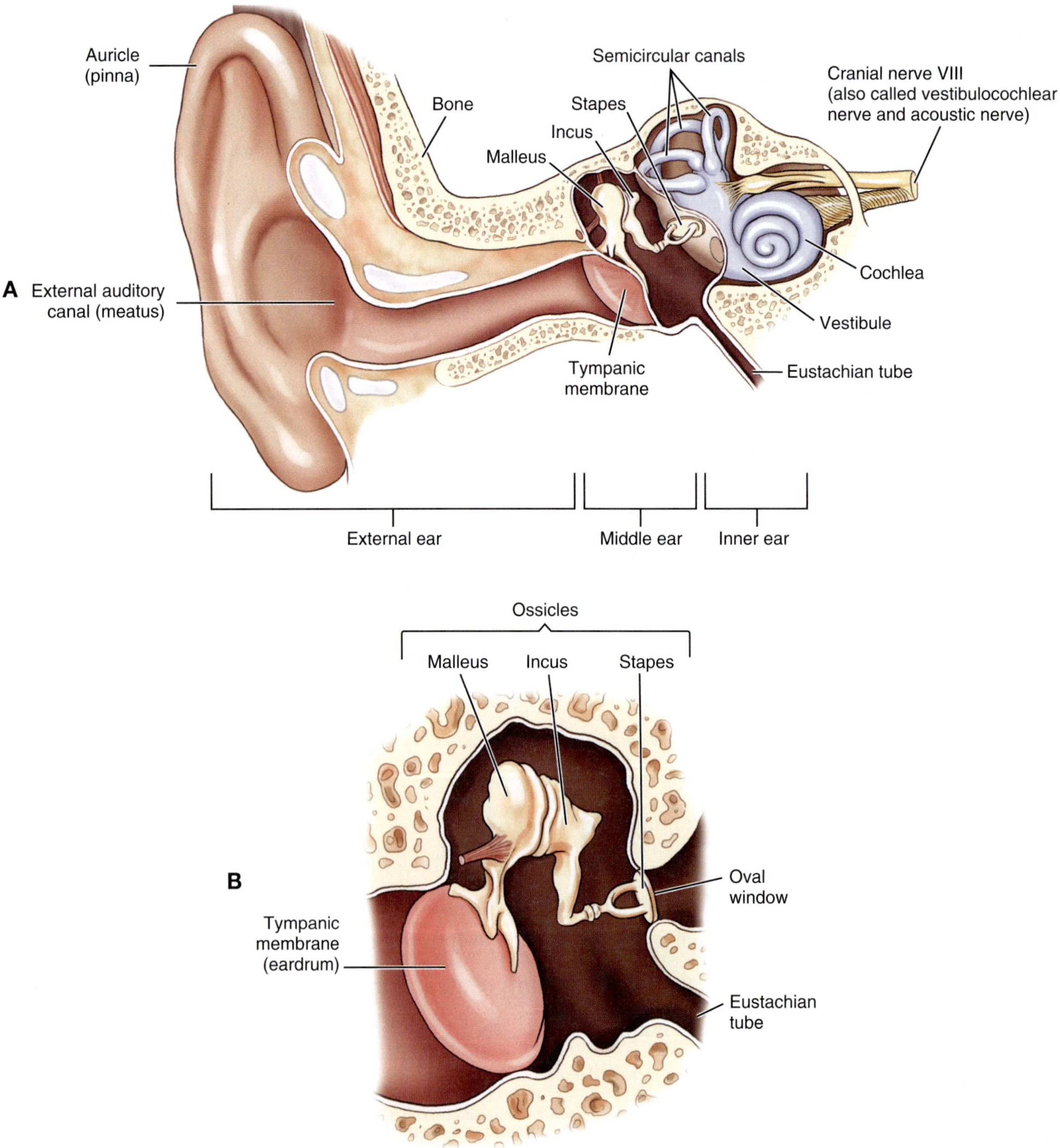

FIGURE 13-1
A, Gross anatomy of the ear. **B,** The middle ear.

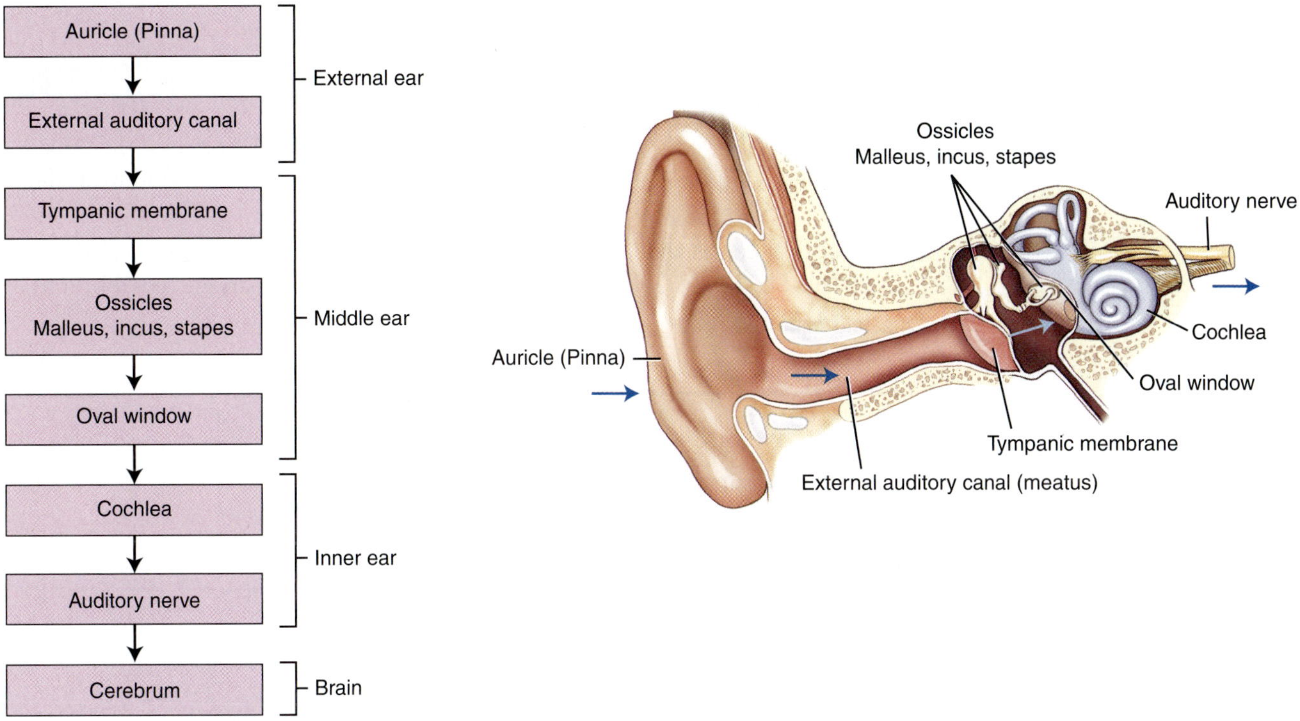

FIGURE 13-2
Pathway of sound.

Structures of the Ear

Term	Definition
external ear	
auricle (pinna)	external structure located on both sides of the head. The auricle directs sound waves into the external auditory canal.
external auditory canal (meatus)	short tube that ends at the tympanic membrane. The inner part lies within the temporal bone of the skull and contains the glands that secrete earwax (cerumen).
middle ear	
tympanic membrane (eardrum)	semitransparent membrane that separates the external auditory canal and the middle ear cavity. The tympanic memrane transmits sound vibrations to the ossicles (See Figure 13-4, B).
eustachian tube	connects the middle ear and the pharynx. It equalizes air pressure on both sides of the eardrum.
ossicles	bones of the middle ear that carry sound vibrations. The ossicles are composed of the **malleus** (hammer), **incus** (anvil), and **stapes** (stirrup). The stapes connects to the **oval window**, which transmits the sound vibrations to the cochlea of the inner ear.
labyrinth (inner ear)	bony spaces within the temporal bone of the skull. It contains the cochlea, semicircular canals, and vestibule.

TYMPANIC MEMBRANE

is derived from the Greek ***tympanon***, meaning ***drum***, because of its resemblance to a drum or tambourine.

STAPES

is Latin for ***stirrup***. The anatomic stapes was so named for its stirruplike shape.

Structures of the Ear—*cont'd*

Term	Definition
cochlea	is snail-shaped and contains the organ of hearing. The cochlea connects to the oval window in the middle ear.
semicircular canals and vestibule	contains receptors and endolymph that help the body maintain its sense of balance (equilibrium)
mastoid bone and cells	located in the skull bone behind the external auditory canal

A & P Booster
For students desiring more anatomy and physiology, go to http://evolve.elsevier.com. Refer to p. 18 for your Evolve Access Information. Select A & P Booster, Chapter 13.

EXERCISE 1

Match the anatomic terms in the first column with the correct definitions in the second column. *To check your answers to the exercises in this chapter, go to Answers, p. 620, at the end of the chapter.*

______ 1. auricle
______ 2. cochlea
______ 3. eustachian tube
______ 4. external auditory meatus
______ 5. labyrinth
______ 6. mastoid bone
______ 7. ossicles
______ 8. oval window
______ 9. semicircular canals and vestibule
______ 10. tympanic membrane

a. contains receptors and endolymph, which help maintain equilibrium
b. equalizes air pressure on both sides of the eardrum
c. separates the external auditory canal and middle ear cavity
d. malleus, incus, and stapes
e. transmits sound vibration to the inner ear
f. contains glands that secrete earwax
g. external structure located on each side of the head
h. bony spaces within the temporal bone
i. relays messages to the brain
j. contains the organ of hearing
k. located in the skull behind the external auditory canal

WORD PARTS

Word parts you need to learn to complete this chapter are listed below. The exercises at the end of each list will help you learn their definitions and spellings.

Use the flashcards accompanying this text or electronic flashcards to assist you in memorizing the word parts for this chapter.

To use electronic flashcards, go to http://evolve.elsevier.com. Refer to p. 18 for your Evolve Access Information. Select Flashcards, Chapter 13.

Combining Forms of the Ear

Combining Form	Definition
audi/o	hearing
aur/i, aur/o, ot/o	ear
cochle/o	cochlea
labyrinth/o	labyrinth (inner ear)
mastoid/o	mastoid bone
myring/o	tympanic membrane (eardrum)
staped/o	stapes (middle ear bone)
tympan/o	tympanic membrane (eardrum), middle ear
vestibul/o	vestibule

Refer to **Appendix A** and **Appendix B** for a complete list of word parts.

EXERCISE FIGURE A

Fill in the blanks with combining forms in this diagram of the ear. *To check your answers, go to p. 620.*

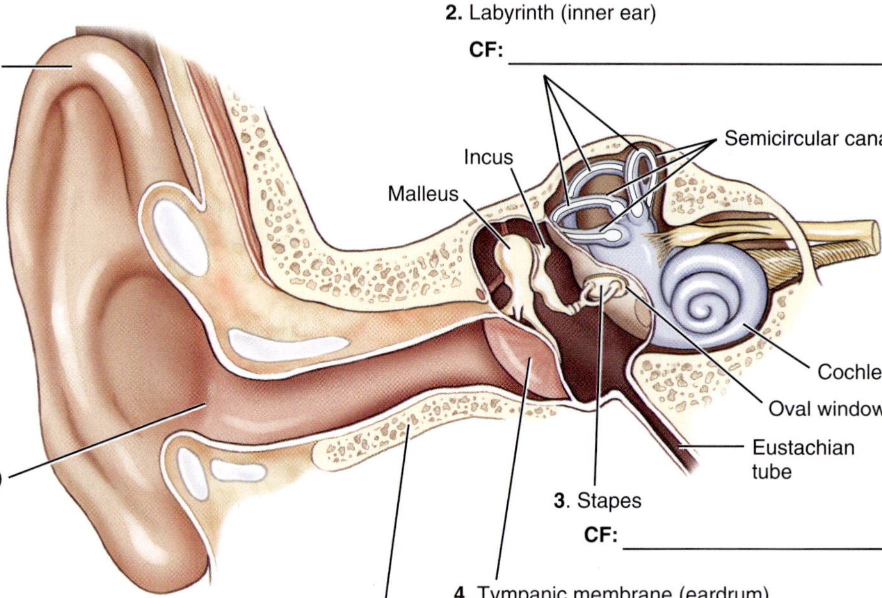

EXERCISE 2

Write the definitions of the following combining forms.

1. staped/o ____________
2. mastoid/o ____________
3. audi/o ____________
4. aur/i, aur/o, ot/o ____________
5. tympan/o ____________
6. vestibul/o ____________
7. labyrinth/o ____________
8. myring/o ____________
9. cochle/o ____________

EXERCISE 3

Write the combining form for each of the following terms.

1. ear a. ______________
   b. ______________
   c. ______________
2. mastoid bone ______________
3. stapes ______________
4. tympanic membrane (eardrum), middle ear ______________
5. labyrinth (inner ear) ______________
6. hearing ______________
7. tympanic membrane (eardrum) ______________
8. cochlea ______________
9. vestibule ______________

MEDICAL TERMS

The terms you need to learn to complete this chapter are listed on the following pages. The exercises following each list will help you learn the definition and spelling of each word.

Disease and Disorder Terms

Built from Word Parts

The following terms are built from word parts you have already learned and can be translated literally to find their meanings. Further explanation of terms beyond the definition of their word parts, if needed, is included in parentheses.

Term	Definition
labyrinthitis (*lab*-i-rin-THĪ-tis)	inflammation of the labyrinth (inner ear) (also called **vestibular neuritis**)
mastoiditis (*mas*-toyd-Ī-tis)	inflammation of the mastoid bone
myringitis (*mir*-in-JĪ-tis)	inflammation of the tympanic membrane (eardrum)
otalgia (ō-TAL-ja)	pain in the ear
otomastoiditis (ō-tō-*mas*-toyd-Ī-tis)	inflammation of the ear and the mastoid bone
otomycosis (ō-tō-mī-KŌ-sis)	abnormal condition of fungus in the ear (usually affects the external auditory canal)
otopyorrhea (ō-tō-*pī*-ō-RĒ-a)	discharge of pus from the ear
otorrhea (ō-tō-RĒ-a)	discharge from the ear (may be serous, bloody, consisting of pus, or containing cerebrospinal fluid)
otosclerosis (ō-tō-skle-RŌ-sis)	hardening of the ear (stapes) (caused by irregular bone development and resulting in hearing loss)

EXERCISE 4

Practice saying aloud each of the disease and disorder terms built from word parts on p. 601.

To hear the terms, go to http://evolve.elsevier.com. Refer to p. 18 for your Evolve Access Information. Select Exercises & Review, Chapter 13, Chapter Exercises, Pronunciation.

☐ Place a check mark in the box when you have completed this exercise.

EXERCISE 5

Analyze and define the following terms.

1. otomycosis ______________________________
2. otomastoiditis ______________________________
3. otalgia ______________________________
4. labyrinthitis ______________________________
5. myringitis ______________________________
6. otosclerosis ______________________________
7. mastoiditis ______________________________
8. otopyorrhea ______________________________
9. otorrhea ______________________________

EXERCISE 6

Build disease and disorder terms for the following definitions with the word parts you have learned.

1. inflammation of the tympanic membrane ________ / ________
   WR / S
2. discharge of pus from the ear ________ / ___ / ________ / ___ / ________
   WR / CV / WR / CV / S
3. inflammation of the mastoid bone ________ / ________
   WR / S
4. pain in the ear ________ / ________
   WR / S
5. hardening of the ear (stapes) ________ / ___ / ________
   WR / CV / S
6. abnormal condition of fungus in the ear ________ / ___ / ________ / ________
   WR / CV / WR / S
7. inflammation of the ear and the mastoid bone ________ / ___ / ________ / ________
   WR / CV / WR / S

8. inflammation of the labyrinth ______ / ______
WR / S

9. discharge from the ear ______ / ___ / ______
WR / CV / S

EXERCISE 7

Spell each of the disease and disorder terms built from word parts on p. 601 by having someone dictate them to you.

To hear and spell the terms, go to http://evolve.elsevier.com. Refer to p. 18 for your Evolve Access Information. Select Exercises & Review, Chapter 13, Chapter Exercises, Spelling.
☐ Place a check mark in the box if you have completed this exercise online.

1. ______________________
2. ______________________
3. ______________________
4. ______________________
5. ______________________
6. ______________________
7. ______________________
8. ______________________
9. ______________________

Disease and Disorder Terms

Not Built from Word Parts

In some of the following terms, you may recognize word parts you have already learned; however, the full meaning of the terms cannot be discerned by the definition of their word parts.

Term	Definition
acoustic neuroma (a-KOOS-tik) (nū-RŌ-ma)	benign tumor within the internal auditory canal growing from the acoustic nerve (cranial nerve VIII, vestibulocochlear nerve); may cause hearing loss and may damage structures of the cerebellum as it grows
ceruminoma (se-*roo*-mi-NŌ-ma)	tumor of a gland that secretes earwax (cerumen)
cholesteatoma (*ko*-le-stē-a-TŌ-ma)	cystlike mass composed of epithelial cells and cholesterol occurring in the middle ear; may be associated with chronic otitis media
Ménière disease (me-NYĀR) (di-ZĒZ)	chronic disease of the inner ear characterized by a sensation of spinning motion (vertigo), ringing in the ear (tinnitus), aural fullness, and fluctuating hearing loss; symptoms are related to a change in volume or composition of fluid within the labyrinth
otitis externa (ō-TĪ-tis) (eks-TER-na)	inflammation of the outer ear (Figure 13-3)

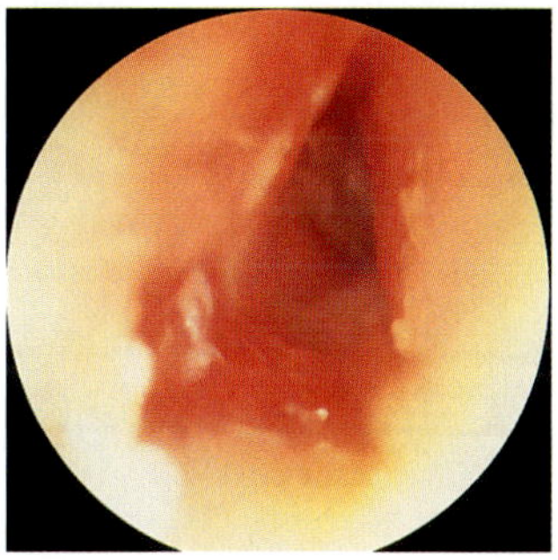

FIGURE 13-3 Otitis externa.

CAM TERM

Biofeedback is learned self-control of physiologic responses using electronic devices to provide monitoring information. Biofeedback, in combination with cognitive behavioral therapy, has been used successfully to treat **tinnitus**.

BENIGN PAROXYSMAL POSITIONAL VERTIGO (BPPV)

is characterized by brief episodes of vertigo associated with a change in the position of the head, such as turning over in bed or sitting up in the morning. In BPPV, normal calcium carbonate crystals called otoconia break loose and shift within the labyrinth, triggering an episode of vertigo.

Disease and Disorder Terms—*cont'd*

Not Built from Word Parts

Term	Definition
otitis media (OM) (ō-TĪ-tis) (MĒ-dē-a)	inflammation of the middle ear (also called **tympanitis**) (Figure 13-4)
presbycusis (*prez*-bi-KŪ-sis)	hearing impairment in old age
tinnitus (tin-NĪ-tus)	ringing in the ears
vertigo (VER-ti-gō)	a sense that either one's own body (subjective vertigo) or the environment (objective vertigo) is revolving; may indicate inner ear disease

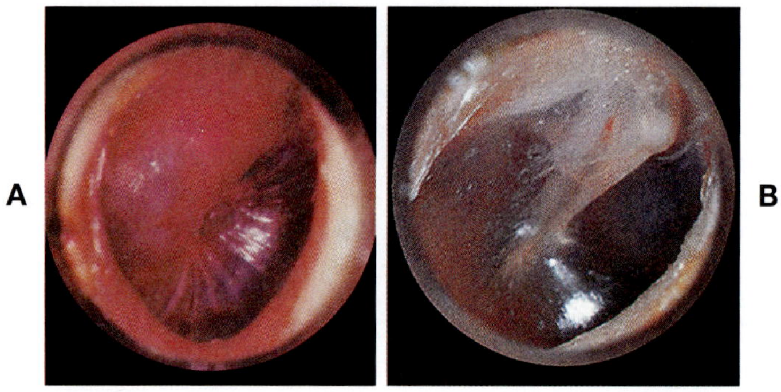

FIGURE 13-4
Otitis media. Signs include bulging, perforated, reddened, or retracted tympanic membrane. **A,** Tympanic membrane demonstrating acute otitis media (AOM). **B,** Normal tympanic membrane.

EXERCISE 8

Practice saying aloud each of the disease and disorder terms not built from word parts on pp. 603-604.

To hear the terms, go to http://evolve.elsevier.com. Refer to p. 18 for your Evolve Access Information. Select Exercises & Review, Chapter 13, Chapter Exercises, Pronunciation.

☐ Place a check mark in the box when you have completed this exercise.

EXERCISE 9

Fill in the blanks with the correct terms.

1. The patient reported that her body seemed to be revolving, or ____________, and ringing in the ears, or ____________.
2. A chronic ear disease characterized by vertigo, tinnitus, aural fullness, and fluctuating hearing loss is called ______________________________ disease.
3. Inflammation of the middle ear is called ____________ ____________.
4. ________________________ is the name given to a tumor of a gland that secretes earwax.
5. ____________ ____________ means inflammation of the outer ear.
6. A benign tumor arising from the acoustic nerve is called a(n) ____________ ____________.
7. ____________________________________ is hearing impairment in old age.
8. ________________________ may be associated with chronic otitis media.

EXERCISE 10

Match the terms in the first column with the correct definitions in the second column.

______ 1. vertigo	a. inflammation of the middle ear
______ 2. ceruminoma	b. tumor of a gland that secretes earwax
______ 3. tinnitus	c. chronic ear problem characterized by vertigo, tinnitus, and fluctuating hearing loss
______ 4. Ménière disease	d. benign tumor arising from the acoustic nerve
______ 5. otitis externa	e. sense of revolving of one's own body or the environment
______ 6. acoustic neuroma	f. hardening of the oval window
______ 7. otitis media	g. ringing in the ears
______ 8. presbycusis	h. inflammation of the outer ear
______ 9. cholesteatoma	i. hearing impairment in old age
	j. mass composed of epithelial cells and cholesterol

EXERCISE 11

Spell each of the disease and disorder terms not built from word parts on pp. 603-604 by having someone dictate them to you.

To hear and spell the terms, go to http://evolve.elsevier.com. Refer to p. 18 for your Evolve Access Information. Select Exercises & Review, Chapter 13, Chapter Exercises, Spelling.

☐ Place a check mark in the box if you have completed this exercise online.

1. ____________________
2. ____________________
3. ____________________
4. ____________________
5. ____________________
6. ____________________
7. ____________________
8. ____________________
9. ____________________

Surgical Terms

Built from Word Parts

The following terms are built from word parts you have already learned and can be translated literally to find their meanings. Further explanation of terms beyond the definition of their word parts, if needed, is included in parentheses.

Term	Definition
cochlear implant (KŌK-lē-ar) (IM-plant)	pertaining to the cochlea implant (surgically inserted prosthetic device that uses electrical currents to stimulate the auditory nerve and provide hearing)
labyrinthectomy (*lab*-i-rin-THEK-to-mē)	excision of the labyrinth
mastoidectomy (*mas*-toy-DEK-to-mē)	excision of the mastoid bone
mastoidotomy (*mas*-toy-DOT-o-mē)	incision into the mastoid bone
myringoplasty (mi-RING-gō-*plas*-tē)	surgical repair of the tympanic membrane
myringotomy (*mir*-ing-GOT-o-mē)	incision into the tympanic membrane (performed to release pus or fluid and relieve pressure in the middle ear) (also called **tympanocentesis**) (Exercise Figure B)
stapedectomy (*stā*-pe-DEK-to-mē)	excision of the stapes (performed to restore hearing in cases of otosclerosis; the stapes is replaced by a prosthesis) (Figure 13-5)
tympanoplasty (TIM-pa-nō-*plas*-tē)	surgical repair (of the hearing mechanism) of the middle ear (including the tympanic membrane and the ossicles)

EXERCISE FIGURE B

Fill in the blanks to complete labeling of the diagram.

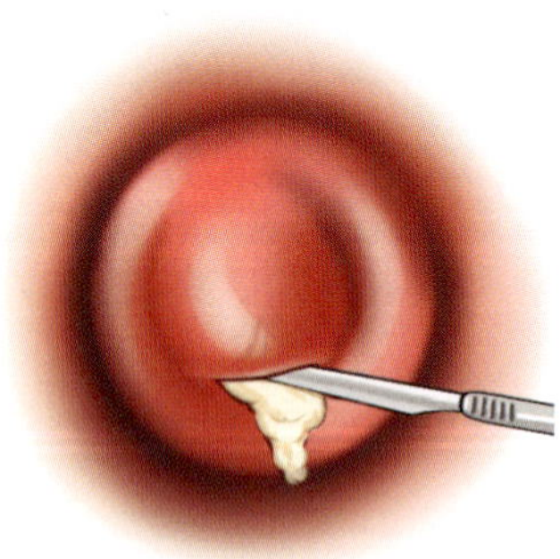

_____ / cv / _____
tympanic membrane / cv / incision

is performed to release pus from the middle ear through the tympanic membrane to treat acute otitis media.

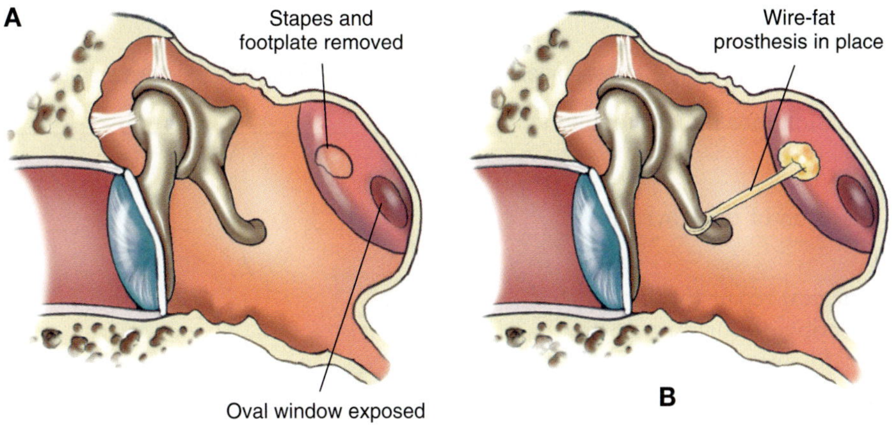

FIGURE 13-5
Stapedectomy. **A,** Stapes is removed. **B,** Prosthesis is in place.

EXERCISE 12

Practice saying aloud each of the surgical terms built from word parts on p. 606.

To hear the terms, go to http://evolve.elsevier.com. Refer to p. 18 for your Evolve Access Information. Select Exercises & Review, Chapter 13, Chapter Exercises, Pronunciation.

☐ Place a check mark in the box when you have completed this exercise.

EXERCISE 13

Analyze and define the following surgical terms.

1. mastoidectomy ____________________
2. myringotomy ____________________
3. labyrinthectomy ____________________
4. mastoidotomy ____________________
5. tympanoplasty ____________________
6. myringoplasty ____________________
7. stapedectomy ____________________
8. cochlear implant ____________________

EXERCISE 14

Build surgical terms for the following definitions by using the word parts you have learned.

1. incision into the mastoid bone ______ / ______ / ______
   WR / CV / S
2. excision of the labyrinth ______ / ______
   WR / S
3. surgical repair (of the hearing mechanism) of the middle ear ______ / ______ / ______
   WR / CV / S
4. excision of the mastoid bone ______ / ______
   WR / S
5. incision into the tympanic membrane ______ / ______ / ______
   WR / CV / S
6. surgical repair of the tympanic membrane ______ / ______ / ______
   WR / CV / S
7. excision of the stapes ______ / ______
   WR / S
8. pertaining to the cochlea ______ / ______ implar
   WR / S

EXERCISE 15

Spell each of the surgical terms built from word parts on p. 606 by having someone dictate them to you.

To hear and spell the terms, go to http://evolve.elsevier.com. Refer to p. 18 for your Evolve Access Information. Select Exercises & Review, Chapter 13, Chapter Exercises, Spelling.

☐ Place a check mark in the box if you have completed this exercise online.

1. ______
2. ______
3. ______
4. ______
5. ______
6. ______
7. ______
8. ______

Diagnostic Terms

Built from Word Parts

The following terms are built from word parts you have already learned and can be translated literally to find their meanings. Further explanation of terms beyond the definition of their word parts, if needed, is included in parentheses.

Term	Definition
audiogram (AW-dē-ō-*gram*)	(graphic) record of hearing (Figure 13-6)
audiometer (*aw*-dē-OM-e-ter)	instrument used to measure hearing
audiometry (*aw*-dē-OM-e-trē)	measurement of hearing
electrocochleography (ē-*lek*-trō-*kok*-lē-OG-ra-fē)	process of recording the electrical activity in the cochlea (in response to sound)
otoscope (Ō-tō-skōp)	instrument used for visual examination of the ear (Exercise Figure C)
otoscopy (ō-TOS-ko-pē)	visual examination of the ear (Exercise Figure C)
tympanometer (*tim*-pa-NOM-e-ter)	instrument used to measure middle ear (function)
tympanometry (*tim*-pa-NOM-e-trē)	measurement (of movement) of the tympanic membrane

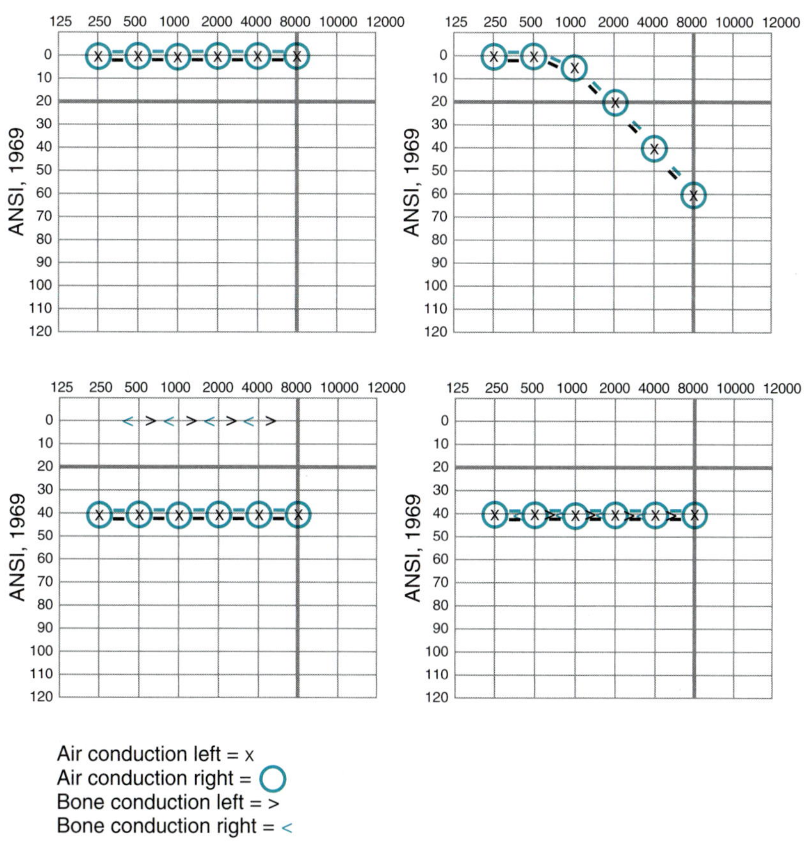

FIGURE 13-6

Audiogram. Although hearing is within normal limits, the results of this audiologic evaluation indicate a mild hearing loss in the left ear.

EXERCISE FIGURE C

Fill in the blanks to label the diagram.

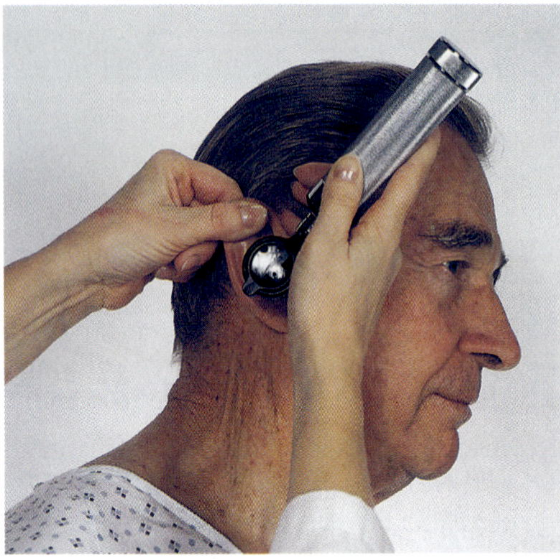

_____ / _____ / _____ performed with an _____ / _____ / _____
ear / cv / visual examination ear / cv / instrument used for visual examination

EXERCISE 16

Practice saying aloud each of the diagnostic terms built from word parts on p. 609.

To hear the terms, go to http://evolve.elsevier.com. Refer to p. 18 for your Evolve Access Information. Select Exercises & Review, Chapter 13, Chapter Exercises, Pronunciation.

☐ Place a check mark in the box when you have completed this exercise.

EXERCISE 17

Analyze and define the following diagnostic terms.

1. otoscope _____
2. audiometry _____
3. audiogram _____
4. otoscopy _____
5. audiometer _____
6. tympanometry _____
7. tympanometer _____
8. electrocochleography _____

EXERCISE 18

Build diagnostic terms that correspond to the following definitions by using the word parts you have learned.

1. measurement (of movement) of the tympanic membrane ______ WR / CV / ______ S
2. instrument used to measure hearing ______ WR / CV / ______ S
3. visual examination of the ear ______ WR / CV / ______ S
4. (graphic) record of hearing ______ WR / CV / ______ S
5. instrument used for visual examination of the ear ______ WR / CV / ______ S
6. measurement of hearing ______ WR / CV / ______ S
7. instrument used to measure middle ear (function) ______ WR / CV / ______ S
8. process of recording the electrical activity in the cochlea ______ WR / CV / ______ WR / CV / ______ S

EXERCISE 19

Spell each of the diagnostic terms built from word parts on p. 609 by having someone dictate them to you.

To hear and spell the terms, go to http://evolve.elsevier.com. Refer to p. 18 for your Evolve Access Information. Select Exercises & Review, Chapter 13, Chapter Exercises, Spelling.

☐ Place a check mark in the box if you have completed this exercise online.

1. ______________________
2. ______________________
3. ______________________
4. ______________________
5. ______________________
6. ______________________
7. ______________________
8. ______________________

Complementary Terms

Built from Word Parts

The following terms are built from word parts you have already learned and can be translated literally to find their meanings. Further explanation of terms beyond the definition of their word parts, if needed, is included in parentheses.

Term	Definition
audiologist (*aw*-dē-OL-o-jist)	one who studies and specializes in hearing
audiology (*aw*-dē-OL-o-jē)	study of hearing
aural (AW-rul)	pertaining to the ear
cochlear (KOK-lē-ar)	pertaining to the cochlea
otologist (ō-TOL-o-jist)	physician who studies and treats diseases of the ear
otology (ō-TOL-o-jē)	study of the ear (a branch of medicine that deals with diseases of the ear)
otorhinolaryngologist (*ō*-tō-*rī*-nō-*lar*-ing-GOL-o-jist)	physician who studies and treats diseases of the ear, nose, and larynx (throat) (also called **otolaryngologist**)
vestibular (ves-TIB-ū-lar)	pertaining to the vestibule
vestibulocochlear (ves-*tib*-ū-lo-KOK-lē-ar)	pertaining to the vestibule and the cochlea

Refer to **Appendix D** for pharmacology terms related to the ear.

EXERCISE 20

Practice saying aloud each of the complementary terms built from word parts above.

To hear the terms, go to http://evolve.elsevier.com. Refer to p. 18 for your Evolve Access Information. Select Exercises & Review, Chapter 13, Chapter Exercises, Pronunciation.

☐ Place a check mark in the box when you have completed this exercise.

EXERCISE 21

Analyze and define the following complementary terms.

1. otology ______________________________
2. audiologist ______________________________
3. otorhinolaryngologist ______________________________
4. audiology ______________________________
5. otologist ______________________________
6. aural ______________________________
7. cochlear ______________________________
8. vestibular ______________________________
9. vestibulocochlear ______________________________

EXERCISE 22

Build the complementary terms for the following definitions by using the word parts you have learned.

1. study of hearing ______ WR /CV/ S
2. physician who studies and treats diseases of the ear, nose, and larynx (throat) ______ WR /CV/ WR /CV/ WR /CV/ S
3. study of the ear ______ WR /CV/ S
4. one who studies and specializes in hearing ______ WR /CV/ S
5. physician who studies and treats diseases of the ear ______ WR /CV/ S
6. pertaining to the ear ______ WR / S
7. pertaining to the vestibule and the cochlea ______ WR /CV/ WR / S
8. pertaining to the vestibule ______ WR / S
9. pertaining to the cochlea ______ WR / S

EXERCISE 23

Spell each of the complementary terms built from word parts on p. 612 by having someone dictate them to you.

To hear and spell the terms, go to http://evolve.elsevier.com. Refer to p. 18 for your Evolve Access Information. Select Exercises & Review, Chapter 13, Chapter Exercises, Spelling.
☐ Place a check mark in the box if you have completed this exercise online.

1. ______________________
2. ______________________
3. ______________________
4. ______________________
5. ______________________
6. ______________________
7. ______________________
8. ______________________
9. ______________________

Abbreviations

AOM	acute otitis media
EENT	eyes, ears, nose, and throat
ENT	ears, nose, throat
OM	otitis media

EXERCISE 24

Write the meaning of the following abbreviations.

1. ENT ____________ ____________ ____________
2. EENT ____________ ____________ ____________ and ____________
3. OM ____________ ____________
4. AOM ____________ ____________ ____________

PRACTICAL APPLICATION

EXERCISE 25 *Interact with Medical Documents*

A. Complete the progress note by writing the medical terms in the blanks. Use the list of definitions with the corresponding numbers.

University Hospital and Medical Center
4700 North Main Street • Wellness, Arizona 54321 • (987) 555-3210

PATIENT NAME: Jimmy Tohe **CASE NUMBER:** 99665-AUD
DATE OF BIRTH: 03/04/19XX **DATE:** 09/04/20XX

PROGRESS NOTE

SUBJECTIVE DATA: Jimmy Tohe is a 62-year-old Native American male, appearing younger than his stated age. He was brought into the 1. ________________ clinic by his daughter, who states that he is unable to hear what is being said to him by family members. She states that this problem has existed for at least 30 years but that it appears to be getting markedly worse. The patient states he had several episodes of ear infections as a child and young adult. He denies any 2. ________________ or 3. ________________. Patient states he is allergic to Demerol.

OBJECTIVE DATA: Temperature, 99.4. Pulse, 72. Respirations, 20. Blood pressure, 136/76 mm Hg. Weight, 162 pounds. Patient ambulates without difficulty. Alert and oriented ×3. 4. ________________ reveals scarring of the tympanic membranes bilaterally. Auditory canals appear normal bilaterally.

ASSESSMENT:
1. Severe loss of hearing bilaterally, probably caused by 5.________________ ________________ as a child.
2. Recent exacerbation of hearing loss most likely attributable to 6. ________________.

PLAN:
1. Patient referred to 7. ________________ for complete 8. ________________ workup.

____

Bridey McKeegan, MD

BM/mcm

1. abbreviation for ears, nose, and throat
2. ringing in the ears
3. a sense of one's own body or the environment revolving
4. visual examination of the ear
5. inflammation of the middle ear
6. hearing impairment in old age
7. one who studies and specializes in hearing
8. measurement of hearing

B. Read the clinical notes report and answer the questions following it.

028464 MARIEB, PAULINA

File Patient Navigate Custom Fields Help

Patient Chart | Lab | Rad | Notes | Documents | Rx | Scheduling | Images | Billing

Name: **MARIEB, PAULINA** MR#: **028464** DOB: **3/24/19XX** Sex: **Female**

CLINICAL NOTES REPORT

ENCOUNTER DATE: 1/7/20XX
PURPOSE OF VISIT: Referred by Dr. Helene Bryce for itching ears.

HISTORY: The patient is a 65-year-old female who has had about six months difficulty with itching in her outer ears. She was seen by an internist who has given her Cortaid cream to use in this area. She denies otorrhea or otalgia or aural fullness, congestion, vertigo, or hearing changes. She denies any ear surgeries or previous ear infections.

PHYSICAL EXAMINATION: Under the operating microscope, the left ear was examined. The external ear shows no edema, no involvement of cartilage. There is no chondritis or edema noted, but along the conchal bowl there is some dry scaling of the skin. There was some cerumen which was removed with suction. Inspection of the right ear revealed more of the same. There are no fissures forming. There was no postauricular dermatitis noted on either ear. There was no lymphadenopathy or adenopathy.

IMPRESSION: Chronic otitis externa.

PLAN: Continue with the cream twice a day until itching symptoms resolve and then to use the cream once a day. The patient has been educated as to the importance of keeping her ears dry. We would be happy to see her back as needed if her symptoms worsen or persist.

Electronically signed by: David Lee, MD 1/7/20XX 4:24 PM

DL/slh

Start | Log On/Off | Print | Edit

1. The patient has been experiencing:
   a. itchiness
   b. hearing loss
   c. otalgia
   d. vertigo

2. In the patient's left ear, suction removed:
   a. scaling
   b. cerumen
   c. chondritis
   d. otorrhea

3. The patient's condition has been diagnosed as chronic:
   a. abnormal condition of fungus in the ear
   b. inflammation of the tympanic membrane
   c. hardening of the stapes
   d. inflammation of the outer ear

EXERCISE 26 Interpret Medical Terms

To test your understanding of the terms introduced in this chapter, circle the words that correctly complete the sentences. The italicized phrase is the definition of the term.

1. *Inflammation of the eardrum* is (**labyrinthitis, mastoiditis, myringitis**).
2. The patient reported *ringing in the ears*, or (**tinnitus, vertigo, tympanitis**).
3. The patient seeking a *physician who studies and treats diseases of the ear* for labyrinthitis consulted an (**optometrist, audiologist, otologist**).
4. The physician planned to release the pus from the middle ear by making an *incision in the tympanic membrane*, or performing a (**mastoidotomy, myringotomy, labyrinthectomy**).
5. Tinnitus, fluctuating hearing loss, and vertigo in *chronic disease of the inner ear* (**mastoiditis, Ménière disease, presbycusis**) usually occur in episodes that can last for several days.
6. Manifestations of *benign tumor within the auditory canal growing from cranial nerve VIII* (**acoustic neuroma, ceruminoma, cholesteatoma**) often begin with tinnitus and gradual hearing loss.
7. A *cystlike mass composed of epithelial cells and cholesterol* (**acoustic neuroma, ceruminoma, cholesteatoma**) may destroy adjacent bones, including the ossicles.
8. Thought to be caused by a viral infection, *inflammation of the inner ear* (**labyrinthitis, mastoiditis, myringitis**) may cause sudden intense *sensation of revolving* (**tinnitus, vertigo, presbycusis**), nausea, vomiting, and imbalance.
9. *Process of recording electrical activity in the cochlea in response to sound* (**audiology, electrocochleography, otoscopy**) may be used in the diagnosis of Ménière disease.

EXERCISE 27 Read Medical Terms in Use

Practice pronunciation of terms by reading the following information on acute otitis media. Use the pronunciation key following the medical term to assist you in saying the words.

To hear these terms, go to http://evolve.elsevier.com. Refer to p. 18 for your Evolve Access Information. Select Exercises & Review, Chapter 13, Chapter Exercises, Read Medical Terms in Use.

ACUTE OTITIS MEDIA

Acute **otitis media** (ō-TĪ-tis) (MĒ-dē-a) is one of the most common pediatric infections. Most middle ear infections are caused by bacteria, and some by viruses. Symptoms include **otalgia** (ō-TAL-ja), **otorrhea** (ō-tō-RĒ-a), ear pulling, and irritability. The tympanic membrane will be bulging, red in color, with a thickened appearance and reduced translucency. Antibiotics may be ordered if the infection does not resolve on its own. If unresponsive to antibiotic treatment, a **myringotomy** (mir-ing-GOT-o-mē) may be performed to identify the causative pathogen, allowing for the appropriate antibiotic treatment to be prescribed.

EXERCISE 28 Comprehend Medical Terms in Use

Test your comprehension of terms in the previous passage by answering T for true and F for false.

______ 1. Inflammation of the outer ear is one of the most common pediatric infections.

______ 2. Pain and discharge from the ear are symptoms of acute otitis media.

______ 3. Surgical repair of the tympanic membrane may be performed to identify causative organisms.

CHAPTER REVIEW

ONLINE CHAPTER REVIEW

To access the Evolve website, go to http://evolve.elsevier.com. Refer to p. 18 for your Evolve Access Information. Select Exercises & Review, Chapter 13, then select Chapter Exercises, Practice Activities, Animations, or Games. Place a check mark in the box when you have completed an exercise or activity, watched an animation, or played a game. Have fun!

Chapter Exercises

Exercises in this section of your Evolve resources correlate to exercises in your textbook. You may have completed them as you worked through the chapter.

- ☐ Pronunciation
- ☐ Spelling
- ☐ Read Medical Terms in Use

Practice Activities

Practice in study mode, then test your learning in assessment mode. Keep track of your scores from assessment mode if you wish.

	SCORE
☐ Picture It	______
☐ Define Word Parts	______
☐ Build Medical Terms	______
☐ Word Shop	______
☐ Define Medical Terms	______
☐ Use It	______
☐ Hear It and Type It: Clinical Vignettes	______

Animations

- ☐ Pathway of Sound

Games

- ☐ Name that Word Part
- ☐ Term Storm
- ☐ Term Explorer
- ☐ Termbusters
- ☐ Medical Millionaire
- ☐ Crossword Puzzle

REVIEW OF WORD PARTS

Can you define and spell the following word parts?

Combining Forms

audi/o	myring/o
aur/i	ot/o
aur/o	staped/o
cochle/o	tympan/o
labyrinth/o	vestibul/o
mastoid/o	

REVIEW OF TERMS

Can you build, analyze, define, pronounce, and spell the following terms *built from word parts?*

Diseases and Disorders	Surgical	Diagnostic	Complementary
labyrinthitis	cochlear implant	audiogram	audiologist
mastoiditis	labyrinthectomy	audiometer	audiology
myringitis	mastoidectomy	audiometry	aural
otalgia	mastoidotomy	electrocochleography	cochlear
otomastoiditis	myringoplasty	otoscope	otologist
otomycosis	myringotomy	otoscopy	otology
otopyorrhea	stapedectomy	tympanometer	otorhinolaryngologist
otorrhea	tympanoplasty	tympanometry	vestibular
otosclerosis			vestibulocochlear

Can you define, pronounce, and spell the following terms not *built from word parts?*

Diseases and Disorders

acoustic neuroma
ceruminoma
cholesteatoma
Ménière disease
otitis externa
otitis media (OM)
presbycusis
tinnitus
vertigo

ANSWERS

Exercise Figures

Exercise Figure

A. 1. ear: aur/i, aur/o, ot/o
2. labyrinth: labyrinth/o
3. stapes: staped/o
4. tympanic membrane: myring/o, tympan/o
5. mastoid bone: mastoid/o

Exercise Figure

B. myring/o/tomy

Exercise Figure

C. ot/o/scopy, ot/o/scope

Exercise 1

1. g
2. j
3. b
4. f
5. h
6. k
7. d
8. e
9. a
10. c

Exercise 2

1. stapes
2. mastoid bone
3. hearing
4. ear
5. tympanic membrane (eardrum), middle ear
6. vestibule
7. labyrinth
8. tympanic membrane (eardrum)
9. cochlea

Exercise 3

1. a. aur/i
   b. aur/o
   c. ot/o
2. mastoid/o
3. staped/o
4. tympan/o
5. labyrinth/o
6. audi/o
7. myring/o
8. cochle/o
9. vestibul/o

Exercise 4

Pronunciation Exercise

Exercise 5

1. WR CV WR S
   ot/o/myc/osis
   CF
   abnormal condition of fungus in the ear
2. WR CV WR S
   ot/o/mastoid/itis
   CF
   inflammation of the ear and the mastoid bone
3. WR S
   ot/algia
   pain in the ear
4. WR S
   labyrinth/itis
   inflammation of the labyrinth
5. WR S
   myring/itis
   inflammation of the tympanic membrane
6. WR CV S
   ot/o/sclerosis
   CF
   hardening of the ear (stapes)
7. WR S
   mastoid/itis
   inflammation of the mastoid bone
8. WR CV WR CV S
   ot /o/ py / o / rrhea
   CF CF
   discharge of pus from the ear
9. WR CV S
   ot/o/rrhea
   CF
   discharge from the ear

Exercise 6

1. myring/itis
2. ot/o/py/o/rrhea
3. mastoid/itis
4. ot/algia
5. ot/o/sclerosis
6. ot/o/myc/osis
7. ot/o/mastoid/itis
8. labyrinth/itis
9. ot/o/rrhea

Exercise 7

Spelling Exercise; see text p. 601.

Exercise 8

Pronunciation Exercise

Exercise 9

1. vertigo; tinnitus
2. Ménière
3. otitis media
4. ceruminoma
5. otitis externa
6. acoustic neuroma
7. presbycusis
8. cholesteatoma

Exercise 10

1. e
2. b
3. g
4. c
5. h
6. d
7. a
8. i
9. j

Exercise 11

Spelling Exercise; see text pp. 603-604.

Exercise 12

Pronunciation Exercise

Exercise 13

1. WR S
   mastoid/ectomy
   excision of the mastoid bone
2. WR CV S
   myring/o/tomy
   CF
   incision into the tympanic membrane
3. WR S
   labyrinth/ectomy
   excision of the labyrinth
4. WR CV S
   mastoid/o/tomy
   CF
   incision into the mastoid bone
5. WR CV S
   tympan/o/plasty
   CF
   surgical repair of the middle ear
6. WR CV S
   myring/o/plasty
   CF
   surgical repair of the tympanic membrane
7. WR S
   staped/ectomy
   excision of the stapes
8. WR S
   cochle/ar implant
   pertaining to the cochlea implant

Exercise 14
1. mastoid/o/tomy
2. labyrinth/ectomy
3. tympan/o/plasty
4. mastoid/ectomy
5. myring/o/tomy
6. myring/o/plasty
7. staped/ectomy
8. cochle/ar implant

Exercise 15
Spelling Exercise; see text p. 606.

Exercise 16
Pronunciation Exercise

Exercise 17
1. WR CV S
   ot/o/scope
   CF
   instrument used for visual examination of the ear
2. WR CV S
   audi/o/metry
   CF
   measurement of hearing
3. WR CV S
   audi/o/gram
   CF
   (graphic) record of hearing
4. WR CV S
   ot/o/scopy
   CF
   visual examination of the ear
5. WR CV S
   audi/o/meter
   CF
   instrument used to measure hearing
6. WR CV S
   tympan/o/metry
   CF
   measurement (of movement) of the tympanic membrane
7. WR CV S
   tympan/o/meter
   CF
   instrument used to measure middle ear (function)
8. WR CV WR CV S
   electr/o/cochle/o/graphy
   CF CF
   process of recording the electrical activity in the cochlea

Exercise 18
1. tympan/o/metry
2. audi/o/meter
3. ot/o/scopy
4. audi/o/gram
5. ot/o/scope
6. audi/o/metry
7. tympan/o/meter
8. electr/o/cochle/o/graphy

Exercise 19
Spelling Exercise; see text p. 609.

Exercise 20
Pronunciation Exercise

Exercise 21
1. WR CV S
   ot/o/logy
   CF
   study of the ear
2. WR CV S
   audi/o/logist
   CF
   one who studies and specializes in hearing
3. WR CV WR CV WR CV S
   ot/o/rhin/o/laryng/o/logist
   CF CF CF
   physician who studies and treats diseases of the ear, nose, and larynx (throat)
4. WR CV S
   audi/o/logy
   CF
   study of hearing
5. WR CV S
   ot/o/logist
   CF
   physician who studies and treats diseases of the ear
6. WR S
   aur/al
   pertaining to the ear
7. WR S
   cochle/ar
   pertaining to the cochlea
8. WR S
   vestibul/ar
   pertaining to the vestibule
9. WR CV WR S
   vestibul/o/cochle/ar
   CF
   pertaining to the vestibule and cochlea

Exercise 22
1. audi/o/logy
2. ot/o/rhin/o/laryng/o/logist
3. ot/o/logy
4. audi/o/logist
5. ot/o/logist
6. aur/al
7. vestibul/o/cochle/ar
8. vestibul/ar
9. cochle/ar

Exercise 23
Spelling Exercise; see text p. 612.

Exercise 24
1. ears, nose, throat
2. eyes, ears, nose, and throat
3. otitis media
4. acute otitis media

Exercise 25
A. 1. ENT
2. tinnitus
3. vertigo
4. otoscopy
5. otitis media
6. presbycusis
7. audiologist
8. audiometry

B. 1. a
2. b
3. d

Exercise 26
1. myringitis
2. tinnitus
3. otologist
4. myringotomy
5. Ménière disease
6. acoustic neuroma
7. cholesteatoma
8. labyrinthitis, vertigo
9. electrocochleography

Exercise 27
Reading Exercise

Exercise 28
1. *F*, inflammation of the middle ear (otitis media) is the most common pediatric infection.
2. *T*
3. *F*, myringotomy, incision into the tympanic membrane would be performed.

Chapter 14

Musculoskeletal System

OUTLINE

OBJECTIVES

Upon completion of this chapter you will be able to:

1. Identify organs and structures of the musculoskeletal system.
2. Identify and define types of body movement.
3. Define and spell word parts related to the musculoskeletal system.
4. Define, pronounce, and spell disease and disorder terms related to the musculoskeletal system.
5. Define, pronounce, and spell surgical terms related to the musculoskeletal system.
6. Define, pronounce, and spell diagnostic terms related to the musculoskeletal system.
7. Define, pronounce, and spell complementary terms related to the musculoskeletal system.
8. Interpret the meaning of abbreviations related to the musculoskeletal system.
9. Interpret, read, and comprehend medical language in simulated medical statements and documents.

PERIOSTEUM

is composed of the prefix **peri-,** meaning **surrounding,** and the word root **oste,** meaning **bone.**

ENDOSTEUM

is composed of the prefix **endo-,** meaning **within,** and the word root **oste,** meaning **bone.**

DIAPHYSIS

comes from the Greek **diaphusis,** meaning **state of growing between.**

EPIPHYSIS

has been used in the English language since the 1600s and retains the meaning given to it by a Greco-Roman physician. It means a **portion of bone attached for a time to another bone by a cartilage, but that later combines with the principal bone.** During the period of growth, the epiphysis is separated from the main portion of the bone by cartilage.

ANATOMY

The musculoskeletal system consists of muscles, bones (Figure 14-1), bone marrow, joints, cartilage, and bursae. The body contains 206 bones (Figure 14-2 and Figure 14-3, *A* and *B*) and more than 600 muscles. Joints are located any place that two or more bones meet, and contain cartilage and bursae.

Function

The functions of the muscular system are movement, posture, joint stability, and heat production. The functions of the skeletal system are to provide a framework for the body, protect the soft body parts such as the brain, store calcium, and produce blood cells. The organs and structures of the musculoskeletal system work together to protect, support, and move the body.

Bone Structure

Term	Definition
periosteum	outermost layer of the bone, made up of fibrous tissue
compact bone	dense, hard layers of bone tissue that lie underneath the periosteum
cancellous (spongy) bone	contains little spaces like a sponge and is encased in the layers of compact bone
endosteum	membranous lining of the hollow cavity of the bone
diaphysis	shaft of the long bones (Figure 14-1)
epiphysis (*pl.* epiphyses)	end of each long bone (Figure 14-1)
bone marrow	material found in the cavities of bones
red marrow	thick, bloodlike material found in flat bones and the ends of long bones; location of blood cell formation
yellow marrow	soft, fatty material found in the medullary cavity of long bones

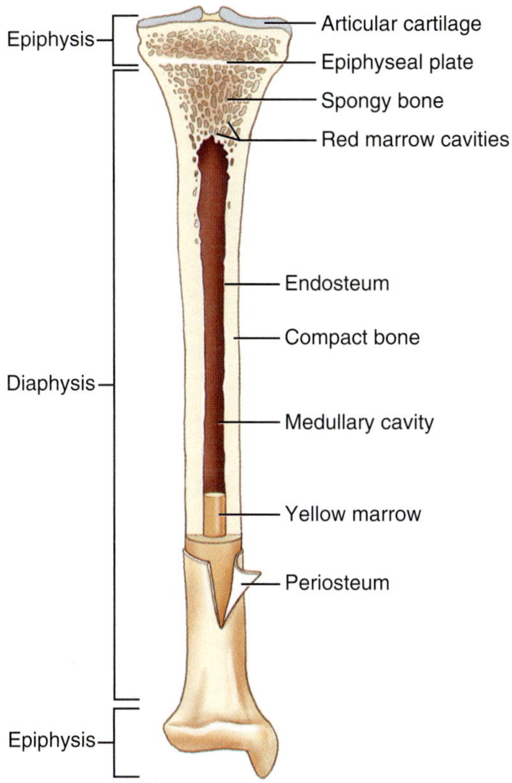

FIGURE 14-1
Bone structure.

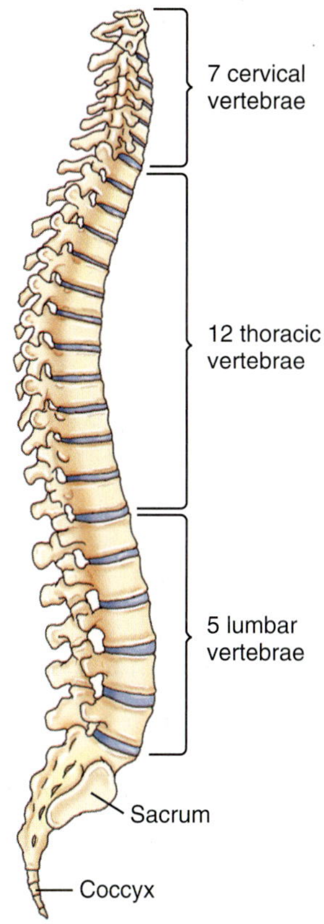

FIGURE 14-2
Vertebral column.

Skeletal Bones

Term	Definition
maxilla	upper jawbone
mandible	lower jawbone
vertebral column	made up of bones called **vertebrae** *(pl.)* or **vertebra** *(sing.)* through which the spinal cord runs. The vertebral column protects the spinal cord, supports the head, and provides points of attachment for ribs and muscles (Figure 14-2).
cervical vertebrae (C1 to C7)	first set of seven bones, forming the neck
thoracic vertebrae (T1 to T12)	second set of 12 vertebrae. They articulate with the 12 pairs of ribs to form the outward curve of the spine.
lumbar vertebrae (L1 to L5)	third set of five larger vertebrae, which forms the inward curve of the spine
sacrum	next five vertebrae, which fuse together to form a triangular bone positioned between the two hip bones
coccyx	four vertebrae fused together to form the tailbone
lamina (*pl.* laminae)	part of the vertebral arch

COCCYX

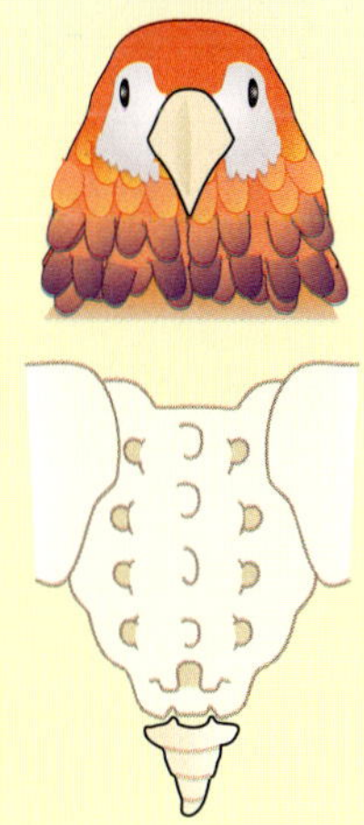

Coccyx is derived from the Greek word *cuckoo* because of its resemblance to a cuckoo's beak.

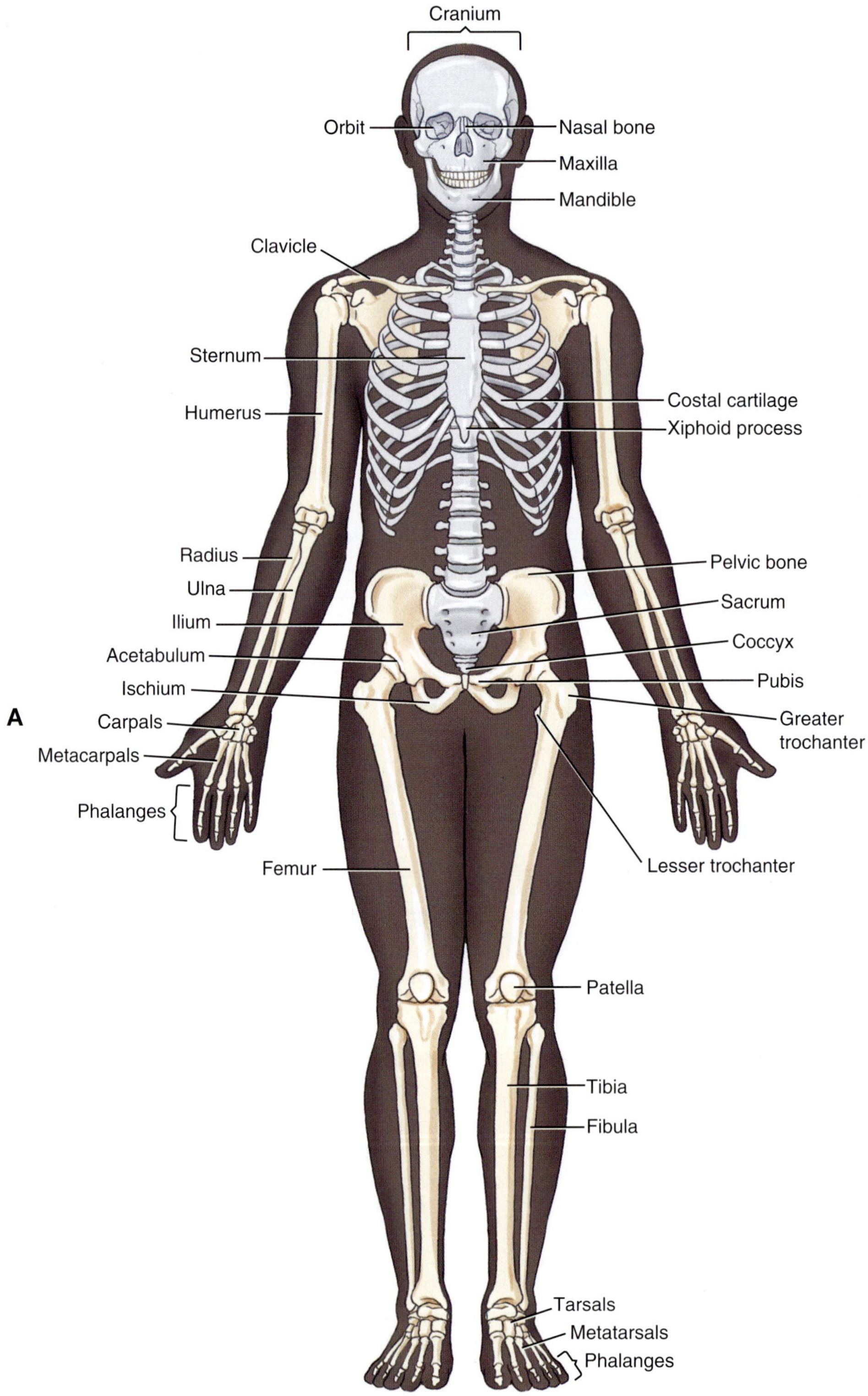

FIGURE 14-3

A, Anterior view of the skeleton.

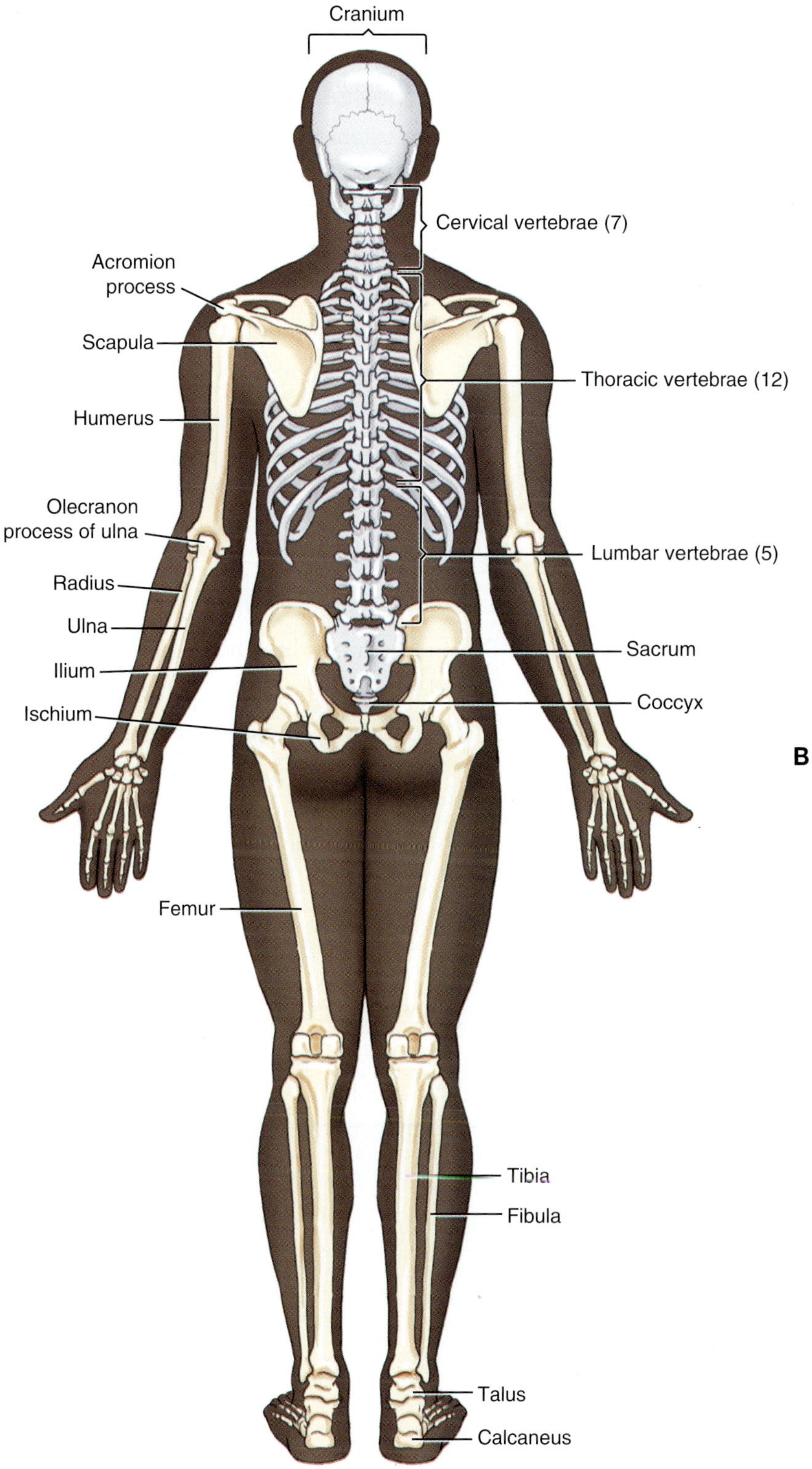

FIGURE 14-3, cont'd
B, Posterior view of the skeleton.

Skeletal Bones—*cont'd*

Term	Definition
clavicle	collarbone
scapula	shoulder blade
acromion process	extension of the scapula, which forms the high point of the shoulder
sternum	breastbone
xiphoid process	lower portion of the sternum
humerus	upper arm bone
ulna and radius	lower arm bones
olecranon process	projection at the upper end of the ulna that forms the bony point of the elbow
carpal bones	wrist bones
metacarpal bones	hand bones
phalanges (*sing.* phalanx)	finger and toe bones
pelvic bone, hip bone	made up of three bones fused together
ischium	lower, rear portion on which one sits
ilium	upper, wing-shaped part on each side
pubis	anterior portion of the pelvic bone
acetabulum	large socket in the pelvic bone for the head of the femur
femur	upper leg bone
tibia and fibula	lower leg bones
patella (*pl.* patellae)	kneecap
tarsal bones	ankle bones
calcaneus	heel bone
metatarsal bones	foot bones

EXERCISE 1

Match the definitions in the first column with the correct terms in the second column. *To check your answers to the exercises in this chapter, go to Answers, p. 687, at the end of the chapter.*

______	1. shaft of a long bone	a.	lamina
______	2. hard layer of bone tissue	b.	cancellous bone
______	3. outermost layer of bone	c.	acetabulum
______	4. found in bone cavities	d.	diaphysis
______	5. lining of the bone cavity	e.	endometrium
______	6. end of each long bone	f.	calcaneus
______	7. contains little spaces	g.	epiphysis
______	8. socket in the pelvic bone	h.	periosteum
______	9. heel bone	i.	compact bone
______	10. part of the arch of the vertebra	j.	endosteum
		k.	bone marrow

EXERCISE 2

Write the name of the bone to match the definition.

1. shoulder blade ______________________
2. breastbone ______________________
3. lower jawbone ______________________
4. collarbone ______________________
5. upper arm bone ______________________
6. lower arm bones a. ______________________
   b. ______________________
7. ankle bones ______________________
8. finger, toe bones ______________________
9. foot bones ______________________
10. hand bones ______________________
11. upper leg bone ______________________
12. lower leg bones a. ______________________
    b. ______________________
13. kneecap ______________________
14. neck ______________________
15. third set of vertebrae ______________________
16. anterior portion of the pelvic bone ______________________
17. five vertebrae fused together ______________________

18. lower rear portion of the pelvic bone ______________________
19. tailbone ______________________
20. upper, wing-shaped part of the pelvic bone ______________________
21. wrist bones ______________________

Joints

Joints, also called **articulations**, hold our bones together and make movement possible (in most joints) (Figure 14-4).

Term	Definition
articular cartilage	smooth layer of firm, fibrous tissue covering the contacting surface of joints
meniscus	crescent-shaped cartilage found in the knee
intervertebral disk	cartilaginous pad found between the vertebrae in the spine
pubic symphysis	cartilaginous joint at which two pubic bones come together
synovia	fluid secreted by the synovial membrane and found in joint cavities
bursa (*pl.* bursae)	fluid-filled sac that allows for easy movement of one part of a joint over another
ligament	flexible, tough band of fibrous connective tissue that attaches one bone to another at a joint
tendon	band of fibrous connective tissue that attaches muscle to bone
aponeurosis	strong sheet of tissue that acts as a tendon to attach muscles to bone

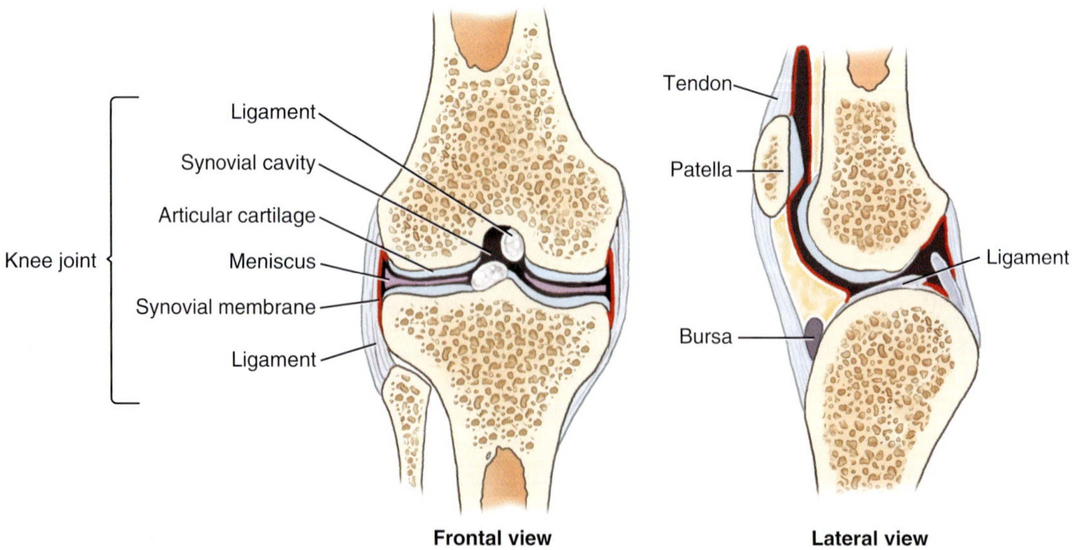

FIGURE 14-4
Knee joint.

Muscles

Term	Definition
skeletal muscles (also known as *striated muscles*)	attached to bones by tendons and make body movement possible. Skeletal muscles produce action by pulling and by working in pairs. They are also known as **voluntary muscles** because we have control over these muscles (Figure 14-5, *A* and *B*, and Figure 14-6).
smooth muscles (also known as *unstriated muscles*)	located in internal organs such as the walls of blood vessels and the digestive tract. They are also called **involuntary muscles** because they respond to impulses from the autonomic nerves and are not controlled voluntarily (see Figure 14-6).
cardiac muscle (known as *myocardium*)	forms most of the wall of the heart. Its involuntary contraction produces the heartbeat (see Figure 14-6).

A & P Booster
For students desiring more anatomy and physiology, go to http://evolve.elsevier.com. Refer to p. 18 for your Evolve Access Information. Select A & P Booster, Chapter 14.

EXERCISE 3

Match the definitions in the first column with the correct terms in the second column.

_____ 1. attaches muscle to bone	a. skeletal muscles
_____ 2. fluid-filled sac	b. aponeurosis
_____ 3. smooth layer of fibrous tissue	c. bursa
_____ 4. voluntary muscles	d. smooth muscles
_____ 5. fluid	e. cartilage
_____ 6. located in the internal organs	f. intervertebral disk
_____ 7. attaches bone to bone	g. cardiac muscles
_____ 8. cartilage found in the knee	h. ligament
_____ 9. pubic bone joint	i. meniscus
_____ 10. acts as a tendon	j. periosteum
_____ 11. found between each vertebra	k. pubic symphysis
_____ 12. produces heartbeat	l. synovia
	m. tendon

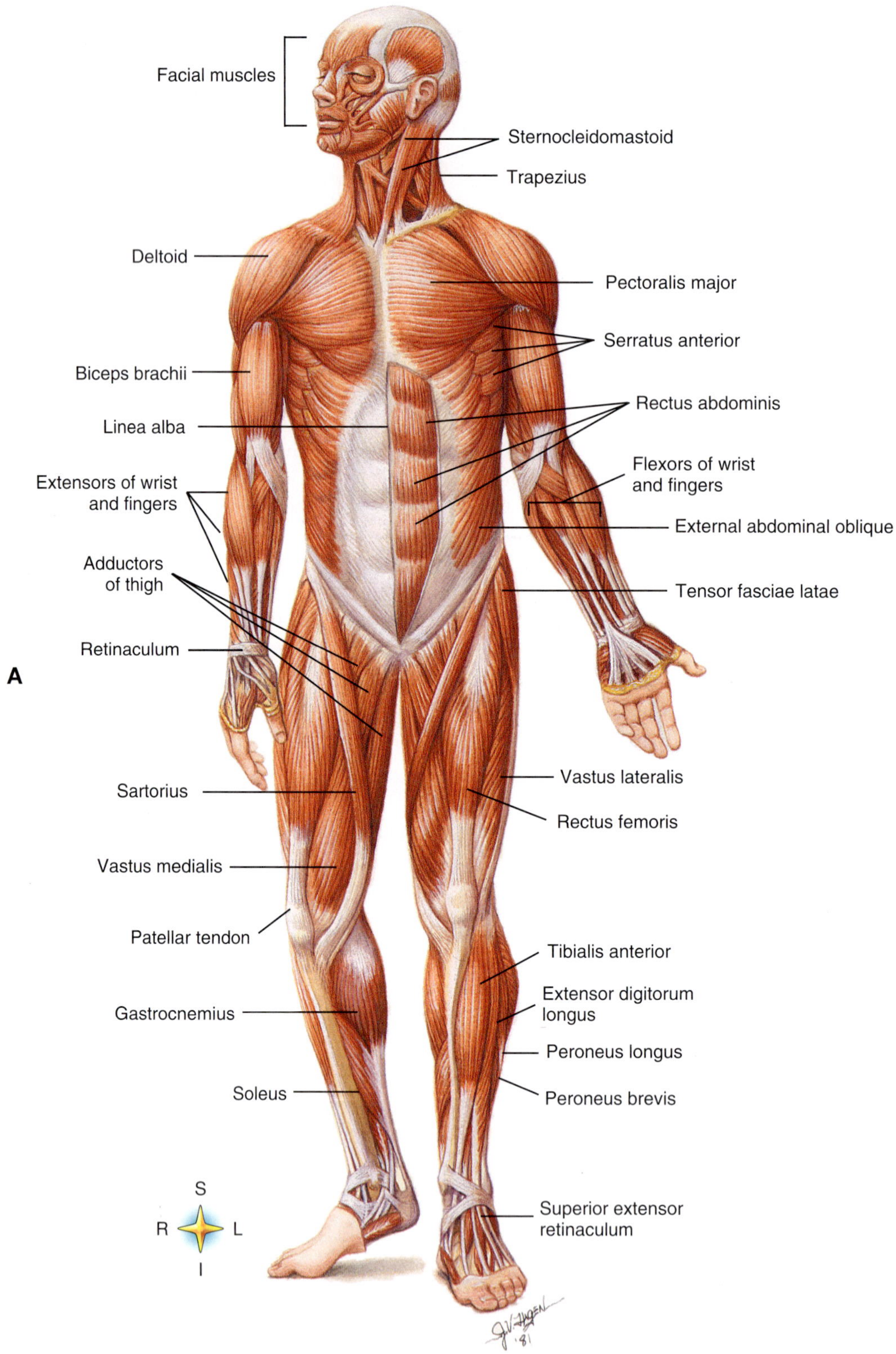

FIGURE 14-5
A, Anterior view of the muscular system.

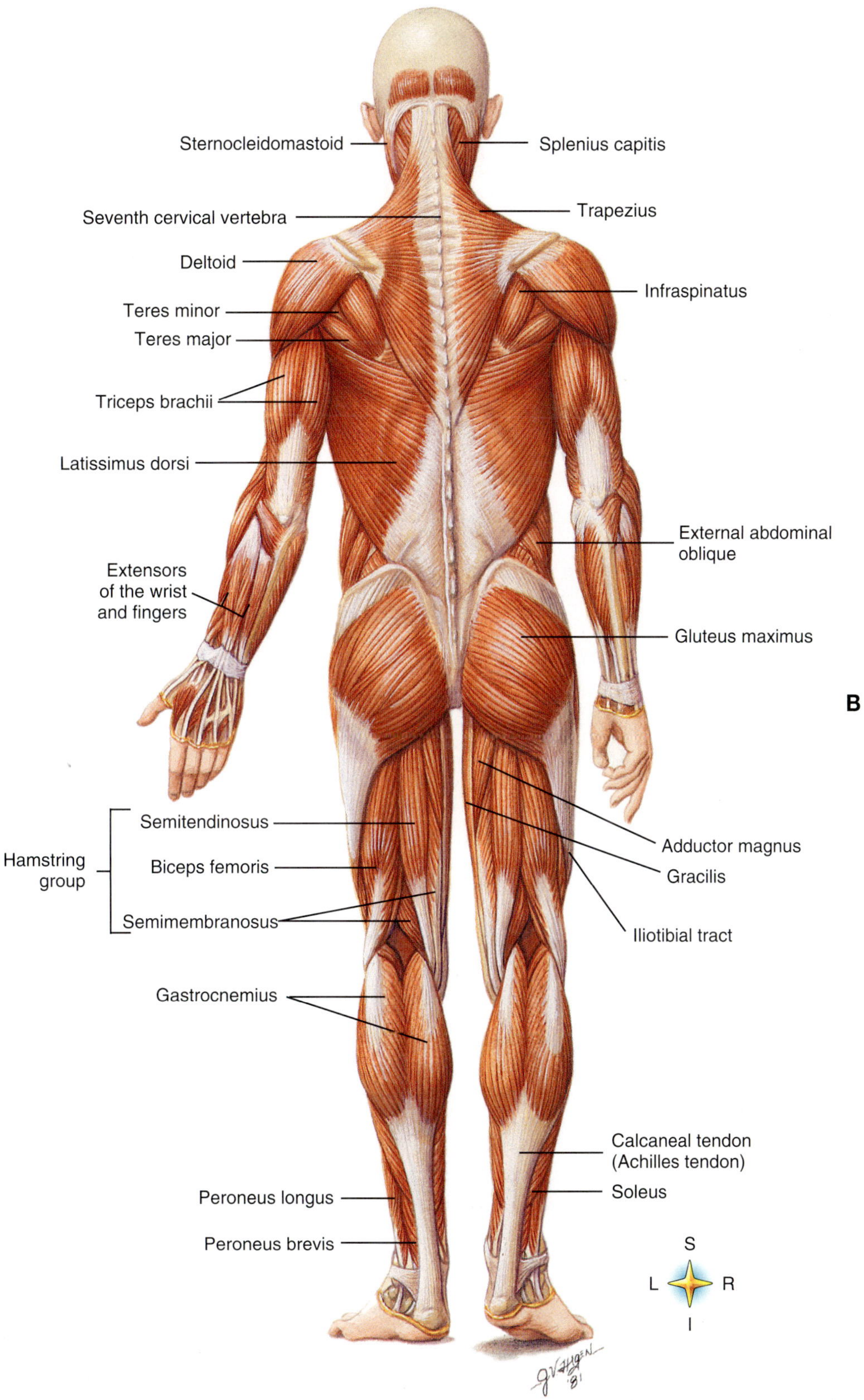

FIGURE 14-5, cont'd
B, Posterior view of the muscular system.

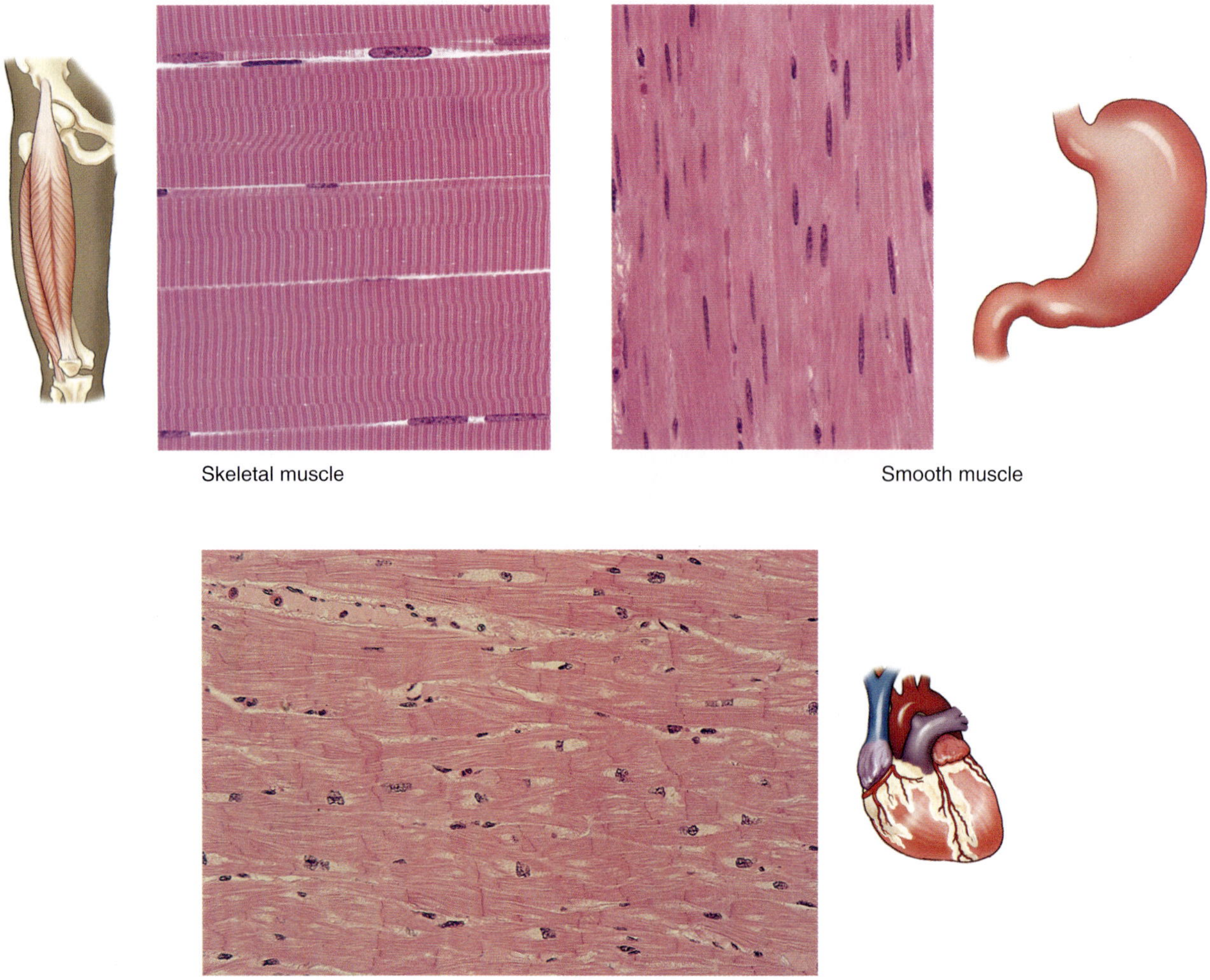

Skeletal muscle

Smooth muscle

Cardiac muscle

FIGURE 14-6
Types of muscle tissue.

TYPES OF BODY MOVEMENT

Bones and muscles work together to produce various types of body movement. Some are listed below (Figure 14-7).

> **MIDLINE VS. MIDDLE**
>
> The two terms are synonyms, both describing an imaginary line that separates the body, or body part, into equal halves. In medical language, *midline* is the preferred term and is used as a common reference point.

Term	Definition
abduction (ab-DUK-shun)	moving away from the midline
adduction (ad-DUK-shun)	moving toward the midline
inversion (in-VER-zhun)	turning inward
eversion (ē-VER-zhun)	turning outward
extension (ek-STEN-shun)	movement in which a limb is placed in a straight position

Term	Definition
flexion (FLEK-shun)	movement in which a limb is bent
pronation (prō-NĀ-shun)	movement that turns the palm down
supination (sū-pi-NĀ-shun)	movement that turns the palm up
rotation (rō-TĀ-shun)	turning around its own axis

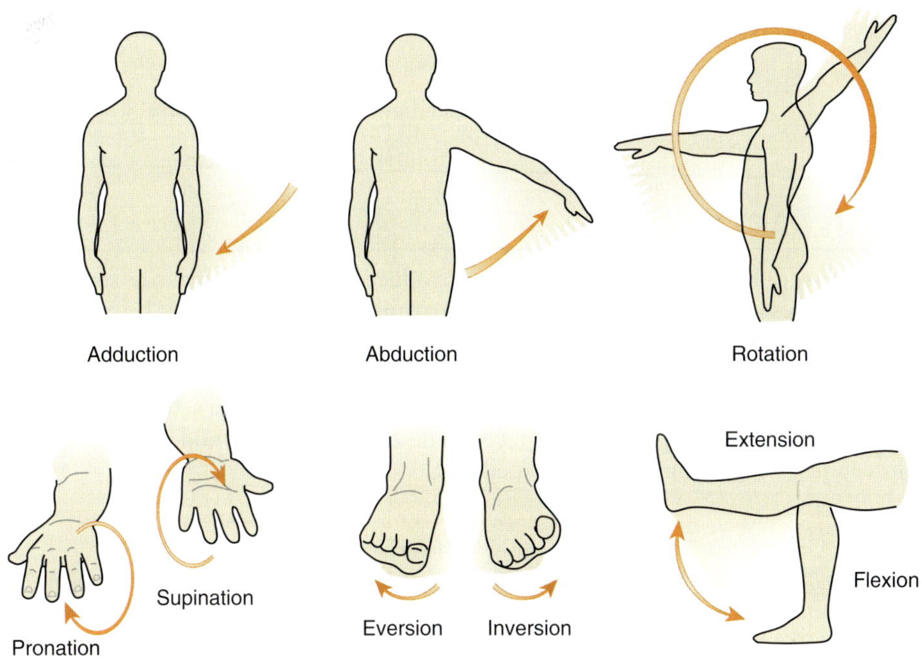

FIGURE 14-7
Types of body movements.

EXERCISE 4

Write the definitions of the following terms.

1. abduction ______________________
2. pronation ______________________
3. supination ______________________
4. rotation ______________________
5. extension ______________________
6. eversion ______________________
7. adduction ______________________
8. flexion ______________________
9. inversion ______________________

EXERCISE 5

Match the terms in the first column with the correct definitions in the second column.

_____ 1. abduction
_____ 2. adduction
_____ 3. pronation
_____ 4. rotation
_____ 5. eversion
_____ 6. extension
_____ 7. flexion
_____ 8. inversion
_____ 9. supination

a. movement in which the limb is placed in a straight position
b. movement that turns the palm up
c. turning outward
d. moving toward the midline
e. conveying toward the center
f. turning inward
g. movement in which the limb is bent
h. moving away from the midline
i. movement that turns the palm down
j. turning around its own axis

WORD PARTS

At first glance the number of word parts introduced in this chapter may seem overwhelming, but notice that many of them are names for bones already learned in the anatomic section. The definitions of the word parts include both anatomic terms and commonly used words. For example, both *carpal* and *wrist bone* are given as the definition of the combining form *carp/o.* Word parts you need to learn to complete this chapter are listed on the following pages. The exercises at the end of each list will help you learn their definitions and spellings.

Use the flashcards accompanying this text or electronic flashcards to assist you in memorizing the word parts for this chapter.

To use electronic flashcards, go to http://evolve.elsevier.com. Refer to p. 18 for your Evolve Access Information. Select Flashcards, Chapter 14.

Combining Forms of the Musculoskeletal System

Combining Form	Definition
carp/o	carpals (wrist bones)
clavic/o, clavicul/o	clavicle (collarbone)
cost/o	rib
crani/o	cranium (skull)
femor/o	femur (upper leg bone) (NOTE: The "u" in fem<u>u</u>r changes to an "o" in the word root fem<u>o</u>r/.)
fibul/o	fibula (lower leg bone) (perone/o is also a word root for fibula)
humer/o	humerus (upper arm bone)
ili/o	ilium
ischi/o	ischium
lumb/o	loin, lumbar region of the spine

METACARPUS

literally means **beyond the wrist.** It is composed of the prefix **meta-,** meaning **beyond,** and **carpus,** meaning **wrist.**

Combining Form	Definition
mandibul/o	mandible (lower jawbone)
maxill/o	maxilla (upper jawbone)
patell/o	patella (kneecap)
pelv/i, pelv/o (NOTE: the combining vowels *i* and *o* are used with the word root **pelv/**.)	pelvis, pelvic bone (also covered in Chapter 9)
phalang/o	phalanges (finger or toe bones)
pub/o	pubis
rachi/o	spine, vertebral column
radi/o	radius (lower arm bone)
sacr/o	sacrum
scapul/o	scapula (shoulder blade)
spondyl/o, vertebr/o	vertebra
stern/o	sternum (breastbone)
tars/o	tarsals (ankle bones)
tibi/o	tibia (lower leg bone)
uln/o	ulna (lower arm bone)

EXERCISE 6

Write the definitions of the following combining forms.

1. clavic/o ______________________
2. cost/o ______________________
3. crani/o ______________________
4. femor/o ______________________
5. clavicul/o ______________________
6. humer/o ______________________
7. ili/o ______________________
8. ischi/o ______________________
9. carp/o ______________________
10. fibul/o ______________________
11. mandibul/o ______________________
12. lumb/o ______________________
13. pelv/o ______________________

EXERCISE FIGURE A

Fill in the blanks with combining forms in this diagram of the skeleton, anterior view. *To check your answers, go to p. 687.*

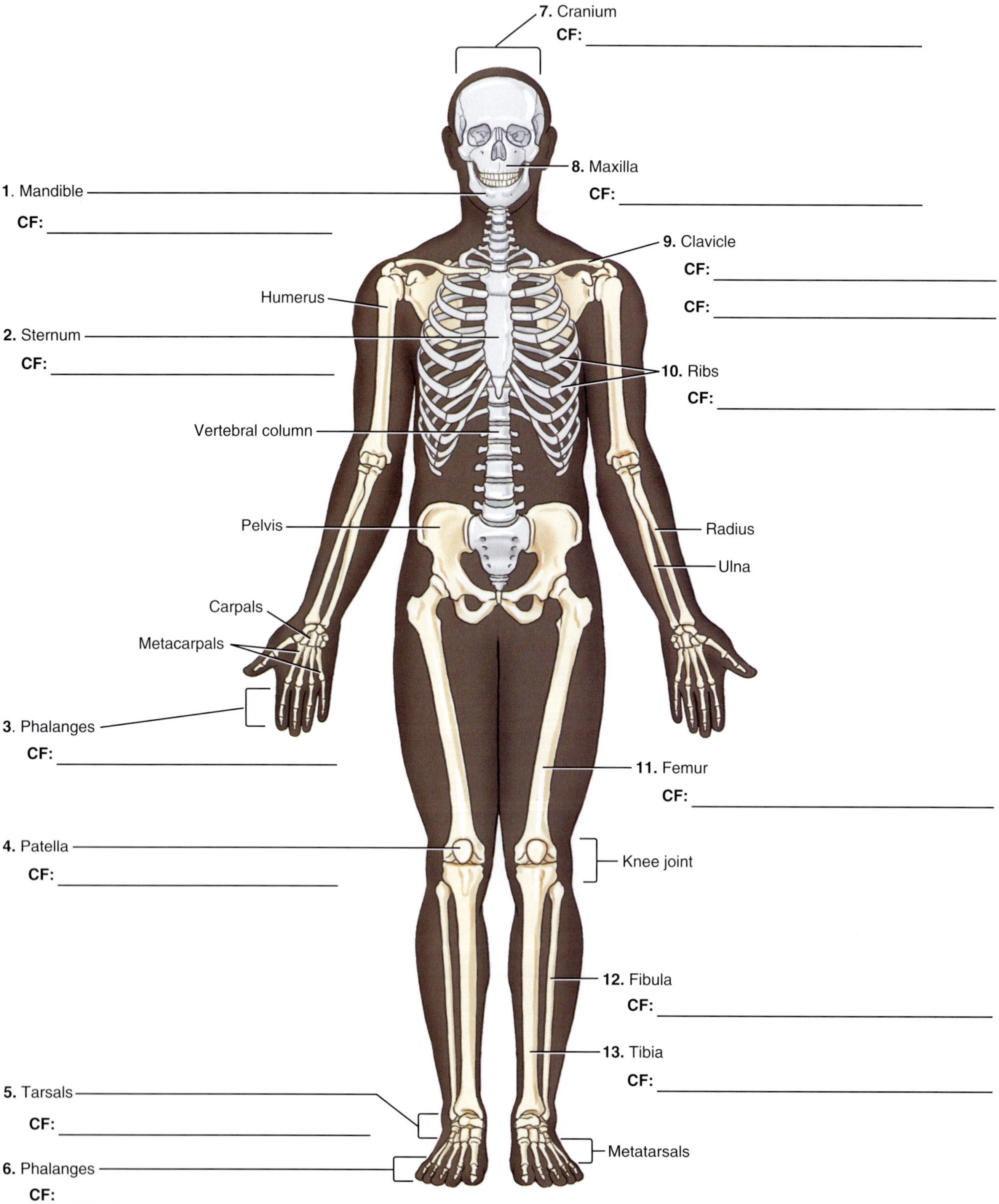

EXERCISE FIGURE B

Fill in the blanks with combining forms in this diagram of the skeleton, posterior view, and the pelvis.

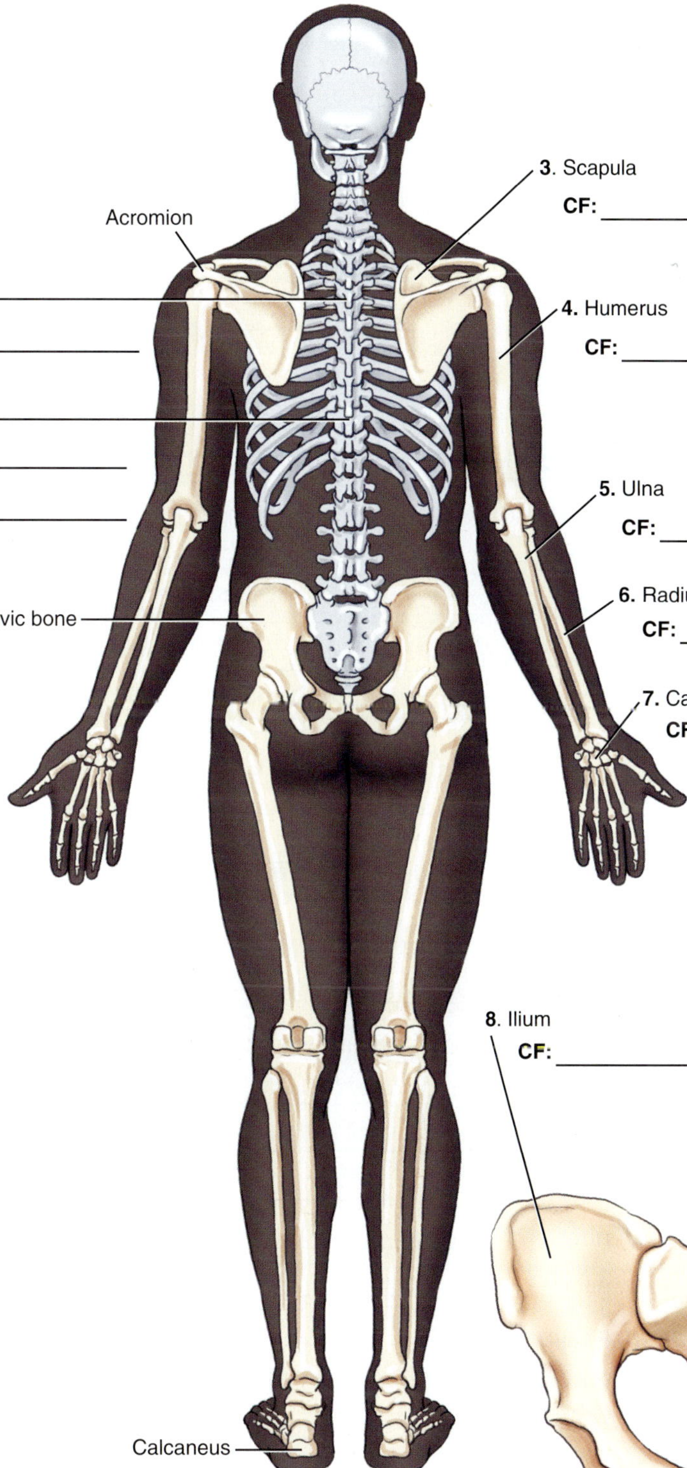

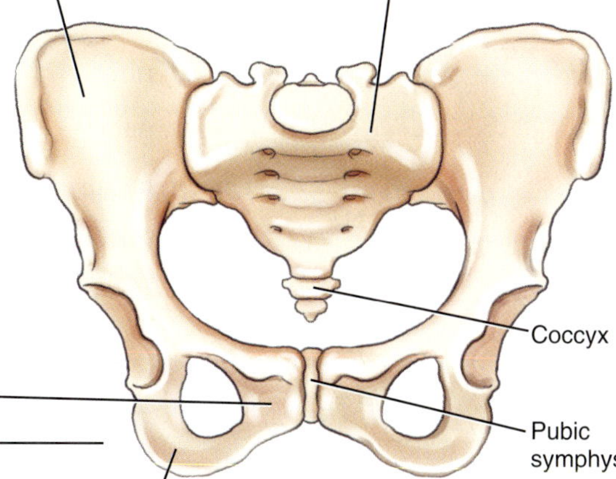

EXERCISE 7

Write the combining form for each of the following terms.

1. clavicle a. ______________
   b. ______________
2. rib ______________
3. cranium ______________
4. femur ______________
5. humerus ______________
6. carpals ______________
7. ischium ______________
8. fibula ______________
9. ilium ______________
10. mandible ______________
11. loin, lumbar region of the spine ______________
12. pelvis, pelvic bone a. ______________
    b. ______________

EXERCISE 8

Write the definitions of the following combining forms.

1. rachi/o ______________________
2. patell/o ______________________
3. spondyl/o ______________________
4. maxill/o ______________________
5. phalang/o ______________________
6. uln/o ______________________
7. radi/o ______________________
8. tibi/o ______________________
9. pub/o ______________________
10. tars/o ______________________
11. scapul/o ______________________
12. stern/o ______________________
13. vertebr/o ______________________
14. sacr/o ______________________

EXERCISE 9

Write the combining form for each of the following terms.

1. maxilla ______________
2. ulna ______________
3. radius ______________
4. tibia ______________
5. pubis ______________
6. tarsals ______________
7. vertebra a. ______________
   b. ______________
8. sternum ______________
9. scapula ______________
10. patella ______________
11. phalanges ______________
12. sacrum ______________
13. vertebral column, spine ______________

Combining Forms of Joints

Combining Form	Definition
aponeur/o	aponeurosis
arthr/o	joint
burs/o	bursa (cavity)
chondr/o	cartilage
disk/o	intervertebral disk
menisc/o	meniscus (crescent)
synovi/o	synovia, synovial membrane
ten/o, tend/o, tendin/o	tendon

DISK

is from the Greek ***diskos,*** meaning flat plate. A variant spelling, ***disc,*** is also used, though chiefly in ophthalmology.

EXERCISE FIGURE C

Fill in the blanks with combining forms on these diagrams of the knee joint.

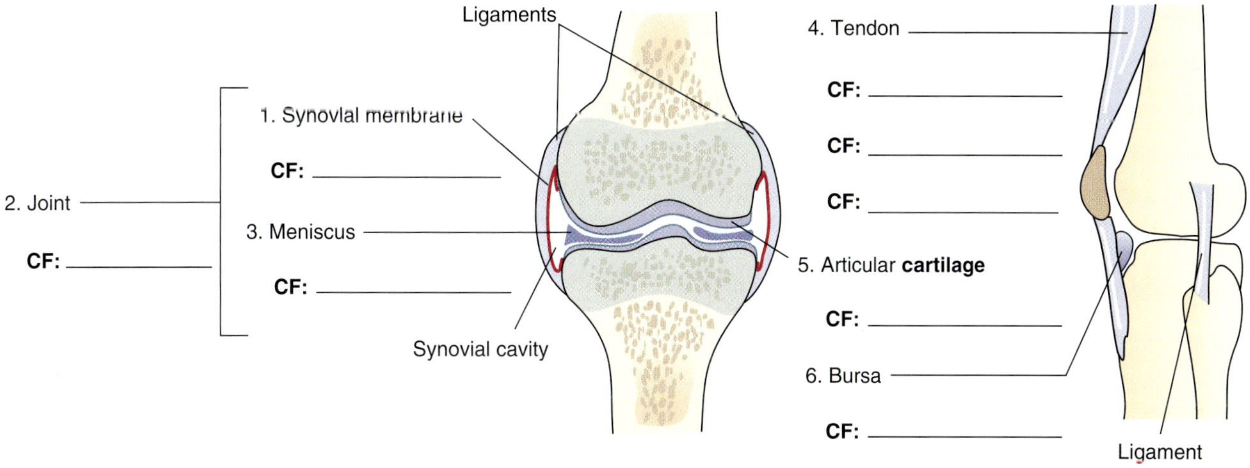

EXERCISE 10

Write the definitions of the following combining forms.

1. arthr/o ____________________
2. aponeur/o ____________________
3. menisc/o ____________________
4. tendin/o ____________________
5. chondr/o ____________________
6. ten/o ____________________
7. burs/o ____________________
8. tend/o ____________________
9. synovi/o ____________________
10. disk/o ____________________

EXERCISE 11

Write the combining form for each of the following terms.

1. meniscus ____________
2. aponeurosis ____________
3. joint ____________
4. cartilage ____________
5. tendon a. ____________
   b. ____________
   c. ____________
6. bursa ____________
7. synovia, synovial membrane ____________
8. intervertebral disk ____________

Combining Forms Commonly Used with Musculoskeletal System Terms

Combining Form	Definition
ankyl/o	crooked, stiff, bent
kinesi/o	movement, motion
kyph/o	hump (increased convexity of the spine)
lamin/o	lamina (thin, flat plate or layer)
lord/o	bent forward (increased concavity of the spine)
myel/o (NOTE: *myel/o* also means *spinal cord;* see Chapter 15.)	bone marrow (also covered in Chapter 10)
my/o, myos/o (NOTE: *my/o* was introduced in Chapter 2.)	muscle
oste/o	bone
petr/o (NOTE: *lith/o*, also a combining form for *stone*, was introduced in Chapter 6.)	stone
scoli/o	crooked, curved

EXERCISE 12

Write the definitions of the following combining forms.

1. my/o ______________________
2. petr/o ______________________
3. kinesi/o ______________________
4. oste/o ______________________
5. lamin/o ______________________
6. myel/o ______________________
7. kyph/o ______________________
8. ankyl/o ______________________
9. scoli/o ______________________
10. myos/o ______________________
11. lord/o ______________________

EXERCISE 13

Write the combining form for each of the following.

1. muscle a. ____________
   b. ____________
2. stone ____________
3. movement, motion ____________
4. bone ____________
5. lamina ____________
6. bone marrow ____________
7. hump ____________
8. crooked, stiff, bent ____________
9. crooked, curved ____________
10. bent forward ____________

Prefixes

Prefix	Definition
inter-	between
supra-	above
sym-, syn-	together, joined

EXERCISE 14

Write the definition of the following prefixes.

1. supra- ______________________________________
2. sym-, syn- ______________________________________
3. inter- ______________________________________

EXERCISE 15

Write the prefix for each of the following definitions.

1. together, joined a. ____________________
   b. ____________________
2. between ____________________
3. above ____________________

Suffixes

Suffix	Definition
-asthenia	weakness
-clasia, -clasis, -clast	break
-desis	surgical fixation, fusion
-physis	growth
-schisis	split, fissure

EXERCISE 16

Write the definitions of the following suffixes.

1. -physis ____________________
2. -clasis ____________________
3. -desis ____________________
4. -clast ____________________
5. -schisis ____________________
6. -clasia ____________________
7. -asthenia ____________________

EXERCISE 17

Write the suffix for each of the following definitions.

1. growth ____________________
2. weakness ____________________
3. break a. ____________________
   b. ____________________
   c. ____________________
4. surgical fixation, fusion ____________________
5. split, fissure ____________________

MEDICAL TERMS

Disease and Disorder Terms

Built from Word Parts

The following terms are built from word parts you have already learned and can be translated literally to find their meanings. Further explanation of terms beyond the definition of their word parts, if needed, is included in parentheses.

Term	Definition
ankylosis (*ang*-ki-LŌ-sis)	abnormal condition of stiffness (often referring to fixation of a joint, such as the result of chronic rheumatoid arthritis)
arthritis (ar-THRĪ-tis)	inflammation of a joint. (The most common forms of arthritis are osteoarthritis and rheumatoid arthritis.) (Figure 14-8)
bursitis (ber-SĪ-tis)	inflammation of a bursa
chondromalacia (*kon*-drō-ma-LĀ-sha)	softening of cartilage
cranioschisis (*krā*-nē-OS-ki-sis)	fissure of the skull (congenital)
diskitis (dis-KĪ-tis)	inflammation of an intervertebral disk (also spelled **discitis**)
fibromyalgia (*fī*-brō-mī-AL-ja)	pain in the fibrous tissues and muscles (a common condition characterized by widespread pain and stiffness of muscles, fatigue, and disturbed sleep)
kyphosis (kī-FŌ-sis)	abnormal condition of a hump (increased convexity of the thoracic spine as viewed from the side) (also called **hunchback** or **humpback**) (Exercise Figure D)
lordosis (lōr-DŌ-sis)	abnormal condition of bending forward (increased concavity of the lumbar spine as viewed from the side) (also called **swayback**) (Exercise Figure D)
maxillitis (*mak*-si-LĪ-tis)	inflammation of the maxilla
meniscitis (*men*-i-SĪ-tis)	inflammation of a meniscus
myasthenia (*mī*-as-THĒ-nē-a)	muscle weakness
myeloma (*mī*-e-LŌ-ma)	tumor of the bone marrow (malignant)
osteitis (*os*-tē-Ī-tis)	inflammation of the bone

Disease and Disorder Terms—*cont'd*

Built from Word Parts

Term	Definition
osteoarthritis (OA) (*os*-tē-ō-ar-THRĪ-tis)	inflammation of the bone and joint (Figure 14-8)
osteochondritis (*os*-tē-ō-kon-DRĪ-tis)	inflammation of the bone and cartilage
osteofibroma (*os*-tē-ō-fī-BRŌ-ma)	tumor of the bone and fibrous tissue (benign)
osteomalacia (*os*-tē-ō-ma-LĀ-sha)	softening of bones
osteomyelitis (*os*-tē-ō-*mī*-e-LĪ-tis)	inflammation of the bone and bone marrow (caused by bacterial infection)
osteopenia (*os*-tē-ō-PĒ-nē-a)	abnormal reduction of bone mass (caused by inadequate replacement of bone lost to normal bone lysis and can lead to osteoporosis)

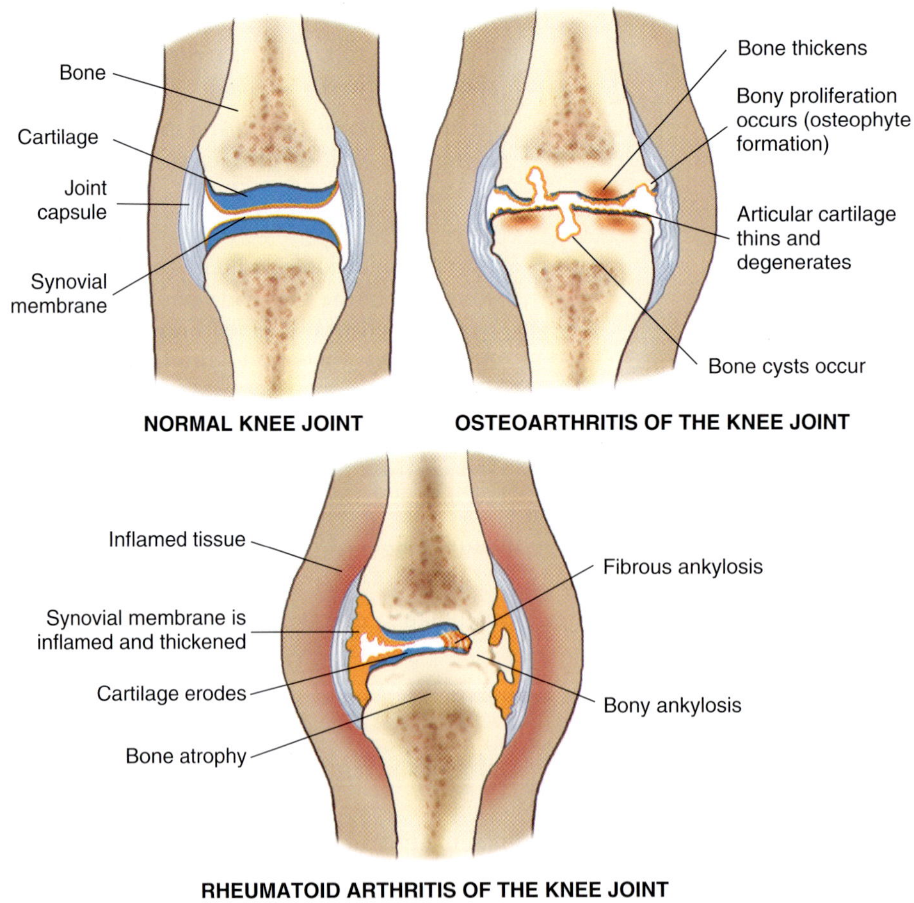

FIGURE 14-8
Normal and arthritic knee joints.

Term	Definition
osteopetrosis (*os*-tē-ō-pe-TRŌ-sis)	abnormal condition of stonelike bones (marblelike bones caused by increased formation of bone)
osteosarcoma (*os*-tē-ō-sar-KŌ-ma)	malignant tumor of the bone
polymyositis (*pol*-ē-*mī*-ō-SĪ-tis)	inflammation of many muscles
rachischisis (ra-KIS-ki-sis)	fissure of the vertebral column (congenital) (also called **spina bifida**) (see Exercise Figure C in Chapter 15)
rhabdomyolysis (*rab*-dō-mī-OL-i-sis)	dissolution of striated muscle (The severity of the condition and the degree of weakness and pain vary. Some causes of the illness are trauma, extreme exertion, and drug toxicity; in severe cases renal failure can result.)
sarcopenia (*sar*-kō-PĒ-nē-a)	abnormal reduction of connective tissue (such as loss of skeletal muscle mass in the elderly)
scoliosis (*skō*-lē-Ō-sis)	abnormal condition of (lateral) a curved (spine) (Figure 14-9) (Exercise Figure D)
spondylarthritis (*spon*-dil-ar-THRĪ-tis)	inflammation of the vertebral joints
spondylosis (*spon*-di-LŌ-sis)	abnormal condition of the vertebra (a general term used to describe changes to the spine from osteoarthritis or ankylosis)
synoviosarcoma (si-*nō*-vē-ō-sar-KŌ-ma)	malignant tumor of the synovial membrane
tendinitis (*ten*-di-NĪ-tis)	inflammation of a tendon (also spelled **tendonitis**)
tenosynovitis (*ten*-ō-*sin*-ō-VI-tis) (NOTE: the *i* in *synovi* is dropped because the suffix begins with an *i*.)	inflammation of the tendon and synovial membrane

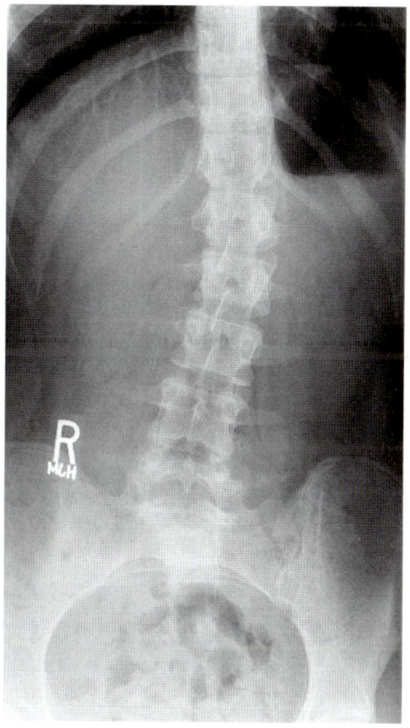

FIGURE 14-9
AP lumbar spine radiograph demonstrating congenital scoliosis.

EXERCISE 18

Practice saying aloud each of the disease and disorder terms built from word parts on pp. 645-647.

To hear the terms, go to http://evolve.elsevier.com. Refer to p. 18 for your Evolve Access Information. Select Exercises & Review, Chapter 14, Chapter Exercises, Pronunciation.

☐ Place a check mark in the box when you have completed this exercise.

EXERCISE FIGURE D

Fill in the blanks to label the diagram.

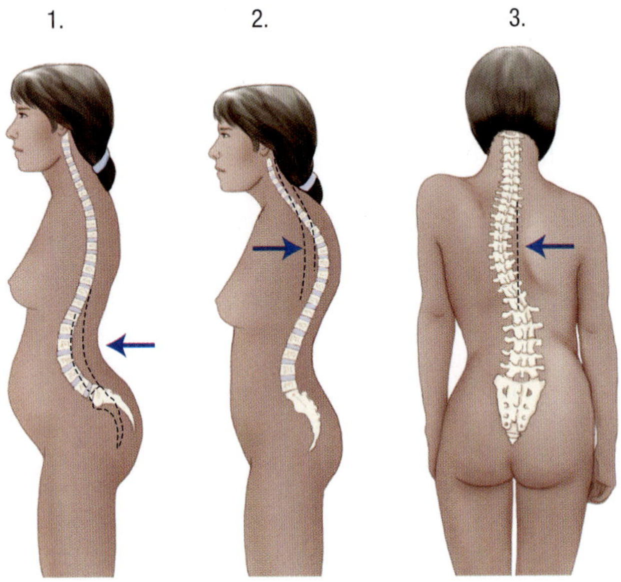

1. ______________ / ______________.
   bent forward / abnormal condition.
2. ______________ / ______________.
   hump / abnormal condition.
3. ______________ / ______________.
   curve (of the spine) / abnormal condition.

EXERCISE 19

Analyze and define the following disease and disorder terms.

1. osteitis ______________
2. osteomyelitis ______________
3. osteopetrosis ______________
4. osteomalacia ______________
5. osteochondritis ______________
6. osteofibroma ______________
7. arthritis ______________

8. rhabdomyolysis ______________________________
9. myeloma ______________________________
10. tendinitis ______________________________
11. osteopenia ______________________________
12. spondylosis ______________________________
13. bursitis ______________________________
14. spondylarthritis ______________________________
15. ankylosis ______________________________
16. kyphosis ______________________________
17. scoliosis ______________________________
18. cranioschisis ______________________________
19. maxillitis ______________________________
20. meniscitis ______________________________
21. rachischisis ______________________________
22. myasthenia ______________________________
23. osteosarcoma ______________________________
24. chondromalacia ______________________________
25. synoviosarcoma ______________________________
26. tenosynovitis ______________________________
27. polymyositis ______________________________
28. diskitis ______________________________
29. lordosis ______________________________
30. osteoarthritis ______________________________
31. fibromyalgia ______________________________
32. sarcopenia ______________________________

EXERCISE 20

Build disease and disorder terms for the following definitions with the word parts you have learned.

1. inflammation of the bone and cartilage ______ / ______ / ______ / ______
   WR / CV / WR / S
2. tumor of the bone and fibrous tissue ______ / ______ / ______ / ______
   WR / CV / WR / S
3. inflammation of a joint ______ / ______
   WR / S
4. dissolution of striated muscle ______ / ______ / ______ / ______ / ______
   WR / CV / WR / CV / S
5. tumor of the bone marrow ______ / ______
   WR / S
6. inflammation of a tendon ______ / ______
   WR / S
7. abnormal condition of the vertebra ______ / ______
   WR / S
8. abnormal reduction of bone mass ______ / ______ / ______
   WR / CV / S
9. inflammation of the bursa ______ / ______
   WR / S
10. inflammation of the vertebral joints ______ / ______ / ______
    WR / WR / S
11. abnormal condition of stiffness ______ / ______
    WR / S
12. abnormal condition of a hump (increased convexity of thoracic spine) ______ / ______
    WR / S
13. abnormal condition of a (lateral) curved (spine) ______ / ______
    WR / S
14. fissure of the skull ______ / ______ / ______
    WR / CV / S
15. inflammation of the maxilla ______ / ______
    WR / S
16. inflammation of the meniscus ______ / ______
    WR / S

17. fissure of the vertebral column
_______ / _______
WR / S

18. muscle weakness
_______ / _______
WR / S

19. inflammation of the bone
_______ / _______
WR / S

20. inflammation of the bone and bone marrow
_______ /CV/ _______ / _______
WR /CV/ WR / S

21. abnormal condition of stonelike bones (marblelike bones)
_______ /CV/ _______ / _______
WR /CV/ WR / S

22. softening of bones
_______ /CV/ _______
WR /CV/ S

23. inflammation of the tendon and synovial membrane
_______ /CV/ _______ / _______
WR /CV/ WR / S

24. malignant tumor of the synovial membrane
_______ /CV/ _______
WR /CV/ S

25. malignant tumor of the bone
_______ /CV/ _______
WR /CV/ S

26. softening of cartilage
_______ /CV/ _______
WR /CV/ S

27. inflammation of an intervertebral disk
_______ / _______
WR / S

28. inflammation of many muscles
_______ / _______ / _______
P / WR / S

29. abnormal condition of bending forward (increased concavity of lumbar spine)
_______ / _______
WR / S

30. inflammation of the bone and joint
_______ /CV/ _______ / _______
WR /CV/ WR / S

31. pain in the fibrous tissues and muscles
_______ /CV/ _______ / _______
WR /CV/ WR / S

32. abnormal reduction of connective tissue
_______ /CV/ _______
WR /CV/ S

EXERCISE 21

Spell each of the disease and disorder terms built from word parts on pp. 645-647 by having someone dictate them to you.

To hear and spell the terms, go to http://evolve.elsevier.com. Refer to p. 18 for your Evolve Access Information. Select Exercises & Review, Chapter 14, Chapter Exercises, Spelling.
☐ Place a check mark in the box if you have completed this exercise online.

1. ______________________
2. ______________________
3. ______________________
4. ______________________
5. ______________________
6. ______________________
7. ______________________
8. ______________________
9. ______________________
10. ______________________
11. ______________________
12. ______________________
13. ______________________
14. ______________________
15. ______________________
16. ______________________
17. ______________________
18. ______________________
19. ______________________
20. ______________________
21. ______________________
22. ______________________
23. ______________________
24. ______________________
25. ______________________
26. ______________________
27. ______________________
28. ______________________
29. ______________________
30. ______________________
31. ______________________
32. ______________________

Disease and Disorder Terms

Not Built from Word Parts

In some of the following terms, you may recognize word parts you have already learned; however, the full meaning of the terms cannot be discerned by the definition of their word parts.

Term	Definition
ankylosing spondylitis (*ang*-ki-LŌ-sing) (*spon*-di-LĪ-tis)	form of arthritis that first affects the spine and adjacent structures and that, as it progresses, causes a forward bend of the spine (also called **Strümpell-Marie arthritis** or **disease,** or **rheumatoid spondylitis**)
bunion (BUN-yun)	abnormal prominence of the joint at the base of the great toe. It is a common problem, often hereditary or caused by poorly fitted shoes (also called **hallux valgus**) (Figure 14-10).
carpal tunnel syndrome (CTS) (KAR-pl) (TUN-el) (SIN-drōm)	a common nerve entrapment disorder of the wrist caused by compression of the median nerve. Symptoms include pain and paresthesia in portions of the hand and fingers (Figure 14-11).
Colles fracture (KOL-ēz) (FRAK-chur)	a type of wrist fracture. The fracture is at the distal end of the radius, the distal fragment being displaced backward. (Figure 14-12 and Figure 14-20, p. 668)
exostosis (*ek*-sos-TŌ-sis)	abnormal benign growth on the surface of a bone (also called **spur**)
fracture (fx) (FRAK-chūr)	broken bone (Figure 14-12)

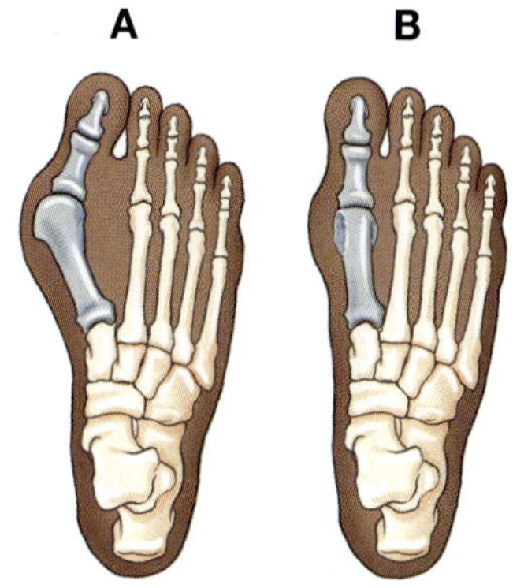

FIGURE 14-10
A, Bunion. **B,** Following a bunionectomy.

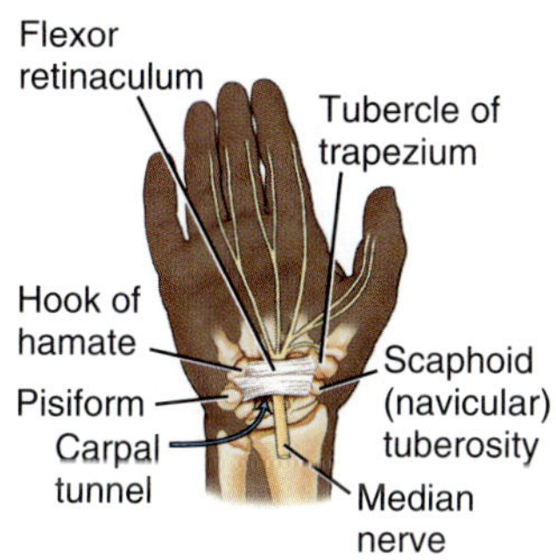

FIGURE 14-11
Structures involved with **carpal tunnel syndrome**, which is caused by compression of the median nerve. **Palmar uniportal endoscopic carpal tunnel release,** also called **Mirza,** is used surgically to treat this condition.

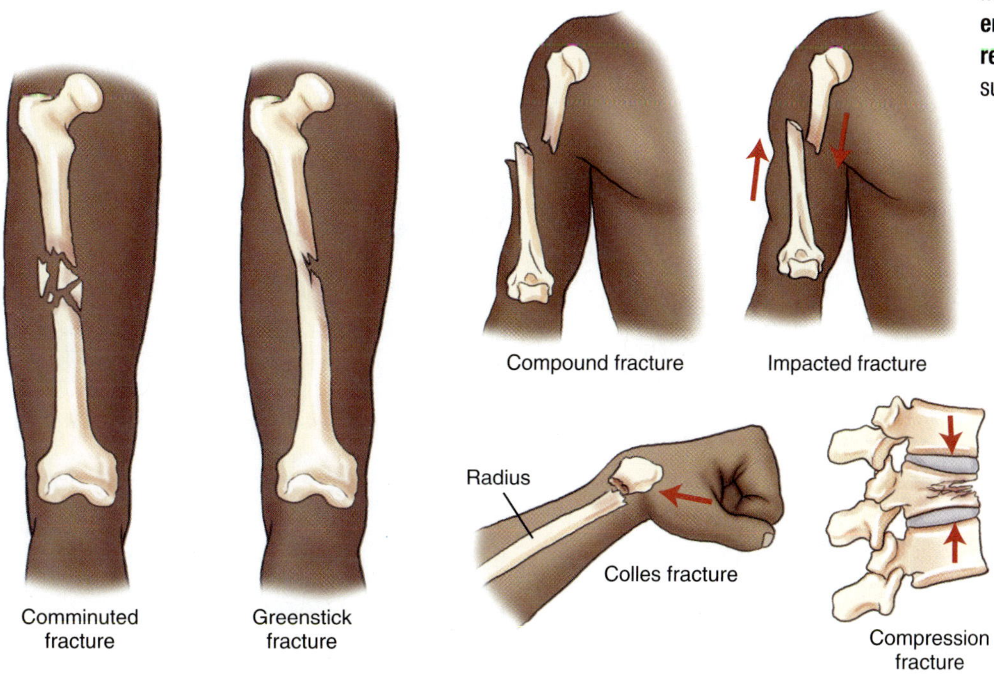

FIGURE 14-12
Types of fractures.

Disease and Disorder Terms—*cont'd*

Not Built from Word Parts

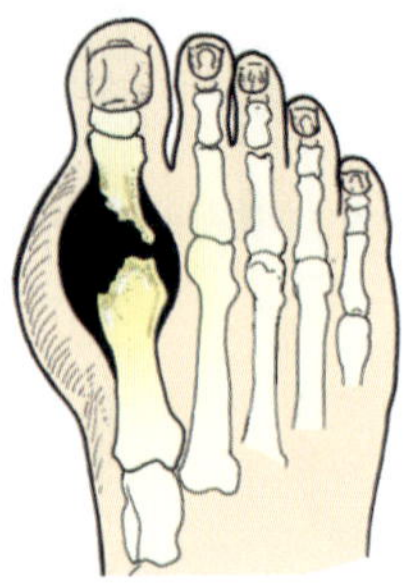

FIGURE 14-13
Gout.

Term	Definition
gout (gowt)	disease in which an excessive amount of uric acid in the blood causes sodium urate crystals (**tophi**) to be deposited in the joints, especially that of the great toe, producing arthritis (Figure 14-13)
herniated disk (HER-nē-*āt*-ed) (disk)	rupture of the intervertebral disk cartilage, which allows the contents to protrude through it, putting pressure on the spinal nerve roots (also called **slipped disk, ruptured disk, herniated intervertebral disk,** or **herniated nucleus pulposus [HNP]**) (Figure 14-14)
Lyme disease (līm) (di-ZĒZ)	an infection caused by a bacteria *(Borrelia burgdorferi)* carried by deer ticks and transmitted to humans by the bite of an infected tick. Symptoms, caused by the body's immune response to the bacteria, vary and may include a rash at the site of the tick bite and flulike symptoms such as fever, headache, joint pain, and fatigue. Lyme disease was first reported in Lyme, Conn., in 1975. The primary treatment is antibiotics. Left untreated, Lyme disease can mimic several musculoskeletal diseases mentioned in this chapter (Figure 14-15).

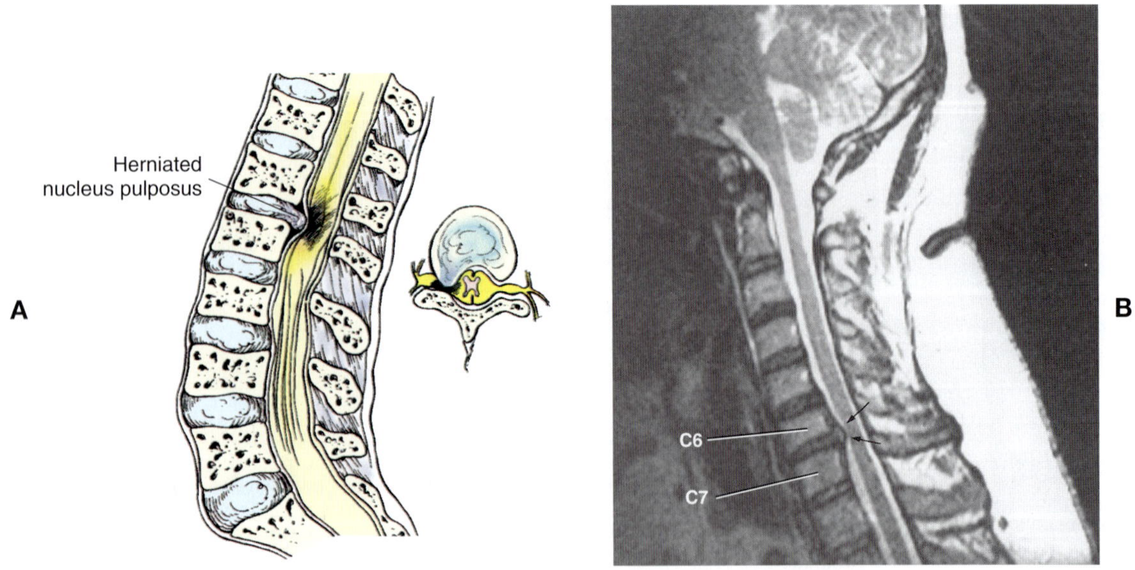

FIGURE 14-14
A, Herniated disk. **B,** MRI image of cervical spine, demonstrating herniated disk between C6 and C7.

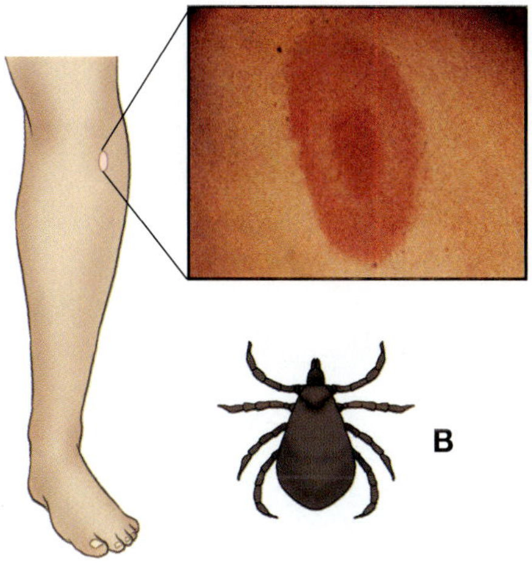

FIGURE 14-15
A, Target lesion of Lyme disease. **B,** Tick that causes Lyme disease.

Term	Definition
muscular dystrophy (MD) (MUS-kū-lar) (DIS-tro-fē)	group of hereditary diseases characterized by degeneration of muscle and weakness
myasthenia gravis (MG) (*mī*-as-THĒ-nē-a) (GRA-vis)	chronic disease characterized by muscle weakness and thought to be caused by a defect in the transmission of impulses from nerve to muscle cell. The face, larynx, and throat are frequently affected; no true paralysis of the muscles exists.
osteoporosis (*os*-tē-ō-po-RŌ-sis)	abnormal loss of bone density that may lead to an increase in fractures of the ribs, thoracic and lumbar vertebrae, hips, and wrists after slight trauma (occurs predominantly in postmenopausal women) (Figure 14-16)
rheumatoid arthritis (RA) (RŪ-ma-toid) (ar-THRĪ-tis)	a chronic systemic disease characterized by autoimmune inflammatory changes in the connective tissue throughout the body (see Figure 14-8)
spinal stenosis (SPĪ-nal) (ste-NŌ-sis)	narrowing of the spinal canal with compression of nerve roots. The condition is either congenital or due to spinal degeneration. Symptoms are pain radiating to the thigh or lower legs and numbness or tingling in the lower extremities (Figure 14-17).
spondylolisthesis (*spon*-di-lō-lis-THĒ-sis)	forward slipping of one vertebra over another (Figure 14-17)

REPETITIVE MOTION SYNDROME

is an increasingly common and somewhat controversial diagnosis in which pain develops in the hand and forearm in the course of normal work activities. Permanent injury is not common. This condition is also referred to as **repetitive strain syndrome.**

EXERCISE 22

Practice saying aloud each of the disease and disorder terms not built from word parts on pp. 653-655.

To hear the terms, go to http://evolve.elsevier.com. Refer to p. 18 for your Evolve Access Information. Select Exercises & Review, Chapter 14, Chapter Exercises, Pronunciation.

☐ Place a check mark in the box when you have completed this exercise.

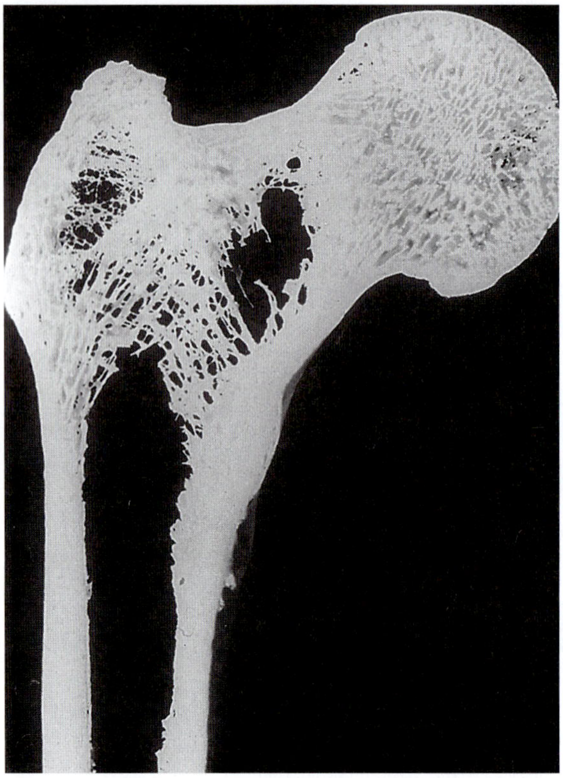

FIGURE 14-16
This thin section of the femur shows the loss of bone seen in patients with osteoporosis. Fractures can occur from slight trauma because the bone is porous and brittle.

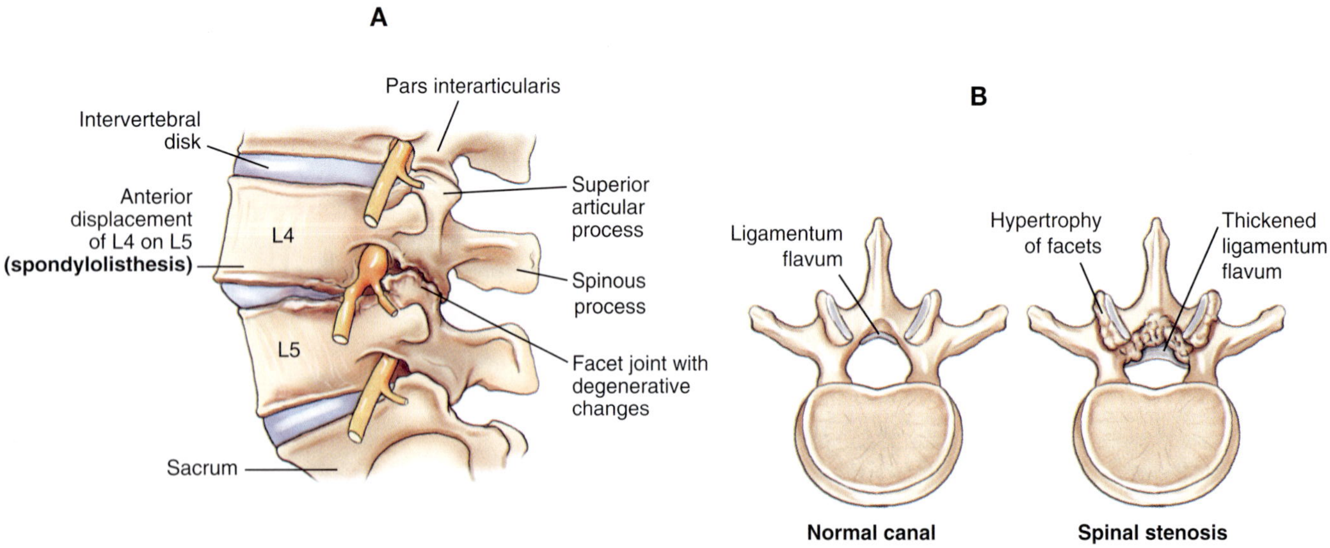

FIGURE 14-17
A, Spondylolisthesis showing degenerative changes in the disk and joint. **B,** Normal canal compared with spinal stenosis. Spondylolisthesis may occur with or without spinal stenosis.

EXERCISE 23

Write the term for each of the following definitions.

1. abnormal benign growth on the surface of a bone ____________________
2. group of hereditary diseases characterized by degeneration of muscle and weakness __________ __________
3. chronic disease characterized by muscle weakness and thought to be caused by a defect in the transmission of impulses from nerve to muscle cell __________ __________
4. abnormal prominence of the joint at the base of the great toe ____________________
5. form of arthritis that first affects the spine and adjacent structures __________ __________
6. disease in which an excessive amount of uric acid in the blood causes sodium urate crystals (tophi) to be deposited in the joints ____________________
7. rupture of the intervertebral disk cartilage, which allows the contents to protrude through it, putting pressure on the spinal nerve roots __________ __________
8. broken bone ____________________
9. abnormal loss of bone density ____________________

10. a disorder of the wrist caused by compression of the median nerve ____________ ____________ ____________
11. a type of fractured wrist ____________ ____________
12. form of arthritis characterized by inflammatory changes in the connective tissue throughout the body ____________ ____________
13. forward slipping of one vertebra over another ________________________
14. an infection transmitted to humans by a deer tick ____________ ____________
15. narrowing of the spinal column with compression of nerve roots ____________ ____________

EXERCISE 24

Write the definitions of the following terms.

1. exostosis ________________________
2. muscular dystrophy ________________________
3. myasthenia gravis ________________________
4. bunion ________________________
5. ankylosing spondylitis ________________________
6. osteoporosis ________________________
7. gout ________________________
8. herniated disk ________________________
9. fracture ________________________
10. carpal tunnel syndrome ________________________
11. Colles fracture ________________________
12. rheumatoid arthritis ________________________
13. Lyme disease ________________________
14. spondylolisthesis________________________
15. spinal stenosis ________________________

ANKYLOSING SPONDYLITIS

was first described in 1884 by Adolf von Strümpell (1853–1925). It became known as **Strümpell-Marie disease** after von Strümpell and French physician Pierre Marie.

COLLES FRACTURE

was first described in 1814 by Irish surgeon and anatomist **Abraham Colles** (1773–1843). In 1804 Colles was appointed Professor of Anatomy and Surgery at the Irish College of Surgeons.

EXERCISE 25

Spell each of the disease and disorder terms not built from word parts on pp. 653-655 by having someone dictate them to you.

To hear and spell the terms, go to http://evolve.elsevier.com. Refer to p. 18 for your Evolve Access Information. Select Exercises & Review, Chapter 14, Chapter Exercises, Spelling.
☐ Place a check mark in the box if you have completed this exercise online.

1. ______________________
2. ______________________
3. ______________________
4. ______________________
5. ______________________
6. ______________________
7. ______________________
8. ______________________
9. ______________________
10. ______________________
11. ______________________
12. ______________________
13. ______________________
14. ______________________
15. ______________________

Surgical Terms

Built from Word Parts

The following terms are built from word parts you have already learned and can be translated literally to find their meanings. Further explanation of terms beyond the definition of their word parts, if needed, is included in parentheses.

Term	Definition
aponeurorrhaphy (*ap*-ō-nū-ROR-a-fē)	suture of an aponeurosis
arthrocentesis (*ar*-thrō-sen-TĒ-sis)	surgical puncture of a joint to aspirate fluid
arthroclasia (*ar*-thrō-KLĀ-zha)	(surgical) breaking of a (stiff) joint
arthrodesis (*ar*-thrō-DĒ-sis)	surgical fixation of a joint (also called **joint fusion**)
arthroplasty (AR-thrō-*plas*-tē)	surgical repair of a joint (Table 14-1)
bursectomy (bur-SEK-to-mē)	excision of a bursa
carpectomy (kar-PEK-to-mē)	excision of a carpal bone
chondrectomy (kon-DREK-to-mē)	excision of a cartilage

TABLE 14-1

Types of Arthroplasty

Total hip replacement arthroplasty (THA) is indicated for degenerative joint disease or rheumatoid arthritis. The operation commonly involves replacement of the hip joint with a metallic femoral head and a plastic-coated acetabulum.

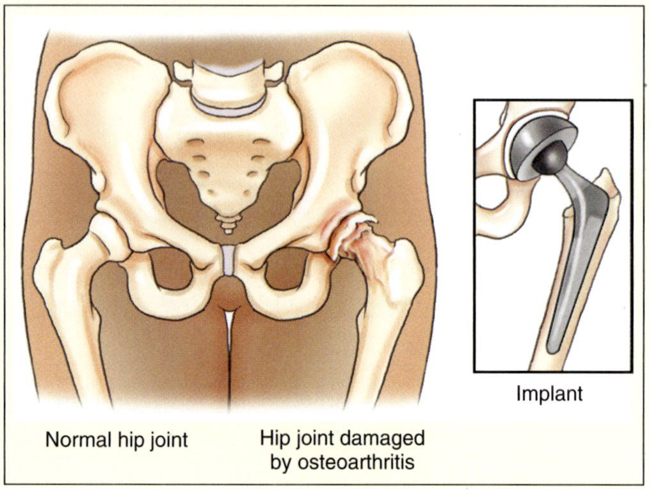

Birmingham hip resurfacing is a procedure that provides an option for younger, active patients needing a total hip arthroplasty. The procedure requires the removal of a few millimeters of bone from the femoral head instead of the removal of the entire femoral head required in total hip arthroplasty. A metal cap is then placed on top of the femur, and smooth metal is placed in the acetabulum.

Total knee joint replacement arthroplasty (TKA) is designed to replace worn surfaces of the knee joint. Various prostheses are used.

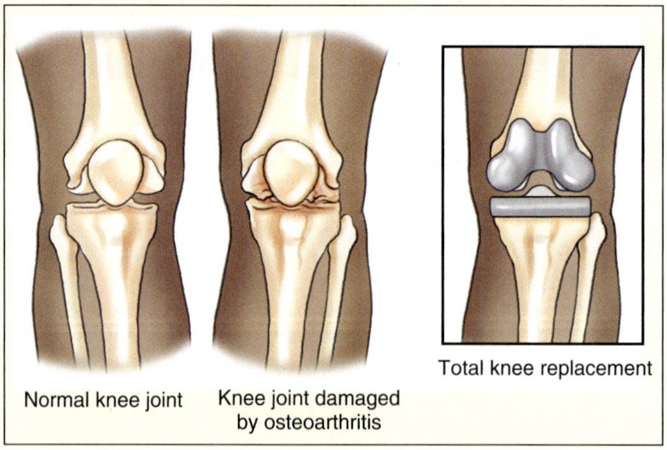

Metatarsal arthroplasty is used to treat deformities associated with rheumatoid arthritis or hallux valgus and to treat painful or unstable joints.

Surgical Terms—*cont'd*

Built from Word Parts

Term	Definition
chondroplasty (KON-drō-*plas*-tē)	surgical repair of a cartilage
costectomy (kos-TEK-to-mē)	excision of a rib
cranioplasty (KRĀ-nē-ō-*plas*-tē)	surgical repair of the skull
craniotomy (*krā*-nē-OT-o-mē)	incision of the skull (as for surgery of the brain)
diskectomy (dis-KEK-to-mē)	excision of an intervertebral disk (a portion of the disk is removed to relieve pressure on nerve roots) (also spelled **discectomy**) (Figure 14-18)
laminectomy (*lam*-i-NEK-to-mē)	excision of a lamina (often performed to relieve pressure on the nerve roots in the lower spine caused by a herniated disk and other conditions)
maxillectomy (*mak*-si-LEK-to-mē)	excision of the maxilla
meniscectomy (*men*-i-SEK-to-mē)	excision of the meniscus (performed for a torn cartilage)
myorrhaphy (mī-OR-a-fē)	suture of a muscle
ostectomy (os-TEK-to-mē) (NOTE: the *e* is dropped from oste.)	excision of bone
osteoclasis (*os*-tē-OK-la-sis)	(surgical) breaking of a bone (to correct a deformity)
patellectomy (*pat*-e-LEK-to-mē)	excision of the patella
phalangectomy (*fal*-an-JEK-to-mē)	excision of a finger or toe bone
rachiotomy (*rā*-kē-OT-o-mē)	incision into the vertebral column
spondylosyndesis (*spon*-di-lō-sin-DĒ-sis) (NOTE: the prefix *syn*-appears in the middle of the term.)	fusing together of the vertebrae (also called **spinal fusion**)
synovectomy (*sin*-ō-VEK-to-mē) (NOTE: the *i* in *synovi* is dropped because the suffix begins with a vowel.)	excision of the synovial membrane (of a joint)
tarsectomy (tar-SEK-to-mē)	excision of (one or more) tarsal bones

MICROENDOSCOPIC DISKECTOMY (MED)

is a minimally-invasive procedure that uses a fluoroscope and special dilating instrumentation to create a small tunnel to the affected disk area. An endoscopic tool allows the surgeon to visualize and remove the thick, sticky nucleus of the herniated disk. The disk then softens and contracts, relieving severe low back and leg pain. Recovery time is significantly quicker than open diskectomy because of a small incision and less trauma to surrounding tissues.

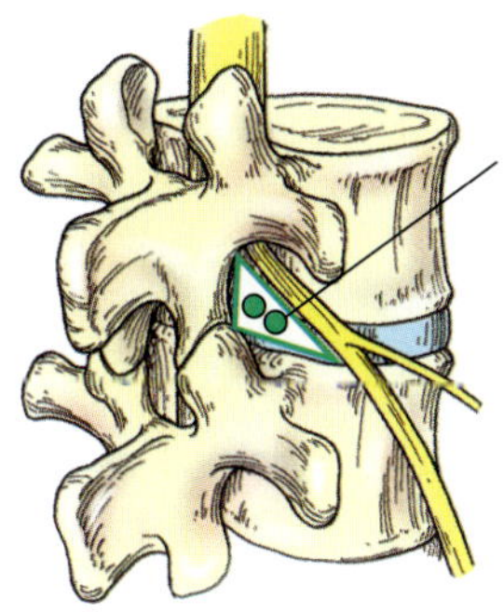

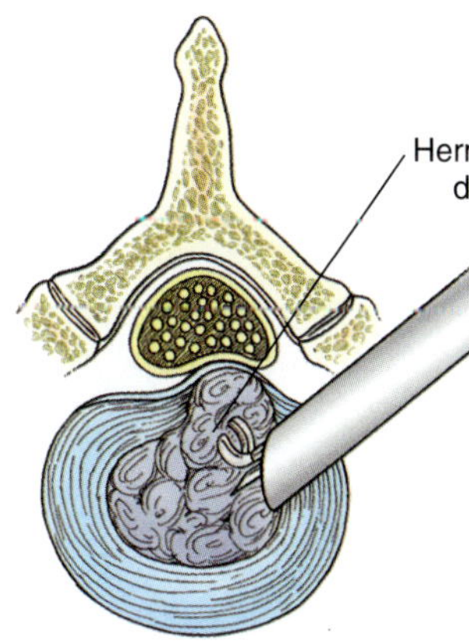

FIGURE 14-18
Microendoscopic diskectomy.

Surgical Terms—*cont'd*

Built from Word Parts

Term	Definition
tenomyoplasty (*ten*-ō-MĪ-ō-*plas*-tē)	surgical repair of the tendon and muscle
tenorrhaphy (ten-NOR-a-fē)	suture of a tendon
vertebroplasty (VER-te-brō-*plas*-tē)	surgical repair of the vertebra (Table 14-2)

TABLE 14-2

Procedures for Treatment of Compression Fractures Caused by Osteoporosis

Percutaneous vertebroplasty (PV) is a minimally invasive operation in which an interventional radiologist places a needle through the skin into the damaged vertebra. A special liquid cement called polymethylmethacrylate is injected into the area through the needle to fill the holes left by osteoporosis. The liquid takes 20 minutes to harden, sealing and stabilizing the fracture and relieving pain. Vertebroplasties were first performed in 1984 and are currently being performed in select health care centers in the United States.

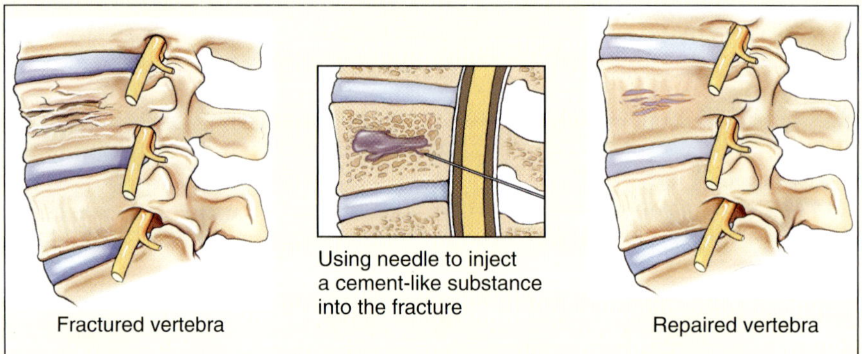

Percutaneous vertebroplasty

Kyphoplasty was approved in 1998 by the Food and Drug Administration. Kyphoplasty is similar to vertebroplasty except a balloonlike device is used to expand the compressed vertebra before the cement is injected.

EXERCISE 26

Practice saying aloud each of the surgical terms built from word parts on pp. 659-662.

To hear the terms, go to http://evolve.elsevier.com. Refer to p. 18 for your Evolve Access Information. Select Exercises & Review, Chapter 14, Chapter Exercises, Pronunciation.

☐ Place a check mark in the box when you have completed this exercise.

EXERCISE 27

Analyze and define the following surgical terms.

1. osteoclasis ______
2. ostectomy ______
3. arthroclasia ______
4. arthrodesis ______
5. arthroplasty ______
6. chondrectomy ______
7. chondroplasty ______
8. myorrhaphy ______
9. tenomyoplasty ______
10. tenorrhaphy ______
11. costectomy ______
12. patellectomy ______
13. aponeurorrhaphy ______
14. carpectomy ______
15. phalangectomy ______
16. meniscectomy ______
17. spondylosyndesis ______
18. laminectomy ______
19. bursectomy ______
20. craniotomy ______
21. cranioplasty ______
22. maxillectomy ______
23. rachiotomy ______
24. tarsectomy ______
25. synovectomy ______
26. diskectomy ______
27. vertebroplasty ______
28. arthrocentesis ______

EXERCISE 28

Build surgical terms for the following definitions by using the word parts you have learned.

1. (surgical) breaking of a bone (to correct a deformity) ________ WR / CV / S
2. excision of bone ________ WR / S
3. (surgical) breaking of a (stiff) joint ________ WR / CV / S
4. surgical fixation of a joint ________ WR / CV / S
5. surgical repair of a joint ________ WR / CV / S
6. excision of cartilage ________ WR / S
7. surgical repair of cartilage ________ WR / CV / S
8. suture of a muscle ________ WR / CV / S
9. surgical repair of a tendon and muscle ________ WR / CV / WR / CV / S
10. suture of a tendon ________ WR / CV / S
11. excision of a rib ________ WR / S
12. excision of the patella ________ WR / S
13. suture of an aponeurosis ________ WR / CV / S
14. excision of a carpal bone ________ WR / S

15. excision of a finger or toe bone

_______ / _______
WR / S

16. excision of a meniscus

_______ / _______
WR / S

17. fusing together of the vertebrae

_______ /CV/ _______ / _______
WR /CV/ P / S

18. excision of a lamina

_______ / _______
WR / S

19. excision of a bursa

_______ / _______
WR / S

20. incision of the skull

_______ /CV/ _______
WR /CV/ S

21. surgical repair of the skull

_______ /CV/ _______
WR /CV/ S

22. excision of the maxilla

_______ / _______
WR / S

23. incision of the vertebral column

_______ /CV/ _______
WR /CV/ S

24. excision of (one or more) tarsal bones

_______ / _______
WR / S

25. excision of the synovial membrane

_______ / _______
WR / S

26. excision of an intervertebral disk

_______ / _______
WR / S

27. surgical repair of the vertebra

_______ /CV/ _______
WR /CV/ S

28. surgical puncture of a joint to aspirate fluid

_______ /CV/ _______
WR /CV/ S

EXERCISE 29

Spell each of the surgical terms built from word parts on pp. 659-662 by having someone dictate them to you.

To hear and spell the terms, go to http://evolve.elsevier.com. Refer to p. 18 for your Evolve Access Information. Select Exercises & Review, Chapter 14, Chapter Exercises, Spelling.
☐ Place a check mark in the box if you have completed this exercise online.

1.	______	15.	______
2.	______	16.	______
3.	______	17.	______
4.	______	18.	______
5.	______	19.	______
6.	______	20.	______
7.	______	21.	______
8.	______	22.	______
9.	______	23.	______
10.	______	24.	______
11.	______	25.	______
12.	______	26.	______
13.	______	27.	______
14.	______	28.	______

Diagnostic Terms

Built from Word Parts

The following terms are built from word parts you have already learned and can be translated literally to find their meanings. Further explanation of terms beyond the definition of their word parts, if needed, is included in parentheses.

Term	Definition
DIAGNOSTIC IMAGING	
arthrography (ar-THROG-ra-fē)	radiographic imaging of a joint (with contrast media). (Magnetic resonance imaging [MRI] has mostly replaced arthrography as the imaging technique for diarthrodial [movable] joints such as the knee, wrist, hip, and shoulder. Arthrography is still used for specialized functions such as when metal is present in the body.)

Term	Definition
ENDOSCOPY	
arthroscopy (ar-THROS-ko-pē)	visual examination of a joint (used for a diarthrodial [movable] joint) (Exercise Figure E)
OTHER	
electromyogram (EMG) (ē-*lek*-trō-MĪ-ō-gram)	record of the (intrinsic) electrical activity in a (skeletal) muscle (Figure 14-19)

EXERCISE FIGURE E

Fill in the blanks to complete labeling of the diagram.

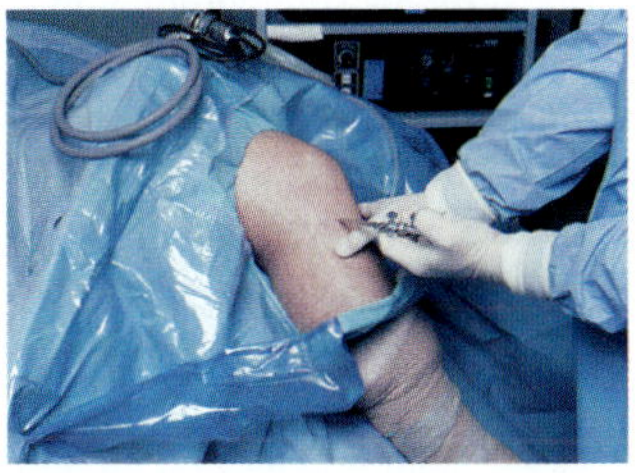

_____ / _____ / _____
joint / cv / visual examination

of the knee performed for diagnostic purposes or for surgical repair of ligaments or meniscus.

EXERCISE 30

Practice saying aloud each of the diagnostic terms built from word parts on these two pages.

To hear the terms, go to http://evolve.elsevier.com. Refer to p. 18 for your Evolve Access Information. Select Exercises & Review, Chapter 14, Chapter Exercises, Pronunciation.

☐ Place a check mark in the box when you have completed this exercise.

EXERCISE 31

Analyze and define the following diagnostic terms.

1. electromyogram _____
2. arthrography _____
3. arthroscopy _____

EXERCISE 32

Build diagnostic terms for the following definitions using word parts you have learned.

1. radiographic imaging of a joint _____ / _____ / _____
WR / CV / S
2. visual examination of a joint _____ / _____ / _____
WR / CV / S
3. record of the electrical activity of a muscle _____ / _____ / _____ / _____ / _____
WR / CV / WR / CV / S

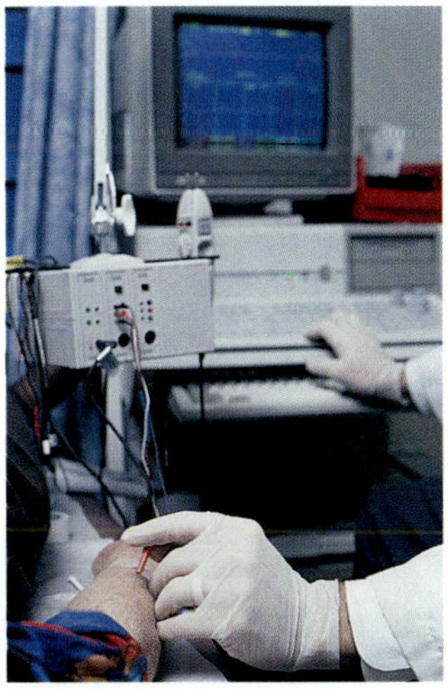

FIGURE 14-19
Patient having an electromyogram (EMG) of the forearm.

TABLE 14-3

Diagnostic imaging Procedures Used for the Musculoskeletal System

The following diagnostic imaging procedures are commonly used for diagnosing diseases, fractures, strains, and other conditions of the musculoskeletal system.

Radiography (radiographic imaging) of the bones and joints is used to identify fractures or tumors, monitor healing, or identify abnormal structures (Figure 14-20).

Computed tomography (CT) of the bones and joints gives accurate definition of bone structure and demonstrates subtle changes such as linear fractures (Figure 14-21).

Magnetic resonance imaging (MRI) is used to evaluate the soft tissue of the knee, spinal stenosis, spinal cord defects, and degenerative disk changes (Figure 14-22).

Bone scan (nuclear medicine test) is used to detect the presence of metastatic disease of the bone and to monitor degenerative bone disease (Figure 14-23).

Single-photon emission computed tomography (SPECT) of the bone is an even more sensitive nuclear method for detecting bone abnormalities.

Bone densitometry is a method of determining the density of bone by radiographic techniques used to diagnose osteoporosis. **DEXA (dual-energy X-ray absorptiometry)** is commonly used for this test.

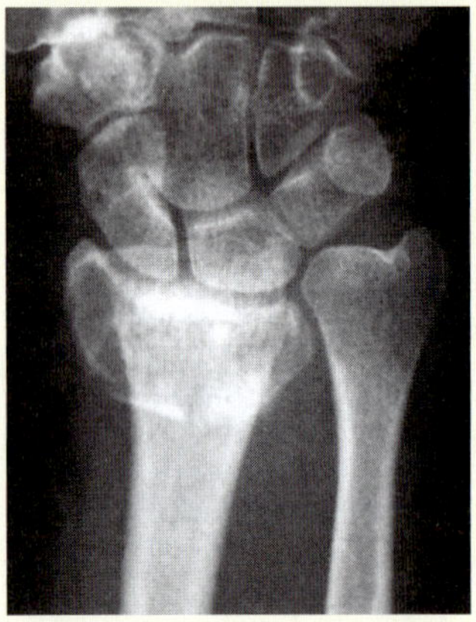

FIGURE 14-20
Radiograph showing a Colles fracture.

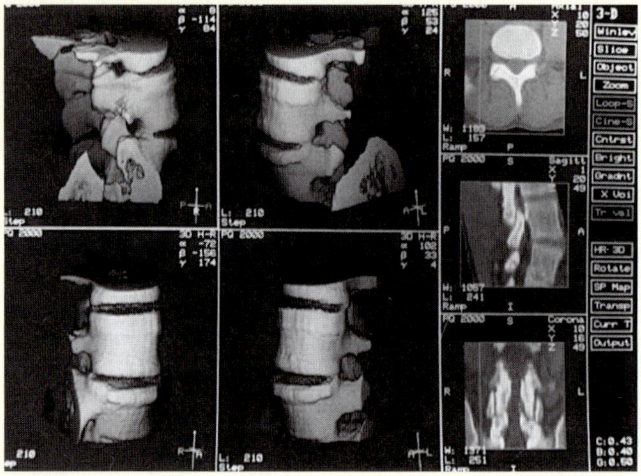

FIGURE 14-21
CT scan showing three-dimensional reconstruction images of the lumbar spine.

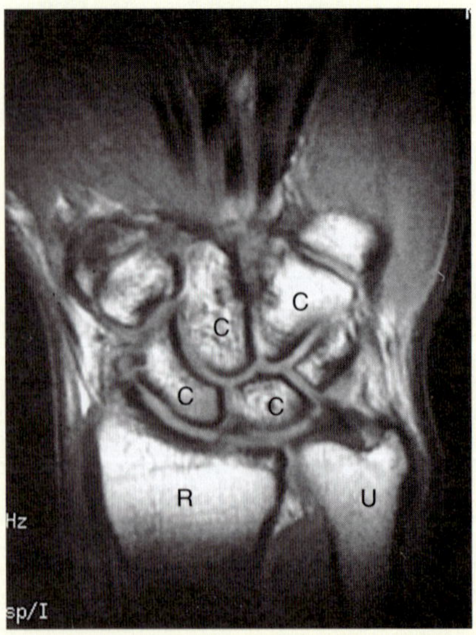

FIGURE 14-22
Coronal MRI of the wrist. Marrow within the carpal bones *(C)*, radius *(R)*, and ulna *(U)*.

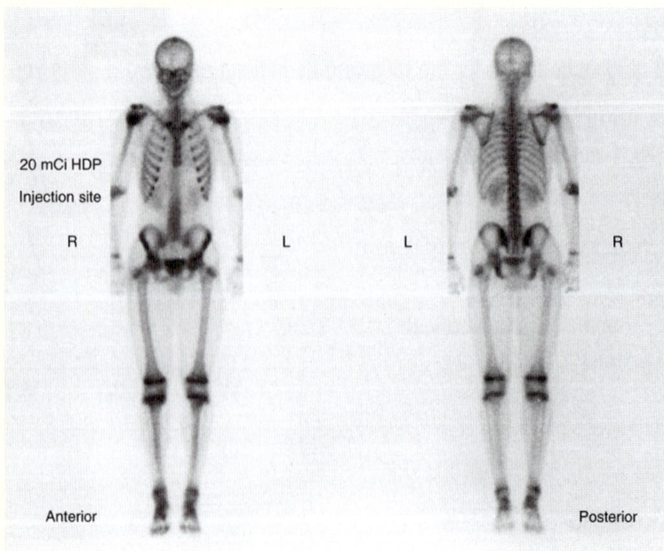

FIGURE 14-23
Whole-body nuclear medicine bone scan.

EXERCISE 33

Spell each of the diagnostic terms built from word parts on pp. 666-667 by having someone dictate them to you.

To hear and spell the terms, go to http://evolve.elsevier.com. Refer to p. 18 for your Evolve Access Information. Select Exercises & Review, Chapter 14, Chapter Exercises, Spelling.
☐ Place a check mark in the box if you have completed this exercise online.

1. ______________________ 3. ______________________
2. ______________________

Complementary Terms

Built from Word Parts

The following terms are built from word parts you have already learned and can be translated literally to find their meanings. Further explanation of terms beyond the definition of their word parts, if needed, is included in parentheses.

Term	Definition
arthralgia (ar-THRAL-ja)	pain in the joint
atrophy (AT-ro-fē)	without development (wasting)
bradykinesia (*brad*-ē-ki-NĒ-zha)	slow movement
carpal (CAR-pal)	pertaining to the wrist
clavicular (kla-VIK-ū-lar)	pertaining to the clavicle
cranial (KRĀ-nē-al)	pertaining to the cranium
dyskinesia (*dis*-ki-NĒ-zha)	difficult movement
dystrophy (DIS-tro-fē)	abnormal development
femoral (FEM-or-al)	pertaining to the femur
humeral (HŪ-mer-al)	pertaining to the humerus
hyperkinesia (*hī*-per-ki-NĒ-zha)	excessive movement (overactive)
hypertrophy (hī-PER-tro-fē)	excessive development
iliofemoral (*il*-ē-ō-FEM-or-al)	pertaining to the ilium and femur

Complementary Terms—*cont'd*

Built from Word Parts

Term	Definition
intercostal (*in*-ter-KOS-tal)	pertaining to between the ribs
intervertebral (*in*-ter-VER-te-bral)	pertaining to between the vertebrae
intracranial (*in*-tra-KRĀ-nē-al)	pertaining to within the cranium
ischiofibular (*is*-kē-ō-FIB-ū-lar)	pertaining to the ischium and fibula
ischiopubic (*is*-kē-ō-PŪ-bik)	pertaining to the ischium and pubis
lumbar (LUM-bar)	pertaining to the loins (the part of the back between the thorax and pelvis)
lumbocostal (*lum*-bō-KOS-tal)	pertaining to the loins and the ribs
lumbosacral (*lum*-bō-SĀ-kral)	pertaining to the lumbar regions (loin) and the sacrum
osteoblast (OS-tē-ō-*blast*)	developing bone cell
osteocyte (OS-tē-ō-*sīt*)	bone cell
osteonecrosis (*os*-tē-ō-ne-KRŌ-sis)	abnormal death of bone (tissues)
pelvic (PEL-vik)	pertaining to the pelvis
pelvisacral (*pel*-vi-SĀ-kral)	pertaining to the pelvis and the sacrum
pubic (PŪ-bik)	pertaining to the pubis
pubofemoral (*pū*-bō-FEM-or-al)	pertaining to the pubis and femur
radial (RĀ-dē-al)	pertaining to the radius
sacral (SĀ-kral)	pertaining to the sacrum
sternoclavicular (*ster*-nō-kla-VIK-ū-lar)	pertaining to the sternum and clavicle
sternoid (STER-noyd)	resembling the sternum
subcostal (sub-KOS-tal)	pertaining to below the rib
submandibular (*sub*-man-DIB-ū-lar)	pertaining to below the mandible

Term	Definition
submaxillary (sub-MAK-si-*lar*-ē)	pertaining to below the maxilla
subscapular (sub-SKAP-ū-lar)	pertaining to below the scapula
substernal (sub-STER-nal)	pertaining to below the sternum
suprapatellar (*sū*-pra-pa-TEL-ar)	pertaining to above the patella
suprascapular (*sū*-pra-SKAP-ū-lar)	pertaining to above the scapula
symphysis (SIM-fi-sis)	growing together (as in symphysis pubis)
tibial (TIB-ē-al)	pertaining to the tibia
ulnoradial (ul-nō-RĀ-dē-al)	pertaining to the ulna and radius
vertebrocostal (*ver*-te-brō-KOS-tal)	pertaining to the vertebrae and ribs

EXERCISE 34

Practice saying aloud each of the complementary terms built from word parts on pp. 669-671.

To hear the terms, go to http://evolve.elsevier.com. Refer to p. 18 for your Evolve Access Information. Select Exercises & Review, Chapter 14, Chapter Exercises, Pronunciation.

☐ Place a check mark in the box when you have completed this exercise.

EXERCISE 35

Analyze and define the following complementary terms.

1. symphysis ____________________
2. femoral ____________________
3. humeral ____________________
4. intervertebral ____________________
5. hyperkinesia ____________________
6. dyskinesia ____________________
7. bradykinesia ____________________
8. intracranial ____________________
9. sternoclavicular ____________________
10. iliofemoral ____________________

11. ischiofibular ______________________
12. submaxillary ______________________
13. ischiopubic ______________________
14. submandibular ______________________
15. pubofemoral ______________________
16. suprascapular ______________________
17. subcostal ______________________
18. vertebrocostal ______________________
19. subscapular ______________________
20. osteoblast ______________________
21. osteocyte ______________________
22. osteonecrosis ______________________
23. sternoid ______________________
24. arthralgia ______________________
25. carpal ______________________
26. lumbar ______________________
27. lumbocostal ______________________
28. lumbosacral ______________________
29. sacral ______________________
30. pubic ______________________
31. substernal ______________________
32. suprapatellar ______________________
33. dystrophy ______________________
34. atrophy ______________________
35. hypertrophy ______________________
36. intercostal ______________________
37. cranial ______________________
38. pelvic ______________________
39. pelvisacral ______________________
40. clavicular ______________________
41. tibial ______________________
42. radial ______________________
43. ulnoradial ______________________

EXERCISE 36

Build the complementary terms for the following definitions by using the word parts you have learned.

1. growing together ______ P / ______ S(WR)
2. pertaining to the femur ______ WR / ______ S
3. pertaining to the humerus ______ WR / ______ S
4. pertaining to between the vertebrae ______ P / ______ WR / ______ S
5. excessive movement (overactivity) ______ P / ______ WR / ______ S
6. difficult movement ______ P / ______ WR / ______ S
7. slow movement ______ P / ______ WR / ______ S
8. pertaining to within the cranium ______ P / ______ WR / ______ S
9. pertaining to the sternum and clavicle ______ WR / CV / ______ WR / ______ S
10. pertaining to the ilium and femur ______ WR / CV / ______ WR / ______ S
11. pertaining to the ischium and fibula ______ WR / CV / ______ WR / ______ S
12. pertaining to below the maxilla ______ P / ______ WR / ______ S
13. pertaining to the ischium and pubis ______ WR / CV / ______ WR / ______ S
14. pertaining to below the mandible ______ P / ______ WR / ______ S
15. pertaining to the pubis and femur ______ WR / CV / ______ WR / ______ S
16. pertaining to above the scapula ______ P / ______ WR / ______ S

17. pertaining to below the rib ______ P / ______ WR / ______ S

18. pertaining to the vertebrae and ribs ______ WR / CV / ______ WR / ______ S

19. pertaining to below the scapula ______ P / ______ WR / ______ S

20. developing bone cell ______ WR / CV / ______ WR

21. bone cell ______ WR / CV / ______ S

22. abnormal death of bone (tissues) ______ WR / CV / ______ WR / ______ S

23. resembling the sternum ______ WR / ______ S

24. pain in the joint ______ WR / ______ S

25. pertaining to the wrist ______ WR / ______ S

26. pertaining to the sacrum ______ WR / ______ S

27. pertaining to the loins ______ WR / ______ S

28. pertaining to the pubis ______ WR / ______ S

29. pertaining to the lumbar region (loin) and the sacrum ______ WR / CV / ______ WR / ______ S

30. pertaining to the loins and ribs ______ WR / CV / ______ WR / ______ S

31. pertaining to below the sternum ______ P / ______ WR / ______ S

32. pertaining to above the patella ______ P / ______ WR / ______ S

33. abnormal development ______ P / ______ S(WR)

34. without development ______ P / ______ S(WR)

35. excessive development ______ P / ______ S(WR)

36. pertaining to the cranium ______ WR / ______ S

37. pertaining to between the ribs ______ P / ______ WR / ______ S

38. pertaining to the pelvis ______ WR / ______ S

39. pertaining to the pelvis and sacrum ______ WR / CV / ______ WR / ______ S

40. pertaining to the clavicle ______ WR / ______ S

41. pertaining to the tibia ______ WR / ______ S

42. pertaining to the radius ______ WR / ______ S

43. pertaining to the ulua and radius ______ WR / CV / ______ WR / ______ S

EXERCISE 37

Spell each of the complementary terms built from word parts on pp. 669-671 by having someone dictate them to you.

To hear and spell the terms, go to http://evolve.elsevier.com. Refer to p. 18 for your Evolve Access Information. Select Exercises & Review, Chapter 14, Chapter Exercises, Spelling.
☐ Place a check mark in the box if you have completed this exercise online.

1. ______	15. ______
2. ______	16. ______
3. ______	17. ______
4. ______	18. ______
5. ______	19. ______
6. ______	20. ______
7. ______	21. ______
8. ______	22. ______
9. ______	23. ______
10. ______	24. ______
11. ______	25. ______
12. ______	26. ______
13. ______	27. ______
14. ______	28. ______

29. ______________________
30. ______________________
31. ______________________
32. ______________________
33. ______________________
34. ______________________
35. ______________________
36. ______________________
37. ______________________
38. ______________________
39. ______________________
40. ______________________
41. ______________________
42. ______________________
43. ______________________

Complementary Terms

Not Built from Word Parts

In some of the following terms, you may recognize word parts you have already learned; however, the full meaning of the terms cannot be discerned by the definition of their word parts.

Term	Definition
chiropodist, podiatrist (kī-ROP-o-dist) (pō-DĪ-a-trist)	specialist in treating and diagnosing diseases and disorders of the foot, including medical and surgical treatment
chiropractic (*kī*-rō-PRAK-tik)	system of treatment that consists of manipulation of the vertebral column
chiropractor (KĪ-rō-*prak*-tor)	specialist in chiropractic
crepitus (KREP-i-tus)	the crackling sound heard when two bones rub against each other or grating caused by the rubbing together of dry surfaces of a joint. (Crepitus is also used to describe the crackling sound heard with pneumonia or the sound heard from the discharge of gas from the bowel.) (also called **crepitation**)
orthopedics (ortho) (*or*-thō-PĒ-diks)	branch of medicine dealing with the study and treatment of diseases and abnormalities of the musculoskeletal system
orthopedist (*or*-thō-PĒ-dist)	physician who specializes in orthopedics
orthotics (or-THOT-iks)	making and fitting of orthopedic appliances, such as arch supports, used to support, align, prevent, or correct deformities
orthotist (or-THOT-ist)	a person who specializes in orthotics
osteoclast (OS-tē-ō-*klast*)	type of bone cell involved in absorption and removal of bone minerals. It works in balance with osteoblasts to maintain healthy bone tissue.
osteopath (OS-tē-ō-path)	physician who specializes in osteopathy

Term	Definition
osteopathy (*os*-tē-OP-a-thē)	system of medicine that uses the usual forms of diagnosis and treatment but places greater emphasis on the role of the relation between body organs and the musculoskeletal system; manipulation may be used in addition to other treatments
prosthesis (*pl.* prostheses) (pros-THĒ-sis) (pros-THĒ-sēz)	an artificial substitute for a missing body part such as a leg, eye, or total hip replacement

CAM TERM

Osteopathy combines conventional medical practices with structural manipulation and education about healthful posture and lifestyle to restore balance in the musculoskeletal system. Studies of osteopathic treatment have revealed it to be effective in addressing **neck, TMJ, and lower back pain,** as well as improving motor function in children with **cerebral palsy.**

Refer to **Appendix D** for pharmacology terms related to the musculoskeletal system.

EXERCISE 38

Practice saying aloud each of the complementary terms not built from word parts on these two pages.

To hear the terms, go to http://evolve.elsevier.com. Refer to p. 18 for your Evolve Access Information. Select Exercises & Review, Chapter 14, Chapter Exercises, Pronunciation.

☐ Place a check mark in the box when you have completed this exercise.

EXERCISE 39

Match the definitions in the first column with the correct terms in the second column.

______	1. specialist in manipulation of the vertebral column	a. chiropodist
______	2. branch of medicine dealing with treatment of diseases of the musculoskeletal system	b. chiropractic
______	3. physician who places emphasis on manipulation	c. chiropractor
______	4. foot specialist	d. osteopath
______	5. substitute for a body part	e. osteopathy
______	6. system of treatment	f. orthopedics
______	7. system of medicine	g. orthopedist
______	8. making of orthopedic appliances	h. podiatrist
______	9. skilled in orthotics	i. orthotics
______	10. crackling or grating sound	j. prosthesis
______	11. physician who treats diseases and disorders of the musculoskeletal system	k. orthotist
______	12. maintains healthy bone tissue with osteoblasts	l. crepitus
		m. osteoclast

EXERCISE 40

Write the definitions of the following.

1. chiropractor ______________________
2. chiropractic ______________________
3. orthopedics ______________________
4. orthopedist ______________________
5. chiropodist ______________________
6. podiatrist ______________________
7. osteopath ______________________
8. osteopathy ______________________
9. orthotics ______________________
10. prosthesis ______________________
11. orthotist ______________________
12. crepitus ______________________
13. osteoclast ______________________

EXERCISE 41

Spell each of the complementary terms not built from word parts on pp. 676-677 by having someone dictate them to you.

To hear and spell the terms, go to http://evolve.elsevier.com. Refer to p. 18 for your Evolve Access Information. Select Exercises & Review, Chapter 14, Chapter Exercises, Spelling.
☐ Place a check mark in the box if you have completed this exercise online.

1. ______________________
2. ______________________
3. ______________________
4. ______________________
5. ______________________
6. ______________________
7. ______________________
8. ______________________
9. ______________________
10. ______________________
11. ______________________
12. ______________________
13. ______________________

Abbreviations

C1-C7	cervical vertebrae
CTS	carpal tunnel syndrome
EMG	electromyogram
fx	fracture
HNP	herniated nucleus pulposus
L1-L5	lumbar vertebrae
MD	muscular dystrophy
MG	myasthenia gravis
OA	osteoarthritis
ortho	orthopedics
RA	rheumatoid arthritis
T1-T12	thoracic vertebrae
THA	total hip arthroplasty

Refer to **Appendix C** for a complete list of abbreviations.

EXERCISE 42

Write the meaning of the abbreviations in the following sentences.

1. Vertebrae make up the bones of the spinal column. **C1 to C7** ____________ ____________ are the first set that form the neck. The second set **T1 to T12** ____________ ____________ articulate with the 12 pairs of ribs that form the outward curve of the spine. **L1 to L5** ____________ ____________, the third set, are larger and form the inward curve of the spine.
2. Patients with **RA** ____________ ____________ may experience muscle atrophy and weakness because of inactivity.
3. Water exercise or gentle movement, such as Tai Chi, is recommended for many patients with **OA** ________________________, the most common joint disease.
4. **MG** ____________ ____________ most often affects women and the onset occurs at any age. It is an acquired autoimmune disorder.
5. **EMG** ________________________ is used to evaluate patients with localized or diffuse muscle weakness, such as polymyositis.
6. **CTS** ____________ ____________ ____________ is a common condition in which, for various reasons, the median nerve in the wrist becomes compressed, causing numbness and pain.
7. Nine types of **MD** ____________ ____________ have been identified. Because symptoms of the disease are similar to other muscular disorders, diagnosis is often difficult.
8. **HNP** ____________ ____________ ____________ may also be referred to as slipped or ruptured disk or herniated intervertebral disk.
9. **THA** ____________ ____________ ____________ is used to treat severe osteoarthritis of the hip joints.

PRACTICAL APPLICATION

EXERCISE 43 *Interact with Medical Documents*

Complete the operative report by writing the medical terms in the blanks. Use the list of definitions with the corresponding numbers.

University Hospital and Medical Center
4700 North Main Street • Wellness, Arizona 54321 • (987) 555-3210

PATIENT NAME: William McBride
DATE OF BIRTH: 12/04/19XX

CASE NUMBER: 10003-MKL
DATE: 04/30/20XX

OPERATIVE REPORT

HISTORY: William McBride is a 55-year-old African American male who reports pain in his left knee when walking and golfing. He states that his knees have "been painful" for many years since he quit playing semiprofessional hockey, but the pain has become much more severe in the last 6 months. He was admitted to the Medical Center's Outpatient 1. ______________ Center for an 2. ______________ of his left knee.

PREOPERATIVE DIAGNOSIS: Degenerative 3. ______________ of the left knee, with possible tear of the 4. ______________ meniscus.

OPERATIVE REPORT: After induction of spinal anesthetic, the patient was positioned on the operating table, and a tourniquet was applied over the upper left thigh. After positioning the leg in a circumferential holder, the end of the table was flexed to allow the leg to hang freely. The patient's left leg was prepped and draped in the usual manner. After exsanguination of the leg with an Esmarch bandage, the tourniquet was inflated to 300 mm Hg. The knee was inspected by anterolateral and anteromedial parapatellar portholes.

FINDINGS: The synovium in the 5. ______________ pouch showed moderate to severe inflammatory changes with villi formation and hyperemia. The undersurface of the patella showed loss of normal articular cartilage on the lateral patellar facet with exposed bone in that area and moderate to severe 6. ______________________________ of the medial facet. Similar changes were noted in the intercondylar groove. In the medial compartment, the patient had smooth articular cartilage on the femur and moderate chondromalacia of the tibial plateau. The medial meniscus appeared normal with no evidence of tears and a smooth articular surface on the femoral condyle. No additional 7. ______________ being identified.

The tourniquet was then released and the knee flushed with lactated Ringer solution until the bleeding slowed. The wounds were Steri-Stripped closed, a sterile bandage with an external Ace wrap applied, and the patient returned to the postoperative recovery area in stable condition. The patient tolerated the procedure well.

POSTOPERATIVE DIAGNOSIS: Degenerative arthritis with mild chondromalacia of the left knee.

____

Martin Spencer, DO

MS/mcm

1. branch of medicine dealing with the study and treatment of diseases and abnormalities of the musculoskeletal system
2. visual examination of a joint
3. inflammation of a joint
4. toward the middle or midline
5. pertaining to above the patella
6. softening of the cartilage
7. study of (body changes caused by) disease

B. Read the chart note and answer the questions following it.

011107 TAFT, GRACE

File Patient Navigate Custom Fields Help

Patient Chart | Lab | Rad | Notes | Documents | Rx | Scheduling | Images | Billing

Name: **TAFT, GRACE** MR#: **011107** DOB: **10/17/19XX** Sex: **Female**

CLINICAL NOTE

ENCOUNTER DATE: 04/02/20XX

HISTORY: This 67-year-old woman is seen for a follow-up visit in Orthopedics. She was seen one week ago in the Emergency Department for treatment of Colles fracture of the right wrist. The patient is postmenopausal with a history of cigarette smoking.

PHYSICAL EXAMINATION: The patient is 5′5″ tall and weighs 117 lb. The examination of the right forearm and hand reveals normal color with minimal swelling. Further skeletal evaluation reveals mild dorsal kyphosis.

DIAGNOSTIC STUDIES: Bone-mineral density measurement shows evidence of osteoporosis.

IMPRESSION: Healing distal radial fracture and osteoporosis.

RECOMMENDATIONS: The patient was advised to continue immobilization of the right forearm for another 3 weeks. Calcium and vitamin D therapy were recommended. Fosamax was prescribed as treatment for her osteoporosis. A follow-up visit is scheduled in 3 weeks.

Electronically signed by: Maxwell S. Kline, MD 04/02/20XX 4:30 PM

MSK/kew

Start | Log On/Off | Print | Edit

1. Physical evaluation of the patient revealed:
   a. an abnormal condition of bending forward
   b. an abnormal condition of stiffness
   c. an abnormal hump of the thoracic spine
   d. an abnormal lateral curve of the spine
2. The patient received a diagnosis of:
   a. softening of the cartilage
   b. abnormal reduction of bone mass
   c. stonelike (marblelike) bones
   d. abnormal loss of bone density

EXERCISE 44 *Interpret Medical Terms*

To test your understanding of the terms introduced in this chapter, circle the words that correctly complete the sentences. The italicized words refer to the correct answer.

1. The medical term for *hunchback* is (**kyphosis, ankylosis, scoliosis**).
2. The medical term for *excision of cartilage* is (**carpectomy, chondrectomy, costectomy**).
3. *Difficult movement* is (**hyperkinesia, bradykinesia, dyskinesia**).
4. Vitamin D deficiency in adults may cause *osteomalacia,* or (**muscle weakness, marblelike bones, softening of bones**).
5. The *surgical breaking of a bone* to correct a deformity is called (**osteoclasis, arthroclasia, osteoplasty**).
6. The medical term that means *pertaining to below the rib* is (**subscapular, subcostal, substernal**).
7. The medical term for *growing together* is (**diaphysis, epiphysis, symphysis**).
8. A(n) (**orthopedist, podiatrist, chiropractor**) is *competent to treat* a person with a *fractured femur.*
9. (**Osteoporosis, osteopetrosis, osteomyelitis**) is the *abnormal loss of bone density.*
10. A common *disorder of the wrist caused by compression of the median nerve* is called (**lordosis, carpal tunnel syndrome, synoviosarcoma**).
11. Some patients who are taking statin drugs to lower their cholesterol levels may experience a rather rare side effect, *dissolution of striated muscle,* or (**spondylosis, rhabdomyolysis, spondylolisthesis**).
12. During an examination of the patient's left knee, *a crackling sound* (**osteopenia, exostosis, crepitus**) was noted during flexion, extension, and range of motion of the joint.

EXERCISE 45 *Read Medical Terms in Use*

Practice the pronunciation of terms by reading the following statements. Use the pronunciation key following the medical terms to assist you in saying the word.

To hear these terms, go to http://evolve.elsevier.com. Refer to p. 18 for your Evolve Access Information. Select Exercises & Review, Chapter 14, Chapter Exercises, Read Medical Terms in Use.

1. The **orthopedist** (or-thō-PĒ-dist) recommended Mr. Shah have an **arthrodesis** (ar-thrō-DĒ-sis) to reduce pain caused from an ankle **fracture** (FRAK-chur) he sustained several years ago.
2. Mrs.Diaz severed a tendon by accidentally walking through a glass patio door. A **tenorrhaphy** (ten-OR-a-fē) was performed to repair the tendon.
3. An **electromyogram** (e-*lek*-trō-MĪ-ō-gram) can assist the physician in diagnosing **muscular dystrophy** (MUS-kū-lar) (DIS-trō-fē). **Atrophy** (AT-rō-fē) frequently occurs in patients with this disease.
4. Adjective forms of medical terms are used by health professionals to indicate areas of the body that describe anatomic locations, areas of pain, sites of injections, locations of lesions, and so forth. Below are some examples.
   a. **cranial** (KRĀ-nē-al) laceration
   b. **intercostal** (in-ter-KOS-tal) muscles
   c. pain in the **subcostal** (sub-KŌS-tal) region
   d. herniation of an **intervertebral** (in-ter-VER-te-bral) disk
   e. **intracranial** (in-tra-KRĀ-nē-al) pressure
   f. **femoral** (FEM-or-al) artery
   g. strain of the **ischiopubic** (is-kē-ō-PŪ-bik) area
   h. degenerative disease of the **sternoclavicular** (*ster*-nō-kla-VIK-ū-lar) joint

EXERCISE 46 *Comprehend Medical Terms in Use*

Test your comprehension of terms in the previous statements by circling the correct answer.

1. T F A specialist in treating and diagnosing disorders of the foot recommended Mr. Shah for surgical fixation of the ankle joint.
2. A record of electrical activity of muscles is used in the diagnosis of:
   a. an abnormal benign growth on the surface of the body
   b. a group of hereditary diseases involving muscular degeneration and weakness
   c. wrist fracture
   d. form of arthritis that causes a forward bend of the spine
3. Which of the following is true for statements in number 4?
   a. herniation within the vertebra
   b. degenerative disease of the joint between the scapula and collarbone
   c. laceration of the wrist
   d. pain below the ribs

WEB LINK

For additional information on arthritis, visit the **Arthritis Foundation** at ***www.arthritis.org***.

EXERCISE 47 *Use Plural Endings*

Circle the correct singular or plural term to match the context of the sentence.

1. The (**epiphysis, epiphyses**) are the enlarged ends of the long bone.
2. The distal (**phalanx, phalanges**) of the ring finger was fractured.
3. Osteoporosis was present in four lumbar (**vertebrae, vertebra**).
4. A (**prosthesis, prostheses**) was implanted in the left hip.
5. Many synovial joints contain (**bursa, bursae**).

CHAPTER REVIEW

ONLINE CHAPTER REVIEW

To access the Evolve website, go to http://evolve.elsevier.com. Refer to p. 18 for your Evolve Access Information. Select Exercises & Review, Chapter 14, then select Chapter Exercises, Practice Activities, Animations, or Games. Place a check mark in the box when you have completed an exercise or activity, watched an animation, or played a game. Have fun!

Chapter Exercises

Exercises in this section of your Evolve resources correlate to exercises in your textbook. You may have completed them as you worked through the chapter.

- ☐ Pronunciation
- ☐ Spelling
- ☐ Read Medical Terms in Use

Practice Activities

Practice in study mode, then test your learning in assessment mode. Keep track of your scores from assessment mode if you wish.

	SCORE
☐ Picture It	_____
☐ Define Word Parts	_____
☐ Build Medical Terms	_____
☐ Word Shop	_____
☐ Define Medical Terms	_____
☐ Use It	_____
☐ Hear It and Type It: Clinical Vignettes	_____

Animations

- ☐ Muscle Range of Motion
- ☐ Osteomyelitis
- ☐ Repair of Tibial Plateau Fracture

Games

- ☐ Name that Word Part
- ☐ Term Storm
- ☐ Term Explorer
- ☐ Termbusters
- ☐ Medical Millionaire

REVIEW OF WORD PARTS

Can you define and spell the following word parts?

Combining Forms

ankyl/o
aponeur/o
arthr/o
burs/o
carp/o
chondr/o
clavic/o
clavicul/o
cost/o
crani/o
disk/o
femor/o
fibul/o
humer/o
ili/o
ischi/o
kinesi/o
kyph/o
lamin/o
lord/o
lumb/o
mandibul/o
maxill/o
menisc/o
my/o
myel/o
myos/o
oste/o
patell/o
pelv/i
pelv/o
petr/o
phalang/o
pub/o
rachi/o
radi/o
sacr/o
scapul/o
scoli/o
spondyl/o
stern/o
synovi/o
tars/o
ten/o
tend/o
tendin/o
tibi/o
uln/o
vertebr/o

Prefixes

inter-
supra-
sym-
syn-

Suffixes

-asthenia
-clasia
-clasis
-clast
-desis
-physis
-schisis

REVIEW OF TERMS

Can you define, pronounce, and spell the following terms *built from word parts?*

Diseases and Disorders

ankylosis
arthritis
bursitis
chondromalacia
cranioschisis
diskitis
fibromyalgia
kyphosis
lordosis
maxillitis
meniscitis
myasthenia
myeloma
osteitis
osteoarthritis (OA)
osteochondritis
osteofibroma
osteomalacia
osteomyelitis
osteopenia
osteopetrosis
osteosarcoma
polymyositis
rachischisis
rhabdomyolysis
sarcopenia
scoliosis
spondylarthritis
spondylosis
synoviosarcoma
tendinitis
tenosynovitis

Surgical

aponeurorrhaphy
arthrocentesis
arthroclasia
arthrodesis
arthroplasty
bursectomy
carpectomy
chondrectomy
chondroplasty
costectomy
cranioplasty
craniotomy
diskectomy
laminectomy
maxillectomy
meniscectomy
myorrhaphy
ostectomy
osteoclasis
patellectomy
phalangectomy
rachiotomy
spondylosyndesis
synovectomy
tarsectomy
tenomyoplasty
tenorrhaphy
vertebroplasty

Diagnostic

arthrography
arthroscopy
electromyogram (EMG)

Complementary

arthralgia
atrophy
bradykinesia
carpal
clavicular
cranial
dyskinesia
dystrophy
femoral
humeral
hyperkinesia
hypertrophy
iliofemoral
intercostal
intervertebral
intracranial
ischiofibular
ischiopubic
lumbar
lumbocostal
lumbosacral
osteoblast
osteoclast
osteocyte
osteonecrosis
pelvic
pelvisacral
pubic
pubofemoral
radial
sacral
sternoclavicular
sternoid
subcostal
submandibular
submaxillary
subscapular
substernal
suprapatellar
suprascapular
symphysis
tibial
ulnoradial
vertebrocostal

Can you define, pronounce, and spell the following terms *not built from word parts?*

Types of Body Movements

abduction
adduction
eversion
extension
flexion
inversion
pronation
rotation
supination

Diseases and Disorders

ankylosing spondylitis
bunion
carpal tunnel syndrome (CTS)
Colles fracture
exostosis
fracture (fx)
gout
herniated disk
Lyme disease
muscular dystrophy (MD)
myasthenia gravis (MG)
osteoporosis
rheumatoid arthritis (RA)
spinal stenosis
spondylolisthesis

Complementary

chiropodist
chiropractic
chiropractor
crepitus
orthopedics (ortho)
orthopedist
orthotics
orthotist
osteopath
osteopathy
podiatrist
prosthesis

ANSWERS

Exercise Figures

Exercise Figure

A. 1. mandible: mandibul/o
2. sternum: stern/o
3. phalanges: phalang/o
4. patella: patell/o
5. tarsals: tars/o
6. phalanges: phalang/o
7. cranium: crani/o
8. maxilla: maxill/o
9. clavicle: clavic/o, clavicul/o
10. ribs: cost/o
11. femur: femor/o
12. fibula: fibul/o
13. tibia: tibi/o

Exercise Figure

B. 1. a. vertebral column, spine: rachi/o
2. vertebra: spondyl/o, vertebr/o
3. scapula: scapul/o
4. humerus: humer/o
5. ulna: uln/o
6. radius: radi/o
7. carpals: carp/o
8. ilium: ili/o
9. pubis: pub/o
10. ischium: ischi/o
11. sacrum: sacr/o

Exercise Figure

C. 1. synovial membrane: synovi/o
2. joint: arthr/o
3. meniscus: menisc/o
4. tendon: ten/o, tend/o, tendin/o
5. cartilage: chondr/o
6. bursa: burs/o

Exercise Figure

D. 1. lord/osis
2. kyph/osis
3. scoli/osis

Exercise Figure

E. arthr/o/scopy

Exercise 1

1. d
2. i
3. h
4. k
5. j
6. g
7. b
8. c
9. f
10. a

Exercise 2

1. scapula
2. sternum
3. mandible
4. clavicle
5. humerus
6. a. ulna
   b. radius
7. tarsals
8. phalanges
9. metatarsals
10. metacarpals
11. femur
12. a. fibula
    b. tibia
13. patella
14. cervical vertebrae
15. lumbar
16. pubis
17. sacrum
18. ischium
19. coccyx
20. ilium
21. carpals

Exercise 3

1. m
2. c
3. e
4. a
5. l
6. d
7. h
8. i
9. k
10. b
11. f
12. g

Exercise 4

1. moving away from the midline
2. movement that turns the palm down
3. movement that turns the palm up
4. turning around its own axis
5. movement in which a limb is placed in a straight position
6. turning outward
7. moving toward the midline
8. movement in which a limb is bent
9. turning inward

Exercise 5

1. h
2. d
3. i
4. j
5. c
6. a
7. g
8. f
9. b

Exercise 6

1. clavicle
2. rib
3. cranium (skull)
4. femur
5. clavicle
6. humerus
7. ilium
8. ischium
9. carpals
10. fibula
11. mandible
12. loin, lumbar region of the spine
13. pelvis, pelvic bone

Exercise 7

1. a. clavicul/o
   b. clavic/o
2. cost/o
3. crani/o
4. femor/o
5. humer/o
6. carp/o
7. ischi/o
8. fibul/o
9. ili/o
10. mandibul/o
11. lumb/o
12. a. pelv/i
    b. pelv/o

Exercise 8

1. vertebral column, spine
2. patella
3. vertebra
4. maxilla
5. phalanges
6. ulna
7. radius
8. tibia
9. pubis
10. tarsals
11. scapula
12. sternum
13. vertebra
14. sacrum

Exercise 9

1. maxill/o
2. uln/o
3. radi/o
4. tibi/o
5. pub/o
6. tars/o
7. a. vertebr/o
   b. spondyl/o
8. stern/o
9. scapul/o
10. patell/o
11. phalang/o
12. sacr/o
13. rachi/o

Exercise 10

1. joint
2. aponeurosis
3. meniscus
4. tendon
5. cartilage
6. tendon
7. bursa
8. tendon
9. synovia, synovial membrane
10. intervertebral disk

Exercise 11

1. menisc/o
2. aponeur/o
3. arthr/o
4. chondr/o
5. a. tendin/o
   b. ten/o
   c. tend/o
6. burs/o
7. synovi/o
8. disk/o

Exercise 12

1. muscle
2. stone
3. movement, motion
4. bone
5. lamina
6. bone marrow
7. hump
8. crooked, stiff, bent
9. crooked, curved
10. muscle
11. bent forward

Exercise 13

1. a. my/o
   b. myos/o
2. petr/o
3. kinesi/o
4. oste/o
5. lamin/o
6. myel/o
7. kyph/o
8. ankyl/o
9. scoli/o
10. lord/o

Exercise 14

1. above
2. together, joined
3. between

Exercise 15

1. a. syn-
   b. sym-
2. inter-
3. supra-

Exercise 16

1. growth
2. break
3. surgical fixation, fusion
4. break
5. split, fissure
6. break
7. weakness

Exercise 17

1. -physis
2. -asthenia
3. a. -clasis
   b. -clast
   c. -clasia
4. -desis
5. -schisis

Exercise 18

Pronunciation Exercise

Exercise 19

1. WR S
   oste/itis
   inflammation of the bone
2. WR CV WR S
   oste/o/myel/itis
   CF
   inflammation of the bone and bone marrow
3. WR CV WR S
   oste/o/petr/osis
   CF
   abnormal condition of stonelike bones (marblelike bones)
4. WR CV S
   oste/o/malacia
   CF
   softening of bones
5. WR CV WR S
   oste/o/chondr/itis
   CF
   inflammation of the bone and cartilage
6. WR CV WR S
   oste/o/fibr/oma
   CF
   tumor of the bone and fibrous tissue
7. WR S
   arthr/itis
   inflammation of a joint
8. WR CV WR CV S
   rhabd/o/my/o/lysis
   CF CF
   dissolution of striated muscle
9. WR S
   myel/oma
   tumor of the bone marrow
10. WR S
    tendin/itis
    inflammation of a tendon
11. WR CV S
    oste/o/penia
    CF
    abnormal reduction of bone (mass)
12. WR S
    spondyl/osis
    abnormal condition of the vertebra
13. WR S
    burs/itis
    inflammation of the bursa
14. WR WR S
    spondyl/arthr/itis
    inflammation of the vertebral joints
15. WR S
    ankyl/osis
    abnormal condition of stiffness
16. WR S
    kyph/osis
    abnormal condition of a hump (increased convexity of thoracic spine)
17. WR S
    scoli/osis
    abnormal condition of (lateral) a curved (spine)
18. WR CV S
    crani/o/schisis
    CF
    fissure of the skull
19. WR S
    maxill/itis
    inflammation of the maxilla
20. WR S
    menisc/itis
    inflammation of the meniscus
21. WR S
    rachi/schisis
    fissure of the vertebral column
22. WR S
    my/asthenia
    muscle weakness
23. WR CV S
    oste/o/sarcoma
    CF
    malignant tumor of the bone
24. WR CV S
    chondr/o/malacia
    CF
    softening of cartilage
25. WR CV S
    synovi/o/sarcoma
    CF
    malignant tumor of the synovial membrane
26. WR CV WR S
    ten/o/synov/itis
    CF
    inflammation of the tendon and synovial membrane
27. P WR S
    poly/myos/itis
    inflammation of many muscles
28. WR S
    disk/itis
    inflammation of an intervertebral disk
29. WR S
    lord/osis
    abnormal condition of bending forward (increased concavity of lumbar spine)
30. WR CV WR S
    oste/o/arthr/itis
    CF
    inflammation of bone and joint
31. WR CV WR S
    fibr/o/my/algia
    CF
    pain in the fibrous tissues and muscles
32. WR CV S
    sarc/o/penia
    CF
    abnormal reduction of connective tissue

Exercise 20

1. oste/o/chondr/itis
2. oste/o/fibr/oma
3. arthr/itis
4. rhabd/o/my/o/lysis
5. myel/oma
6. tendin/itis
7. spondyl/osis
8. oste/o/penia
9. burs/itis
10. spondyl/arthr/itis

11. ankyl/osis
12. kyph/osis
13. scoli/osis
14. crani/o/schisis
15. maxill/itis
16. menisc/itis
17. rachi/schisis
18. my/asthenia
19. oste/itis
20. oste/o/myel/itis
21. oste/o/petr/osis
22. oste/o/malacia
23. ten/o/synov/itis
24. synovi/o/sarcoma
25. oste/o/sarcoma
26. chondr/o/malacia
27. disk/itis
28. poly/myos/itis
29. lord/osis
30. oste/o/arthr/itis
31. fibr/o/my/algia
32. sarc/o/penia

Exercise 21
Spelling Exercise; see text pp. 645-647.

Exercise 22
Pronunciation Exercise

Exercise 23
1. exostosis
2. muscular dystrophy
3. myasthenia gravis
4. bunion
5. ankylosing spondylitis
6. gout
7. herniated disk
8. fracture
9. osteoporosis
10. carpal tunnel syndrome
11. Colles fracture
12. rheumatoid arthritis
13. spondylolisthesis
14. Lyme disease
15. spinal stenosis

Exercise 24
1. abnormal benign growth on the surface of a bone
2. group of hereditary diseases characterized by degeneration of muscle and weakness
3. chronic disease characterized by muscle weakness and thought to be caused by a defect in the transmission of impulses from nerve to muscle cell
4. abnormal prominence of the joint at the base of the great toe
5. form of arthritis that first affects the spine and adjacent structures
6. abnormal loss of bone density
7. disease in which an excessive amount of uric acid in the blood causes sodium urate crystals (tophi) to be deposited in the joints
8. rupture of the intervertebral disk cartilage, which allows the contents to protrude through it, putting pressure on the spinal nerve roots
9. broken bone
10. a disorder of the wrist caused by compression of the median nerve
11. a type of fractured wrist
12. a chronic systemic disease characterized by inflammatory changes in the connective tissue throughout the body
13. an infection transmitted to humans by deer ticks
14. forward slipping of one vertebra over another
15. narrowing of the spinal column with compression of nerve roots

Exercise 25
Spelling Exercise; see text pp. 653-655.

Exercise 26
Pronunciation Exercise

Exercise 27
1. WR CV S
oste/o/clasis
CF
(surgical) breaking of a bone
2. WR S
ost/ectomy
excision of bone
3. WR CV S
arthr/o/clasia
CF
(surgical) breaking of a (stiff) joint
4. WR CV S
arthr/o/desis
CF
surgical fixation of a joint
5. WR CV S
arthr/o/plasty
CF
surgical repair of a joint
6. WR S
chondr/ectomy
excision of a cartilage
7. WR CV S
chondr/o/plasty
CF
surgical repair of a cartilage
8. WR CV S
my/o/rrhaphy
CF
suture of a muscle
9. WR CV WR CV S
ten/o/my/o/plasty
CF CF
surgical repair of the tendon and muscle
10. WR CV S
ten/o/rrhaphy
CF
suture of a tendon
11. WR S
cost/ectomy
excision of a rib
12. WR S
patell/ectomy
excision of the patella
13. WR CV S
aponeur/o/rrhaphy
CF
suture of an aponeurosis
14. WR S
carp/ectomy
excision of a carpal bone
15. WR S
phalang/ectomy
excision of a finger or toe bone
16. WR S
menisc/ectomy
excision of the meniscus
17. WR CV P S
spondyl/o/syn/desis
CF
fusing together of the vertebrae
18. WR S
lamin/ectomy
excision of the lamina
19. WR S
burs/ectomy
excision of a bursa
20. WR CV S
crani/o/tomy
CF
incision into the skull
21. WR CV S
crani/o/plasty
CF
surgical repair of the skull
22. WR S
maxill/ectomy
excision of the maxilla
23. WR CV S
rachi/o/tomy
CF
incision into the vertebral column

24. WR S
tars/ectomy
excision of (one or more) tarsal bones
25. WR S
synov/ectomy
excision of the synovial membrane
26. WR S
disk/ectomy
excision of an intervertebral disk
27. WR CV S
vertebr/o/plasty
CF
surgical repair of a vertebra
28. WR CV S
arthr/o/centesis
CF
surgical puncture of a joint to aspirate fluid

Exercise 28

1. oste/o/clasis
2. ost/ectomy
3. arthr/o/clasia
4. arthr/o/desis
5. arthr/o/plasty
6. chondr/ectomy
7. chondr/o/plasty
8. my/o/rrhaphy
9. ten/o/my/o/plasty
10. ten/o/rrhaphy
11. cost/ectomy
12. patell/ectomy
13. aponeur/o/rrhaphy
14. carp/ectomy
15. phalang/ectomy
16. menisc/ectomy
17. spondyl/o/syn/desis
18. lamin/ectomy
19. burs/ectomy
20. crani/o/tomy
21. crani/o/plasty
22. maxill/ectomy
23. rachi/o/tomy
24. tars/ectomy
25. synov/ectomy
26. disk/ectomy
27. vertebr/o/plasty
28. arthr/o/centesis

Exercise 29

Spelling Exercise; see text pp. 659-662.

Exercise 30

Pronunciation Exercise

Exercise 31

1. WR CV WR CV S
electr/o/my/o/gram
CF CF
record of the electrical activity in a muscle
2. WR CV S
arthr/o/graphy
CF
radiographic imaging of a joint
3. WR CV S
arthr/o/scopy
CF
visual examination of a joint

Exercise 32

1. arthr/o/graphy
2. arthr/o/scopy
3. electr/o/my/o/gram

Exercise 33

Spelling Exercise; see text pp. 666-667.

Exercise 34

Pronunciation Exercise

Exercise 35

1. P S(WR)
sym/physis
growing together
2. WR S
femor/al
pertaining to the femur
3. WR S
humer/al
pertaining to the humerus
4. P WR S
inter/vertebr/al
pertaining to between the vertebrae
5. P WR S
hyper/kinesi/a
excessive movement (overactivity)
6. P WR S
dys/kinesi/a
difficult movement
7. P WR S
brady/kinesi/a
slow movement
8. P WR S
intra/crani/al
pertaining to within the cranium
9. WR CV WR S
stern/o/clavicul/ar
CF
pertaining to the sternum and clavicle
10. WR CV WR S
ili/o/femor/al
CF
pertaining to the ilium and femur
11. WR CV WR S
ischi/o/fibul/ar
CF
pertaining to the ischium and fibula
12. P WR S
sub/maxill/ary
pertaining to below the maxilla
13. WR CV WR S
ischi/o/pub/ic
CF
pertaining to the ischium and pubis
14. P WR S
sub/mandibul/ar
pertaining to below the mandible
15. WR CV WR S
pub/o/femor/al
CF
pertaining to the pubis and femur
16. P WR S
supra/scapul/ar
pertaining to above the scapula
17. P WR S
sub/cost/al
pertaining to below the rib
18. WR CV WR S
vertebr/o/cost/al
CF
pertaining to the vertebrae and ribs
19. P WR S
sub/scapul/ar
pertaining to below the scapula
20. WR CV WR
oste/o/blast
CF
developing bone (cell)
21. WR CV S
oste/o/cyte
CF
bone cell
22. WR CV WR S
oste/o/necr/osis
CF
abnormal death of bone (tissues)
23. WR S
stern/oid
resembling the sternum
24. WR S
arthr/algia
pain in the joint
25. WR S
carp/al
pertaining to the wrist

26. WR S
lumb/ar
pertaining to the loins
27. WR CV WR S
lumb/o/cost/al
CF
pertaining to the loins and to the ribs
28. WR CV WR S
lumb/o/sacr/al
CF
pertaining to the lumbar region (loin) and the sacrum
29. WR S
sacr/al
pertaining to the sacrum
30. WR S
pub/ic
pertaining to the pubis
31. P WR S
sub/stern/al
pertaining to below the sternum
32. P WR S
supra/patell/ar
pertaining to above the patella
33. P S(WR)
dys/trophy
abnormal development
34. P S(WR)
a/trophy
without development
35. P S(WR)
hyper/trophy
excessive development
36. P WR S
inter/cost/al
pertaining to between the ribs
37. WR S
crani/al
pertaining to the cranium
38. WR S
pelv/ic
pertaining to the pelvis
39. WR CV WR S
pelv/i/sacr/al
CF
pertaining to the pelvis and sacrum
40. WR S
clavicul/ar
pertaining to the clavicle
41. WR S
tibi/al
pertaining to the tibia
42. WR S
radi/al
pertaining to the radius
43. WR CV WR S
uln/o/radi/al
pertaining to the ulna and radius

Exercise 36
1. sym/physis
2. femor/al
3. humer/al
4. inter/vertebr/al
5. hyper/kinesi/a
6. dys/kinesi/a
7. brady/kinesi/a
8. intra/crani/al
9. stern/o/clavicul/ar
10. ili/o/femor/al
11. ischi/o/fibul/ar
12. sub/maxill/ary
13. ischi/o/pub/ic
14. sub/mandibul/ar
15. pub/o/femor/al
16. supra/scapul/ar
17. sub/cost/al
18. vertebr/o/cost/al
19. sub/scapul/ar
20. oste/o/blast
21. oste/o/cyte
22. oste/o/necr/osis
23. stern/oid
24. arthr/algia
25. carp/al
26. sacr/al
27. lumb/ar
28. pub/ic
29. lumb/o/sacr/al
30. lumb/o/cost/al
31. sub/stern/al
32. supra/patell/ar
33. dys/trophy
34. a/trophy
35. hyper/trophy
36. crani/al
37. inter/cost/al
38. pelv/ic
39. pelv/i/sacr/al
40. clavicul/ar
41. tibi/al
42. radi/al
43. uln/o/radi/al

Exercise 37
Spelling Exercise; see text pp. 669-671.

Exercise 38
Pronunciation Exercise

Exercise 39
1. c
2. f
3. d
4. a, h
5. j
6. b
7. e
8. i
9. k
10. l
11. g
12. m

Exercise 40
1. specialist in chiropractic
2. system of treatment that consists of manipulation of the vertebral column
3. branch of medicine dealing with the study and treatment of diseases and abnormalities of the musculoskeletal system
4. physician who specializes in orthopedics
5. specialist in treating and diagnosing foot diseases and disorders
6. specialist in treating and diagnosing diseases and disorders of the foot
7. physician who specializes in osteopathy
8. system of medicine in which emphasis is on the relation between body organs and the musculoskeletal system
9. making and fitting of orthopedic appliances
10. an artificial substitute for a missing body part
11. a person who is skilled in orthotics
12. crackling sound heard when two bones rub against each other or grating caused by rubbing together of dry surfaces
13. type of bone cell involved in absorption and removal of bone minerals

Exercise 41
Spelling Exercise; see text pp. 676-677.

Exercise 42
1. cervical vertebrae; thoracic vertebrae; lumbar vertebrae
2. rheumatoid arthritis
3. osteoarthritis
4. myasthenia gravis
5. electromyogram
6. carpal tunnel syndrome
7. muscular dystrophy
8. herniated nucleus pulposus
9. total hip arthroplasty

Exercise 43
A. 1. orthopedic
2. arthroscopy
3. arthritis
4. medial
5. suprapatellar
6. chondromalacia
7. pathology

B. 1. c
2. d

Exercise 44
1. kyphosis
2. chondrectomy
3. dyskinesia
4. softening of bones
5. osteoclasis
6. subcostal
7. symphysis
8. orthopedist
9. osteoporosis
10. carpal tunnel syndrome
11. rhabdomyolysis
12. crepitus

Exercise 45
Reading Exercise

Exercise 46
1. *F*, an orthopedist and not a podiatrist is treating Mr. Shah.
2. b
3. d

Exercise 47
1. epiphyses
2. phalanx
3. vertebrae
4. prosthesis
5. bursae

NOTES

Chapter 15

Nervous System and Behavioral Health

OUTLINE

OBJECTIVES

Upon completion of this chapter you will be able to:

1. Identify organs and structures of the nervous system.
2. Define and spell word parts related to the nervous system.
3. Define, pronounce, and spell disease and disorder terms related to the nervous system.
4. Define, pronounce, and spell surgical terms related to the nervous system.
5. Define, pronounce, and spell diagnostic terms related to the nervous system.
6. Define, pronounce, and spell complementary terms related to the nervous system.
7. Define, pronounce, and spell behavioral health terms.
8. Interpret the meaning of abbreviations related to the nervous system.
9. Interpret, read, and comprehend medical language in simulated medical statements and documents.

ANATOMY

The nervous system consists of the brain, spinal cord, and nerves and may be divided into two parts: the **central nervous system** (CNS) and the **peripheral nervous system** (PNS) (Figures 15-1 and 15-2). The central nervous system consists of the brain and spinal cord. The peripheral nervous system is made up of cranial nerves, which carry impulses between the brain and neck and head, and spinal nerves, which carry messages between the spinal cord and abdomen, limbs, and chest.

Function

The nervous system forms a complex communication system allowing for the coordination of body functions and activities. As a whole, the nervous system is designed to detect changes inside and outside the body, to evaluate this sensory information, and to send directions to muscles or glands in response. This system also provides for mental activities such as thought, memory, and emotions.

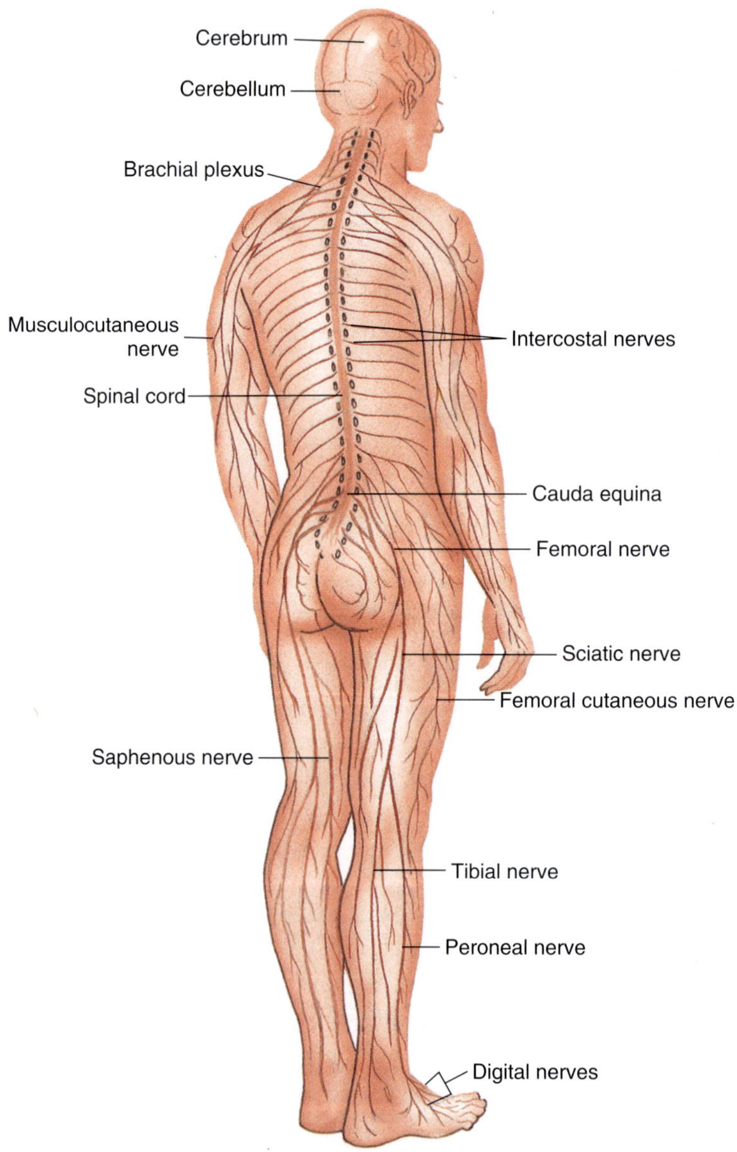

FIGURE 15-1
Simplified view of the nervous system.

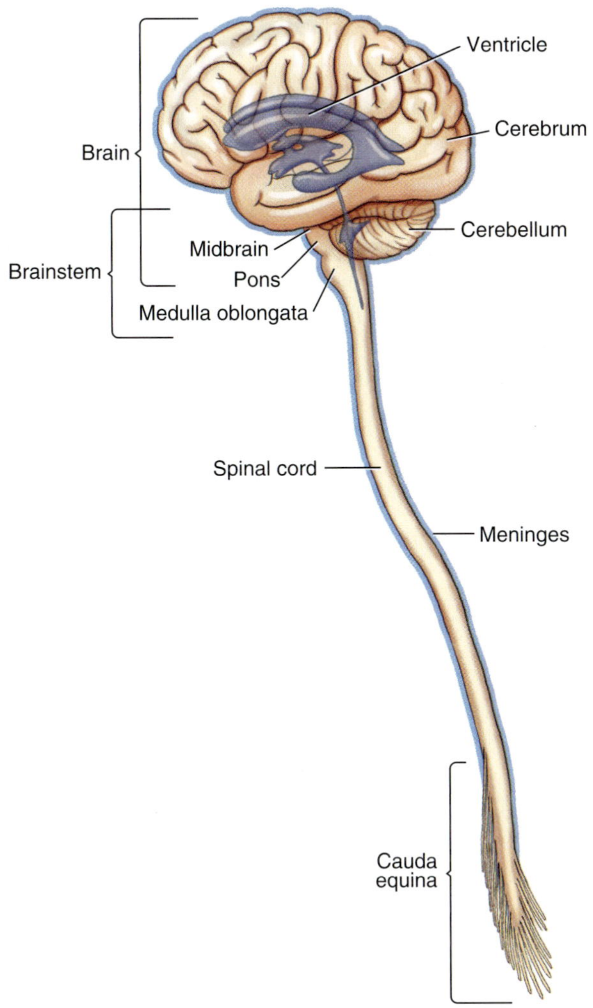

FIGURE 15-2
Brain and spinal cord.

Organs of the Central Nervous System

Term	Definition
brain	contained within the cranium, the center for coordinating body activities (Figure 15-2)
cerebrum	largest portion of the brain, divided into left and right hemispheres. The cerebrum controls the skeletal muscles, interprets general senses (such as temperature, pain, and touch), and contains centers for sight and hearing. Intellect, memory, and emotional reactions also take place in the cerebrum.
ventricles	spaces within the brain that contain a fluid called **cerebrospinal fluid.** The cerebrospinal fluid flows through the subarachnoid space around the brain and spinal cord.
cerebellum	located under the posterior portion of the cerebrum. Its function is to assist in the coordination of skeletal muscles and to maintain balance (also called **hindbrain**).

CEREBELLUM

was named in the third century BC by Erasistratus, who also named the cerebrum. ***Cerebellum*** literally means **little brain** and is the diminutive of ***cerebrum,*** meaning **brain.** Although it was named long ago, its function was not understood until the nineteenth century.

Organs of the Central Nervous System—*cont'd*

Term	Definition
brainstem	stemlike portion of the brain that connects with the spinal cord. Ten of the 12 cranial nerves originate in the brainstem.
pons	literally means **bridge**. It connects the cerebrum with the cerebellum and brainstem.
medulla oblongata	located between the pons and spinal cord. It contains centers that control respiration, heart rate, and the muscles in the blood vessel walls, which assist in determining blood pressure.
midbrain	most superior portion of the brainstem
cerebrospinal fluid (CSF)	clear, colorless fluid contained in the ventricles that flows through the subarachnoid space around the brain and spinal cord. It cushions the brain and spinal cord from shock, transports nutrients, and clears metabolic waste.
spinal cord	passes through the vertebral canal extending from the medulla oblongata to the level of the second lumbar vertebra. The spinal cord conducts nerve impulses to and from the brain and initiates reflex action to sensory information without input from the brain.
meninges	three layers of membrane that cover the brain and spinal cord (Figure 15-3)
dura mater	tough outer layer of the meninges
arachnoid	delicate middle layer of the meninges. The arachnoid membrane is loosely attached to the pia mater by weblike fibers, which allow for the **subarachnoid space**.
pia mater	thin inner layer of the meninges

MENINGES

were first named by a Persian physician in the tenth century. When translated into Latin, they became **dura mater**, meaning **hard mother** (because it is a tough membrane), and **pia mater**, meaning **soft mother** (because it is a delicate membrane). **Mater** was used because the Arabians believed that the meninges were the mother of all other body membranes.

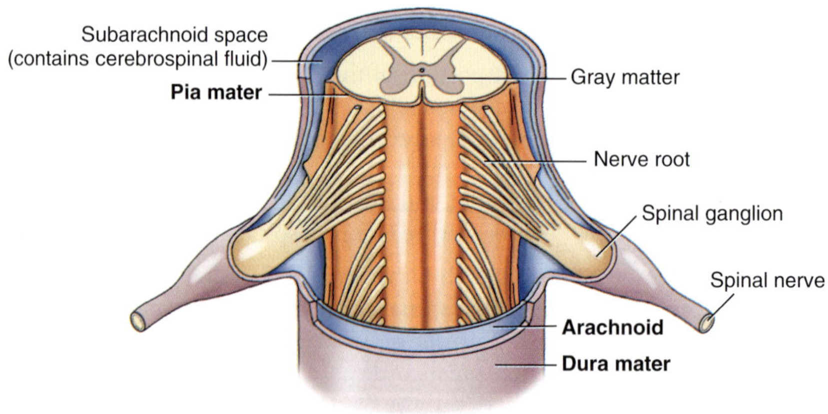

FIGURE 15-3
Layers of meninges.

Organs of the Peripheral Nervous System

Term	Definition
nerve	cordlike structure made up of fibers that carries impulses from one part of the body to another. There are 12 pairs of cranial nerves and 31 pairs of spinal nerves (see Figures 15-1 and 15-4).
ganglion (*pl.* **ganglia**)	group of nerve cell bodies located outside the central nervous system
glia	specialized cells that support and nourish nervous tissue. Some cells assist in the secretion of cerebrospinal fluid and others assist with phagocytosis. They do not conduct impulses. Three types of glia are **astroglia, oligodendroglia,** and **microglia.** (also called **neuroglia**)
neuron	a nerve cell that conducts nerve impulses to carry out the function of the nervous system. Destroyed neurons cannot be replaced.

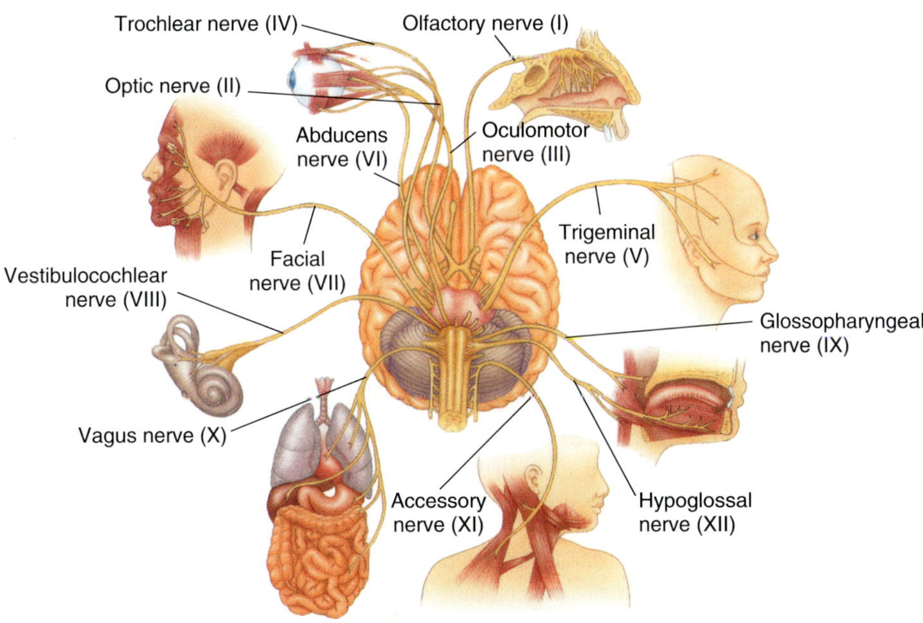

FIGURE 15-4
Cranial nerves.

A & P Booster
For students desiring more anatomy and physiology, go to http://evolve.elsevier.com. Refer to p. 18 for your Evolve Access Information. Select A & P Booster, Chapter 15.

EXERCISE 1

Fill in the blanks with the correct terms. *To check your answers to the exercises in this chapter, go to Answers, p. 746, at the end of the chapter.*

The layer of membrane that covers the brain and spinal cord is called the (1) ____________________. Three layers that comprise this membrane are called (2) ____________________ ____________________, (3) ____________________, and (4) ____________________ ____________________. Below the middle layer is a space called the (5) ____________________ ____________________ through which the (6) ____________________ ____________________ flows around the brain and spinal cord.

EXERCISE 2

Match the definitions in the first column with the correct terms in the second column.

_____ 1. maintains balance
_____ 2. connects the cerebrum with the cerebellum and brainstem
_____ 3. spaces within the brain
_____ 4. contains the control center for respiration
_____ 5. carries impulses from one part of the body to another
_____ 6. conducts impulses to and from the brain and initiates reflex action to sensory information
_____ 7. group of nerve cell bodies outside the central nervous system
_____ 8. colorless fluid contained in the ventricles
_____ 9. supports and nourishes nervous tissue

a. nerve
b. ganglion
c. cerebrospinal fluid
d. cerebellum
e. medulla oblongata
f. pons
g. ventricles
h. spinal cord
i. pia mater
j. glia

WORD PARTS

Word parts you need to learn to complete this chapter are listed on the following pages. The exercises at the end of each list will help you learn their definitions and spellings.

Use the flashcards accompanying this text or electronic flashcards to assist you in memorizing the word parts for this chapter.

To use electronic flashcards, go to http://evolve.elsevier.com. Refer to p. 18 for your Evolve Access Information. Select Flashcards, Chapter 15.

Combining Forms of the Nervous System

Combining Form	Definition
cerebell/o	cerebellum
cerebr/o	cerebrum, brain
dur/o	hard, dura mater
encephal/o	brain
gangli/o, ganglion/o	ganglion

Combining Form	Definition
gli/o	glia, gluey substance
mening/o, meningi/o	meninges
myel/o (NOTE: *myel/o* also means *bone marrow;* see Chapter 14.)	spinal cord
neur/o (NOTE: *neur/o* was introduced in Chapter 2.)	nerve
radic/o, radicul/o, rhiz/o	nerve root (proximal end of a peripheral nerve, closest to the spinal cord)

EXERCISE FIGURE A

Fill in the blanks with combining forms in this diagram of the brain and spinal cord. *To check your answers, go to p. 746.*

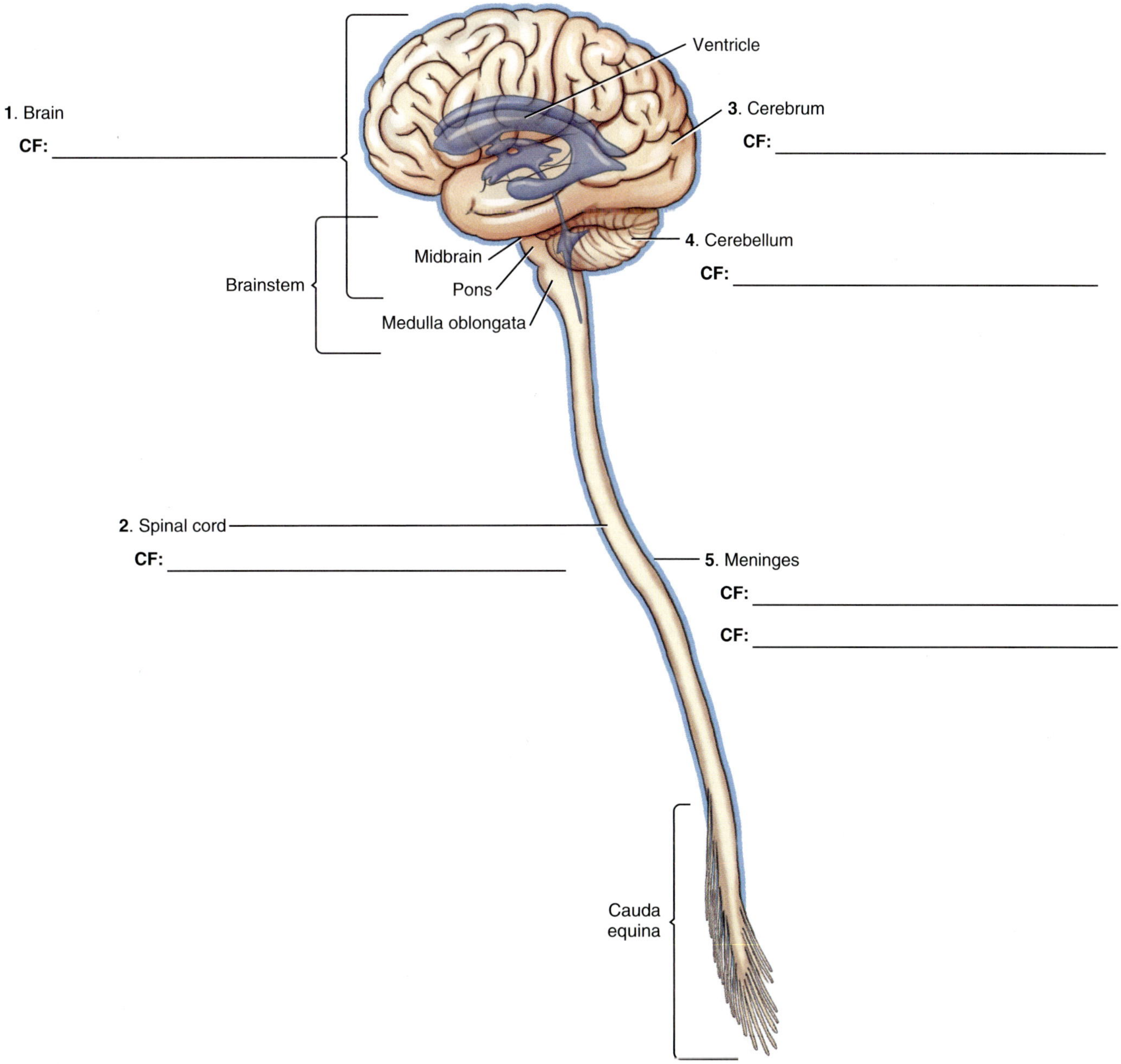

EXERCISE FIGURE B

Fill in the blanks with combining forms in this diagram of the spinal cord and layers of meninges.

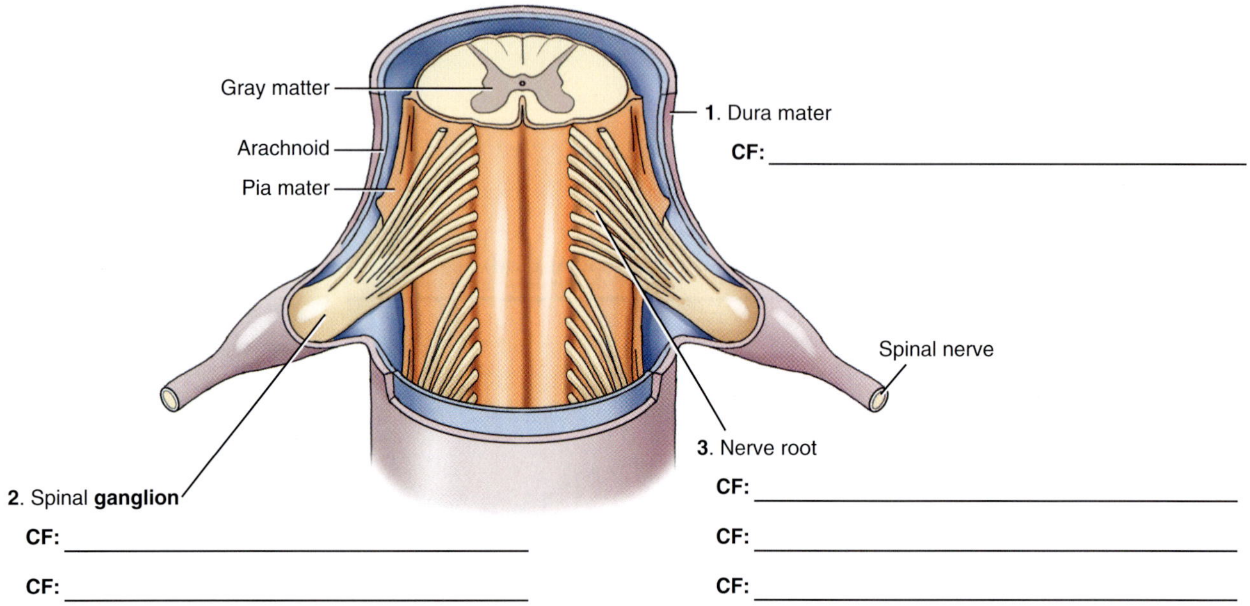

EXERCISE 3

Write the definitions of the following combining forms.

1. cerebell/o ______
2. neur/o ______
3. myel/o ______
4. meningi/o, mening/o ______
5. encephal/o ______
6. cerebr/o ______
7. radicul/o ______
8. gangli/o ______
9. radic/o ______
10. dur/o ______
11. ganglion/o ______
12. rhiz/o ______
13. gli/o ______

EXERCISE 4

Write the combining form for each of the following terms.

1. cerebellum ______________
2. nerve ______________
3. spinal cord ______________
4. meninges a. ______________
   b. ______________
5. brain ______________
6. cerebrum, brain ______________
7. nerve root a. ______________
   b. ______________
   c. ______________
8. hard, dura mater ______________
9. ganglion a. ______________
   b. ______________
10. glia, gluey substance ______________

Combining Forms Commonly Used with Nervous System Terms

Combining Form	Definition
esthesi/o	sensation, sensitivity, feeling
ment/o, psych/o	mind
mon/o	one, single
phas/o	speech
poli/o	gray matter
quadr/i (NOTE: an *i* is the combining vowel in *quadr/i*.)	four

EXERCISE 5

Write the definitions of the following combining forms.

1. mon/o ______________
2. psych/o ______________
3. quadr/i ______________
4. ment/o ______________
5. phas/o ______________
6. esthesi/o ______________
7. poli/o ______________

EXERCISE 6

Write the combining form for each of the following.

1. four ______________
2. one, single ______________
3. mind a. ______________ b. ______________
4. speech ______________
5. gray matter ______________
6. sensation, sensitivity, feeling ______________

Suffixes

Suffix	Definition
-iatrist	specialist, physician (*-logist* also means specialist)
-iatry	treatment, specialty
-ictal	seizure, attack
-paresis	slight paralysis (*-plegia*, meaning *paralysis*, was covered in Chapter 12)

EXERCISE 7

Write the definitions of the following suffixes.

1. -paresis ______________________________
2. -iatry ______________________________
3. -ictal ______________________________
4. -iatrist ______________________________

EXERCISE 8

Write the suffix for each of the following.

1. slight paralysis ______________________________
2. treatment, specialty ______________________________
3. seizure, attack ______________________________
4. specialist, physician ______________________________

MEDICAL TERMS

Disease and Disorder Terms

Built from Word Parts

The following terms are built from word parts you have already learned and can be translated literally to find their meanings. Further explanation of terms beyond the definition of their word parts, if needed, is included in parentheses.

Term	Definition
cerebellitis (*ser*-e-bel-Ī-tis)	inflammation of the cerebellum
cerebral thrombosis (se-RĒ-bral) (throm-BŌ-sis)	pertaining to the cerebrum, abnormal condition of a clot (blood clot in a blood vessel of the brain). (Onset of symptoms may appear from minutes to days after an obstruction occurs; a cause of **ischemic stroke**) (see Figure 15-12).
duritis (dū-RĪ-tis)	inflammation of the dura mater
encephalitis (en-*sef*-a-LĪ-tis)	inflammation of the brain
encephalomalacia (en-*sef*-a-lō-ma-LĀ-sha)	softening of the brain
encephalomyeloradiculitis (en-*sef*-a-lō-*mī*-e-lō-ra-*dik*-ū-LĪ-tis)	inflammation of the brain, spinal cord, and nerve roots
gangliitis (*gang*-glē-Ī-tis)	inflammation of a ganglion
glioblastoma (*glī*-ō-blas-TŌ-ma)	tumor composed of developing glial tissue (the most malignant and most common primary tumor of the brain) (Figure 15-5)
glioma (glī-Ō-ma)	tumor composed of the glial tissue (glioma is used to describe all primary neoplasms of the brain and spinal cord)
meningioma (me-*nin*-jē-Ō-ma)	tumor of the meninges (benign and slow growing)
meningitis (*men*-in-JĪ-tis)	inflammation of the meninges
meningocele (me-NING-gō-sēl)	protrusion of the meninges (through a defect in the skull or vertebral arch)
meningomyelocele (me-*ning*-gō-MĪ-e-lō-*sēl*)	protrusion of the meninges and spinal cord (through a neural arch defect in the vertebral column) (also called **myelomeningocele**)
mononeuropathy (*mon*-ō-nū-ROP-a-thē)	disease affecting a single nerve (such as carpal tunnel syndrome)
neuralgia (nū-RAL-ja)	pain in a nerve
neurasthenia (*nū*-ras-THĒ-nē-a)	nerve weakness

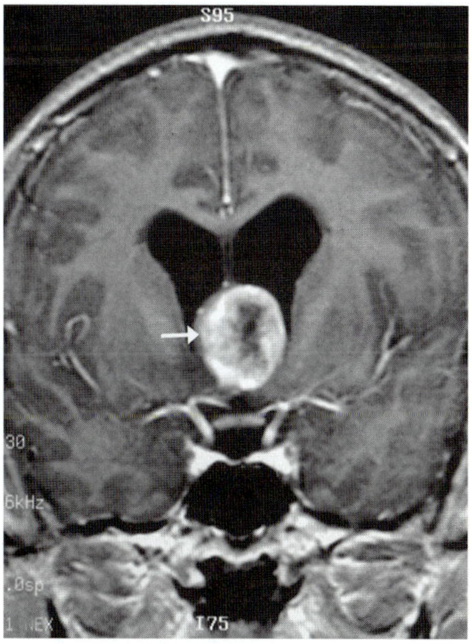

FIGURE 15-5
MRI image of brain demonstrating glioblastoma (arrow).

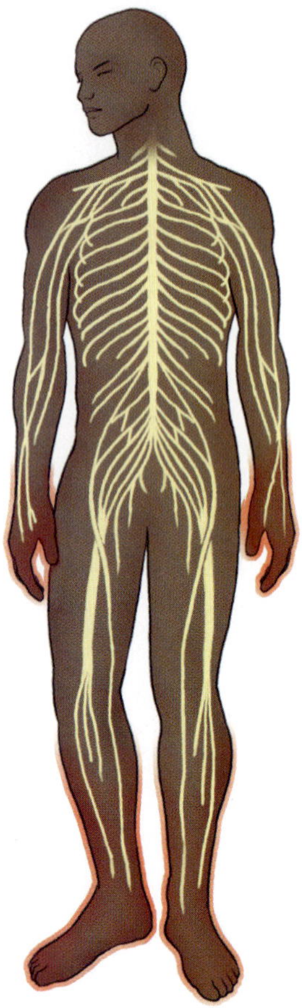

FIGURE 15-6
Peripheral neuropathy.

Disease and Disorder Terms—*cont'd*

Built from Word Parts

Term	Definition
neuritis (nū-RĪ-tis)	inflammation of a nerve
neuroarthropathy (*nū*-rō-ar-THROP-a-thē)	disease of nerves and joints
neuroma (nū-RŌ-ma)	tumor made up of nerve (cells)
neuropathy (nū-ROP-a-thē)	disease of the nerves (peripheral) (Figure15-6)
poliomyelitis (*pō*-lē-ō-*mī*-e-LĪ-tis)	inflammation of the gray matter of the spinal cord. (This infectious disease, commonly referred to as *polio*, is caused by one of three polio viruses.)
polyneuritis (*pol*-ē-nū-RĪ-tis)	inflammation of many nerves
polyneuropathy (*pol*-ē-nū-ROP-a-thē)	disease of many nerves (most often occurs as a side effect of diabetes mellitus, but may also occur as a result of drug therapy, critical illness such as sepsis, or carcinoma; exhibiting symptoms of weakness, distal sensory loss, and burning)
radiculitis (ra-*dik*-ū-LĪ-tis)	inflammation of the nerve roots
radiculopathy (ra-*dik*-ū-LOP-a-thē)	disease of the nerve roots
rhizomeningomyelitis (*rī*-zō-me-*ning*-gō-*mī*-ē-LĪ-tis)	inflammation of the nerve root, meninges, and spinal cord
subdural hematoma (sub-DŪ-ral) (*hē*-ma-TŌ-ma)	pertaining to below the dura mater, tumor of blood (*hematoma*, translated literally, means *blood tumor*; however, a hematoma is a collection of blood resulting from a broken blood vessel) (Figure 15-7)

PERIPHERAL NEUROPATHY

refers to disorders of the peripheral nervous system, including **radiculopathy, neuropathy,** and **mononeuropathy.** The term is often used synonymously with **polyneuropathy.** Signs and symptoms vary and usually begin gradually, starting with tingling and numbness in the toes and spreading to the feet and upwards. Symptoms may be felt only at night, be constant, or be barely noticed by the patient. Other symptoms include numbness, loss of balance, tingling, burning or freezing sensation, and muscle weakness.

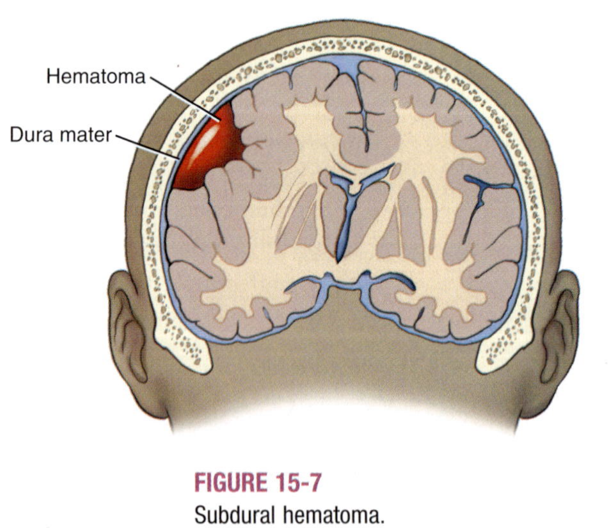

FIGURE 15-7
Subdural hematoma.

EXERCISE 9

Practice saying aloud each of the disease and disorder terms built from word parts on pp. 705-706.

To hear the terms, go to http://evolve.elsevier.com. Refer to p. 18 for your Evolve Access Information. Select Exercises & Review, Chapter 15, Chapter Exercises, Pronunciation.

☐ Place a check mark in the box when you have completed this exercise.

EXERCISE 10

Analyze and define the following terms.

1. neuritis ______
2. neuroma ______
3. neuralgia ______
4. neuroarthropathy ______
5. meningioma ______
6. neurasthenia ______
7. encephalomalacia ______
8. encephalitis ______
9. encephalomyeloradiculitis ______
10. meningitis ______
11. meningocele ______
12. meningomyelocele ______
13. radiculitis ______
14. cerebellitis ______
15. gangliitis ______
16. duritis ______
17. polyneuritis ______
18. poliomyelitis ______
19. cerebral thrombosis ______
20. subdural hematoma ______
21. rhizomeningomyelitis ______

22. mononeuropathy ______________________
23. neuropathy ______________________
24. radiculopathy ______________________
25. glioma ______________________
26. glioblastoma ______________________
27. polyneuropathy ______________________

EXERCISE 11

Build disease and disorder terms for the following definitions with the word parts you have learned.

1. inflammation of the nerve ______ / ______ (WR / S)
2. tumor made up of nerve (cells) ______ / ______ (WR / S)
3. pain in a nerve ______ / ______ (WR / S)
4. disease of nerves and joints ______ / ______ / ______ / ______ / ______ (WR / CV / WR / CV / S)
5. disease of the nerve roots ______ / ______ / ______ (WR / CV / S)
6. nerve weakness ______ / ______ (WR / S)
7. softening of the brain ______ / ______ / ______ (WR / CV / S)
8. inflammation of the brain ______ / ______ (WR / S)
9. inflammation of the brain, spinal cord, and nerve roots ______ / ______ / ______ / ______ / ______ / ______ (WR / CV / WR / CV / WR / S)
10. inflammation of the meninges ______ / ______ (WR / S)
11. protrusion of the meninges (through a defect in the skull or vertebral column) ______ / ______ / ______ (WR / CV / S)
12. protrusion of the meninges and spinal cord (through the vertebral column) ______ / ______ / ______ / ______ / ______ (WR / CV / WR / CV / S)

13. inflammation of the (spinal) nerve roots

_____ / _____
WR / S

14. inflammation of the cerebellum

_____ / _____
WR / S

15. inflammation of the ganglion

_____ / _____
WR / S

16. inflammation of the dura mater

_____ / _____
WR / S

17. inflammation of many nerves

_____ / _____ / _____
P / WR / S

18. inflammation of the gray matter of the spinal cord

_____ /CV/ _____ / _____
WR / CV / WR / S

19. pertaining to the cerebrum; abnormal condition of a clot

_____ / _____ ; _____ / _____
WR / S ; WR / S

20. pertaining to below the dura mater; tumor of blood

_____ / _____ / _____ ; _____ / _____
P / WR / S ; WR / S

21. inflammation of the nerve root, meninges, and spinal cord

_____ /CV/ _____ /CV/ _____ / _____
WR / CV / WR / CV / WR / S

22. tumor of the meninges

_____ / _____
WR / S

23. disease affecting a single nerve

_____ /CV/ _____ /CV/ _____
WR / CV / WR / CV / S

24. disease of the nerves

_____ /CV/ _____
WR / CV / S

25. tumor composed of glial tissue

_____ / _____
WR / S

26. tumor composed of developing glial tissue

_____ /CV/ _____ / _____
WR / CV / WR / S

27. disease of many nerves

_____ / _____ /CV/ _____
P / WR / CV / S

EXERCISE 12

Spell each of the disease and disorder terms built from word parts on pp. 705-706 by having someone dictate them to you.

To hear and spell the terms, go to http://evolve.elsevier.com. Refer to p. 18 for your Evolve Access Information. Select Exercises & Review, Chapter 15, Chapter Exercises, Spelling.
☐ Place a check mark in the box if you have completed this exercise online.

1. ____________
2. ____________
3. ____________
4. ____________
5. ____________
6. ____________
7. ____________
8. ____________
9. ____________
10. ____________
11. ____________
12. ____________
13. ____________
14. ____________
15. ____________
16. ____________
17. ____________
18. ____________
19. ____________
20. ____________
21. ____________
22. ____________
23. ____________
24. ____________
25. ____________
26. ____________
27. ____________

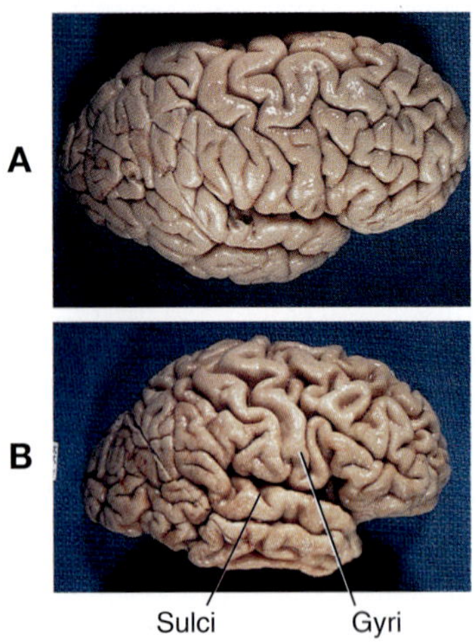

FIGURE 15-8
Alzheimer disease. **A,** Normal brain, age matched. **B,** Brain showing changes of Alzheimer disease. Note the brain is smaller, the gyri are narrower, and the sulci are wider than the normal brain.

Disease and Disorder Terms

Not Built from Word Parts

In some of the following terms, you may recognize word parts you have already learned; however, the full meaning of the terms cannot be discerned by the definition of their word parts.

Term	Definition
Alzheimer disease (AD) (AWLZ-hī-mer) (di-ZĒZ)	disease characterized by early dementia, confusion, loss of recognition of persons or familiar surroundings, restlessness, and impaired memory (Figure 15-8)
amyotrophic lateral sclerosis (ALS) (a-mī-ō-TRŌ-fik) (LAT-er-al) (skle-RŌ-sis)	progressive muscle atrophy caused by degeneration and scarring of neurons along the lateral columns of the spinal cord that control muscles (also called **Lou Gehrig disease**)

Term	Definition
Bell palsy (bel) (PAWL-zē)	paralysis of muscles on one side of the face, usually a temporary condition. Signs include a sagging mouth on the affected side and nonclosure of the eyelid (Figure 15-9).
cerebral aneurysm (se-RĒ-bral) (AN-ū-rizm)	aneurysm in the cerebrum (See Figure 15-12)
cerebral embolism (se-RĒ-bral) (EM-bō-lizm)	an embolus (usually a blood clot or a piece of atherosclerotic plaque arising from a distant site) lodges in a cerebral artery, causing sudden blockage of blood supply to the brain tissue. A common cause of cerebral embolism, a type of **ischemic stroke,** is atrial fibrillation (See Figure 15-12).
cerebral palsy (CP) (se-RĒ-bral) (PAWL-zē)	condition characterized by lack of muscle control and partial paralysis, caused by a brain defect or lesion present at birth or shortly after
dementia (de-MEN-sha)	cognitive impairment characterized by a loss of intellectual brain function. Patients have difficulty in various ways, including difficulty in performing complex tasks, reasoning, learning and retaining new information, orientation, word finding, and behavior. Dementia has several causes and is not considered part of normal aging.
epilepsy (EP-i-lep-sē)	condition characterized by recurrent seizures; a general term given to a group of neurologic disorders, all characterized by abnormal electrical activity in the brain
hydrocephalus (*hī*-drō-SEF-a-lus)	increased amount of cerebrospinal fluid in the ventricles of the brain, which can cause enlargement of the cranium in infants

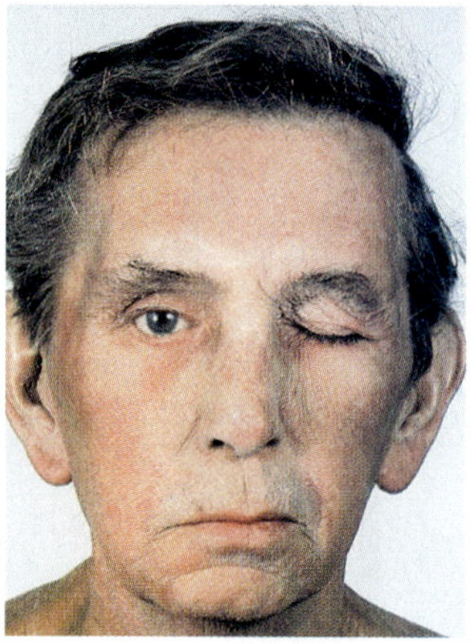

FIGURE 15-9
Bell palsy.

BELL PALSY

is named after **Sir Charles Bell,** a Scottish physician (1774-1842) who demonstrated sensory function of the fifth cranial nerve and the cause of facial palsy.

EPILEPSY

was written about by Hippocrates, in 400 BC, in a book titled **Sacred Disease.** It was believed at one time that epilepsy was a punishment for offending the gods. The Greek **epilepsia** meant **seizure** and is derived from **epi,** meaning **upon,** and **lambaneia,** meaning **to seize.** The term literally means **seized upon** (by the gods).

HYDROCEPHALUS

literally means **water in the head** and is made of the word parts **hydro,** meaning **water,** and **cephal,** meaning **head.** The condition was first described around 30 AD in the book **De Medicina.**

TYPES OF DEMENTIA

Alzheimer disease is the most common type of dementia, making up 60% to 80% of all cases. The disease, the cause of which is unknown, is a progressive neurodegenerative disorder characterized by diffuse brain atrophy and the presence of senile plaques and neurofibrillary tangles within the brain cortex. Women are affected more than men, and the disease usually occurs after the age of 60. The disease is slowly progressive and usually results in profound dementia in 5 to 10 years.

Vascular or multiple infarct dementia affects approximately 10% to 20% of patients with dementia. It is secondary to cerebrovascular disease and usually occurs in older patients.

Central nervous system infection dementia may be caused by herpes simplex encephalitis or AIDS.

Lewy body dementia is usually a rapidly progressive form of dementia with Parkinson syndrome.

Parkinson disease dementia may develop in patients with advanced disease.

Wernicke-Korsakoff syndrome is a form of dementia found in chronic alcoholism.

Normal pressure hydrocephalus may cause dementia in elderly individuals and can be treated with a ventricular peritoneal shunt.

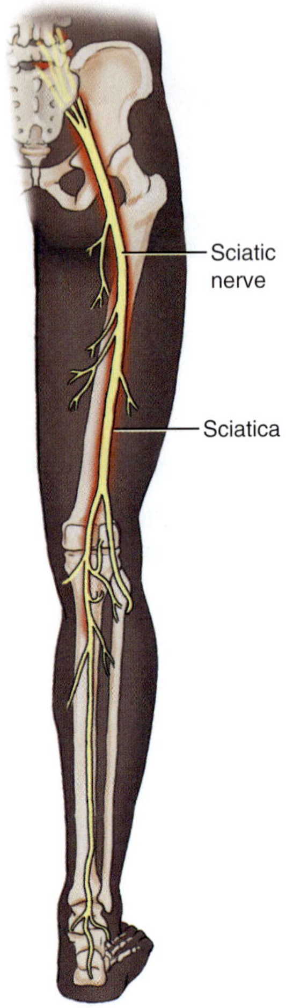

FIGURE 15-10
Sciatica. The sciatic nerve, the longest in the body, travels through the hip from the spine to the thigh and continues with branches throughout the lower leg and foot. Sciatica is the inflammation of the nerve along its course.

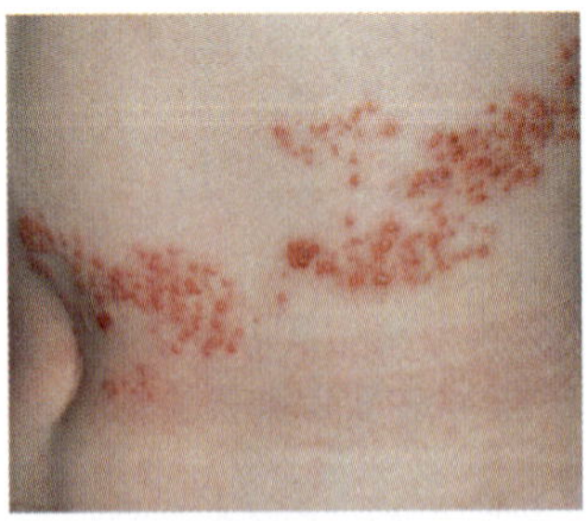

FIGURE 15-11
Shingles.

POSTHERPETIC NEURALGIA

is a complication of **shingles** (herpes zoster) and is caused by damage to the nerve fibers. Severe pain and hyperesthesia persist after the skin lesions disappear and may last months or even years.

Disease and Disorder Terms—*cont'd*

Not Built from Word Parts

Term	Definition
intracerebral hemorrhage (*in*-tra-SER-e-bral) (HEM-o-rij)	bleeding into the brain as a result of a ruptured blood vessel within the brain. Symptoms vary depending on the location of the hemorrhage; acute symptoms include dyspnea, dysphagia, aphasia, diminished level of consciousness, and hemiparesis. The symptoms often develop suddenly. Intracerebral hemorrhage, a cause of **hemorrhagic stroke,** is frequently associated with high blood pressure (See Figure 15-12).
multiple sclerosis (MS) (MUL-ti-pl) (skle-RŌ-sis)	degenerative disease characterized by sclerotic patches along the brain and spinal cord. Signs and symptoms are variable and fluctuate over the course of the disease. More common symptoms include fatigue, balance and coordination impairments, numbness, and vision problems.
Parkinson disease (PD) (PAR-kin-sun) (di-ZĒZ)	chronic degenerative disease of the central nervous system. Signs and symptoms include resting tremors of the hands and feet, rigidity, expressionless face, and shuffling gait. It usually occurs after the age of 50 years.
sciatica (sī-AT-i-ka)	inflammation of the sciatic nerve, causing pain that travels from the thigh through the leg to the foot and toes; can be caused by injury, infection, athritis, herniated disk, or from prolonged pressure on the nerve from sitting for long periods (Figure 15-10)
shingles (SHING-gelz)	viral disease that affects the peripheral nerves and causes blisters on the skin that follow the course of the affected nerves (also called **herpes zoster** [Figure 15-11])
stroke (strōk)	occurs when there is an interruption of blood supply to a region of the brain, depriving nerve cells in the affected area of oxygen and nutrients. The cells cannot perform and may be damaged or die within minutes. The parts of the body controlled by the involved cells will experience dysfunction. Speech, movement, memory, and other CNS functions may be affected in varying degrees. **Ischemic stroke** is a result of a blocked blood vessel. **Hemorrhagic stroke** is a result of bleeding. (also called **cerebrovascular accident [CVA],** or **brain attack** [Figure 15-12])

Term	Definition
subarachnoid hemorrhage (*sub*-e-RAK-noid) (HEM-o-rij)	bleeding caused by a ruptured blood vessel just outside the brain (usually a ruptured cerebral aneurysm) that rapidly fills the space between the brain and skull (subarachnoid space) with blood. The patient may experience an intense, sudden headache accompanied by nausea, vomiting, and neck pain (a cause of **hemorrhagic stroke**) (Figure 15-12).
transient ischemic attack (TIA) (TRAN-sē-ent) (is-KĒ-mik) (a-TAK)	sudden deficient supply of blood to the brain lasting a short time. The symptoms may be similar to those of stroke, but with TIA the symptoms are temporary and the usual outcome is complete recovery. TIAs are often warning signs for eventual occurrence of a stroke (Figure 15-13).

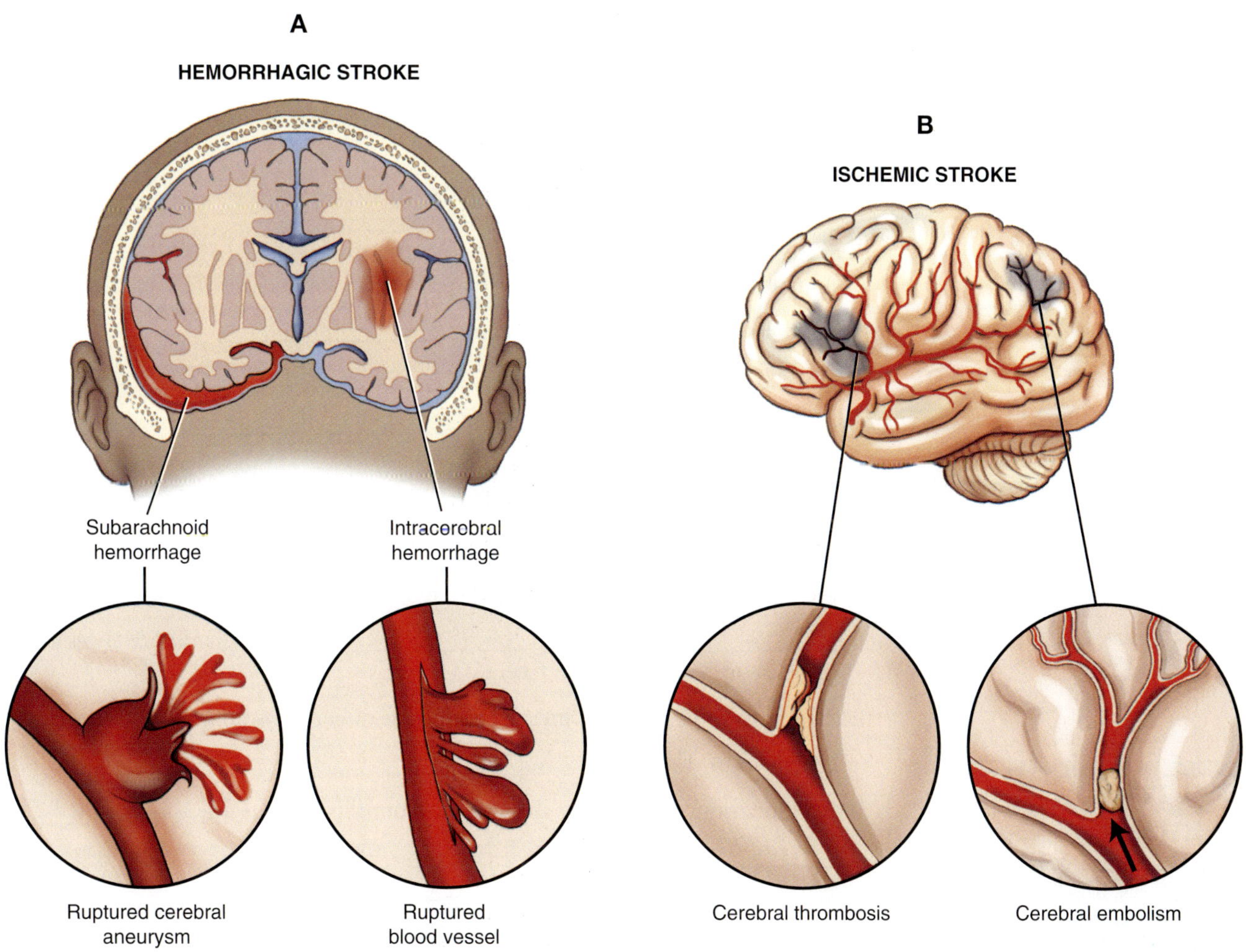

FIGURE 15-12

Causes of stroke. **A,** Hemorrhagic stroke is the result of bleeding caused by a **subarachnoid hemorrhage** or an **intracerebral hemorrhage,** usually a result of a ruptured cerebral aneurysm or ruptured blood vessel. **B,** Ischemic stroke is the result of a blocked blood vessel caused by a **cerebral thrombosis** or **cerebral embolism.**

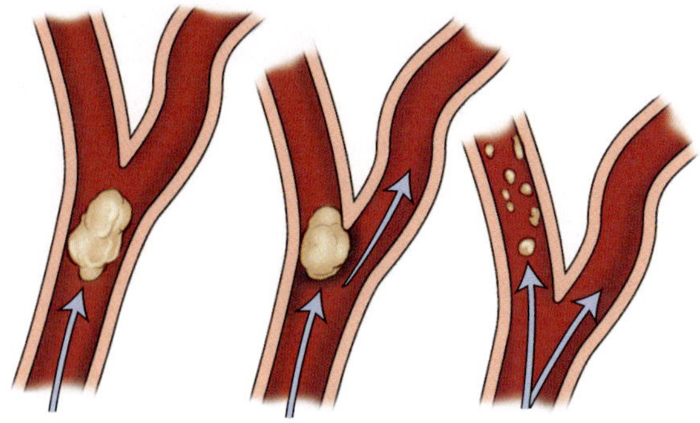

FIGURE 15-13
Transient ischemic attack (TIA).

EXERCISE 13

Practice saying aloud each of the disease and disorder terms not built from word parts on pp. 710-713.

To hear the terms, go to http://evolve.elsevier.com. Refer to p. 18 for your Evolve Access Information. Select Exercises & Review, Chapter 15, Chapter Exercises, Pronunciation.

☐ Place a check mark in the box when you have completed this exercise.

EXERCISE 14

Fill in the blanks with correct terms.

1. A stroke occurs when there is a disruption of blood supply to a region of the brain. Four causes of stroke are a) ______________________ ______________________, b) ______________________ ______________________, c) ______________________ ______________________, and d) ______________________ ______________________.
2. A ruptured ______________________ ______________________ is often the cause of a subarachnoid hemorrhage.
3. ______________________ ______________________ is the paralysis of muscles on one side of the face.
4. The term to describe an increased amount of cerebrospinal fluid in the ventricles of the brain is ______________________.
5. Inflammation of the nerve that travels from the thigh to the toes is called ______________________.
6. A viral disease that affects peripheral nerves is ______________________.
7. The symptoms of a ______________________ ______________________ ______________________ are similar to a stroke but temporary and the patient usually experiences complete recovery.
8. A degenerative disease of the nervous system usually occurring after the age of 50 years is called ______________________ ______________________.

> **PARKINSON DISEASE**
> is also called **parkinsonism, paralysis agitans,** and **shaking palsy.** Since James Parkinson, an English professor, described the disease in 1817 in his *Essay on the Shaking Palsy,* it has often been referred to as **Parkinson disease.**

9. A condition with the main symptom being recurring seizures is ______________________.

10. ______________________ ______________________ ______________________ is caused by degeneration and scarring of the nerve tissue along the lateral columns of the spinal cord.

11. ______________________ ______________________ is characterized by early dementia, confusion, impaired memory, and loss of recognition.

12. ______________________ ______________________ is characterized by lack of muscle coordination and partial paralysis and is present at birth or shortly after.

13. A disease characterized by sclerotic patches along the brain and spinal cord is called ______________________ ______________________.

14. A type of cognitive impairment that is not considered part of normal aging is called ______________________.

EXERCISE 15

Match the diseases in the first column with the corresponding phrases in the second column.

______ 1. cerebral embolism
______ 2. sciatica
______ 3. transient ischemic attack
______ 4. Parkinson disease
______ 5. cerebral palsy
______ 6. hydrocephalus
______ 7. dementia
______ 8. stroke
______ 9. Alzheimer disease
______ 10. intracerebral hemorrhage
______ 11. epilepsy
______ 12. multiple sclerosis
______ 13. shingles
______ 14. amyotrophic lateral sclerosis
______ 15. Bell palsy
______ 16. cerebral aneurysm
______ 17. subarachnoid hemorrhage

a. causes pain from the thigh to the toes
b. blocking of a cerebral artery by a blood clot or plaque
c. paralysis of muscles on one side of the face
d. sclerotic patches scattered along the brain and spinal cord
e. cognitive impairment
f. aneurysm in the cerebrum
g. occurs when there is an interruption of blood supply to the brain
h. blisters on the skin
i. disease charaterized by early dementia
j. resting tremors of the hands and feet and rigidity
k. inflammation of the spinal cord
l. lack of muscle control
m. bleeding within the brain tissue
n. deficient supply of blood to the brain
o. also called Lou Gehrig disease
p. increased amount of cerebrospinal fluid in the ventricles of the brain
q. recurring seizures
r. bleeding that fills space between the brain and skull

EXERCISE 16

Spell each of the disease and disorder terms not built from word parts on pp. 710-713 by having someone dictate them to you.

To hear and spell the terms, go to http://evolve.elsevier.com. Refer to p. 18 for your Evolve Access Information. Select Exercises & Review, Chapter 15, Chapter Exercises, Spelling.
☐ Place a check mark in the box if you have completed this exercise online.

1. ______________________
2. ______________________
3. ______________________
4. ______________________
5. ______________________
6. ______________________
7. ______________________
8. ______________________
9. ______________________
10. ______________________
11. ______________________
12. ______________________
13. ______________________
14. ______________________
15. ______________________
16. ______________________
17. ______________________

EXERCISE FIGURE C

Fill in the blanks to complete labeling of this diagram.

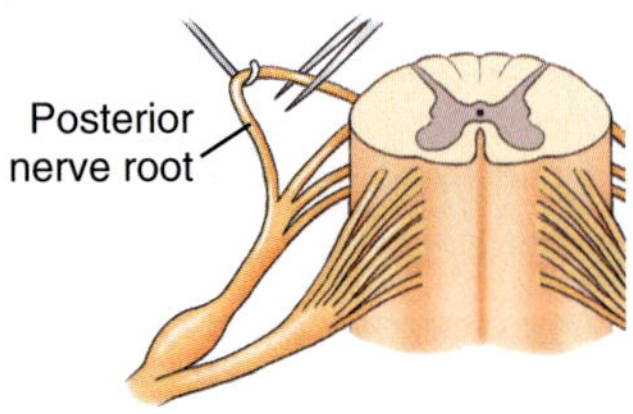

______ / ______ / ______
nerve root / cv / incision

OR

______ / ______ / ______
nerve root / cv / incision

after posterior laminectomy

Surgical Terms

Built from Word Parts

The following terms are built from word parts you have already learned and can be translated literally to find their meanings. Further explanation of terms beyond the definition of their word parts, if needed, is included in parentheses.

Term	Definition
ganglionectomy (*gang*-glē-o-NEK-to-mē)	excision of a ganglion (also called **gangliectomy**)
neurectomy (nū-REK-to-mē)	excision of a nerve
neurolysis (nū-ROL-i-sis)	separating a nerve (from adhesions)
neuroplasty (NŪR-ō-*plas*-tē)	surgical repair of a nerve
neurorrhaphy (nū-ROR-a-fē)	suture of a nerve
neurotomy (nū-ROT-o-mē)	incision into a nerve
radicotomy, rhizotomy (*rad*-i-KOT-o-mē) (rī-ZOT-o-mē)	incision into a nerve root (Exercise Figure C)

EXERCISE 17

Practice saying aloud each of the surgical terms built from word parts on p. 716.

To hear the terms, go to http://evolve.elsevier.com. Refer to p. 18 for your Evolve Access Information. Select Exercises & Review, Chapter 15, Chapter Exercises, Pronunciation.

☐ Place a check mark in the box when you have completed this exercise.

EXERCISE 18

Analyze and define the following surgical terms.

1. radicotomy ______
2. neurectomy ______
3. neurorrhaphy ______
4. ganglionectomy ______
5. neurotomy ______
6. neurolysis ______
7. neuroplasty ______
8. rhizotomy ______

EXERCISE 19

Build surgical terms for the following definitions by using the word parts you have learned.

1. incision into a nerve root
   a. ______ / ______ / ______
   WR / CV / S
   b. ______ / ______ / ______
   WR / CV / S
2. excision of a nerve ______ / ______
   WR / S
3. suture of a nerve ______ / ______ / ______
   WR / CV / S
4. excision of a ganglion ______ / ______
   WR / S
5. incision into a nerve ______ / ______ / ______
   WR / CV / S

STEREOTACTIC RADIOSURGERY

is used to treat patients with **brain tumors or arteriovenous malformations (AVMs).** A special frame is mounted on the patient's head. Images of the brain are produced by MRI. A high-powered computer uses the images to design a plan for high-intensity radiation that matches the exact size and shape of the tumor. Radiation is then delivered directly to the tumor only, sparing surrounding tissue. This procedure may also be called **Gamma-knife radiosurgery**.

6. separating a nerve (from adhesions) ____ / CV / ____
   WR / CV / S

7. surgical repair of a nerve ____ / CV / ____
   WR / CV / S

EXERCISE 20

Spell each of the surgical terms built from word parts on p. 716 by having someone dictate them to you.

To hear and spell the terms, go to http://evolve.elsevier.com. Refer to p. 18 for your Evolve Access Information. Select Exercises & Review, Chapter 15, Chapter Exercises, Spelling.

☐ Place a check mark in the box if you have completed this exercise online.

1. ____________________
2. ____________________
3. ____________________
4. ____________________
5. ____________________
6. ____________________
7. ____________________
8. ____________________

Diagnostic Terms

Built from Word Parts

The following terms are built from word parts you have already learned and can be translated literally to find their meanings. Further explanation of terms beyond the definition of their word parts, if needed, is included in parentheses.

Term	Definition
DIAGNOSTIC IMAGING	
cerebral angiography (se-RĒ-bral) (*an*-jē-OG-ra-fē)	radiographic imaging of the blood vessels in the brain (after an injection of contrast medium)
CT myelography (*mī*-e-LOG-ra-fē)	process of recording (scan) the spinal cord (after an injection of a contrast agent into the subarachnoid space by lumbar puncture. Size, shape, and position of the spinal cord and nerve roots are demonstrated.) (Exercise Figure D)
NEURODIAGNOSTIC PROCEDURES	
electroencephalogram (EEG) (ē-*lek*-trō-en-SEF-a-lō-gram)	record of the electrical impulses of the brain
electroencephalograph (ē-*lek*-trō-en-SEF-a-lō-graf)	instrument used to record the electrical impulses of the brain
electroencephalography (ē-*lek*-trō-en-*sef*-a-LOG-ra-fē)	process of recording the electrical impulses of the brain

EXERCISE FIGURE D

Fill in the blanks to complete labeling of the diagram.

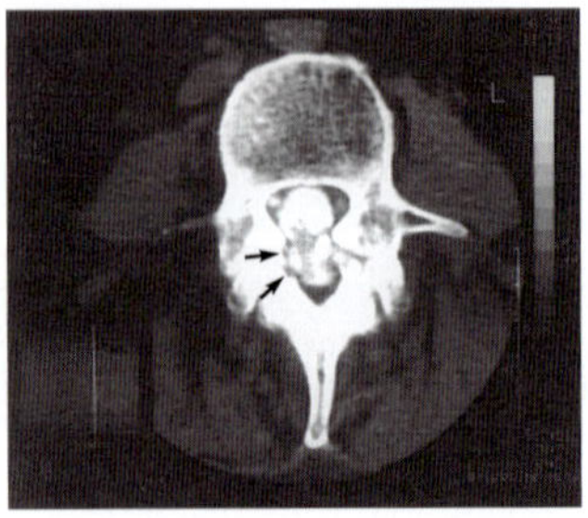

CT ____ / cv / ____
spinal cord / cv / process of recording

EXERCISE 21

Practice saying aloud each of the diagnostic terms built from word parts on p. 718.

To hear the terms, go to http://evolve.elsevier.com. Refer to p. 18 for your Evolve Access Information. Select Exercises & Review, Chapter 15, Chapter Exercises, Pronunciation.

☐ Place a check mark in the box when you have completed this exercise.

EXERCISE 22

Analyze and define the following diagnostic terms.

1. electroencephalogram ______________________
2. electroencephalograph ______________________
3. electroencephalography ______________________
4. CT myelography ______________________
5. cerebral angiography ______________________

EXERCISE 23

Build diagnostic terms that correspond to the following definitions by using the word parts you have learned.

1. record of the electrical impulses of the brain
   ______ / ___ / ______ / ___ / ______
   WR / CV / WR / CV / S

2. instrument used for recording the electrical impulses of the brain
   ______ / ___ / ______ / ___ / ______
   WR / CV / WR / CV / S

3. process of recording the electrical impulses of the brain
   ______ / ___ / ______ / ___ / ______
   WR / CV / WR / CV / S

4. process of recording (scan) the spinal cord
   CT ______ / ___ / ______
   WR / CV / S

5. radiographic imaging of the blood vessels in the brain
   ______ / ______ ______ / ___ / ______
   WR / S WR / CV / S

EXERCISE 24

Spell each of the diagnostic terms built from word parts on p. 718 by having someone dictate them to you.

To hear and spell the terms, go to http://evolve.elsevier.com. Refer to p. 18 for your Evolve Access Information. Select Exercises & Review, Chapter 15, Chapter Exercises, Spelling.

☐ Place a check mark in the box if you have completed this exercise online.

1. ______________________
2. ______________________
3. ______________________
4. ______________________
5. ______________________

Diagnostic Terms

Not Built from Word Parts

Term	Definition
DIAGNOSTIC IMAGING	
computed tomography of the brain (CT scan) (com-PŪ-td) (tō-MOG-ra-fē)	process that includes the use of a computer to produce a series of brain tissue images at any desired depth. The procedure is painless and particularly useful in diagnosing brain tumors (Figure 15-14).
magnetic resonance imaging of the brain or spine (MRI scan) (mag-NET-ik) (REZ-ō-nans) (IM-a-jing)	a noninvasive technique that produces sectional images of soft tissues of the brain or spine through a strong magnetic field. Unlike a CT scan, MRI produces images without use of radiation. It is used to visualize tumors, edema, multiple sclerosis, and herniated disks (Figure 15-15).

The **first full-scale CT unit** for head scanning was installed in a hospital in **Wimbledon,** United Kingdom in **1971**. Its ability to provide neurological diagnostic information gained rapid recognition. The first units in the **United States** were used in **1973**. The first scanner for visualizing sections of the body other than the brain was developed in **1974** by Dr. Robert Ledly at Georgetown University Medical Center.

A **magnetic resonance imaging (MRI) scanner** was first used in the **United States in 1981**. The scanner was developed in England and installed there in 1975.

A

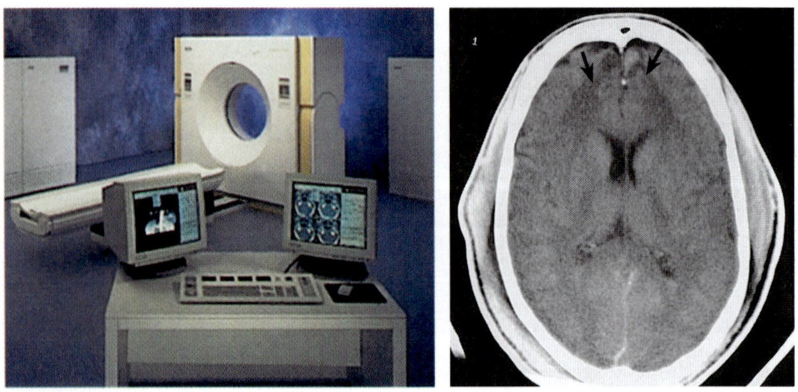

B

FIGURE 15-14

A, CT scanner. **B,** CT scan of the brain demonstrating bilateral temporal lobe brain contusions *(arrows)* caused by trauma.

Term	Definition
positron emission tomography of the brain (PET scan) (POZ-i-tron) (ē-MISH-un) (tō-MOG-ra-fē)	nuclear medicine imaging technique with a radioactive substance that produces sectional imaging of the brain to examine blood flow and metabolic activity. Images are projected on a viewing screen (Figure 15-16).
NEURODIAGNOSTIC PROCEDURES	
evoked potential studies (EP studies) (i-VŌKD) (pō-TEN-shal)	a group of diagnostic tests that measure changes and responses in brain waves elicited by visual, auditory, or somatosensory stimuli. Visual evoked response (VER) is a response to visual stimuli. Auditory evoked response (AER) is a response to auditory stimuli.
OTHER	
lumbar puncture (LP) (LUM-bar) (PUNK-chur)	insertion of a needle into the subarachnoid space usually between the third and fourth lumbar vertebrae. It is performed for many reasons, including the removal of cerebrospinal fluid for diagnostic purposes (also called **spinal tap**) (Figure 15-17).

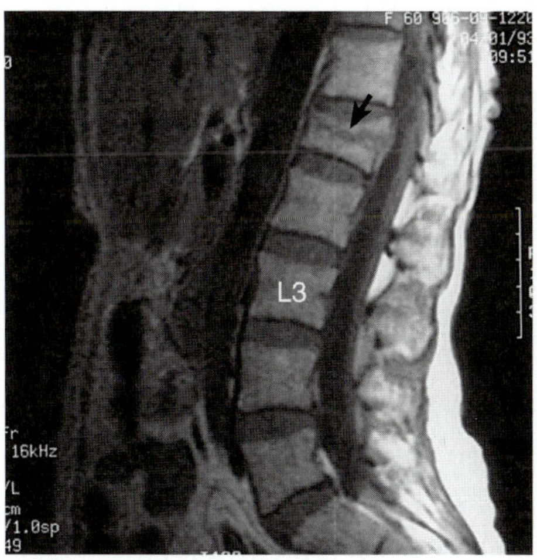

FIGURE 15-15
Sagittal MRI section of the lumbar spine demonstrating a compression fracture of L1 caused by trauma. (arrow)

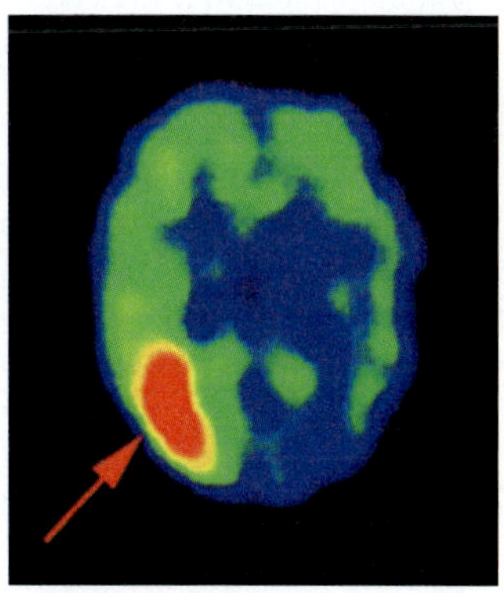

FIGURE 15-16
Positron emission tomography (PET) brain scan of an infant with seizures. The arrow points to the area of increased brain metabolism, indicating the seizure focus.

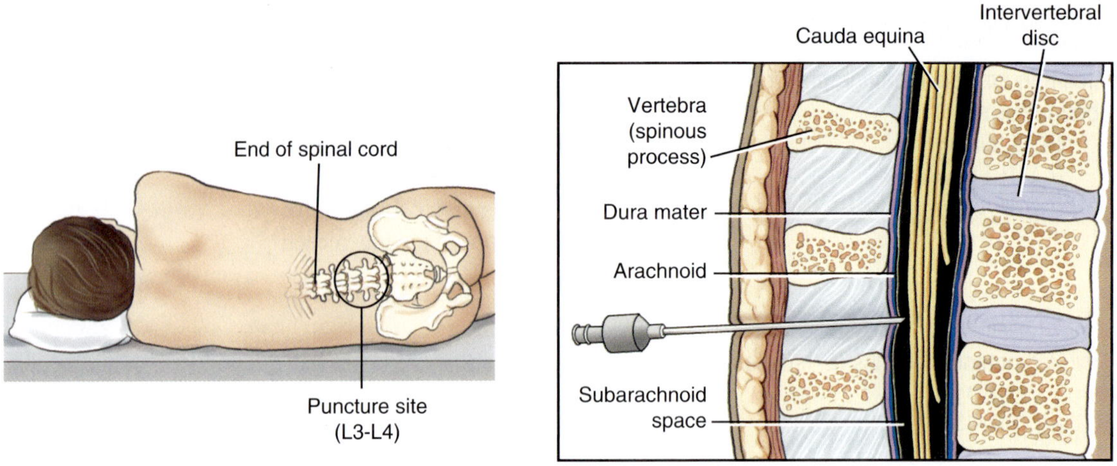

FIGURE 15-17
Lumbar puncture (spinal tap).

EXERCISE 25

Practice saying aloud each of the diagnostic terms not built from word parts on pp. 720-721.

To hear the terms, go to http://evolve.elsevier.com. Refer to p. 18 for your Evolve Access Information. Select Exercises & Review, Chapter 15, Chapter Exercises, Pronunciation.

☐ Place a check mark in the box when you have completed this exercise.

EXERCISE 26

Fill in the blanks with the correct terms.

1. A computer is used to produce images during ______________________ ______________________ of the brain.
2. A needle is inserted into the subarachnoid space during a(n) ______________________ ______________________.
3. ______________________ ______________________ ______________________ produces images to examine blood flow and metabolic activity of the brain.
4. Uses a strong magnetic field to produce images of the brain or spine: ______________________ ______________________ ______________________.
5. Measures responses in brain waves from stimuli: ______________________ ______________________ ______________________.

EXERCISE 27

Write the definitions of the following terms.

1. lumbar puncture ____

____

2. computed tomography of the brain ______________________________

____

3. magnetic resonance imaging of the brain or spine ________________

____

4. positron emission tomography of the brain ______________________

____

5. evoked potential studies ______________________________________

____

EXERCISE 28

Spell each of the diagnostic terms not built from word parts on pp. 720-721 by having someone dictate them to you.

To hear and spell the terms, go to http://evolve.elsevier.com. Refer to p. 18 for your Evolve Access Information. Select Exercises & Review, Chapter 15, Chapter Exercises, Spelling.
☐ Place a check mark in the box if you have completed this exercise online.

1. ______________________ 4. ______________________
2. ______________________ 5. ______________________
3. ______________________

Complementary Terms

Built from Word Parts

The following terms are built from word parts you have already learned and can be translated literally to find their meanings. Further explanation of terms beyond the definition of their word parts, if needed, is included in parentheses.

Term	Definition
anesthesia (*an*-es-THĒ-zha)	without (loss of) feeling or sensation
aphasia (a-FĀ-zha)	condition of without speaking (loss or impairment of the ability to speak)
cephalalgia (*sef*-el-AL-ja)	pain in the head (headache) (also called **cephalgia**)
cerebral (se-RĒ-bral)	pertaining to the cerebrum
craniocerebral (*krā*-nē-ō-su-RĒ-bral)	pertaining to the cranium and cerebrum
dysphasia (dis-FĀ-zha)	condition of difficulty speaking

HEADACHES

Migraine, tension headache, and **cluster** headaches account for nearly 90% of all headaches. Other types of headaches include **posttraumatic headaches, giant cell (temporal) arteritis, sinus headaches, brain tumor, and chronic daily headache.**

EXERCISE FIGURE E

Fill in the blanks to complete labeling of these diagrams of types of paralysis.

1
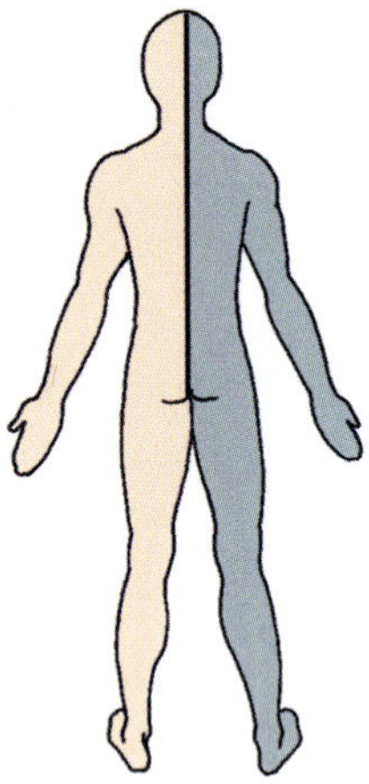

1. ______ / ______
half / paralysis

2
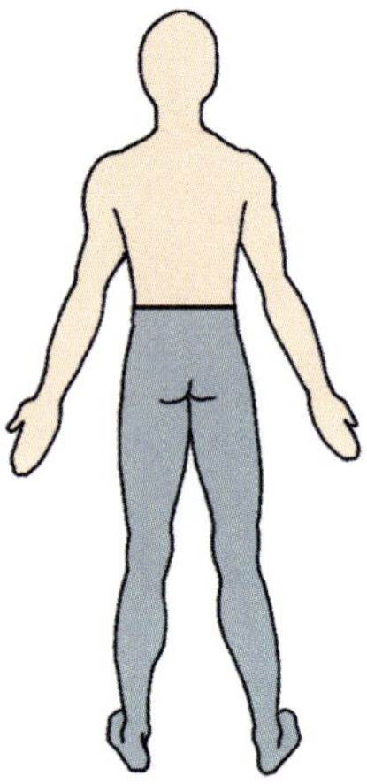

2. Paraplegia

3
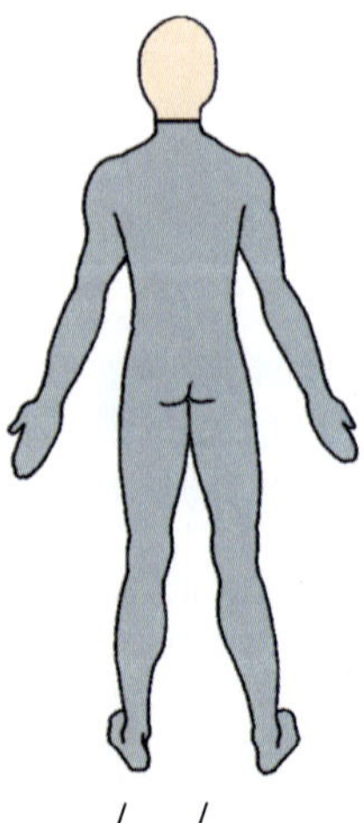

3. ______ / ______ / ______
four / cv / paralysis

Complementary Terms—*cont'd*

Built from Word Parts

Term	Definition
encephalosclerosis (en-*sef*-a-lō-skle-RŌ-sis)	hardening of the brain
gliocyte (GLI-ō-sīt)	glial cell
hemiparesis (*hem*-ē-pa-RĒ-sis)	slight paralysis of half (right or left side of the body)
hemiplegia (*hem*-ē-PLĒ-ja)	paralysis of half (right or left side of the body); stroke is the most common cause of hemiplegia (Exercise Figure E)
hyperesthesia (*hī*-per-es-THĒ-zha)	excessive sensitivity (to stimuli)
interictal (*in*-ter-IK-tal)	(occurring) between seizures or attacks
intracerebral (*in*-tra-SER-e-bral)	pertaining to within the cerebrum
mental (MEN-tel)	pertaining to the mind
monoparesis (*mon*-ō-pa-RĒ-sis)	slight paralysis of one (limb)
monoplegia (*mon*-ō-PLĒ-ja)	paralysis of one (limb)
myelomalacia (*mī*-e-lō-ma-LĀ-sha)	softening of the spinal cord
neuroid (NŪ-royd)	resembling a nerve
neurologist (nū-ROL-o-jist)	physician who studies and treats diseases of the nerves (nervous system)
neurology (nū-ROL-o-jē)	study of nerves (branch of medicine dealing with diseases of the nervous system)
panplegia (pan-PLĒ-ja)	total paralysis (also spelled **pamplegia**)
paresthesia (*par*-es-THĒ-zha) (Note: the *a* is dropped from the prefix *para*)	abnormal sensation (such as burning, prickling, or tingling sensation, often in the extremities; may be caused by nerve damage or peripheral neuropathy)
postictal (pōst-IK-tal)	(occurring) after a seizure or attack
preictal (prē-IK-tal)	(occurring) before a seizure or attack
quadriplegia (*kwod*-ri-PLĒ-ja)	paralysis of four (limbs) (see Exercise Figure E)
subdural (sub-DŪ-ral)	pertaining to below the dura mater

EXERCISE 29

Practice saying aloud each of the complementary terms built from word parts on pp. 723-724.

To hear the terms, go to http://evolve.elsevier.com. Refer to p. 18 for your Evolve Access Information. Select Exercises & Review, Chapter 15, Chapter Exercises, Pronunciation.

☐ Place a check mark in the box when you have completed this exercise.

EXERCISE 30

Analyze and define the following complementary terms.

1. hemiplegia ______
2. paresthesia ______
3. neurologist ______
4. neurology ______
5. neuroid ______
6. quadriplegia ______
7. cerebral ______
8. monoplegia ______
9. aphasia ______
10. dysphasia ______
11. hemiparesis ______
12. anesthesia ______
13. hyperesthesia ______
14. subdural ______
15. cephalalgia ______
16. craniocerebral ______
17. myelomalacia ______
18. encephalosclerosis ______
19. postictal ______
20. panplegia ______
21. interictal ______
22. monoparesis ______
23. preictal ______
24. intracerebral ______
25. gliocyte ______
26. mental ______

EXERCISE 31

Build the complementary terms for the following definitions by using the word parts you have learned.

1. slight paralysis of half (right or left side of the body)
   ______ P / ______ S(WR)
2. without (loss of) feeling or sensation
   ______ P / ______ WR / ______ S
3. excessive sensitivity (to stimuli)
   ______ P / ______ WR / ______ S
4. pertaining to below the dura mater
   ______ P / ______ WR / ______ S
5. pain in the head (headache)
   ______ WR / ______ S
6. pertaining to the cranium and cerebrum
   ______ WR / CV / ______ WR / ______ S
7. softening of the spinal cord
   ______ WR / CV / ______ S
8. hardening of the brain
   ______ WR / CV / ______ S
9. paralysis of half (left or right side) of the body
   ______ P / ______ S(WR)
10. physician who studies and treats diseases of the nervous system
    ______ WR / CV / ______ S
11. study of nerves (branch of medicine dealing with diseases of the nervous system)
    ______ WR / CV / ______ S
12. resembling a nerve
    ______ WR / ______ S

13. paralysis of four (limbs) ______ / ______ / ______
WR / CV / S

14. pertaining to the cerebrum ______ / ______
WR / S

15. paralysis of one (limb) ______ / ______ / ______
WR / CV / S

16. condition of without speaking (loss or impairment of the ability to speak) ______ / ______ / ______
P / WR / S

17. condition of difficulty speaking ______ / ______ / ______
P / WR / S

18. (occurring) before a seizure or attack ______ / ______
P / S(WR)

19. slight paralysis of one (limb) ______ / ______ / ______
WR / CV / S

20. (occurring) after a seizure ______ / ______
P / S(WR)

21. total paralysis ______ / ______
P / S(WR)

22. (occurring) between seizures or attacks ______ / ______
P / S(WR)

23. pertaining to within the cerebrum ______ / ______ / ______
P / WR / S

24. glial cell ______ / ______ / ______
WR / CV / S

25. abnormal sensation ______ / ______ / ______
P / WR / S

26. pertaining to the mind ______ / ______
WR / S

EXERCISE 32

Spell each of the complementary terms built from word parts on pp. 723-724 by having someone dictate them to you.

To hear and spell the terms, go to http://evolve.elsevier.com. Refer to p. 18 for your Evolve Access Information. Select Exercises & Review, Chapter 15, Chapter Exercises, Spelling.

☐ Place a check mark in the box if you have completed this exercise online.

1.	________	14.	________
2.	________	15.	________
3.	________	16.	________
4.	________	17.	________
5.	________	18.	________
6.	________	19.	________
7.	________	20.	________
8.	________	21.	________
9.	________	22.	________
10.	________	23.	________
11.	________	24.	________
12.	________	25.	________
13.	________	26.	________

TYPES OF COGNITIVE IMPAIRMENT

Mild cognitive impairment (MCI) is the presence of significant memory difficulty when adjusted for age-related norms. The patient usually has little difficulty performing activities of daily living. This condition may be an early manifestation of Alzheimer disease.

Age-associated memory impairment is when memory function tends to decline with aging when compared with young adults. This is not necessarily a forerunner of dementia.

Delirium is potentially reversible acute disturbance of consciousness with impairment of cognition. A number of conditions can cause delirium by interfering with brain metabolism. Drugs, alcohol, systemic infections, head trauma, hypoglycemia, and electrolyte disturbances are common examples.

Pseudodementia is a disorder resembling dementia but is not caused by a brain disease. This can be found in mental illness, such as major depression, and can be reversible with treatment.

Complementary Terms

Not Built from Word Parts

In some of the following terms you may recognize word parts you have already learned; however, the full meaning of the terms cannot be discerned by the definition of their word parts.

Term	Definition
afferent (AF-er-ent)	conveying toward a center (for example, afferent nerves carry impulses to the central nervous system)
ataxia (a-TAK-sē-a)	lack of muscle coordination
cognitive (COG-ni-tiv)	pertaining to the mental processes of comprehension, judgment, memory, and reason
coma (KŌ-ma)	state of profound unconsciousness

Term	Definition
concussion (kon-KUSH-un)	injury to the brain caused by major or minor head trauma; symptoms include vertigo, headache, and possible loss of consciousness
conscious (KON-shus)	awake, alert, aware of one's surroundings
convulsion (kun-VUL-zhun)	sudden, involuntary contraction of a group of muscles; may be present during a seizure
disorientation (dis-*or*-ē-en-TĀ-shun)	a state of mental confusion as to time, place, or identity
dysarthria (dis-AR-thrē-a)	the inability to use speech that is distinct and connected because of a loss of muscle control after damage to the peripheral or central nervous system
efferent (EF-er-ent)	conveying away from the center (for example, efferent nerves carry information away from the central nervous system)
gait (gāt)	a manner or style of walking
incoherent (*in*-kō-HĒR-ent)	unable to express one's thoughts or ideas in an orderly, intelligible manner
paraplegia (*par* a PLĒ ja)	paralysis from the waist down caused by damage to the lower level of the spinal cord (see Exercise Figure E)
seizure (SĒ-zher)	sudden surge of abnormal electrical activity in the brain, resulting in involuntary body movements or behaviors
shunt (shunt)	tube implanted in the body to redirect the flow of a fluid
syncope (SINK-o-pē)	fainting or sudden loss of consciousness caused by lack of blood supply to the cerebrum
unconsciousness (un-KON-shus-nes)	state of being unaware of surroundings and incapable of responding to stimuli as a result of injury, shock, illness, or drugs

PARAPLEGIA

is composed of the Greek **para**, meaning **beside**, and **plegia**, meaning **paralysis**. It has been used since Hippocrates' time and at first meant paralysis of any limb or side of the body. Since the nineteenth century, it has been used to mean paralysis from the waist down.

EXERCISE 33

Practice saying aloud each of the complementary terms not built from word parts on pp. 728-729.

To hear the terms, go to http://evolve.elsevier.com. Refer to p. 18 for your Evolve Access Information. Select Exercises & Review, Chapter 15, Chapter Exercises, Pronunciation.

☐ Place a check mark in the box when you have completed this exercise.

EXERCISE 34

Write the term for each of the following definitions.

1. injury to the brain caused by head trauma ____________________
2. state of being unaware of surroundings and incapable of responding to stimuli as a result of injury, shock, illness, or drugs ____________________
3. awake, alert, aware of one's surroundings ____________________
4. sudden surge of abnormal electrical activity in the brain ____________________
5. sudden, involuntary contraction of a group of muscles ____________________
6. tube implanted in the body to redirect the flow of a fluid ____________________
7. paralysis from the waist down caused by damage to the lower level of the spinal cord ____________________
8. state of profound unconsciousness ____________________
9. fainting or sudden loss of consciousness ____________________

10. lack of muscle coordination ________________
11. a manner or style of walking ________________
12. inability to use speech that is distinctive and connected ________________
13. unable to express one's thoughts or ideas in an orderly, intelligible manner ________________
14. a state of mental confusion as to time, place, or identity ________________
15. pertaining to the mental processes of comprehension, judgment, memory, and reason ________________
16. conveying toward the center ________________
17. conveying away from the center ________________

EXERCISE 35

Write the definitions for the following terms.

1. shunt ________________
2. paraplegia ________________
3. coma ________________
4. concussion ________________
5. unconsciousness ________________
6. conscious ________________
7. seizure ________________
8. convulsion ________________
9. syncope ________________
10. ataxia ________________
11. dysarthria ________________
12. gait ________________
13. cognitive ________________
14. disorientation ________________
15. incoherent ________________
16. efferent ________________
17. afferent ________________

EXERCISE 36

Spell each of the complementary terms not built from word parts on pp. 728-729 by having someone dictate them to you.

To hear and spell the terms, go to http://evolve.elsevier.com. Refer to p. 18 for your Evolve Access Information. Select Exercises & Review, Chapter 15, Chapter Exercises, Spelling.

☐ Place a check mark in the box if you have completed this exercise online.

1. ____________________
2. ____________________
3. ____________________
4. ____________________
5. ____________________
6. ____________________
7. ____________________
8. ____________________
9. ____________________
10. ____________________
11. ____________________
12. ____________________
13. ____________________
14. ____________________
15. ____________________
16. ____________________
17. ____________________

Behavioral Health

Although the terms below are listed as behavioral health terms, medications, physical changes, substance abuse, and illness may contribute to these conditions.

Built from Word Parts

The following terms are built from word parts you have already learned and can be translated literally to find their meanings. Further explanation of terms beyond the definition of their word parts, if needed, is included in parentheses.

PSYCHIATRIST

is a **physician** who has had **additional training** and experience in prevention, diagnosis, and treatment of mental disorders.

CLINICAL PSYCHOLOGIST

is one who has had **graduate study** in **psychology** and training in clinical psychology and who provides testing and counseling for mental and emotional disorders. A psychologist cannot prescribe medication or medical tests and treatments.

Term	Definition
psychiatrist (sī-KĪ-a-trist)	a physician who studies and treats disorders of the mind
psychiatry (sī-KĪ-a-trē)	specialty of the mind (branch of medicine that deals with the treatment of mental disorders)
psychogenic (sī-*kō*-JEN-ik)	originating in the mind
psychologist (sī-KOL-o-jist)	specialist of the mind
psychology (sī-KOL-o-jē)	study of the mind (a profession that involves dealing with the mind and mental processes in relation to human behavior)

Term	Definition
psychopathy (sī-KOP-a-thē)	(any) disease of the mind
psychosis (*pl.* psychoses) (sī-KO-sis) (sī-KO-sēz)	abnormal condition of the mind (major mental disorder characterized by extreme derangement, often with delusions and hallucinations)
psychosomatic (*sī*-kō-sō-MAT-ik)	pertaining to the mind and body (interrelations of)

EXERCISE 37

Practice saying aloud each of the behavioral health terms built from word parts on these two pages.

To hear the terms, go to http://evolve.elsevier.com. Refer to p. 18 for your Evolve Access Information. Select Exercises & Review, Chapter 15, Chapter Exercises, Pronunciation.

☐ Place a check mark in the box when you have completed this exercise.

EXERCISE 38

Build the behavioral health terms for the following definitions by using the word parts you have learned.

1. specialty of the mind (branch of medicine that deals with the treatment of mental disorders) ________ / ________
   WR / S
2. abnormal condition of the mind ________ / ________
   WR / S
3. study of the mind (a profession that involves dealing with the mind and mental processes in relation to human behavior) ________ / ____ / ________
   WR / CV / S
4. originating in the mind ________ / ____ / ________
   WR / CV / S
5. a physician who studies and treats disorders of the mind ________ / ________
   WR / S

6. specialist of the mind ________ / CV / ________
WR CV S

7. pertaining to the mind and body ________ / CV / ________ / ________
WR CV WR S

8. disease of the mind ________ / CV / ________
WR CV S

EXERCISE 39

Analyze and define the following terms.

1. psychosomatic ____________________
2. psychopathy ____________________
3. psychology ____________________
4. psychiatry ____________________
5. psychologist ____________________
6. psychogenic ____________________
7. psychiatrist ____________________
8. psychosis ____________________

EXERCISE 40

Spell each of the behavioral health terms built from word parts on pp. 732-733 by having someone dictate them to you.

To hear and spell the terms, go to http://evolve.elsevier.com. Refer to p. 18 for your Evolve Access Information. Select Exercises & Review, Chapter 15, Chapter Exercises, Spelling.
☐ Place a check mark in the box if you have completed this exercise online.

1. ____________________
2. ____________________
3. ____________________
4. ____________________
5. ____________________
6. ____________________
7. ____________________
8. ____________________

Behavioral Health

Not Built from Word Parts

In some of the following terms, you may recognize word parts you have already learned; however, the full meaning of the terms cannot be discerned by the definition of their word parts.

Term	Definition
anorexia nervosa (*an*-ō-REK-sē-a) (ner-VŌ-sa)	an eating disorder characterized by a disturbed perception of body image resulting in failure to maintain body weight, intensive fear of gaining weight, pronounced desire for thinness, and, in females, amenorrhea (introduced in Chapter 11)
anxiety disorder (ang-ZĪ-e-tē) (dis-OR-der)	an emotional disorder characterized by feelings of apprehension, tension, or uneasiness arising typically from the anticipation of unreal or imagined danger
attention deficit hyperactivity disorder (ADHD) (a-TEN-shun) (DEF-i-sit) (*hī*-per-ak-TIV-i-tē)	a disorder of learning and behavioral problems characterized by marked inattention, distractability, impulsiveness, and hyperactivity
autism (AW-tizm)	a spectrum of mental disorders, the features of which include onset during infancy or childhood, preoccupation with subjective mental activity, inability to interact socially, and impaired communication (also referred to as **Autism Spectrum Disorders** [ASD] or **Pervasive Developmental Disorders** [PDD])
bipolar disorder (bī-PŌ-lar) (dis-OR-der)	a major psychological disorder typified by a disturbance in mood. The disorder is manifested by manic and depressive episodes that may alternate or elements of both may occur simultaneously.
bulimia nervosa (bū-LĒ-mē-a) (ner-VŌ-sa)	an eating disorder characterized by uncontrolled binge eating followed by purging (induced vomiting) (introduced in Chapter 11)
major depression (MĀ-jor) (dē-PRESH-un)	a mood disturbance characterized by feelings of sadness, despair, discouragement, hopelessness, lack of joy, altered sleep patterns, and difficulty with decision making and daily function. Depression ranges from normal feelings of sadness (resulting from and proportional to personal loss or tragedy), through dysthymia (chronic depressive neurosis), to major depression (also referred to as **clinical depression, mood disorder**).

CAM TERM

Music therapy is the use of music within a therapeutic relationship to address physical, emotional, cognitive, and social needs of individuals. Current research suggests that music therapy is an effective modality for reducing the **anxiety, stress,** and **pain** often associated with medical procedures, as well as improving activation of the motor cortex after a stroke.

Behavioral Health—*cont'd*

Not Built from Word Parts

Term	Definition
obsessive-compulsive disorder (OCD) (ob-SES-iv-kom-PUL-siv) (dis-OR-der)	a disorder characterized by intrusive, unwanted thoughts that result in the tendency to perform repetitive acts or rituals (compulsions), usually as a means of releasing tension or anxiety
panic attack (PAN-ik) (a-TAK)	an episode of sudden onset of acute anxiety, occurring unpredictably, with feelings of acute apprehension, dyspnea, dizziness, sweating, and/or chest pain, depersonalization, paresthesia and fear of dying, loss of mind or control
phobia (FŌ-bē-a)	a marked and persistent fear that is excessive or unreasonable cued by the presence or anticipation of a specific situation or object (such as claustrophobia, the abnormal fear of being in enclosed spaces)
pica (PĪ-ka)	compulsive eating of nonnutritive substances such as clay or ice. This condition is often a result of an iron deficiency. When iron deficiency is the cause of pica the condition will disappear in 1 or 2 weeks when treated with iron therapy.
posttraumatic stress disorder (PTSD) (*pōst*-tra-MAT-ik) (stres) (dis-OR-der)	a disorder characterized by an acute emotional response to a traumatic event perceived as life threatening or severe emotional stress such as an airplane crash, repeated physical or emotional trauma, or military combat. Symptoms include anxiety, sleep disturbance, nightmares, difficulty concentrating, and depression.
schizophrenia (*skit*-sō-FRĒ-nē-a)	any one of a large group of psychotic disorders characterized by gross distortions of reality, disturbance of language and communication, withdrawal from social interaction, and the disorganization and fragmentation of thought, perception, and emotional reaction
somatoform disorders (sō-MAT-ō-form)	disorders characterized by physical symptoms for which no known physical cause exists

Refer to **Appendix D** for pharmacology terms related to the nervous system and behavioral health.

To learn more behavioral health terms, go to http://evolve.elsevier.com. Refer to p. 18 for your Evolve Access Information. Select **Appendices, Appendix H, Behavioral Health Terms.**

EXERCISE 41

Practice saying aloud each of the behavioral health terms not built from word parts on pp. 735-736.

To hear the terms, go to http://evolve.elsevier.com. Refer to p. 18 for your Evolve Access Information. Select Exercises & Review, Chapter 15, Chapter Exercises, Pronunciation.

☐ Place a check mark in the box when you have completed the exercise.

EXERCISE 42

Match the definitions in the first column with the correct terms in the second column.

_____ 1. manifested by manic and depressive episodes

_____ 2. an episode of acute anxiety

_____ 3. characterized by feelings of apprehension and tension

_____ 4. a disorder of learning and behavioral problems

_____ 5. a mood disturbance characterized by feelings of sadness, despair, and discouragement

_____ 6. a marked and persistent fear that is excessive or unreasonable

_____ 7. binge eating followed by purging

_____ 8. physical symptoms for which no known physical cause exists

_____ 9. eating of nonnutritive substances, such as ice

_____ 10. failure to maintain body weight

_____ 11. characterized by gross distortions of reality and disturbance of language and communication

_____ 12. preoccupation with subjective mental activity, inability to interact socially, and impaired communication

_____ 13. acute emotional response to a traumatic event

_____ 14. intrusive unwanted thoughts that result in rituals and/or repetitive acts

a. phobia

b. anxiety disorder

c. attention deficit hyperactivity disorder

d. somatoform disorders

e. schizophrenia

f. anorexia nervosa

g. bulimia nervosa

h. pica

i. bipolar disorder

j. major depression

k. obsessive-compulsive disorder

l. posttraumatic stress disorder

m. panic attack

n. autism

EXERCISE 43

Spell each of the behavioral health terms not built from word parts on pp. 735-736 by having someone dictate them to you.

To hear and spell the terms, go to http://evolve.elsevier.com. Refer to p. 18 for your Evolve Access Information. Select Exercises & Review, Chapter 15, Chapter Exercises, Spelling.
☐ Place a check mark in the box if you have completed this exercise online.

1. ______________________ 8. ______________________
2. ______________________ 9. ______________________
3. ______________________ 10. ______________________
4. ______________________ 11. ______________________
5. ______________________ 12. ______________________
6. ______________________ 13. ______________________
7. ______________________ 14. ______________________

Abbreviations

AD	Alzheimer disease
ADHD	attention deficit hyperactivity disorder
ALS	amyotrophic lateral sclerosis
CNS	central nervous system
CP	cerebral palsy
CSF	cerebrospinal fluid
CVA	cerebrovascular accident
EEG	electroencephalogram
EP studies	evoked potential studies
LP	lumbar puncture
MRI scan	magnetic resonance imaging scan
MS	multiple sclerosis
OCD	obsessive-compulsive disorder
PD	Parkinson disease
PET scan	positron emission tomography scan
PNS	peripheral nervous system
PTSD	posttraumatic stress disorder
TIA	transient ischemic attack

Refer to **Appendix C** for a complete list of abbreviations.

EXERCISE 44

Write the meaning of the abbreviations in the following sentences.

1. Diagnostic tests used to diagnose patients with diseases of the nervous system include **EEG** ____________________________, **MRI scan** ________________ ________________ ________________ ________________, **PET scan** ________________ ________________ ________________ ________________, **EP studies** ________________ ________________ ________________, and **LP** ________________ ________________.
2. Diseases that affect the nervous system are **AD** ________________ ________________, **ALS** ________________ ________________ ________________, **CP** ________________ ________________, **MS** ________________ ________________, and **PD** ________________ ________________.
3. Stroke is the disruption of normal blood supply to the brain. It often occurs suddenly. Because of this, Hippocrates used the term *apoplexy*, which literally means *struck down*, to describe the condition. The term *stroke* grew out of the term *apoplexy*. The term *brain attack* is a fairly new term used to signify that a stroke is in progress and an emergency situation exists. **CVA** ________________ ________________ is also used to describe a stroke. An ischemic stroke, which is caused by a thrombosis or embolus, is frequently preceded by a **TIA** ________________ ________________ ________________.
4. The examination of **CSF** ____________________________ ________________ may assist in the diagnosis of cerebral hemorrhage, meningitis, encephalitis, and other diseases.
5. Three common psychiatric disorders are **PTSD**, ____________________________ ________________ ________________, **OCD** ____________________________ ______________________________________, and **ADHD** ________________ ________________ ______________________________ ________________.
6. The nervous system may be divided into the **CNS** ________________ ________________ ________________, and the **PNS** ________________ ________________ ________________.

PRACTICAL APPLICATION

EXERCISE 45 *Interact with Medical Documents*

A. Complete the progress note by writing the medical terms in the blanks. Use the list of definitions with the corresponding numbers.

University Hospital and Medical Center
4700 North Main Street • Wellness, Arizona 54321 • (987) 555-3210

PATIENT NAME: Eldon Drake **CASE NUMBER:** 71086-NUR
DATE OF BIRTH: 08/12/19XX **DATE OF ADMISSION:** 01/02/20XX

PROGRESS NOTE

HISTORY: Eldon Drake is an 85-year-old Caucasian male who was admitted to the hospital on 01/02/20XX for fever and confusion. Mr. Drake was in his usual state of good health until 3 days before admission, when he began to show signs of confusion and 1. ________________ accompanied by a fever of 38.5° C. His fever continued, and he showed a steady decline in 2. ________________ function. He developed expressive 3. ________________.
OBJECTIVE FINDINGS: On physical examination the patient was 4. ________________ and alert but disoriented to time and place. Blood pressure was 160/80 mm Hg. Pulse, 96. Respirations, 20. Temperature 38.8° C. There were no focal neurologic deficits. Chest radiograph, urinalysis, and blood cultures were negative. A 5. ________________ consultation was obtained. consultation was obtained. 6. ________________ ________________ ________________ of the brain was performed, which disclosed 7. ________________. An 8. ________________ was markedly abnormal for his age.

TREATMENT SUMMARY: The patient was given acyclovir by intravenous infusion. On the second hospital day, the patient developed a generalized 9. ________________. He was placed on intravenous Dilantin and lorazepam. He later lapsed into a semicomatose state. He responded to tactile and verbal stimuli but was completely 10. ________________. A nasogastric tube was placed, and enteral feedings were begun. After 14 days of IV acyclovir, the patient slowly began to improve and by the third week of his illness, he was talking normally and taking nourishment.

____
Rashid Maitryi MD

RM/mcm

1. a state of mental confusion as to time, place, or identity
2. pertaining to the mental processes of comprehension, judgment, memory, and reason
3. loss of the ability to speak
4. awake, alert, and aware of one's surroundings
5. study of nerves (branch of medicine dealing with diseases of the nervous system)
6. noninvasive technique that produces cross-sectional and sagittal images of the brain by magnetic waves
7. inflammation of the brain
8. record of electrical impulses of the brain
9. sudden surge of abnormal electrical activity in the brain
10. unable to express one's thoughts or ideas in an orderly, intelligible manner

EXERCISE 45 *Interact with Medical Documents—cont'd*

B. Read the consultation report and answer the questions following it.

32463 CASTILLA, ALANZE

File Patient Navigate Custom Fields Help

Patient Chart | Lab | Rad | Notes | Documents | Rx | Scheduling | Images | Billing

Name: **CASTILLA, ALANZE** MR#: **32463** Sex: **F**
DOB: **04/11/19XX**

NEUROLOGY CONSULTATION

ENCOUNTER DATE: 06/04/20XX

HISTORY: The patient is a 63-year-old Hispanic female referred to Neurology because of persistent low back and right leg pain and paresthesias of 6 months duration. The pain is described as dull and aching and is rated 6/10. The discomfort is worse when standing and intensifies after walking about a block. The pain improves when the patient is sitting or when bending over. Her general health is good and there has been no weight loss.

NEUROLOGIC EXAM: The gait is somewhat wide based. Balance is normal. No muscle atrophy is present. Muscle strength is normal for age. The right Achilles reflex is absent. Sensation to pin prick is diminished over the right S1 dermatome.

LAB AND IMAGING: CBC and sed rate are normal. Fasting blood sugar is 106 mg/dL. A lumbosacral spine radiograph shows spondylosis and spondylolisthesis of L5 over S1. A CT scan shows a moderate degree of facet joint arthropathy and bulging discs at L2-3 and L4-5 levels along with narrowing of the spinal canal at these levels.

IMPRESSION: Lumbar spinal stenosis with radiculopathy of the S1 nerve root.

RECOMMENDATION: Referral to neuroanesthesia for a series of epidural steroid injections. Physical therapy is also advised. Surgical referral is not necessary at this time.

Electronically signed by: Susan Rand, MD 06/04/20XX 6:15 PM

SR/dlb

Start | Log On/Off | Print | Edit

1. Spinal stenosis causes compression of nerve roots demonstrated by which of the following symptoms for the patient?
   a. total paralysis
   b. abnormal sensation of prickling and tingling
   c. paralysis of one limb
   d. slight paralysis

2. The patient's diagnosis is spinal stenosis with:
   a. disease of the nerve roots
   b. disease of peripheral nerves
   c. disease affecting a single nerve
   d. disease of many nerves

EXERCISE 46 *Interpret Medical Terms*

To test your understanding of the terms introduced in this chapter, circle the words that correctly complete the sentences. The italicized words refer to the correct answer.

1. *Paralysis of all four limbs* is (**paraplegia, monoplegia, hemiplegia, quadriplegia**).
2. The *inability to speak* or (**dysarthria, aphasia, dysphasia, dysphagia**) may be an after-effect of cerebrovascular accident.
3. A symptom of brain concussion that may cause a patient to be *unaware of his or her surroundings and unable to respond to stimuli* is (**subconscious, unconscious, convulsive**).
4. The newborn had *meninges protruding through a defect in his skull,* or a (**meningocele, myelomeningocele, myelomalacia**).
5. *The branch of medicine that deals with the treatment of mental disorders* is (**neurology, psychology, psychiatry**).
6. *Multiple sclerosis* is a disease of the nervous system; it is characterized by (**seizures, sclerotic patches along the brain and spinal cord, muscular tremors**).
7. *The process of recording of electrical impulses of the brain*, or (**electroencephalogram, electroencephalograph, electroencephalography**), is used to study brain function and is valuable for diagnosing epilepsy, tumors, and other brain diseases.
8. Cerebral *thrombosis*, or abnormal condition of a(n) (**blood clot, infection, hardened patches**), may cause a stroke.
9. The patient was admitted to the neurology unit of the hospital with a diagnosis of stroke. The physician ordered *a diagnostic procedure to examine blood flow and metabolic activity* or (**computed tomography, positron emission tomography, magnetic resonance imaging**).
10. The patient was diagnosed with (**ganglion, ganglia**) on both wrists.
11. Following a burn injury to the right hand, the patient developed paresthesia of the ring finger related to scarring. Surgery to *separate the nerve from adhesions* (**neurolysis, neuralgia, rhizotomy**) was performed to improve function and provide pain relief.
12. Herpes zoster virus is the cause of chickenpox and *viral disease affecting peripheral nerves* (**sciatica, shingles, polyneuritis**).

EXERCISE 47 Read Medical Terms in Use

Practice pronunciation of terms by reading the following document. Use the pronunciation key following the medical term to assist you in saying the word.

To hear these terms, go to http://evolve.elsevier.com. Refer to p. 18 for your Evolve Access Information. Select Exercises & Review, Chapter 15, Chapter Exercises, Read Medical Terms in Use.

A 78-year-old right-handed male presented to the Emergency Department with a right **hemiparesis** (*hem*-ē-pa-RĒ-sis), expressive **aphasia** (a-FĀ-zha), and no apparent **cognitive** (COG-ni-tiv) decline. He has a history of hypertension and 2 years ago had a **transient ischemic** (is-KĒ-mik) **attack.** A **computed tomography** (tō-MOG-ra-fē) **scan of the brain** was negative for an **intracerebral** (in-tra-SER-e-bral) hemorrhage. A **neurologist** (nū-ROL-o-jist) was consulted. She confirmed the diagnosis of an **ischemic stroke** (strōk) after **magnetic resonance imaging** (mag-NET-ik) (REZ-ō-nans) (IM-a-jing) **of the brain** demonstrated an ischemic area of the left **cerebral** (se-RĒ-bral) cortex caused by a **cerebral embolism** (se-RĒ-bral) (EM-bō-lizm).

EXERCISE 48 Comprehend Medical Terms in Use

Test your comprehension of terms in the previous medical document by circling the correct answer.

1. While in the emergency department, the patient had:
   a. inability to swallow and paralysis from the waist down
   b. inability to speak and slight paralysis of the right side of the body
   c. inability to swallow and slight paralysis of the right side of the body
   d. inability to speak and paralysis from the waist down
2. T F A diagnosis of stroke was made after an MRI of the brain was performed.
3. The patient had a history of:
   a. sudden deficient supply of blood to the brain
   b. sudden loss of consciousness
   c. slight paralysis of one side
   d. a clot in the cerebrum

CHAPTER REVIEW

ONLINE CHAPTER REVIEW

To access the Evolve website, go to http://evolve.elsevier.com. Refer to p. 18 for your Evolve Access Information. Select Exercises & Review, Chapter 15, then select Chapter Exercises, Practice Activities, Animations, or Games. Place a check mark in the box when you have completed an exercise or activity, watched an animation, or played a game. Have fun!

Chapter Exercises

Exercises in this section of your Evolve resources correlate to exercises in your textbook. You may have completed them as you worked through the chapter.

- ☐ Pronunciation
- ☐ Spelling
- ☐ Read Medical Terms in Use

Practice Activities

Practice in study mode, and then test your learning in assessment mode. Keep track of your scores from assessment mode if you wish.

	SCORE
☐ Picture It	_____
☐ Define Word Parts	_____
☐ Build Medical Terms	_____
☐ Word Shop	_____
☐ Define Medical Terms	_____
☐ Use It	_____
☐ Hear It and Type It: Clinical Vignettes	_____

Animations

- ☐ Brain Blood Clot Leading to Stroke
- ☐ Hemiparesis
- ☐ Quadriplegia
- ☐ Subdural Hematoma

games

- ☐ Name that Word Part
- ☐ Term Storm
- ☐ Term Explorer
- ☐ Termbusters
- ☐ Medical Millionaire
- ☐ Crossword Puzzle

REVIEW OF WORD PARTS

Can you define and spell the following word parts?

Combining Forms

cerebell/o
cerebr/o
dur/o
encephal/o
esthesi/o
gangli/o
ganglion/o
gli/o
mening/i
meningi/o
ment/o
mon/o
myel/o
neur/o
phas/o
poli/o
psych/o
quadr/i
radic/o
radicul/o
rhiz/o

Suffixes

-iatrist
-iatry
-ictal
-paresis

REVIEW OF TERMS

Can you build, analyze, define, pronounce, and spell the following terms *built from word parts?*

Diseases and Disorders

cerebellitis
cerebral thrombosis
duritis
encephalitis
encephalomalacia
encephalomyeloradiculitis
gangliitis
glioblastoma
glioma
meningioma
meningitis
meningocele
meningomyelocele
mononeuropathy
neuralgia
neurasthenia
neuritis
neuroarthropathy
neuroma
neuropathy
poliomyelitis
polyneuritis
polyneuropathy
radiculitis
radiculopathy
rhizomeningomyelitis
subdural hematoma

Surgical

ganglionectomy
neurectomy
neurolysis
neuroplasty
neurorrhaphy
neurotomy
radicotomy
rhizotomy

Diagnostic

cerebral angiography
CT myelography
electroencephalogram (EEG)
electroencephalograph
electroencephalography

Complementary

anesthesia
aphasia
cephalalgia
cerebral
craniocerebral
dysphasia
encephalosclerosis
gliocyte
hemiparesis
hemiplegia
hyperesthesia
interictal
intracerebral
mental
monoparesis
monoplegia
myelomalacia
neuroid
neurologist
neurology
panplegia
paresthesia
postictal
preictal
quadriplegia
subdural

Behavioral health

psychiatrist
psychiatry
psychogenic
psychologist
psychology
psychopathy
psychosis
psychosomatic

Can you define, pronounce, and spell the following terms *not built from word parts?*

Diseases and Disorders

Alzheimer disease (AD)
amyotrophic lateral sclerosis (ALS)
Bell palsy
cerebral aneurysm
cerebral embolism
cerebral palsy (CP)
dementia
epilepsy
hydrocephalus
intracerebral hemorrhage
multiple sclerosis (MS)
Parkinson disease (PD)
sciatica
shingles
stroke
subarachnoid hemorrhage
transient ischemic attack (TIA)

Diagnostic

computed tomography of the brain (CT scan)
evoked potential studies (EP)
lumbar puncture (LP)
magnetic resonance imaging of the brain or spine (MRI scan)
positron emission tomography of the brain (PET scan)

Complementary

afferent
ataxia
cognitive
coma
concussion
conscious
convulsion
disorientation
dysarthria
efferent
gait
incoherent
paraplegia
seizure
shunt
syncope
unconsciousness

Behavioral health

anorexia nervosa
anxiety disorder
attention deficit hyperactivity disorder (ADHD)
autism
bipolar disorder
bulimia nervosa
major depression
obsessive-compulsive disorder (OCD)
panic attack
phobia
pica
posttraumatic stress disorder (PTSD)
schizophrenia
somatoform disorders

ANSWERS

Exercise Figures

Exercise Figure

A. 1. brain: encephal/o
2. spinal cord: myel/o
3. cerebrum: cerebr/o
4. cerebellum: cerebell/o
5. meninges: meningi/o, mening/o

Exercise Figure

B. 1. dura mater: dur/o
2. ganglion: gangli/o, ganglion/o
3. nerve root: radic/o, radicul/o, rhiz/o

Exercise Figure

C. rhiz/o/tomy or radic/o/tomy

Exercise Figure

D. myel/o/graphy

Exercise Figure

E. 1. hemi/plegia
3. quadr/i/plegia

Exercise 1

1. meninges
2. dura mater
3. arachnoid
4. pia mater
5. subarachnoid space
6. cerebrospinal fluid

Exercise 2

1. d
2. f
3. g
4. e
5. a
6. h
7. b
8. c
9. j

Exercise 3

1. cerebellum
2. nerve
3. spinal cord
4. meninges
5. brain
6. cerebrum, brain
7. nerve root
8. ganglion
9. nerve root
10. hard, dura mater
11. ganglion
12. nerve root
13. glia, gluey substance

Exercise 4

1. cerebell/o
2. neur/o
3. myel/o
4. a. mening/o
   b. meningi/o
5. encephal/o
6. cerebr/o
7. a. radicul/o
   b. radic/o
   c. rhiz/o
8. dur/o
9. a. gangli/o
   b. ganglion/o
10. gli/o

Exercise 5

1. one, single
2. mind
3. four
4. mind
5. speech
6. sensation, sensitivity, feeling
7. gray matter

Exercise 6

1. quadr/i
2. mon/o
3. a. psych/o
   b. ment/o
4. phas/o
5. poli/o
6. esthesi/o

Exercise 7

1. slight paralysis
2. treatment, specialty
3. seizure, attack
4. specialist, physician

Exercise 8

1. -paresis
2. -iatry
3. -ictal
4. -iatrist

Exercise 9

Pronunciation Exercise

Exercise 10

1. WR S
neur/itis
inflammation of a nerve
2. WR S
neur/oma
tumor made up of nerve (cells)
3. WR S
neur/algia
pain in a nerve
4. WR CV WR CV S
neur/o/arthr/o/pathy
CF CF
disease of nerves and joints
5. WR S
meningi/oma
tumor of the meninges
6. WR S
neur/asthenia
nerve weakness
7. WR CV S
encephal/o/malacia
CF
softening of the brain
8. WR S
encephal/itis
inflammation of the brain
9. WR CV WR CV WR S
encephal/o/myel/o/radicul/itis
CF CF
inflammation of the brain, spinal cord, and nerve roots
10. WR S
mening/itis
inflammation of the meninges
11. WR CV S
mening/o/cele
CF
protrusion of the meninges
12. WR CV WR CV S
mening/o/myel/o/cele
CF CF
protrusion of the meninges and spinal cord
13. WR S
radicul/itis
inflammation of the nerve roots
14. WR S
cerebell/itis
inflammation of the cerebellum
15. WR S
gangli/itis
inflammation of a ganglion
16. WR S
dur/itis
inflammation of the dura mater
17. P WR S
poly/neur/itis
inflammation of many nerves
18. WR CV WR S
poli/o/myel/itis
CF
inflammation of the gray matter of the spinal cord
19. WR S WR S
cerebr/al thromb/osis
pertaining to the cerebrum, abnormal condition of a clot

20. P WR S WR S
sub/dur/al hemat/oma
CF
pertaining to below the dura mater; tumor of blood

21. WR CV WR CV WR S
rhiz/o/mening/o/myel/itis
CF CF
inflammation of the nerve root, meninges, and spinal cord

22. WR CV WR CV S
mon/o/neur/o/pathy
CF CF
disease affecting a single nerve

23. WR CV S
neur/o/pathy
CF
disease of the nerves (peripheral)

24. WR CV S
radicul/o/pathy
CF
disease of the nerve roots

25. WR S
gli/oma
tumor composed of glial tissue

26. WR CV WR S
gli/o/blast/oma
CF
tumor composed of developing glial tissue

27. P WR CV S
poly/neur/o/pathy
CF
disease of many nerves

Exercise 11

1. neur/itis
2. neur/oma
3. neur/algia
4. neur/o/arthr/o/pathy
5. radicul/o/pathy
6. neur/asthenia
7. encephal/o/malacia
8. encephal/itis
9. encephal/o/myel/o/radicul/itis
10. mening/itis
11. mening/o/cele
12. mening/o/myel/o/cele
13. radicul/itis
14. cerebell/itis
15. gangli/itis
16. dur/itis
17. poly/neur/itis
18. poli/o/myel/itis
19. cerebr/al thromb/osis
20. sub/dur/al hemat/oma
21. rhiz/o/mening/o/myel/itis
22. meningi/oma
23. mon/o/neur/o/pathy
24. neur/o/pathy
25. gli/oma
26. gli/o/blast/oma
27. poly/neur/o/pathy

Exercise 12

Spelling Exercise; see text pp. 705-706.

Exercise 13

Pronunciation Exercise

Exercise 14

1. a. intracerebral hemorrhage
   b. cerebral embolism
   c. subarachnoid hemorrhage
   d. cerebral thrombosis
2. cerebral aneurysm
3. Bell palsy
4. hydrocephalus
5. sciatica
6. shingles
7. transient ischemic attack
8. Parkinson disease
9. epilepsy
10. amyotrophic lateral sclerosis
11. Alzheimer disease
12. cerebral palsy
13. multiple sclerosis
14. dementia

Exercise 15

1. b
2. a
3. n
4. j
5. l
6. p
7. e
8. g
9. i
10. m
11. q
12. d
13. h
14. o
15. c
16. f
17. r

Exercise 16

Spelling Exercise; see text pp. 710-713.

Exercise 17

Pronunciation Exercise

Exercise 18

1. WR CV S
radic/o/tomy
CF
incision into a nerve root

2. WR S
neur/ectomy
excision of a nerve

3. WR CV S
neur/o/rrhaphy
CF
suture of a nerve

4. WR S
ganglion/ectomy
excision of a ganglion

5. WR CV S
neur/o/tomy
CF
incision into a nerve

6. WR CV S
neur/o/lysis
CF
separating a nerve (from adhesions)

7. WR CV S
neur/o/plasty
CF
surgical repair of a nerve

8. WR CV S
rhiz/o/tomy
CF
incision into a nerve root

Exercise 19

1. a. radic/o/tomy
   b. rhiz/o/tomy
2. neur/ectomy
3. neur/o/rrhaphy
4. ganglion/ectomy
5. neur/o/tomy
6. neur/o/lysis
7. neur/o/plasty

Exercise 20

Spelling Exercise; see text p. 716.

Exercise 21

Pronunciation Exercise

Exercise 22

1. WR CV WR CV S
electr/o/encephal/o/gram
CF CF
record of the electrical impulses of the brain

2. WR CV WR CV S
electr/o/encephal/o/graph
CF CF
instrument used to record the electrical impulses of the brain

3. WR CV WR CV S
electr/o/encephal/o/graphy
CF CF
process of recording the electrical impulses of the brain

4. WR CV S
CT myel/o/graphy
CF
process of recording (scan) the spinal cord

5. WR S WR CV S
cerebr/al angi/o/graphy
CF
radiographic imaging of the blood vessels in the brain

Exercise 23

1. electr/o/encephal/o/gram
2. electr/o/encephal/o/graph
3. electr/o/encephal/o/graphy
4. CT myel/o/graphy
5. cerebr/al angi/o/graphy

Exercise 24

Spelling Exercise; see text p. 718.

Exercise 25

Pronunciation Exercise

Exercise 26

1. computed tomography
2. lumbar puncture
3. positron emission tomography
4. magnetic resonance imaging
5. evoked potential studies

Exercise 27

1. insertion of a needle into the subarachnoid space
2. process that includes the use of a computer to produce a series of images of the brain tissues at any desired depth
3. produces sectional images of the brain or spine by a strong magnetic field
4. a technique that produces sectional imaging of the brain to examine blood flow and metabolic activity
5. a group of diagnostic tests that measure changes and responses in brain waves from stimuli

Exercise 28

Spelling Exercise; see text pp. 720-721.

Exercise 29

Pronunciation Exercise

Exercise 30

1. P S(WR)
hemi/plegia
paralysis of half (left or right side of the body)
2. P WR S
par/esthesi/a
abnormal sensation
3. WR CV S
neur/o/logist
CF
physician who studies and treats diseases of the nerves (nervous system)
4. WR CV S
neur/o/logy
CF
study of nerves (branch of medicine dealing with diseases of the nervous system)
5. WR S
neur/oid
resembling a nerve
6. WR CV S
quadr/i/plegia
CF
paralysis of four (limbs)
7. WR S
cerebr/al
pertaining to the cerebrum
8. WR CV S
mon/o/plegia
CF
paralysis of one (limb)
9. P WR S
a/phas/ia
condition of without speaking
10. P WR S
dys/phas/ia
condition of difficulty speaking
11. P S(WR)
hemi/paresis
slight paralysis of half (right or left side of the body)
12. P WR S
an/esthesi/a
without (loss of) feeling or sensation
13. P WR S
hyper/esthesi/a
excessive sensitivity (to stimuli)
14. P WR S
sub/dur/al
pertaining to below the dura mater
15. WR S
cephal/algia
pain in the head (headache)
16. WR CV WR S
crani/o/cerebr/al
CF
pertaining to the cranium and cerebrum
17. WR CV S
myel/o/malacia
CF
softening of the spinal cord
18. WR CV S
encephal/o/sclerosis
CF
hardening of the brain
19. P S(WR)
post/ictal
(occurring) after a seizure or attack
20. P S(WR)
pan/plegia
total paralysis
21. P S(WR)
inter/ictal
(occurring) between seizures or attacks
22. WR CV S
mon/o/paresis
CF
slight paralysis of one (limb)
23. P S(WR)
pre/ictal
(occurring) before a seizure or attack
24. P WR S
intra/cerebr/al
pertaining to within the cerebrum
25. WRCV S
gli/o/cyte
CF
glial cell
26. WR S
ment/al
pertaining to the mind

Exercise 31

1. hemi/paresis
2. an/esthesi/a
3. hyper/esthesi/a
4. sub/dur/al
5. cephal/algia
6. crani/o/cerebr/al
7. myel/o/malacia
8. encephal/o/sclerosis
9. hemi/plegia
10. neur/o/logist
11. neur/o/logy
12. neur/oid
13. quadr/i/plegia
14. cerebr/al
15. mon/o/plegia
16. a/phas/ia
17. dys/phas/ia
18. pre/ictal
19. mon/o/paresis
20. post/ictal
21. pan/plegia
22. inter/ictal
23. intra/cerebr/al
24. gli/o/cyte
25. par/esthesi/a
26. ment/al

Exercise 32
Spelling Exercise; see text pp. 723-724.

Exercise 33
Pronunciation Exercise

Exercise 34
1. concussion
2. unconsciousness
3. conscious
4. seizure
5. convulsion
6. shunt
7. paraplegia
8. coma
9. syncope
10. ataxia
11. gait
12. dysarthria
13. incoherent
14. disorientation
15. cognitive
16. afferent
17. efferent

Exercise 35
1. tube implanted in the body to redirect the flow of a fluid
2. paralysis from the waist down caused by damage to the lower level of the spinal cord
3. state of profound unconsciousness
4. injury to the brain caused by head trauma
5. state of being unaware of surroundings and incapable of responding to stimuli as a result of injury, shock, or illness
6. awake, alert, aware of one's surroundings
7. sudden surge of abnormal electrical activity in the brain
8. sudden involuntary contraction of a group of muscles
9. fainting, or sudden loss of consciousness
10. lack of muscle coordination
11. the inability to use speech that is distinct and connected
12. a manner or style of walking
13. pertaining to the mental processes of comprehension, judgment, memory, and reasoning
14. a state of mental confusion regarding time, place, and identity
15. unable to express one's thoughts or ideas in an orderly, intelligible manner
16. conveying away from the center
17. conveying toward the center

Exercise 36
Spelling Exercise; see text pp. 728-729.

Exercise 37
Pronunciation Exercise

Exercise 38
1. psych/iatry
2. psych/osis
3. psych/o/logy
4. psych/o/genic
5. psych/iatrist
6. psych/o/logist
7. psych/o/somat/ic
8. psych/o/pathy

Exercise 39
1. WR CV WR S
   psych/o/somat/ic
   CF
   pertaining to the mind and body
2. WR CV S
   psych/o/pathy
   CF
   (any) disease of the mind
3. WR CV S
   psych/o/logy
   CF
   study of the mind
4. WR S
   psych/iatry
   specialty of the mind (branch of medicine that deals with the treatment of mental disorders)
5. WR CV S
   psych/o/logist
   CF
   specialist of the mind
6. WR CV S
   psych/o/genic
   CF
   originating in the mind
7. WR S
   psych/iatrist
   a physician who studies and treats disorders of the mind
8. WR S
   psych/osis
   abnormal condition of the mind

Exercise 40
Spelling Exercise; see text p. 734.

Exercise 41
Pronunciation Exercise

Exercise 42
1. i
2. m
3. b
4. c
5. j
6. a
7. g
8. d
9. h
10. f
11. e
12. n
13. l
14. k

Exercise 43
Spelling Exercise; see text p. 738.

Exercise 44
1. electroencephalogram, magnetic resonance imaging scan, positron emission tomography scan, evoked potential studies, lumbar puncture
2. Alzheimer disease, amyotrophic lateral sclerosis, cerebral palsy, multiple sclerosis, Parkinson disease
3. cerebrovascular accident, transient ischemic attack
4. cerebrospinal fluid
5. posttraumatic stress disorder, obsessive-compulsive disorder, attention deficit hyperactivity disorder
6. central nervous system, peripheral nervous system

Exercise 45
A.
1. disorientation
2. cognitive
3. aphasia
4. conscious
5. neurology
6. magnetic resonance imaging
7. encephalitis
8. electroencephalogram
9. seizure
10. incoherent

B.
1. b
2. a

Exercise 46
1. quadriplegia
2. aphasia
3. unconscious
4. meningocele
5. psychiatry
6. sclerotic patches along brain and spinal cord
7. electroencephalography
8. blood clot
9. positron emission tomography
10. ganglia
11. neurolysis
12. shingles

Exercise 47
Reading Exercise

Exercise 48
1. b
2. *T*
3. a

Chapter 16

Endocrine System

OUTLINE

OBJECTIVES

Upon completion of this chapter you will be able to:

1. Identify organs and structures of the endocrine system.
2. Define and spell word parts related to the endocrine system.
3. Define, pronounce, and spell disease and disorder terms related to the endocrine system.
4. Define, pronounce, and spell surgical terms related to the endocrine system.
5. Define, pronounce, and spell diagnostic terms related to the endocrine system.
6. Define, pronounce, and spell complementary terms related to the endocrine system.
7. Interpret the meaning of abbreviations related to the endocrine system.
8. Interpret, read, and comprehend medical language in simulated medical statements and documents.

ANATOMY

The endocrine system is composed of endocrine glands distributed throughout the body. The endocrine glands are: pituitary, thyroid, parathyroid, adrenal, pancreas, gonads (ovaries and testes), and thymus.

Function

The endocrine system regulates body activities through the use of chemical messengers called *hormones*, which when released into the bloodstream influence metabolic activities, growth, and development (Figure 16-1). The nervous system also regulates body activities but does so through electrical impulses and activation of glandular secretions. *Hormones* secreted by the *endocrine glands* that make up the endocrine system go directly into the bloodstream and are transported throughout the body. They are referred to as *ductless glands* because they do not have ducts to carry their secretions. In contrast, the *exocrine* or *duct glands* have ducts that carry their secretions from the producing gland to other parts of the body. An example is the parotid gland, which produces saliva that flows through the parotid duct into the mouth. Only those terms related to the major endocrine glands—pituitary, thyroid, parathyroids, adrenals, and the islets of Langerhans in the pancreas—are presented in this chapter. The thymus and the male and female sex glands were discussed in previous chapters.

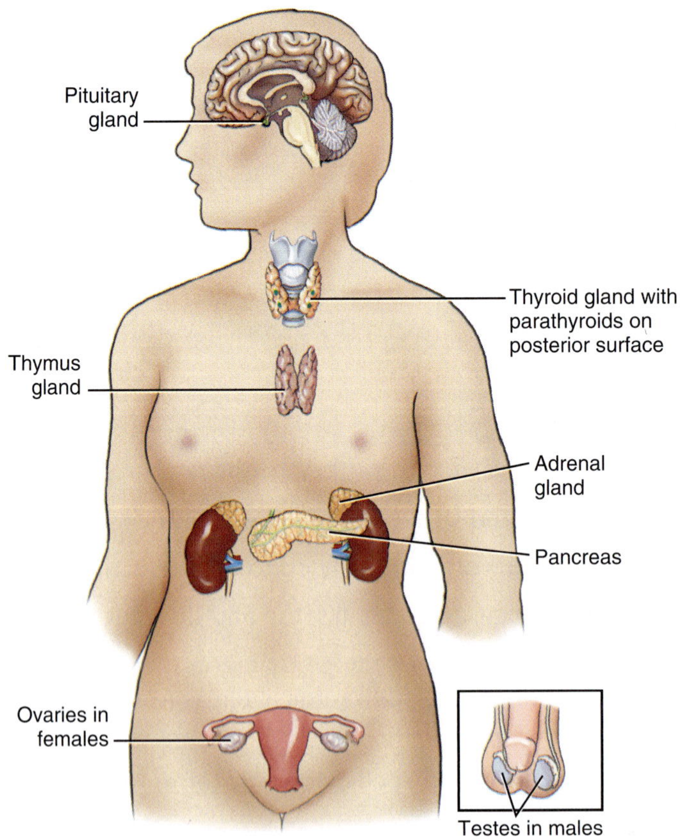

FIGURE 16-1
The endocrine system.

Endocrine Glands

Term	Definition
pituitary gland or hypophysis cerebri	approximately the size of a pea and located at the base of the brain. The pituitary is divided into two lobes. It is often referred to as the master gland because it produces hormones that stimulate the function of other endocrine glands (Figure 16-2).
anterior lobe or adenohypophysis	produces and secretes the following hormones:
growth hormone (GH)	regulates the growth of the body
adrenocorticotropic hormone (ACTH)	stimulates the adrenal cortex
thyroid-stimulating hormone (TSH)	stimulates the thyroid gland
gonadotropic hormones	affect the male and female reproductive systems
follicle-stimulating hormone (FSH), luteinizing hormone (LH)	regulate development, growth, and function of the ovaries and testes
prolactin-releasing hormone (PRH), lactogenic hormone	promotes development of glandular tissue during pregnancy and produces milk after birth of an infant
posterior lobe or neurohypophysis	stores and releases antidiuretic hormone and oxytocin
antidiuretic hormone (ADH)	stimulates the kidney to reabsorb water
oxytocin	stimulates uterine contractions during labor and postpartum
hypothalamus	located superior to the pituitary gland in the brain. The hypothalamus secretes "releasing" hormone that functions to stimulate or inhibit the release of pituitary gland hormones.
thyroid gland	largest endocrine gland. It is located anteriorly in the neck below the larynx and comprises bilateral lobes connected by an isthmus (see Figure 16-3). The thyroid gland secretes the hormones triiodothyronine (T3) and thyroxine (T4), which require iodine for their production. Thyroxine is necessary for body cell metabolism.

A & P Booster
For students desiring more anatomy and physiology, go to http://evolve.elsevier.com. Refer to p. 18 for your Evolve Access Information. Select A & P Booster, Chapter 16.

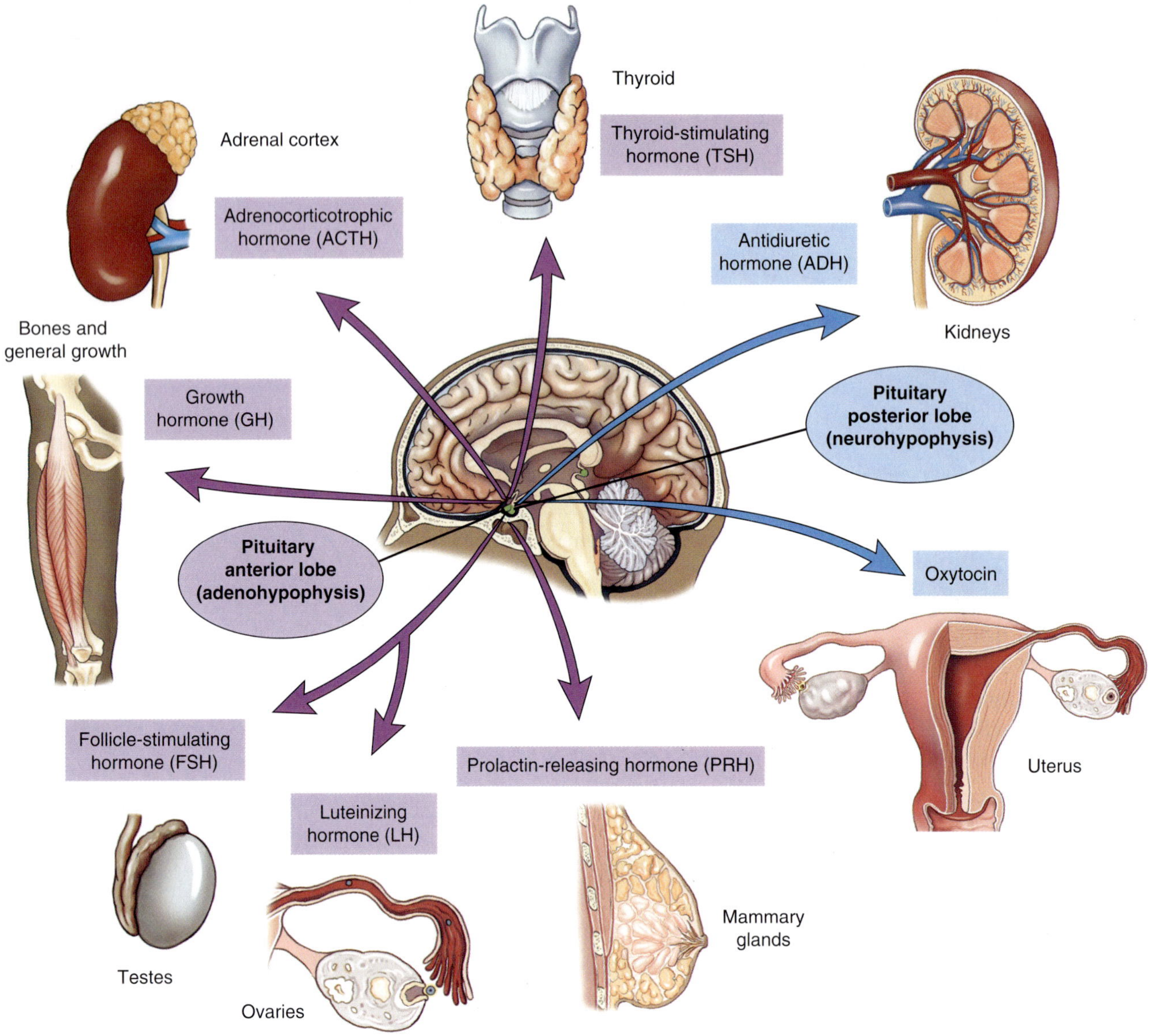

FIGURE 16-2
Pituitary gland, hormones secreted, and target organs.

Endocrine Glands—*cont'd*

Term	Definition
parathyroid glands	four small bodies embedded in the posterior aspect of the lobes of the thyroid gland (Figure 16-3). Parathormone (PTH), the hormone produced by the glands, helps maintain the level of calcium in the blood.
islets of Langerhans	clusters of endocrine tissue found throughout the pancreas, made up of different cell types that secrete various hormones, including insulin and glucagon. Non-endocrine cells found throughout the pancreas produce enzymes that facilitate digestion (Figure 16-4).

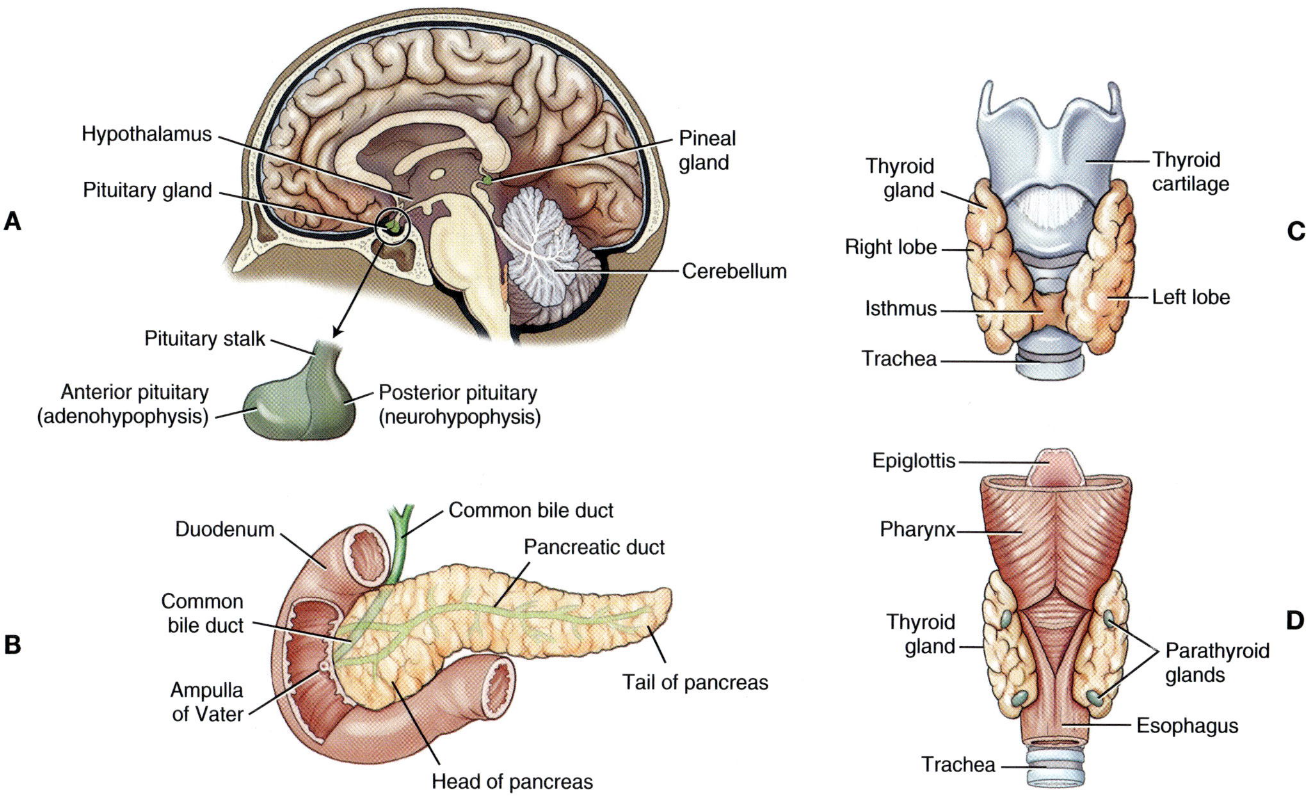

FIGURE 16-3

A, Pituitary and pineal glands. **B,** Pancreas. **C,** Thyroid gland, anterior view. **D,** Parathyroid glands, posterior view.

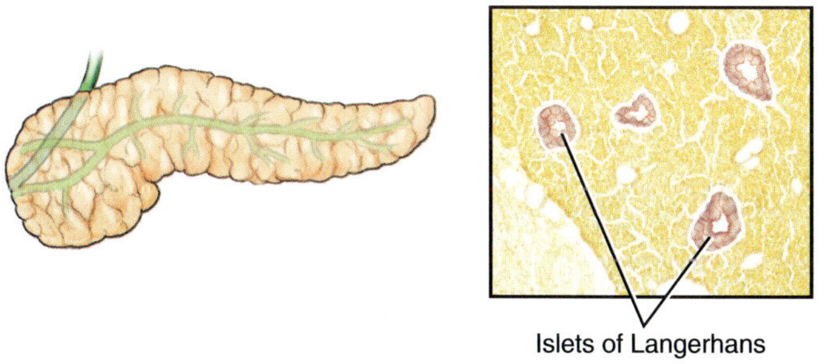

FIGURE 16-4

Pancreas, with islets of Langerhans.

Term	Definition
adrenal glands or suprarenals	paired glands, one of which is located above each kidney. The outer portion is called the **adrenal cortex,** and the inner portion is called the **adrenal medulla.** The following hormones are secreted by the adrenal glands:
cortisol	secreted by the adrenal cortex. It aids the body during stress by increasing glucose levels to provide energy (also called **hydrocortisone**).

Endocrine Glands—*cont'd*

Term	Definition
aldosterone	secreted by the adrenal cortex. Electrolytes (mineral salts) that are necessary for normal body function are regulated by this hormone.
epinephrine (adrenaline), norepinephrine (noradrenaline)	secreted by the adrenal medulla. These hormones help the body to deal with stress by increasing the blood pressure, heartbeat, and respirations.

EXERCISE 1

Match the terms in the first column with the correct definitions in the second column. *To check your answers to the exercises in this chapter, go to Answers, p. 784, at the end of the chapter.*

_____ 1. adrenal cortex
_____ 2. adrenal glands
_____ 3. adrenaline
_____ 4. adrenal medulla
_____ 5. adrenocorticotropic hormone
_____ 6. adenohypophysis
_____ 7. aldosterone

a. hormone that stimulates the adrenal cortex
b. tissue that secretes cortisol and aldosterone
c. anterior lobe of pituitary that secretes growth hormone and thyroid-stimulating hormone
d. another name for epinephrine
e. assists in regulating body electrolytes
f. another name for norepinephrine
g. located above each kidney
h. secretes epinephrine and norepinephrine

EXERCISE 2

Match the terms in the first column with the correct phrases in the second column.

_____ 1. antidiuretic hormone
_____ 2. islets of Langerhans
_____ 3. neurohypophysis
_____ 4. parathyroid glands
_____ 5. pituitary gland
_____ 6. thyroid gland

a. portions of the pancreas that secrete insulin
b. glands that maintain the blood calcium level
c. gland located anteriorly in the neck that secretes thyroxine
d. hormone secreted by posterior lobe of the pituitary
e. gland that stores and releases antidiuretic hormone and oxytocin
f. another name for the anterior lobe of the pituitary
g. gland located at the base of the brain

WORD PARTS

Word parts you need to learn to complete this chapter are listed on the following pages. The exercises at the end of each list will help you learn their definitions and spellings.

Use the flashcards accompanying this text or electronic flashcards to assist you in memorizing the word parts for this chapter.

To use electronic flashcards, go to http://evolve.elsevier.com. Refer to p. 18 for your Evolve Access Information. Select Flashcards, Chapter 16.

Combining Forms of the Endocrine System

Combining Form	Definition
aden/o (NOTE: *aden/o* was introduced in Chapter 2.)	gland
adren/o, adrenal/o	adrenal glands
cortic/o	cortex (the outer layer of a body organ)
endocrin/o	endocrine
parathyroid/o	parathyroid glands
pituitar/o	pituitary gland
thyroid/o, thyr/o	thyroid gland

EXERCISE FIGURE A

Fill in the blanks with combining forms in this diagram of the endocrine glands. *To check your answers, go to p. 784.*

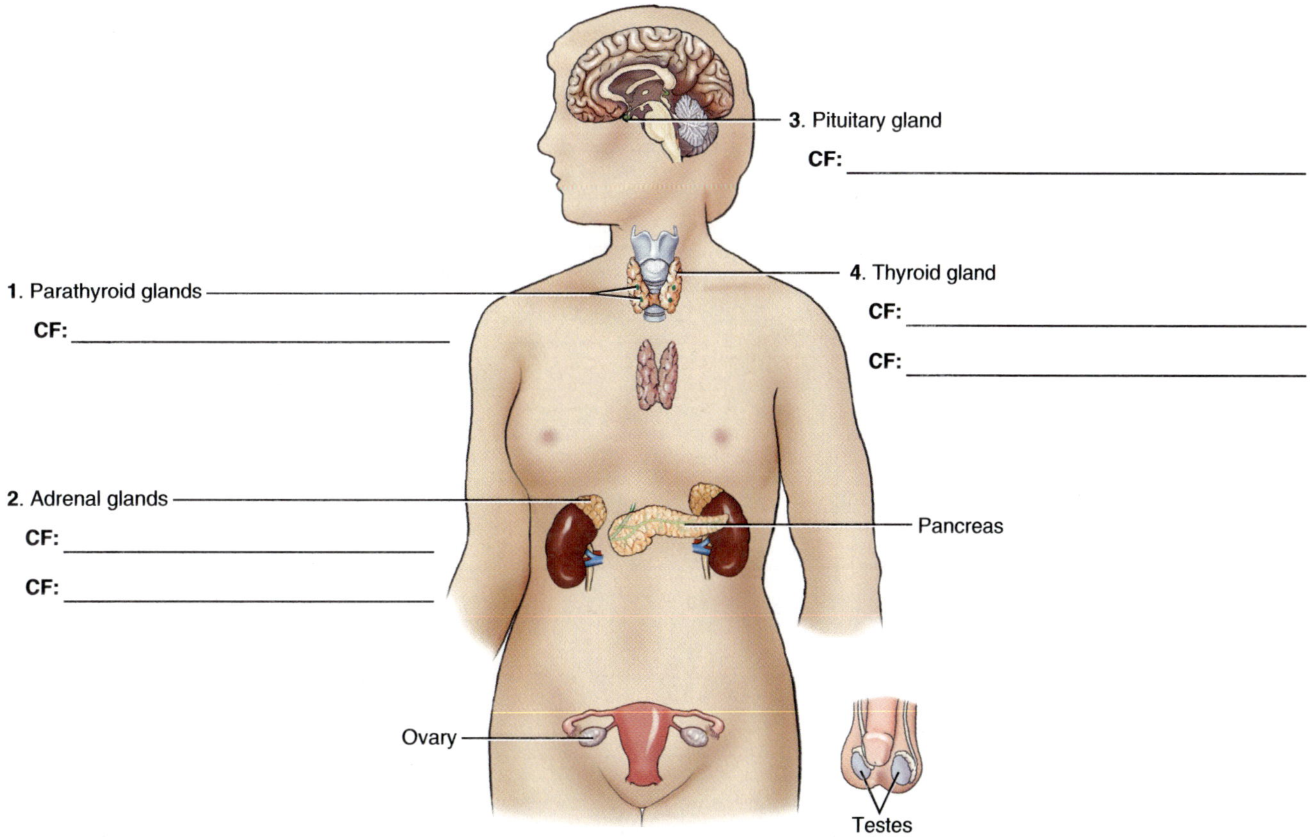

EXERCISE FIGURE B

Fill in the blank with the combining form in this diagram of adrenal glands (with transverse cross-sectional view).

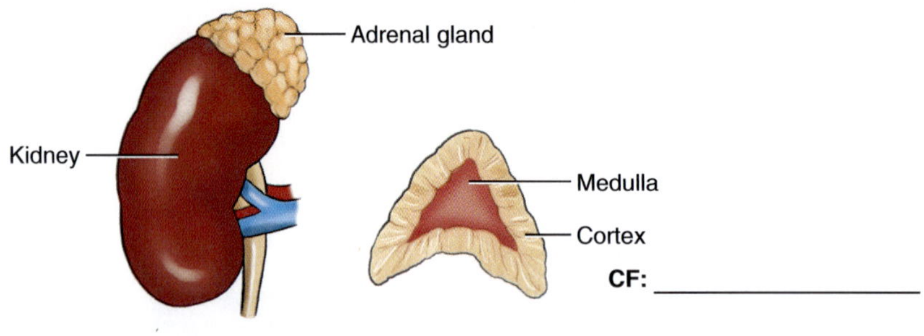

EXERCISE 3

Write the definitions of the following combining forms.

1. cortic/o ________________
2. adren/o ________________
3. parathyroid/o ________________
4. thyroid/o ________________
5. adrenal/o ________________
6. thyr/o ________________
7. endocrin/o ________________
8. aden/o ________________
9. pituitar/o ________________

EXERCISE 4

Write the combining form for each of the following terms.

1. adrenal gland a. ____________
   b. ____________
2. thyroid gland a. ____________
   b. ____________
3. endocrine ____________
4. cortex ____________
5. parathyroid gland ____________
6. gland ____________
7. pituitary gland ____________

Combining Forms Commonly Used with Endocrine System Terms

Combining Form	Definition
acr/o	extremities, height
calc/i (NOTE: The combining vowel is *i*.)	calcium
dips/o	thirst
kal/i (NOTE: the combining vowel is *i*.)	potassium
natr/o	sodium

EXERCISE 5

Write the definitions of the following combining forms.

1. dips/o ______________________
2. kal/i ______________________
3. calc/i ______________________
4. acr/o ______________________
5. natr/o ______________________

EXERCISE 6

Write the combining form for each of the following.

1. extremities, height ______________
2. calcium ______________
3. thirst ______________
4. potassium ______________
5. sodium ______________

Suffix

Suffix	Definition
-drome	run, running

Refer to **Appendix A** and **Appendix B** for a complete list of word parts.

EXERCISE 7

Write the definition of the following word part.

1. -drome ____

EXERCISE 8

Write the suffix for the following.

1. run, running ____

MEDICAL TERMS

The terms you need to learn to complete this chapter are listed below. The exercises following each list will help you learn the definition and spelling of each word.

Disease and Disorder Terms

Built from Word Parts

The following terms are built from word parts you have already learned and can be translated literally to find their meanings. Further explanation of terms beyond the definition of their word parts, if needed, is included in parentheses.

Term	Definition
acromegaly (*ak*-rō-MEG-a-lē)	enlargement of the extremities (and bones of the face, hands, and feet caused by excessive production of the growth hormone by the pituitary gland after puberty) (Exercise Figure C)
adenitis (ad-e-NĪ-tis)	inflammation of a gland
adenomegaly (*ad*-e-nō-MEG-a-lē)	enlargement of a gland
adenosis (*ad*-e-NŌ-sis)	abnormal condition of a gland
adrenalitis (a-*drē*-nal-Ī-tis)	inflammation of the adrenal glands
adrenomegaly (a-*drē*-nō-MEG-a-lē)	enlargement (of one or both) of the adrenal glands
hypercalcemia (*hī*-per-kal-SĒ-mē-a)	excessive calcium in the blood
hyperglycemia (*hī*-per-glī-SĒ-mē-a)	excessive sugar in the blood
hyperkalemia (*hī*-per-ka-LĒ-mē-a)	excessive potassium in the blood
hyperpituitarism (*hī*-per-pi-TOO-i-ta-*rizm*)	state of excessive pituitary gland activity (characterized by excessive secretion of pituitary hormones)
hyperthyroidism (*hī*-per-THĪ-royd-izm)	state of excessive thyroid gland activity (characterized by excessive secretion of thyroid hormones). Signs and symptoms include weight loss, irritability, and heat intolerance.
hypocalcemia (*hī*-pō-kal-SĒ-mē-a)	deficient calcium in the blood
hypoglycemia (*hī*-pō-glī-SĒ-mē-a)	deficient sugar in the blood
hypokalemia (*hī*-pō-ka-LĒ-mē-a)	deficient potassium in the blood

EXERCISE FIGURE C

Fill in the blanks to complete labeling of this photograph.

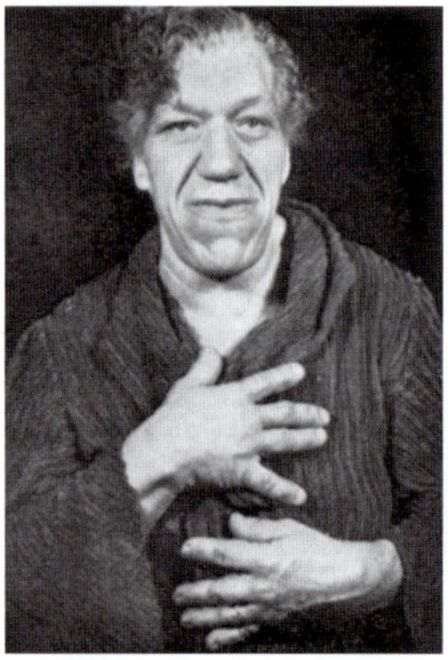

_____ / _____ / _____
extremities / cv / enlargement

a metabolic disorder characterized by marked enlargement of the bones of the face, jaw, and extremities.

HYPOTHYROIDISM

is the state of deficient thyroid gland activity, resulting in the decreased production of the thyroid hormone called thyroxine. A severe form of hypothyroidism in adults is called **myxedema** and in children is called **cretinism** or **congenital hypothyroidism.**

Term	Definition
hyponatremia (*hī*-pō-na-TRĒ-mē-a)	deficient sodium in the blood
hypopituitarism (*hī*-pō-pi-TŪ-i-ta-*rizm*)	state of deficient pituitary gland activity (characterized by decreased secretion of one or more of the pituitary hormones, which can affect the function of the target endocrine gland; for example, hypothyroidism results from decreased secretion of thyroid-stimulating hormone by the pituitary gland)
hypothyroidism (*hī*-pō-THĪ-royd-izm)	state of deficient thyroid gland activity (characterized by decreased secretion of thyroid hormones). Signs and symptoms include fatigue, weight gain, and cold intolerance.
panhypopituitarism (pan-*hī*-po-pi-TŪ-i-ta-*rizm*) (NOTE: two prefixes contained in this term)	state of total deficient pituitary gland activity (characterized by decreased secretion of all the pituitary hormones; this is a more serious condition than hypopituitarism in that it affects the function of all the other endocrine glands)
parathyroidoma (*par*-a-*thī*-royd-Ō-ma)	tumor of a parathyroid gland
thyroiditis (*thī*-royd-Ī-tis)	inflammation of the thyroid gland

EXERCISE 9

Practice saying aloud each of the disease and disorder terms built from word parts on these two pages.

To hear the terms, go to http://evolve.elsevier.com. Refer to p. 18 for your Evolve Access Information. Select Exercises & Review, Chapter 16, Chapter Exercises, Pronunciation.

☐ Place a check mark in the box when you have completed this exercise.

EXERCISE 10

Analyze and define the following terms.

1. adrenalitis ____________________
2. hypocalcemia ____________________
3. hyperthyroidism ____________________
4. hyperkalemia ____________________
5. hyperglycemia ____________________
6. adrenomegaly ____________________

7. adenomegaly ______________________
8. hypothyroidism ______________________
9. hypokalemia ______________________
10. adenitis ______________________
11. parathyroidoma ______________________
12. acromegaly ______________________
13. panhypopituitarism ______________________
14. hypoglycemia ______________________
15. hypercalcemia ______________________
16. hyperpituitarism ______________________
17. hyponatremia ______________________
18. adenosis ______________________
19. thyroiditis ______________________
20. hypopituitarism ______________________

EXERCISE 11

Build disease and disorder terms for the following definitions with the word parts you have learned.

1. enlargement of (one or both) the adrenal glands ______ WR / CV / S
2. state of deficient thyroid gland activity ______ P / WR / S
3. enlargement of the extremities ______ WR / CV / S
4. deficient sugar in the blood ______ P / WR / S
5. excessive potassium in the blood ______ P / WR / S

6. deficient calcium in the blood ______ / ______ / ______
P / WR / S

7. state of excessive thyroid gland activity ______ / ______ / ______
P / WR / S

8. state of deficient pituitary gland activity ______ / ______ / ______
P / WR / S

9. excessive calcium in the blood ______ / ______ / ______
P / WR / S

10. state of excessive pituitary gland activity ______ / ______ / ______
P / WR / S

11. tumor of a parathyroid gland ______ / ______
WR / S

12. excessive sugar in the blood ______ / ______ / ______
P / WR / S

13. abnormal condition of a gland ______ / ______
WR / S

14. deficient potassium in the blood ______ / ______ / ______
P / WR / S

15. inflammation of the adrenal glands ______ / ______
WR / S

16. enlargement of a gland ______ / ______ / ______
WR / CV / S

17. deficient sodium in the blood ______ / ______ / ______
P / WR / S

18. inflammation of a gland ______ / ______
WR / S

19. inflammation of the thyroid gland ______ / ______
WR / S

20. state of total deficient pituitary gland activity ______ / ______ / ______ / ______
P / P / WR / S

EXERCISE 12

Spell each of the disease and disorder terms built from word parts on pp. 760-761 by having someone dictate them to you.

To hear and spell the terms, go to http://evolve.elsevier.com. Refer to p. 18 for your Evolve Access Information. Select Exercises & Review, Chapter 16, Chapter Exercises, Spelling.
☐ Place a check mark in the box if you have completed this exercise online.

1. ____________	11. ____________
2. ____________	12. ____________
3. ____________	13. ____________
4. ____________	14. ____________
5. ____________	15. ____________
6. ____________	16. ____________
7. ____________	17. ____________
8. ____________	18. ____________
9. ____________	19. ____________
10. ____________	20. ____________

ADDISON DISEASE

was named in **1855** for **Thomas Addison,** an English physician and pathologist. He described the disease as a "morbid state with feeble heart action, anemia, irritability of the stomach, and a peculiar change in the color of the skin."

Disease and Disorder Terms

Not Built from Word Parts

In some of the following terms, you may recognize word parts you have already learned; however, the full meaning of the terms cannot be discerned by the definition of their word parts.

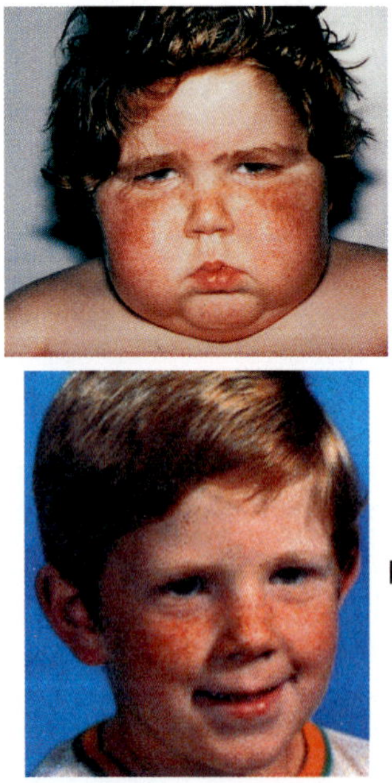

A

B

FIGURE 16-5
Cushing syndrome was named for an American neurosurgeon, **Harvey Williams Cushing** (1869-1939), after he described adrenocortical hyperfunction. **A,** At diagnosis. **B,** Four months after treatment.

Term	Definition
acidosis (*as*-i-DŌ-sis)	condition brought about by an abnormal accumulation of acid products of metabolism such as seen in uncontrolled diabetes mellitus
Addison disease (AD-i-sun) (di-ZĒZ)	chronic syndrome resulting from a deficiency in the hormonal secretion of the adrenal cortex. Signs and symptoms may include weakness, darkening of skin, loss of appetite, depression, and other emotional problems.
cretinism (KRĒ-tin-izm)	condition caused by congenital absence or atrophy (wasting away) of the thyroid gland, resulting in hypothyroidism. The disease is characterized by puffy features, mental deficiency, large tongue, and dwarfism; (also called **congenital hypothyroidism**).
Cushing syndrome (KŪSH-ing) (SIN-drōm)	group of signs and symptoms attributed to the excessive production of cortisol by the adrenal cortices (*pl.* of cortex). This syndrome may be the result of a pituitary tumor or a primary adrenal gland dysfunction. Signs include abnormally pigmented skin, "moon face," pads of fat on the chest and abdomen, "buffalo hump" (fat on the upper back), wasting away of muscle, and hypertension (Figure 16-5).

Term	Definition
diabetes insipidus (DI) (*dī*-a-BĒ-tēz) (in-SIP-i-dus)	result of decreased secretion of antidiuretic hormone by the posterior lobe of the pituitary gland. Symptoms include excessive thirst *(polydipsia)*, large amounts of urine *(polyuria)*, and sodium being excreted from the body.
diabetes mellitus (DM) (*dī*-a-BĒ-tēz) (MEL-li-tus)	chronic disease involving a disorder of carbohydrate metabolism caused by underactivity of the islets of Langerhans and characterized by elevated blood sugar (hyperglycemia). DM can cause chronic renal disease, retinopathy, and neuropathy. In extreme cases the patient may develop ketosis, acidosis, and finally coma.
gigantism (jī-GAN-tizm)	condition brought about by hypersecretion of growth hormone by the pituitary gland before puberty
goiter (GOY-ter)	enlargement of the thyroid gland (Figure 16-6)
Graves disease (grāvz) (di-ZĒZ)	a disorder of the thyroid gland characterized by the presence of hyperthyroidism, goiter, and abnormal protrusion of the eyeballs *(exophthalmos)*
ketosis (kē-TŌ-sis)	condition resulting from uncontrolled diabetes mellitus, in which the body has an abnormal concentration of ketone bodies resulting from excessive fat metabolism
metabolic syndrome (*met*-a-BOL-ik) (SIN-drōm)	group of signs and symptoms including insulin resistance, obesity characterized by excessive fat around the waist and abdomen, hypertension, hyperglycemia, elevated triglycerides, and low levels of the "good" cholesterol HDL. Risks include development of type 2 diabetes, coronary heart disease, or stroke (also called **syndrome X** and **insulin resistance syndrome**).
myxedema (*mik*-se-DĒ-ma)	condition resulting from a deficiency of the thyroid hormone thyroxine; a severe form of hypothyroidism in an adult. Signs include puffiness of the face and hands, coarse and thickened skin, enlarged tongue, slow speech, and anemia (Figure 16-7).
pheochromocytoma (*fe*-ō-*krō*-mō-sī-TŌ-ma)	tumor of the adrenal medulla, which is usually non-malignant and characterized by hypertension, headaches, palpitations, diaphoresis, chest pain, and abdominal pain. Surgical removal of the tumor is the most common treatment. Though usually curable with early detection, it can be fatal if untreated.

GIGANTISM AND ACROMEGALY

are both caused by overproduction of growth hormone. **Gigantism** occurs before puberty and before the growing ends of the bones have closed. If untreated, an individual may reach 8 feet tall in adulthood.

Acromegaly occurs after puberty. The bones most affected are those in the hands, feet, and jaw.

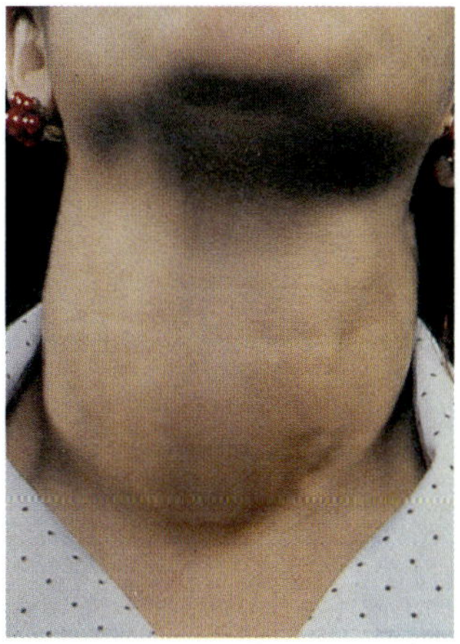

FIGURE 16-6
Goiter. May be caused by Graves disease, thyroiditis, or a thyroid nodule, which is a lump on the thyroid gland. Goiter is a general term for the enlargement of the thyroid gland.

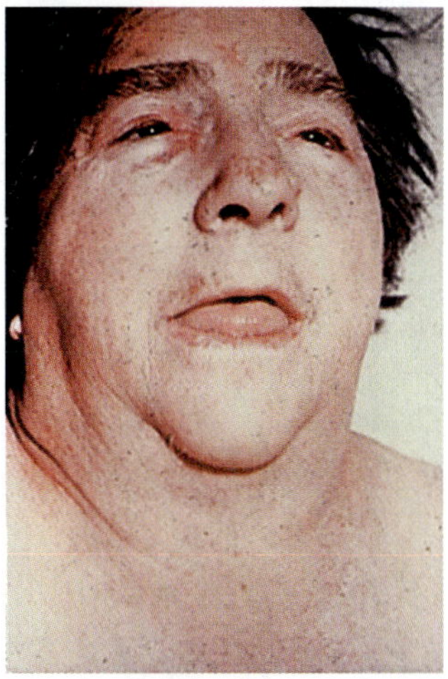

FIGURE 16-7
Myxedema.

Disease and Disorder Terms—*cont'd*

Not Built from Word Parts

Term	Definition
tetany (TET-a-nē)	condition affecting nerves causing muscle spasms as a result of low amounts of calcium in the blood caused by a deficiency of the parathyroid hormone
thyrotoxicosis (*thī*-rō-*tok*-si-KŌ-sis)	a condition caused by excessive thyroid hormones

EXERCISE 13

Practice saying aloud each of the disease and disorder terms not built from word parts on pp. 764-766.

To hear the terms, go to http://evolve.elsevier.com. Refer to p. 18 for your Evolve Access Information. Select Exercises & Review, Chapter 16, Chapter Exercises, Pronunciation.

☐ Place a check mark in the box when you have completed this exercise.

TABLE 16-1

Diabetes Mellitus

Two major forms of diabetes mellitus are **type 1,** previously called *insulin-dependent diabetes mellitus (IDDM)* or *juvenile-onset diabetes,* and **type 2,** previously called *noninsulin-dependent diabetes mellitus (NIDDM)* or *adult-onset diabetes (AODM).* Type 2 diabetes mellitus has reached epidemic proportions and is a major cause of cardiovasular disease.

Type 1 Diabetes Mellitus

Cause the beta cells of the pancreas that produce insulin are destroyed and eventually no insulin is produced

Characteristics abrupt onset, occurs primarily in childhood or adolescence; patients often are thin

Symptoms polyuria, polydipsia, weight loss, hyperglycemia, acidosis, and ketosis

Treatment insulin injections and diet

Type 2 Diabetes Mellitus

Cause resistance of body cells to the action of insulin, which may eventually lead to a decrease in insulin secretion

Characteristics slow onset, usually occurs in middle-aged or elderly adults; most patients are obese

Symptoms fatigue, blurred vision, thirst, and hyperglycemia; may have neural or vascular complications.

Treatment diet, exercise, oral medication, and perhaps insulin

Long-term Complications of Diabetes Mellitus

Macrovasular complications

- coronary artery disease → myocardial infarction
- cerebrovascular disease → stroke
- peripheral artery disease → leg pain when walking (intermittent vascular claudication)

Microvascular complications

- diabetic retinopathy → loss of vision
- diabetic nephropathy → chronic renal disease, kidney failure
- neuropathy → loss of feeling in extremities, amputation

CAM TERM

Tai Chi, often referred to as "meditation in motion," is an ancient Chinese art using slow movements and focused breathing to support mental and physical health. The regular practice of Tai Chi has demonstrated efficacy as an adjunct therapy for addressing glucose control and improving plantar sensation, balance, and quality of life in elderly patients with **type 2 diabetes mellitus**.

EXERCISE 14

Match the terms in the first column with the correct definitions in the second column.

______ 1. acidosis
______ 2. Addison disease
______ 3. cretinism
______ 4. Cushing syndrome
______ 5. diabetes insipidus
______ 6. diabetes mellitus
______ 7. gigantism
______ 8. goiter
______ 9. ketosis
______ 10. myxedema
______ 11. tetany
______ 12. thyrotoxicosis
______ 13. Graves disease
______ 14. pheochromocytoma
______ 15. metabolic syndrome

a. results from a deficiency in the hormonal secretion of the adrenal cortex
b. attributed to the excessive production of cortisol
c. chronic disease involving a disorder of carbohydrate metabolism
d. abnormal accumulation of acid products of metabolism
e. enlargement of the thyroid gland
f. results from low blood calcium
g. caused by excessive thyroid hormones
h. result of a decreased amount of antidiuretic hormone
i. caused by deficiency of the thyroid hormone thyroxine
j. caused by a wasting away of the thyroid gland
k. abnormal concentration of compounds resulting from excessive fat metabolism
l. caused by overproduction of the pituitary growth hormone
m. caused by an excessive amount of parahormone
n. characterized by hyperthyroidism, goiter, and exophthalmos
o. tumor of the adrenal medulla
p. group of signs and symptoms including insulin resistance, excessive fat around the waist and abdomen, hypertension, hyperglycemia, elevated triglycerides, and low HDL

EXERCISE 15

Write the name of the endocrine gland responsible for each of the following conditions.

1. myxedema ______
2. tetany ______
3. ketosis ______
4. gigantism ______
5. goiter ______
6. Addison disease ______
7. diabetes mellitus ______
8. cretinism ______
9. acidosis ______
10. Cushing syndrome ______
11. diabetes insipidus ______
12. Graves disease ______
13. thyrotoxicosis ______
14. pheochromocytoma ______

EXERCISE 16

Spell each of the disease and disorder terms not built from word parts on pp. 764-766 by having someone dictate them to you.

To hear and spell the terms, go to http://evolve.elsevier.com. Refer to p. 18 for your Evolve Access Information. Select Exercises & Review, Chapter 16, Chapter Exercises, Spelling.

☐ Place a check mark in the box if you have completed this exercise online.

1. ______
2. ______
3. ______
4. ______
5. ______
6. ______
7. ______
8. ______
9. ______
10. ______
11. ______
12. ______
13. ______
14. ______
15. ______

Surgical Terms

Built from Word Parts

The following terms are built from word parts you have already learned and can be translated literally to find their meanings. Further explanation of terms beyond the definition of their word parts, if needed, is included in parentheses.

Term	Definition
adenectomy (*ad*-en-EK-to-mē)	excision of a gland
adrenalectomy (ad-*rē*-nal-EK-to-mē)	excision of (one or both) adrenal glands
parathyroidectomy (*par*-a-*thī*-royd-EK-to-mē)	excision of (one or more) parathyroid glands
thyroidectomy (*thī*-royd-EK-to-mē)	excision of the thyroid gland
thyroidotomy (*thī*-royd-OT-o-mē)	incision of the thyroid gland
thyroparathyroidectomy (*thī*-rō-*par*-a-*thī*-royd-EK-to-mē)	excision of the thyroid and parathyroid glands

EXERCISE 17

Practice saying aloud each of the surgical terms built from word parts above.

To hear the terms, go to http://evolve.elsevier.com. Refer to p. 18 for your Evolve Access Information. Select Exercises & Review, Chapter 16, Chapter Exercises, Pronunciation.

☐ Place a check mark in the box when you have completed this exercise.

EXERCISE 18

Analyze and define the following surgical terms.

1. thyroidotomy ______________________________
2. adrenalectomy ______________________________
3. thyroparathyroidectomy ______________________________
4. thyroidectomy ______________________________
5. parathyroidectomy ______________________________
6. adenectomy ______________________________

EXERCISE 19

Build surgical terms for the following definitions by using the word parts you have learned.

1. excision of the thyroid gland ______ / ______
   WR / S
2. excision of the thyroid and parathyroid glands ______ / ______ / ______ / ______
   WR / CV / WR / S
3. excision of (one or both) adrenal glands ______ / ______
   WR / S
4. excision of (one or more) parathyroid glands ______ / ______
   WR / S
5. incision of the thyroid gland ______ / ______ / ______
   WR / CV / S
6. excision of a gland ______ / ______
   WR / S

EXERCISE 20

Spell each of the surgical terms built from word parts on p. 769 by having someone dictate them to you.

To hear and spell the terms, go to http://evolve.elsevier.com. Refer to p. 18 for your Evolve Access Information. Select Exercises & Review, Chapter 16, Chapter Exercises, Spelling.

☐ Place a check mark in the box if you have completed this exercise online.

1. ______
2. ______
3. ______
4. ______
5. ______
6. ______

Diagnostic Terms

Not Built from Word Parts

In some of the following terms, you may recognize word parts you have already learned; however, the full meaning of the terms cannot be discerned by the definition of their word parts.

ULTRASOUND AND COMPUTED TOMOGRAPHY (CT SCANNING)

are also used to diagnose various other conditions of the endocrine system. Examples are CT of the adrenal glands and thyroid ultrasonography.

Term	Definition
DIAGNOSTIC IMAGING	
radioactive iodine uptake (RAIU) (*rā*-dē-ō-AK-tiv) (Ī-ō-dīn)	a nuclear medicine scan that measures thyroid function. Radioactive iodine is given to the patient orally, after which its uptake into the thyroid gland is measured.

Term	Definition
thyroid scan (THĪ-royd)	a nuclear medicine test that shows the size, shape, and function of the thyroid gland. The patient is given a radioactive substance to visualize the thyroid gland. An image is recorded as the scanner is passed over the neck area; used to detect tumors and nodules.
LABORATORY	
fasting blood sugar (FBS)	a blood test performed after the patient has fasted for 8 to 10 hours to determine the amount of glucose (sugar) in the blood at the time of the test. Elevation may indicate diabetes mellitus.
glycosylated hemoglobin (HbA1C) (glī-KŌ-sa-*lāt*-ad) (HĒ-mō-*glō*-bin)	a blood test used to monitor diabetic treatment by measuring the amount of glycosylated hemoglobin (hemoglobin coated with sugar) in the blood. HbA1C provides an indication of blood sugar level over the past three months, covering the 120-day lifespan of the red blood cell (also called **hemoglobin A1C**)
thyroid-stimulating hormone level (TSH) (THĪ-royd)	a blood test that measures the amount of thyroid-stimulating hormone in the blood; used to diagnose hypothyroidism and to monitor patients on thyroid replacement therapy.
thyroxine level (T4) (thī-ROK-sin)	a blood study that gives the direct measurement of the amount of thyroxine in the patient's blood. A greater-than-normal amount indicates hyperthyroidism; a less-than-normal amount indicates hypothyroidism.

EXERCISE 21

Practice saying aloud each of the diagnostic terms not built from word parts on these two pages.

To hear the terms, go to http://evolve.elsevier.com. Refer to p. 18 for your Evolve Access Information. Select Exercises & Review, Chapter 16, Chapter Exercises, Pronunciation.

☐ Place a check mark in the box when you have completed this exercise.

EXERCISE 22

Match the terms in the first column with their correct definitions in the second column.

_____ 1. fasting blood sugar

_____ 2. thyroid scan

_____ 3. thyroxine level

_____ 4. radioactive iodine uptake

_____ 5. thyroid-stimulating hormone level

_____ 6. glycosylated hemoglobin

a. a nuclear medicine test used to determine the size, shape, and function of the thyroid gland

b. determines the amount of glucose in the blood at the time of the test

c. used to determine hypernatremia

d. uses radioactive iodine to measure thyroid function

e. used to diagnose hypothyroidism and to monitor thyroid replacement therapy

f. measures the amount of thyroxine in the blood

g. provides an indication of blood sugar level over the past three months

EXERCISE 23

Write the name of the procedure that measures each of the following.

1. thyroid function _____________________
2. amount of glucose in the blood at the time of the test _____________________
3. amount of thyroid-stimulating hormone in the blood _____________________
4. amount of thyroxine in the blood _____________________
5. size, shape, and function of the thyroid gland _____________________
6. amount of hemoglobin coated with sugar _____________________

EXERCISE 24

Spell each of the diagnostic terms not built from word parts on pp. 770-771 by having someone dictate them to you.

To hear and spell the terms, go to http://evolve.elsevier.com. Refer to p. 18 for your Evolve Access Information. Select Exercises & Review, Chapter 16, Chapter Exercises, Spelling.

☐ Place a check mark in the box if you have completed this exercise online.

1. ______________________ 4. ______________________
2. ______________________ 5. ______________________
3. ______________________ 6. ______________________

Complementary Terms

Built from Word Parts

The following terms are built from word parts you have already learned and can be translated literally to find their meanings. Further explanation of terms beyond the definition of their word parts, if needed, is included in parentheses.

Term	Definition
adrenocorticohyperplasia (a-*drē*-nō-*kōr*-ti-kō-*hī*-per-PLĀ-zha) (NOTE: *hyper,* a prefix, appears within this word.)	excessive development of the adrenal cortex
adrenopathy (*ad*-ren-OP-a-thē)	disease of the adrenal gland
cortical (KŌR-ti-kal)	pertaining to the cortex
corticoid (KŌR-ti-koyd)	resembling the cortex
endocrinologist (*en*-dō-kri-NOL-o-jist)	physician who studies and treats diseases of the endocrine (system)
endocrinology (*en*-dō-kri-NOL-o-jē)	the study of the endocrine (system) (a branch of medicine dealing with diseases of the endocrine system)
endocrinopathy (*en*-dō-kri-NOP-a-thē)	(any) disease of the endocrine (system)
euglycemia (*u*-glī-SĒ-mē-a)	normal (level of) sugar in the blood (within normal range)
euthyroid (ū-THĪ-royd)	resembling a normal thyroid gland (normal thyroid function)
polydipsia (*pol*-ē-DIP-sē-a)	abnormal state of much thirst
syndrome (SIN-drōm)	run together (signs and symptoms occurring together that are characteristic of a specific disorder)

EXERCISE 25

Practice saying aloud each of the complementary terms built from word parts on p. 773.

To hear the terms, go to http://evolve.elsevier.com. Refer to p. 18 for your Evolve Access Information. Select Exercises & Review, Chapter 16, Chapter Exercises, Pronunciation.

☐ Place a check mark in the box when you have completed this exercise.

EXERCISE 26

Analyze and define the following complementary terms.

1. corticoid ______________________
2. syndrome ______________________
3. adrenopathy ______________________
4. endocrinologist ______________________
5. polydipsia ______________________
6. euglycemia ______________________
7. endocrinopathy ______________________
8. adrenocorticohyperplasia ______________________
9. euthyroid ______________________
10. cortical ______________________
11. endocrinology ______________________

EXERCISE 27

Build the complementary terms for the following definitions by using the word parts you have learned.

1. (any) disease of the endocrine (system) ______ / ______ / ______
   WR / CV / S
2. resembling the cortex ______ / ______
   WR / S
3. run together (signs and symptoms occurring together) ______ / ______
   P / S(WR)
4. excessive development of the adrenal cortex ______ / ______ / ______ / ______ / ______ / ______
   WR / CV / WR / CV / P / S

5. the study of the endocrine (system)

________ / CV / ________
WR / CV / S

6. abnormal state of much thirst

________ / ________ / ________
P / WR / S

7. disease of the adrenal gland

________ / CV / ________
WR / CV / S

8. normal (level of) sugar in the blood

________ / ________ / ________
P / WR / S

9. resembling a normal thyroid gland

________ / ________ / ________
P / WR / S

10. pertaining to the cortex

________ / ________
WR / S

11. a physician who studies and treats diseases of the endocrine (system)

________ / CV / ________
WR / CV / S

EXERCISE 28

Spell each of the complementary terms built from word parts on p. 773 by having someone dictate them to you.

To hear and spell the terms, go to http://evolve.elsevier.com. Refer to p. 18 for your Evolve Access Information. Select Exercises & Review, Chapter 16, Chapter Exercises, Spelling.
☐ Place a check mark in the box if you have completed this exercise online.

1. ________________
2. ________________
3. ________________
4. ________________
5. ________________
6. ________________
7. ________________
8. ________________
9. ________________
10. ________________
11. ________________

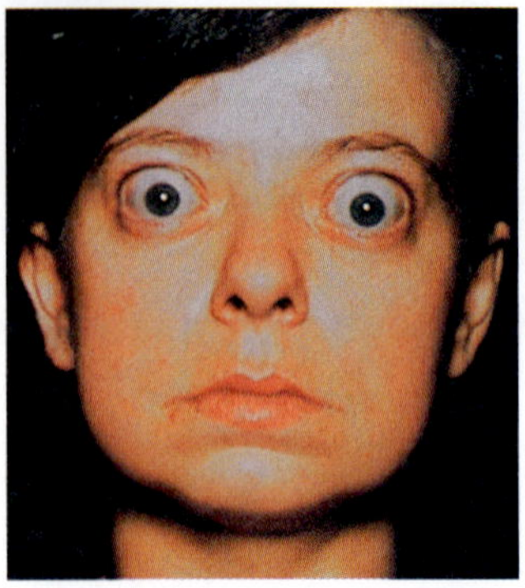

FIGURE 16-8
Abnormal protrusion of eyeballs, exophthalmos, a characteristic of thyroid disease.

EXOPHTHALMOS

is derived from the Greek ***ex***, meaning **outward**, and **ophthalmos**, meaning ***eye***. Protrusion of the eyeball is sometimes a symptom of Graves disease, first described by Dr. Robert Graves, an Irish physician, in 1835.

Complementary Terms

Not Built from Word Parts

In some of the following terms, you may recognize word parts you have already learned; however, the full meaning of the terms cannot be discerned by the definition of their word parts.

Term	Definition
exophthalmos (*ek*-sof-THAL-mos)	abnormal protrusion of the eyeball (Figure 16-8)
hormone (HOR-mōn)	a chemical substance secreted by an endocrine gland that is carried in the blood to a target tissue
isthmus (IS-mus)	narrow strip of tissue connecting two larger parts in the body, such as the isthmus that connects the two lobes of the thyroid gland (see Figure 16-3, *B*)
metabolism (me-TAB-ō-*liz-m*)	sum total of all the chemical processes that take place in a living organism

Refer to **Appendix D** for pharmacology terms related to the endocrine system.

EXERCISE 29

Practice saying aloud each of the complementary terms not built from word parts above.

To hear the terms, go to http://evolve.elsevier.com. Refer to p. 18 for your Evolve Access Information. Select Exercises & Review, Chapter 16, Chapter Exercises, Pronunciation.

☐ Place a check mark in the box when you have completed this exercise.

EXERCISE 30

Fill in the blanks with the correct terms.

1. The total of all the chemical processes that take place in a living organism is called its ________________.
2. A chemical substance secreted by an endocrine gland is called a(n) ________________.
3. A narrow strip of tissue connecting larger parts in the body is called a(n) ________________.
4. Abnormal protrusion of the eyeball is called ________________.

EXERCISE 31

Write the definitions of the following terms.

1. isthmus ________________
2. metabolism ________________
3. hormone ________________
4. exophthalmos ________________

EXERCISE 32

Spell each of the complementary terms not built from word parts on p. 776 by having someone dictate them to you.

To hear and spell the terms, go to http://evolve.elsevier.com. Refer to p. 18 for your Evolve Access Information. Select Exercises & Review, Chapter 16, Chapter Exercises, Spelling.
☐ Place a check mark in the box if you have completed this exercise online.

1. ______________________
2. ______________________
3. ______________________
4. ______________________

Refer to **Appendix D** for pharmacology terms related to the endocrine system.

Abbreviations

ACTH	adrenocorticotropic hormone
ADH	antidiuretic hormone
DI	diabetes insipidus
DM	diabetes mellitus
FBS	fasting blood sugar
FSH	follicle-stimulating hormone
GH	growth hormone
HbA1C	glycosylated hemoglobin
LH	luteinizing hormone
PRH	prolactin-releasing hormone
RAIU	radioactive iodine uptake
TSH	thyroid-stimulating hormone
T4	thyroxine level

Refer to **Appendix C** for a complete list of abbreviations.

EXERCISE 33

Write the meaning of the following abbreviations.

1. RAIU ____________ ____________ ____________
2. FBS ____________ ____________ ____________
3. DM ____________ ____________
4. DI ____________ ____________
5. T4 ____________ ____________
6. HbA1C ____________________ ____________________
7. TSH ____________ ____________ ____________
8. PRH ____________ ____________ ____________
9. LH ____________ ____________
10. GH ____________ ____________
11. FSH ____________ ____________ ____________
12. ADH ____________ ____________
13. ACTH ____________________ ____________________

PRACTICAL APPLICATION

EXERCISE 34 *Interact with Medical Documents*

A. Complete the history and physical by writing the medical terms in the blanks. Use the list of definitions with the corresponding numbers.

University Hospital and Medical Center
4700 North Main Street • Wellness, Arizona 54321 • (987) 555-3210

PATIENT NAME: Jane Nelson
DATE OF BIRTH: 05/21/19XX
CASE NUMBER: 021286-END
DATE: 06/20/20XX

HISTORY AND PHYSICAL

CHIEF COMPLAINT: Jane Nelson is a 33-year-old Caucasian female presenting with an episode of syncope at work, complaining of excessive urination and thirst and fatigue for approximately 1 month.

HISTORY OF PRESENT ILLNESS: For the past 4 weeks she has been having 1. ________________ and 2. ________________, drinking 3 to 4 quarts of water daily for the past 10 days. This has also resulted in nocturia, getting up 2 to 3 times a night to void. She denies anorexia, nausea, vomiting, 3. ________________, or any abdominal pain.

MEDICAL HISTORY: No known allergies. No previous hospitalizations. She does not smoke. She has had no recent illness.

FAMILY HISTORY: Mother died of a 4. ________________ at age 78. Father is still living at the age of 85, but has had 5. ________________ ________________ for 20 years. She has two brothers, both in good health, and no sisters.

SOCIAL HISTORY: Unmarried without children. She does not smoke and uses alcohol rarely.

REVIEW OF SYSTEMS: She denies fever, chills, headache, palpitations, chest pain, or edema.

PHYSICAL EXAM: Temperature, 98.9. Pulse, 80. Respirations, 24. Her blood pressure is 125/80 mm Hg. Her weight is 143 pounds, down 10 pounds since her last routine visit 3 months ago. **HEENT:** Normal. **CHEST:** Clear to auscultation and percussion. **HEART:** Regular rhythm. No murmurs or extra heart sounds. **ABDOMEN:** Soft, nontender, bowel sounds normal, without evidence of organomegaly. **RECTAL:** Unremarkable. **EXTREMITIES:** No 6. ________________, clubbing, or edema. Pedal pulses are intact. **NEUROLOGIC:** Alert and oriented to time, person, and place. Cranial nerves II through XII are grossly intact.

LABORATORY FINDINGS: Random blood sugar was discovered to be greater than 600 mg/dL. Urinalysis showed moderate ketonuria. Guaiac was negative.

ASSESSMENT: Diabetic 7. ________________, most likely caused by type 1 diabetes mellitus.

PLAN: Administer IV fluids and insulin. Schedule 8. ________________ consult for this afternoon for complete diagnosis and treatment.

____
Christina Kraemer, MD

CK/mcm

1. excessive urine
2. excessive thirst
3. vomiting of blood
4. interruption of blood supply to a region of the brain
5. chronic disease involving a disorder of carbohydrate metabolism caused by underactivity of islets of Langerhans and characterized by hyperglycemia
6. abnormal condition of blue (bluish discoloration of skin) caused by inadequate supply of oxygen in the blood
7. abnormal concentration of ketone bodies
8. study of the endocrine system

B. Read the operative report and answer the questions on p. 780

029210 GOMEZ, RUTH

File Patient Navigate Custom Fields Help

Patient Chart | Lab | Rad | Notes | Documents | Rx | Scheduling | Images | Billing

Name: **GOMEZ, RUTH** MR#: **029210** DOB: **5/11/19XX** Sex: **Female**

DATE OF OPERATION: April 10, 20XX

SURGERY PERFORMED: Right laparoscopic adrenalectomy

PREOPERATIVE DIAGNOSIS: Primary hyperaldosteronism (Conn syndrome), adrenal adenoma.

INDICATIONS: The patient is a 39-year-old woman who has a history of hypertension and hypokalemia seen on referral from her endocrinologist. The patient complained of headache and muscle weakness. She underwent a 24-hour urine collection, a general metastatic workup, and evaluation for Cushing syndrome. Laboratory studies indicated elevated plasma and urinary aldosterone levels. CT scan revealed the presence of a 3.5-cm right adrenal mass, and adrenal sampling confirmed that it was an aldosterone-producing adenoma.

PROCEDURE: The procedure was performed with the patient under general endotracheal anesthesia and with an arterial line, a Foley catheter, and a central venous pressure line in place. A Veress needle was inserted into the abdominal cavity between the midclavicular and anterior axillary lines. The abdominal cavity was then insufflated with CO_2. A 10- to 11-mm trocar was placed at the site of the Veress needle, and a 30-degree videotelescope was inserted. A third 10- to 11-mm port was placed 3 to 4 cm behind the posterior axillary line, and a fourth port inserted after mobilization of the right lobe of the liver. The superior pole and lateral border of the adrenal gland were mobilized first, with the dissection proceeding carefully along the lateral edge of the inferior vena cava. The right adrenal vein was ligated with endoscopic clips and divided, freeing the adrenal gland from its surrounding attachments. The gland was placed in an impermeable entrapment sac and removed from the most anterior port site. After evacuation of CO_2, all ports were removed, and the incisions were closed with absorbable sutures.

POSTOPERATIVE DIAGNOSIS: Aldosteronoma

Electronically signed by: Merriam Fitch, MD 4/11/20XX 11:24 AM

MF/abr

Start | Log On/Off | Print | Edit

EXERCISE 34 *Interact with Medical Documents—cont'd*

B.

1. Which procedure was performed during surgery:
   a. excision of a parathyroid gland
   b. surgical repair of the thyroid gland
   c. excision of an adrenal gland
   d. surgical repair of the thymus

2. The patient had a history of:
   a. excessive sugar in the blood
   b. deficient potassium in the blood
   c. excessive sodium in the blood
   d. deficient calcium in the blood

3. The patient was evaluated for a:
   a. group of symptoms from the excessive production of cortisol
   b. condition caused by congenital absence of the thyroid gland
   c. syndrome caused by deficient secretion from the adrenal cortex
   d. condition causing muscle spasms resulting from low amounts of calcium

EXERCISE 35 *Interpret Medical Terms*

To test your understanding of the terms introduced in this chapter, circle the words that correctly complete the sentences. The italicized words refer to the correct answer.

1. A patient who has an *enlargement of the thyroid gland* has (**myxedema, tetany, goiter**).
2. A condition that results from *uncontrolled diabetes mellitus* is (**calcipenia, ketosis, tetany**).
3. *Addison disease* is caused by an *underfunctioning* of the (**adrenal, pituitary, thyroid**) gland.
4. *Decreased secretion* of (**ACTH, antidiuretic hormone, TSH**) may cause diabetes insipidus.
5. *Cushing syndrome* is caused by (**overactivity, underactivity**) of the *adrenal cortices.*
6. A *wasting away of the thyroid gland* may result in (**cretinism, myxedema, tetany**).
7. The primary treatment for *tumor of the adrenal medulla* (**pheochromocytoma, adenomegaly, thyrotoxicosis**) is surgical removal of the tumor by laparoscopic *excision of an adrenal gland* (**adenectomy, adrenalectomy, thyroidectomy**).
8. Unlike *the blood test measuring the amount of glucose in the blood at the time of the test* (**fasting blood sugar, glycosylated hemoglobin, radioactive iodine uptake test**), *the test measuring the amount of hemoglobin coated in sugar over the lifespan of the red blood cell* (**fasting blood sugar, glycosylated hemoglobin, radioactive iodine uptake test**) test results are not altered by eating habits the day before the test.
9. Lifestyle changes such as weight loss, regular exercise, healthy eating, and cessation of smoking are central in the treatment and prevention of *a group of health problems including insulin resistance, obesity, hypertension, hyperglycemia, elevated triglycerides and low levels of HDL* (**euglycemia, Addison disease, metabolic syndrome**).

EXERCISE 36 *Read Medical Terms in Use*

Practice pronunciation of the terms by reading the following medical document. Use the pronunciation key following the medical terms to assist you.

To hear these terms, go to http://evolve.elsevier.com. Refer to p. 18 for your Evolve Access Information. Select Exercises & Review, Chapter 16, Chapter Exercises, Read Medical Terms in Use.

A 55-year-old female patient presented to her doctor because of a 10-pound weight gain, fatigue, hair loss, dry skin, and cold intolerance. She was referred to an **endocrinologist** (en-dō-kri-NOL-o-jist), who established a diagnosis of **hypothyroidism** (*hī*-pō-THĪ-royd-izm) after test results indicated an elevated **thyroid** (THĪ-royd)**-stimulating hormone level** and a low **thyroxine** (thī-ROX-sin) **level.** Thyroid hormone therapy was prescribed. Approximately 20 years ago she was diagnosed with Graves disease characterized by hyperthyroidism, **exophthalmos** (ek-sof-THAL-mos), fatigue, irritability, weight loss, and **goiter** (GOY-ter). At this time she had an increased **radioactive iodine** (ra-dē-ō-AK-tiv) (Ī-ō-dīn) **uptake** (RAIU). Treatment included a **thyroidectomy** (*thī*-royd-EK-to-mē) with subsequent thyroid hormone therapy. She remained in a **euthyroid** (ū-THĪ–royd) state until she stopped taking the medication 6 months ago. Consequently she became hypothyroid and could easily have developed **myxedema** (*mik*-se-DĒ-ma) if she had not sought treatment.

EXERCISE 37 *Comprehend Medical Terms in Use*

Test your comprehension of terms in the previous medical document by circling the correct answer.

1. On a recent visit to the endocrinologist the patient was diagnosed with:
   a. a state of deficient thyroid gland activity
   b. an enlargement of the thyroid gland
   c. a state of excessive thyroid gland activity
   d. Graves disease
2. After a thyroidectomy the patient remained in a state resembling a:
   a. stressed thyroid gland
   b. normal thyroid gland
   c. hyperactive thyroid gland
   d. hypoactive thyroid gland
3. The patient's earlier diagnosis of Graves disease was characterized by:
   a. thirst, excessive thyroid activity, protruding eyes
   b. protruding eyes, spasms, excessive thyroid activity
   c. excessive thyroid activity, enlargement of the thyroid gland, protruding eyes
   d. enlargement of the extremities, excessive thyroid activities, protruding eyes
4. What type of diagnostic procedure was used to assist in diagnosing hypothyroidism?
   a. computed tomography
   b. nuclear medicine
   c. ultrasound
   d. blood test

CHAPTER REVIEW

ONLINE CHAPTER REVIEW

To access the Evolve website, go to http://evolve.elsevier.com. Refer to p. 18 for your Evolve Access Information. Select Exercises & Review, Chapter 16, then select Chapter Exercises, Practice Activities, Animations, or Games. Place a check mark in the box when you have completed an exercise or activity, watched an animation, or played a game. Have fun!

Chapter Exercises

Exercises in this section of your Evolve resources correlate to exercises in your textbook. You may have completed them as you worked through the chapter.

- ☐ Pronunciation
- ☐ Spelling
- ☐ Read Medical Terms in Use

Practice Activities

Practice in study mode, then test your learning in assessment mode. Keep track of your scores from assessment mode if you wish.

	SCORE
☐ Picture It	_____
☐ Define Word Parts	_____
☐ Build Medical Terms	_____
☐ Word Shop	_____
☐ Define Medical Terms	_____
☐ Use It	_____
☐ Hear It and Type It: Clinical Vignettes	_____

Animations

- ☐ Hyperthyroidism
- ☐ Hypothyroidism
- ☐ Type 1 Diabetes
- ☐ Type 2 Diabetes
- ☐ Acidosis

Games

- ☐ Name that Word Part
- ☐ Term Storm
- ☐ Term Explorer
- ☐ Termbusters
- ☐ Medical Millionaire
- ☐ Crossword Puzzle

REVIEW OF WORD PARTS

Can you define and spell the following word parts?

Combining Forms

acr/o
aden/o
adren/o
adrenal/o
calc/i
cortic/o
dips/o
endocrin/o
kal/i
natr/o
parathyroid/o
pituitar/o
thyr/o
thyroid/o

Suffix

-drome

REVIEW OF TERMS

Can you build, analyze, define, pronounce, and spell the following terms *built from word parts?*

Diseases and Disorders

acromegaly
adenitis
adenomegaly
adenosis
adrenalitis
adrenomegaly
hypercalcemia
hyperglycemia
hyperkalemia
hyperpituitarism
hyperthyroidism
hypocalcemia
hypoglycemia
hypokalemia
hyponatremia
hypopituitarism
hypothyroidism
panhypopituitarism
parathyroidoma
thyroiditis

Surgical

adenectomy
adrenalectomy
parathyroidectomy
thyroidectomy
thyroidotomy
thyroparathyroidectomy

Complementary

adrenocorticohyperplasia
adrenopathy
cortical
corticoid
endocrinologist
endocrinology
endocrinopathy
euglycemia
euthyroid
polydipsia
syndrome

Can you define, pronounce, and spell the following terms *not built from word parts?*

Diseases and Disorders

acidosis
Addison disease
cretinism
Cushing syndrome
diabetes insipidus (DI)
diabetes mellitus (DM)
gigantism
goiter
Graves disease
ketosis
metabolic syndrome
myxedema
pheochromocytoma
tetany
thyrotoxicosis

Diagnostic

fasting blood sugar (FBS)
glycosylated hemoglobin (HbA1C)
radioactive iodine uptake (RAIU)
thyroid scan
thyroid-stimulating hormone (TSH) level
thyroxine level (T4)

Complementary

exophthalmos
hormone
isthmus
metabolism

ANSWERS

Exercise Figures

Exercise Figure

A. 1. parathyroid glands: parathyroid/o
2. adrenal glands: adren/o, adrenal/o
3. pituitary gland: pituitar/o
4. thyroid gland: thyroid/o, thyr/o

Exercise Figure

B. cortex: cortic/o

Exercise Figure

C. acr/o/megaly

Exercise 1

1. b
2. g
3. d
4. h
5. a
6. c
7. e

Exercise 2

1. d
2. a
3. e
4. b
5. g
6. c

Exercise 3

1. cortex
2. adrenal glands
3. parathyroid glands
4. thyroid gland
5. adrenal glands
6. thyroid gland
7. endocrine
8. gland
9. pituitary gland

Exercise 4

1. a. adren/o
   b. adrenal/o
2. a. thyroid/o
   b. thyr/o
3. endocrin/o
4. cortic/o
5. parathyroid/o
6. aden/o
7. pituitar/o

Exercise 5

1. thirst
2. potassium
3. calcium
4. extremities, height
5. sodium

Exercise 6

1. acr/o
2. calc/i
3. dips/o
4. kal/i
5. natr/o

Exercise 7

1. run, running

Exercise 8

1. -drome

Exercise 9

Pronunciation Exercise

Exercise 10

1. WR S
   adrenal/itis
   inflammation of the adrenal glands
2. P WR S
   hypo/calc/emia
   deficient calcium in the blood
3. P WR S
   hyper/thyroid/ism
   state of excessive thyroid gland activity
4. P WR S
   hyper/kal/emia
   excessive potassium in the blood
5. P WR S
   hyper/glyc/emia
   excessive sugar in the blood
6. WR CV S
   adren/o/megaly
   CF
   enlargement of the adrenal glands
7. WR CV S
   aden/o/megaly
   CF
   enlargement of a gland
8. P WR S
   hypo/thyroid/ism
   state of deficient thyroid gland activity
9. P WR S
   hypo/kal/emia
   deficient potassium in the blood
10. WR S
    aden/itis
    inflammation of a gland
11. WR S
    parathyroid/oma
    tumor of a parathyroid gland
12. WR CV S
    acr/o/megaly
    CF
    enlargement of the extremities
13. P P WR S
    pan/hypo/pituitar/ism
    a state of total deficient pituitary gland activity
14. P WR S
    hypo/glyc/emia
    deficient sugar in the blood
15. P WR S
    hyper/calc/emia
    excessive calcium in the blood
16. P WR S
    hyper/pituitar/ism
    state of excessive pituitary gland activity
17. P WR S
    hypo/natr/emia
    deficient sodium in the blood
18. WR S
    aden/osis
    abnormal condition of a gland
19. WR S
    thyroid/itis
    inflammation of the thyroid gland
20. P WR S
    hypo/pituitar/ism
    a state of deficient pituitary gland activity

Exercise 11

1. adren/o/megaly
2. hypo/thyroid/ism
3. acr/o/megaly
4. hypo/glyc/emia
5. hyper/kal/emia
6. hypo/calc/emia
7. hyper/thyroid/ism
8. hypo/pituitar/ism
9. hyper/calc/emia
10. hyper/pituitar/ism
11. parathyroid/oma
12. hyper/glyc/emia
13. aden/osis
14. hypo/kal/emia
15. adrenal/itis
16. aden/o/megaly
17. hypo/natr/emia
18. aden/itis
19. thyroid/itis
20. pan/hypo/pituitar/ism

Exercise 12

Spelling Exercise; see text pp. 760-761.

Exercise 13

Pronunciation Exercise

Exercise 14

1. d
2. a
3. j
4. b
5. h
6. c
7. l
8. e
9. k
10. i
11. f
12. g
13. n
14. o
15. p

Exercise 15

1. thyroid
2. parathyroid
3. islets of Langerhans (pancreas)
4. pituitary
5. thyroid
6. adrenal
7. islets of Langerhans (pancreas)
8. thyroid
9. islets of Langerhans (pancreas)
10. adrenal
11. pituitary
12. thyroid
13. thyroid
14. adrenal

Exercise 16

Spelling Exercise; see text pp. 764-766.

Exercise 17

Pronunciation Exercise

Exercise 18

1. WR CV S
   thyroid/o/tomy
   CF
   incision of the thyroid gland
2. WR S
   adrenal/ectomy
   excision of (one or both) adrenal glands
3. WR CV WR S
   thyr/o/parathyroid/ectomy
   CF
   excision of the thyroid and parathyroid glands
4. WR S
   thyroid/ectomy
   excision of the thyroid gland
5. WR S
   parathyroid/ectomy
   excision of (one or more) parathyroid glands
6. WR S
   aden/ectomy
   excision of a gland

Exercise 19

1. thyroid/ectomy
2. thyr/o/parathyroid/ectomy
3. adrenal/ectomy
4. parathyroid/ectomy
5. thyroid/o/tomy
6. aden/ectomy

Exercise 20

Spelling Exercise; see text p. 769.

Exercise 21

Pronunciation Exercise

Exercise 22

1. b
2. a
3. f
4. d
5. e
6. g

Exercise 23

1. radioactive iodine uptake
2. fasting blood sugar
3. thyroid-stimulating hormone level
4. thyroxine level
5. thyroid scan
6. glycosylated hemoglobin

Exercise 24

Spelling Exercise; see text pp. 770-771.

Exercise 25

Pronunciation Exercise

Exercise 26

1. WR S
   cortic/oid
   resembling the cortex
2. P S(WR)
   syn/drome
   run together
3. WR CV S
   adren/o/pathy
   CF
   disease of the adrenal glands
4. WR CV S
   endocrin/o/logist
   CF
   a physician who studies and treats diseases of the endocrine (system)
5. P WR S
   poly/dips/ia
   abnormal state of much thirst
6. P WR S
   eu/glyc/emia
   normal (level of) sugar in the blood
7. WR CV S
   endocrin/o/pathy
   CF
   (any) disease of the endocrine (system)
8. WR CV WR CV P S
   adren/o/cortic/o/hyper/plasia
   CF CF
   excessive development of the adrenal cortex
9. P WR S
   eu/thyr/oid
   resembling normal thyroid gland
10. WR S
    cortic/al
    pertaining to the cortex
11. WR CV S
    endocrin/o/logy
    CF
    study of the endocrine (system)

Exercise 27

1. endocrin/o/pathy
2. cortic/oid
3. syn/drome
4. adren/o/cortic/o/hyper/plasia
5. endocrin/o/logy
6. poly/dips/ia
7. adren/o/pathy
8. eu/glyc/emia
9. eu/thyr/oid
10. cortic/al
11. endocrin/o/logist

Exercise 28

Spelling Exercise; see text p. 773.

Exercise 29

Pronunciation Exercise

Exercise 30

1. metabolism
2. hormone
3. isthmus
4. exophthalmos

Exercise 31

1. narrow strip of tissue connecting two larger parts in the body
2. total of all chemical processes that take place in living organisms
3. a chemical substance secreted by an endocrine gland
4. abnormal protrusion of the eyeball

Exercise 32

Spelling Exercise; see text p. 776.

Exercise 33

1. radioactive iodine uptake
2. fasting blood sugar
3. diabetes mellitus
4. diabetes insipidus
5. thyroxine level
6. glycosylated hemoglobin
7. thyroid-stimulating hormone
8. prolactin-releasing hormone
9. lutenizing hormone
10. growth hormone
11. follicle-stimulating hormone
12. antidiuretic hormone
13. adrenocorticotropic hormone

Exercise 34

A. 1. polyuria
2. polydipsia
3. hematemesis
4. stroke
5. diabetes mellitus
6. cyanosis
7. ketosis
8. endocrinology

B. 1. c
2. b
3. a

Exercise 35

1. goiter
2. ketosis
3. adrenal
4. antidiuretic hormone
5. overactivity
6. cretinism
7. pheochromocytoma, adrenalectomy
8. fasting blood sugar, glycosylated hemoglobin
9. metabolic syndrome

Exercise 36

Reading Exercise

Exercise 37

1. a
2. b
3. c
4. d

APPENDIX A

Combining Forms, Prefixes, and Suffixes Alphabetized According to Word Part

Combining Forms	Definition	Chapter
A		
abdomin/o	abdomen (abdominal cavity)	11
acr/o	extremities, height	16
aden/o	gland	2, 16
adenoid/o	adenoids	5
adren/o	adrenal glands	16
adrenal/o	adrenal glands	16
albumin/o	albumin	6
alveol/o	alveolus	5
amni/o	amnion	9
amnion/o	amnion	9
andr/o	male	7
angi/o	vessel	10
ankyl/o	crooked, stiff, bent	14
an/o	anus	11
anter/o	front	3
antr/o	antrum	11
aort/o	aorta	10
aponeur/o	aponeurosis	14
appendic/o	appendix	11
append/o	appendix	11
arche/o	first, beginning	8
arteri/o	artery	10
arthr/o	joint	14
atel/o	imperfect, incomplete	5
ather/o	yellowish, fatty plaque	10
atri/o	atrium	10
aur/i	ear	13
aur/o	ear	13
aut/o	self	4
azot/o	urea, nitrogen	6
B		
balan/o	glans penis	7
bi/o	life	4
blast/o	developing cell, germ cell	6
blephar/o	eyelid	12
bronch/i	bronchus	5
bronchi/o	bronchus	5
burs/o	bursa (cavity)	14
C		
calc/i	calcium	16
cancer/o	cancer	2
capn/o	carbon dioxide	5
carcin/o	cancer	2
cardi/o	heart	10
carp/o	carpals (wrist bones)	14
caud/o	tail (downward)	3

Combining Forms	Definition	Chapter
cec/o	cecum	11
celi/o	abdomen (abdominal cavity)	11
cephal/o	head	3, 9
cerebell/o	cerebellum	15
cerebr/o	cerebrum, brain	15
cervic/o	cervix	8
cheil/o	lip	11
chlor/o	green	2
cholangi/o	bile duct	11
chol/e	gall, bile	11
choledoch/o	common bile duct	11
chondr/o	cartilage	14
chori/o	chorion	9
chrom/o	color	2
clavic/o	clavicle (collarbone)	14
clavicul/o	clavicle (collarbone)	14
col/o	colon	11
cocle/o	cochlea	13
colon/o	colon	11
colp/o	vagina	8
coni/o	dust	4
conjunctiv/o	conjunctiva	12
cor/o	pupil	12
core/o	cornea	12
corne/o	pupil	12
cortic/o	cortex (outer layer of body organ)	16
cost/o	rib	14
crani/o	cranium (skull)	14
cry/o	cold	12
crypt/o	hidden	4
culd/o	cul-de-sac	8
cutane/o	skin	4
cyan/o	blue	2
cyst/o	bladder, sac	6
cyt/o	cell	2
D		
dacry/o	tear, tear duct	12
dermat/o	skin	4
derm/o	skin	4
diaphragmat/o	diaphragm	5
dipl/o	two, double	12
dips/o	thirst	16
disk/o	intervertebral disk	14
dist/o	away (from the point of attachment of a body part)	3
diverticul/o	diverticulum	11
dors/o	back	3
duoden/o	duodenum	11
dur/o	hard, dura mater	15
E		
ech/o	sound	10
electr/o	electricity, electrical activity	10
embry/o	embryo, to be full	9
encephal/o	brain	15
endocrin/o	endocrine	16
enter/o	intestine	11
epididym/o	epididymis	7
epiglott/o	epiglottis	5

Combining Forms	Definition	Chapter
episi/o	vulva	8
epitheli/o	epithelium	2
erythr/o	red	2
esophag/o	esophagus	9, 11
esthesi/o	sensation, sensitivity, feeling	15
eti/o	cause (of disease)	2
F		
femor/o	femur (upper leg bone)	14
fet/i	fetus, unborn child	9
fet/o	fetus, unborn child	9
fibr/o	fiber	2
fibul/o	fibula (lower leg bone)	14
G		
gangli/o	ganglion	15
ganglion/o	ganglion	15
gastr/o	stomach	11
gingiv/o	gum	11
gli/o	glia, gluey substance	15
glomerul/o	glomerulus	6
gloss/o	tongue	11
glyc/o	sugar	6
glycos/o	sugar	6
gno/o	knowledge	2
gravid/o	pregnancy	9
gynec/o	woman	8
gyn/o	woman	8
H		
hemat/o	blood	5
hem/o	blood	5
hepat/o	liver	11
herni/o	hernia	11
heter/o	other	4
hidr/o	sweat	4
hist/o	tissue	2
humer/o	humerus (upper arm bone)	14
hydr/o	water	6
hymen/o	hymen	8
hyster/o	uterus	8
I		
iatr/o	medicine, physician, (treatment)	2
ile/o	ileum	11
ili/o	ilium	14
infer/o	below	3
irid/o	iris	12
ir/o	iris	12
is/o	equal	12
ischi/o	ischium	14
isch/o	deficiency, blockage	10
J		
jejun/o	jejunum	11
K		
kal/i	potassium	16
kary/o	nucleus	2
kerat/o	cornea	12
kerat/o	horny tissue, hard	4
kinesi/o	movement, motion	14
kyph/o	hump (increased convexity of the spine)	14

Combining Forms	Definition	Chapter
L		
labyrinth/o	labyrinth, (inner ear)	13
lacrim/o	tear, tear duct	12
lact/o	milk	9
lamin/o	lamina (thin, flat plate or layer)	14
lapar/o	abdomen, (abdominal cavity)	11
laryng/o	larynx (voice box)	5
later/o	side	3
lei/o	smooth	2
leuk/o	white	2
lingu/o	tongue	11
lip/o	fat	2
lith/o	stone, calculus	6
lob/o	lobe	5
lord/o	bent forward (increased concavity of the spine)	14
lumb/o	loin (or lumbar region of the spine)	14
lymphaden/o	lymph node	10
lymph/o	lymph, lymph tissue	10
M		
mamm/o	breast	8
mandibul/o	mandible (lower jawbone)	14
mast/o	breast	8
mastoid/o	mastoid bone	13
maxill/o	maxilla (upper jawbone)	14
meat/o	meatus (opening)	6
melan/o	black	2
meningi/o	meninges	15
mening/o	meninges	15
menisc/o	meniscus (crescent)	14
men/o	menstruation	8
ment/o	mind	15
metr/i	uterus	8
metr/o	uterus	8
mon/o	one, single	15
muc/o	mucus	5
myc/o	fungus	4
myel/o	bone marrow	10
myel/o	spinal cord	15
my/o	muscle	2, 14
myos/o	muscle	14
myring/o	tympanic membrane (eardrum)	13
N		
nas/o	nose	5
nat/o	birth	9
necr/o	death (cells, body)	4
nephr/o	kidney	6
neur/o	nerve	2, 15
noct/i	night	6
O		
ocul/o	eye	12
olig/o	scanty, few	6
omphal/o	umbilicus, navel	9
onc/o	tumor, mass	2
onych/o	nail	4
oophor/o	ovary	8
ophthalm/o	eye	12
opt/o	vision	12
orchid/o	testis, testicle	7

Combining Forms	Definition	Chapter
orchi/o	testis, testicle	7
orch/o	testis, testicle	7
organ/o	organ	2
or/o	mouth	11
orth/o	straight	5
oste/o	bone	14
ot/o	ear	13
ox/i	oxygen	5
ox/o	oxygen	5
P		
pachy/o	thick	4
palat/o	palate	11
pancreat/o	pancreas	11
parathyroid/o	parathyroid gland	16
par/o	bear, give birth to, labor	9
part/o	bear, give birth to, labor	9
patell/o	patella (kneecap)	14
path/o	disease	2
pelv/i	pelvis, pelvic bone	9, 14
pelv/o	pelvis, pelvic bone	9, 14
perine/o	perineum	8
peritone/o	peritoneum	11
petr/o	stone	14
phac/o	lens	12
phak/o	lens	12
phalang/o	phalanx (finger or toe bone)	14
pharyng/o	pharynx (throat)	5
phas/o	speech	15
phleb/o	vein	10
phon/o	sound	5
phot/o	light	12
phren/o	diaphragm	5
pituitar/o	pituitary	16
plasm/o	plasma	10
pleur/o	pleura	5
pneumat/o	lung, air	5
pneum/o	lung, air	5
pneumon/o	lung, air	5
poli/o	gray matter	15
polyp/o	polyp, small growth	11
poster/o	back, behind	3
prim/i	first	9
proct/o	rectum	11
prostat/o	prostate gland	7
proxim/o	near (the point of attachment of a body part)	3
pseud/o	false	9
psych/o	mind	15
pub/o	pubis	14
puerper/o	childbirth	9
pulmon/o	lung	5
pupill/o	pupil	12
pyel/o	renal pelvis	6
pylor/o	pylorus (pyloric sphincter)	9, 11
py/o	pus	5
Q		
quadr/i	four	15

Combining Forms	Definition	Chapter
R		
rachi/o	spinal or vertebral column	14
radic/o	nerve root	15
radicul/o	nerve root	15
radi/o	radius (lower arm bone)	14
rect/o	rectum	11
ren/o	kidney	6
retin/o	retina	12
rhabd/o	rod-shaped, striated	2
rhin/o	nose	5
rhiz/o	nerve root	15
rhytid/o	wrinkles	4
S		
sacr/o	sacrum	14
salping/o	uterine (fallopian) tube	8
sarc/o	flesh, connective tissue	2
scapul/o	scapula (shoulder blade)	14
scler/o	sclera	12
scoli/o	crooked, curved	14
seb/o	sebum (oil)	4
sept/o	septum	5
sial/o	saliva	11
sigmoid/o	sigmoid	11
sinus/o	sinus	5
somat/o	body	2
somn/o	sleep	5
son/o	sound	6
sperm/o	spermatozoon, sperm	7
spermat/o	spermatozoon, sperm	7
spir/o	breathe, breathing	5
splen/o	spleen	10
spondyl/o	vertebra	14
staped/o	stapes (middle ear bone)	13
staphyl/o	grapelike clusters	4
stern/o	sternum (breastbone)	14
stomat/o	mouth	11
steat/o	fat	11
strept/o	twisted chains	4
super/o	above	3
synovi/o	synovia, synovial membrane	14
system/o	system	2
T		
tars/o	tarsals (ankle bones)	14
tendin/o	tendon	14
tend/o	tendon	14
ten/o	tendon	14
terat/o	malformations	9
test/o	testis, testicle	7
therm/o	heat	10
thorac/o	thorax (chest)	5
thromb/o	clot	10
thym/o	thymus gland	10
thyroid/o	thyroid gland	16
thyr/o	thyroid gland	16
tibi/o	tibia (lower leg bone)	14
tom/o	cut, section	6
ton/o	tension, pressure	12
tonsill/o	tonsil	5

Combining Forms	Definition	Chapter
T—cont'd		
trache/o	trachea	5
trich/o	hair	4
tympan/o	tympanic membrane (eardrum), middle ear	13
U		
uln/o	ulna (lower arm bone)	14
ungu/o	nail	4
ureter/o	ureter	6
urethr/o	urethra	6
ur/o	urine, urinary tract	6
urin/o	urine, urinary tract	6
uvul/o	uvula	11
V		
vagin/o	vagina	8
valv/o	valve	10
valvul/o	valve	10
vas/o	vessel, duct	7
ven/o	vein	10
ventricul/o	ventricle	10
ventr/o	belly, front	3
vertebr/o	vertebra	14
vesic/o	bladder, sac	6
vesicul/o	seminal vesicles	7
vestibul/o	vestibule	13
viscer/o	internal organs	2
vulv/o	vulva	8
X		
xanth/o	yellow	2
xer/o	dry	4

Prefix	Definition	Chapter
a-	without, absence of	5
an-	without, absence of	5
ante-	before	9
bi-	two	3, 12
bin-	two	12
brady-	slow	10
dia-	through, complete	2
dys-	painful, abnormal, difficult, labored	2
endo-	within	5
epi-	on, upon, over	4
eu-	normal, good	5
hemi-	half	11
hyper-	above, excessive	2
hypo-	below, incomplete, deficient	2
inter-	between	14
intra-	within	4
meta-	after, beyond, change	2
micro-	small	9
multi-	many	9
neo-	new	2
nulli-	none	9
pan-	all, total	5
para-	beside, beyond, around, abnormal	4
per-	through	4
peri-	surrounding (outer)	8
poly-	many, much	5
post-	after	9

Prefix	Definition	Chapter
pre-	before	9
pro-	before	2
sub-	under, below	4
supra-	above	14
sym-	together, joined	14
syn-	together, joined	14
tachy-	fast, rapid	5
trans-	through, across, beyond	4
uni-	one	3

Suffix	Definition	Chapter
-a	no meaning	4
-ac	pertaining to	10
-ad	toward	3
-al	pertaining to	2
-algia	pain	5
-amnios	amniotic fluid, amnion	9
-apheresis	removal	10
-ar	pertaining to	5
-ary	pertaining to	5
-asthenia	weakness	14
-atresia	absence of a normal body opening, occlusion, closure	8
-cele	hernia, protrusion	5
-centesis	surgical puncture to aspirate fluid	5
-clasia	break	14
-clasis	break	14
-clast	break	14
-coccus (*pl.* -cocci)	berry-shaped (a form of bacterium)	4
-cyesis	pregnancy	9
-cyte	cell	2
-desis	surgical fixation, fusion	14
-drome	run, running	16
-eal	pertaining to	5
-ectasis	stretching out, dilation, expansion	5
-ectomy	excision, surgical removal	4
-emia	blood condition	5
-esis	condition	6
-gen	substance or agent that produces or causes	2
-genic	producing, originating, causing	2
-gram	record, radiographic image	6
-graph	instrument used to record; record	10
-graphy	process of recording, radiographic imaging	5
-ia	diseased or abnormal state, condition of	4
-iasis	condition	6
-iatrist	specialist, physician	15
-iatry	treatment, specialty	15
-ic	pertaining to	2
-ictal	seizure, attack	15
-ior	pertaining to	3
-is	no meaning	9
-ism	state of	7
-itis	inflammation	4
-logist	one who studies and treats, specialist, physician	2
-logy	study of	2
-lysis	loosening, dissolution, separating	6
-malacia	softening	4
-megaly	enlargement	6
-meter	instrument used to measure	5

Suffix	Definition	Chapter
-metry	measurement	5
-oid	resembling	2
-oma	tumor, swelling	2
-opia	vision (condition)	12
-opsy	view of, viewing	4
-osis	abnormal condition (means increase when used with blood cell word roots)	2
-ous	pertaining to	2
-paresis	slight paralysis	15
-partum	childbirth, labor	9
-pathy	disease	2
-penia	abnormal reduction (in number)	10
-pepsia	digestion	11
-pexy	surgical fixation, suspension	5
-phagia	eating, swallowing	4
-phobia	abnormal fear of or aversion to specific things	12
-physis	growth	14
-plasia	condition of formation, development, growth	2
-plasm	growth, substance, formation	2
-plasty	surgical repair	4
-plegia	paralysis	12
-pnea	breathing	5
-poiesis	formation	10
-ptosis	drooping, sagging, prolapse	6
-rrhagia	rapid flow of blood	5
-rrhaphy	suturing, repairing	6
-rrhea	flow, discharge	4
-rrhexis	rupture	9
-salpinx	uterine (fallopian) tube	8
-sarcoma	malignant tumor	2
-schisis	split, fissure	14
-sclerosis	hardening	10
-scope	instrument used for visual examination	5
-scopic	pertaining to visual examination	5
-scopy	visual examination	5
-sis	state of	2
-spasm	sudden, involuntary muscle contraction	5
-stasis	control, stop, standing	2
-stenosis	constriction or narrowing	5
-stomy	creation of an artificial opening	5
-thorax	chest	5
-tocia	birth, labor	9
-tome	instrument used to cut	4
-tomy	cut into or incision	5
-tripsy	surgical crushing	6
-trophy	nourishment, development	6
-um	no meaning	9
-uria	urine, urination	6
-us	no meaning	9

APPENDIX B

Combining Forms, Prefixes, and Suffixes Alphabetized According to Definition

Definition	Combining Form	Chapter
A		
abdomen (abdominal cavity)	abdomin/o	11
abdomen (abdominal cavity)	lapar/o	11
abdomen (abdominal cavity)	celi/o	11
above	super/o	3
adenoids	adenoid/o	5
adrenal glands	adren/o	16
adrenal glands	adrenal/o	16
albumin	albumin/o	6
alveolus	alveol/o	5
amnion	amni/o	9
amnion	amnion/o	9
antrum	antr/o	11
anus	an/o	11
aorta	aort/o	10
aponeurosis	aponeur/o	14
appendix	appendic/o	11
appendix	append/o	11
artery	arteri/o	10
atrium	atri/o	10
away (from the point of attachment of a body part)	dist/o	3
B		
back	dors/o	3
back, behind	poster/o	3
bear, give birth to, labor, childbirth	part/o	9
bear, give birth to, labor, childbirth	par/o	9
belly, front	ventr/o	3
below	infer/o	3
bent forward (increased concavity of the spine)	lord/o	14
bile duct	cholangi/o	11
birth	nat/o	9
black	melan/o	2
bladder, sac	cyst/o	6
bladder, sac	vesic/o	6
blood	hemat/o	5
blood	hem/o	5
blue	cyan/o	2
body	somat/o	2
bone	oste/o	14
bone marrow	myel/o	10
brain	encephal/o	15
breast	mamm/o	8
breast	mast/o	8
breathe, breathing	spir/o	5
bronchus	bronch/o	5
bursa (cavity)	burs/o	14

Definition	Combining Form	Chapter
C		
calcium	calc/i	16
cancer	cancer/o	2
cancer	carcin/o	2
carbon dioxide	capn/o	5
carpus (wrist bone)	carp/o	14
cartilage	chondr/o	14
cause (of disease)	eti/o	2
cecum	cec/o	11
cell	cyt/o	2
cerebellum	cerebell/o	15
cerebrum, brain	cerebr/o	15
cervix	cervic/o	8
childbirth	puerper/o	9
chorion	chori/o	9
clavicle (collarbone)	clavic/o	14
clavicle (collarbone)	clavicul/o	14
clot	thromb/o	10
cochlea	cochle/o	13
cold	cry/o	12
colon	col/o, colon/o	11
color	chrom/o	2
common bile duct	choledoch/o	11
conjunctiva	conjunctiv/o	12
cornea	corne/o	12
cornea	kerat/o	12
cortex	cortic/o	16
cranium, skull	crani/o	14
crooked, curved	scoli/o	14
crooked, stiff, bent	ankyl/o	14
cul-de-sac	culd/o	8
cut, section	tom/o	6
D		
death (cells, body)	necr/o	4
deficiency, blockage	isch/o	10
developing cell	blast/o	6
diaphragm	diaphragmat/o	5
disease	path/o	2
diverticulum	diverticul/o	11
dry	xer/o	4
duodenum	duoden/o	11
dust	coni/o	4
E		
ear	ot/o	13
ear	aur/i, aur/o	13
tympanic membrane (eardrum)	myring/o	13
(eardrum), middle ear	tympan/o	13
electricity, electrical activity	electr/o	10
embryo, to be full	embry/o	9
endocrine	endocrin/o	16
epididymis	epididym/o	7
epiglottis	epiglott/o	5
epithelium	epitheli/o	2
equal	is/o	12
esophagus	esophag/o	9, 11
extremities, height	acr/o	16
eye	ophthalm/o	12

Definition	Combining Form	Chapter
eye	ocul/o	12
eyelid	blephar/o	12
F		
false	pseud/o	9
fat	lip/o	2
fat	steat/o	11
femur (upper leg bone)	femor/o	14
fetus, unborn child	fet/o, fet/i	9
fiber	fibr/o	2
fibula (lower leg bone)	fibul/o	14
first	prim/i	9
first, beginning	arche/o	8
flesh, connective tissue	sarc/o	2
four	quadr/i	15
fungus	myc/o	3
G		
gall, bile	chol/e	11
ganglion	gangli/o	15
ganglion	ganglion/o	15
gland	aden/o	2, 16
glans penis	balan/o	7
glia, gluey substance	gli/o	15
glomerulus	glomerul/o	6
grapelike clusters	staphyl/o	4
gray matter	poli/o	15
green	chlor/o	2
gum	gingiv/o	11
H		
hair	trich/o	4
hard, dura mater	dur/o	15
head	cephal/o	3, 9
hearing	audi/o	13
heart	cardi/o	10
heat	therm/o	10
hernia	herni/o	11
hidden	crypt/o	4
horny tissue, hard	kerat/o	4
humerus (upper arm bone)	humer/o	14
hump (increased convexity of the spine)	kyph/o	14
hymen	hymen/o	8
I		
ileum	ile/o	11
ilium	ili/o	14
imperfect, incomplete	atel/o	5
inner ear	labyrinth/o	13
internal organs	viscer/o	2
intervertebral disk	disk/o	14
intestine	enter/o	11
iris	irid/o	12
iris	ir/o	12
ischium	ischi/o	14
J		
jejunum	jejun/o	11
joint	arthr/o	14
K		
kidney	nephr/o	6
kidney	ren/o	6
knowledge	gno/o	2

Definition	Combining Form	Chapter
L		
labyrinth (inner ear)	labyrinth/o	13
lamina (thin, flat plate or layer)	lamin/o	14
larynx	laryng/o	5
lens	phac/o	12
lens	phak/o	12
life	bi/o	4
light	phot/o	12
lip	cheil/o	11
liver	hepat/o	11
lobe	lob/o	5
lung	pulmon/o	5
lung, air	pneumat/o	5
lung, air	pneum/o	5
lung, air	pneumon/o	5
lymph node	lymphaden/o	10
lymph, lymph tissue	lymph/o	10
M		
male	andr/o	7
malformations	terat/o	9
mandible (lower jawbone)	mandibul/o	14
mastoid	mastoid/o	13
maxilla (upper jawbone)	maxill/o	14
meatus (opening)	meat/o	6
medicine (treatment)	iatr/o	2
meninges	mening/o, meningi/o	15
meniscus (crescent)	menisc/o	14
menstruation	men/o	8
middle	medi/o	3
mind	ment/o	15
mind	psych/o	15
mouth	or/o	11
mouth	stomat/o	11
movement, motion	kinesi/o	14
mucus	muc/o	5
muscle	my/o	2, 14
muscle	myos/o	14
N		
nail	ungu/o	4
nail	onych/o	4
near (the point of attachment of a body part)	proxim/o	3
nerve	neur/o	2, 15
nerve root	radicul/o	15
nerve root	radic/o	15
nerve root	rhiz/o	15
night	noct/i	6
nose	rhin/o	5
nose	nas/o	5
nucleus	kary/o	2
O		
one, single	mon/o	15
organ	organ/o	2
other	heter/o	4
ovary	oophor/o	8
oxygen	ox/o, ox/i	5
P		
palate	palat/o	11
pancreas	pancreat/o	11

Definition	Combining Form	Chapter
parathyroid gland	parathyroid/o	16
patella (kneecap)	patell/o	14
pelvis, pelvic bone	pelv/i, pelv/o	14
perineum	perine/o	8
peritoneum	peritone/o	11
phalanx (finger or toe)	phalang/o	14
pharynx	pharyng/o	5
physician (treatment)	iatr/o	2
plasma	plasm/o	10
pleura	pleur/o	5
potassium	kal/i	16
pregnancy	gravid/o	9
prostate gland	prostat/o	7
pubis	pub/o	14
pupil	core/o, cor/o	12
pupil	pupill/o	12
pus	py/o	5
pylorus, pyloric sphincter	pylor/o	9, 11
R		
radius (lower arm bone)	radi/o	14
rectum	proct/o	11
rectum	rect/o	11
red	erythr/o	2
renal pelvis	pyel/o	6
retina	retin/o	12
rib	cost/o	14
rod-shaped, striated	rhabd/o	2
S		
sacrum	sacr/o	14
saliva	sial/o	11
scanty, few	olig/o	6
scapula (shoulder blade)	scapul/o	14
sclera	scler/o	12
sebum (oil)	seb/o	4
self	aut/o	4
seminal vesicles	vesicul/o	7
sensation, sensitivity, feeling	esthesi/o	14
septum	sept/o	5
side	later/o	3
sigmoid	sigmoid/o	11
sinus	sinus/o	5
skin	cutane/o	4
skin	dermat/o	4
skin	derm/o	4
sleep	somn/o	5
small growth	polyp/o	11
smooth	lei/o	2
sound	son/o	6
sound	ech/o	10
speech	phas/o	15
(spermatozoon), sperm	sperm/o	7
(spermatozoon), sperm	spermat/o	7
spinal column	rachi/o	14
spinal cord	myel/o	15
spleen	splen/o	10
stapes (middle ear)	staped/o	13
sternum (breast bone)	stern/o	14
stomach	gastr/o	11
stone	petr/o	14

Definition	Combining Form	Chapter
stone, calculus	lith/o	6
straight	orth/o	5
sugar	glycos/o	6
sugar	glyc/o	6
sweat	hidr/o	4
synovia, synovial membrane	synovi/o	14
system	system/o	2
T		
tail (downward)	caud/o	3
tarsals (ankle bones)	tars/o	14
tear duct, tear	lacrim/o	12
tear duct, tear	dacry/o	12
tendon	ten/o	14
tendon	tendin/o	14
tendon	tend/o	14
tension, pressure	ton/o	12
testis, testicle	orch/o	7
testis, testicle	test/o	7
testis, testicle	orchi/o	7
testis, testicle	orchid/o	7
thick	pachy/o	4
thirst	dips/o	16
thorax (chest)	thorac/o	5
thymus gland	thym/o	10
thyroid gland	thyroid/o	16
thyroid gland	thyr/o	16
tibia (lower leg bone)	tibi/o	14
tissue	hist/o	2
tongue	lingu/o	11
tongue	gloss/o	11
tonsils	tonsill/o	5
trachea	trache/o	5
tumor	onc/o	2
twisted chains	strept/o	4
two, double	dipl/o	12
U		
ulna (lower arm bone)	uln/o	14
umbilicus, navel	omphal/o	9
urea, nitrogen	azot/o	6
ureter	ureter/o	6
urethra	urethr/o	6
urinary bladder	vesic/o, cyst/o	6
urine, urinary tract	urin/o	6
urine, urinary tract	ur/o	6
uterine (fallopian) tube	salping/o	8
uterus	metr/o, metr/i	8
uterus	hyster/o	8
uvula	uvul/o	11
V		
vagina	vagin/o	8
vagina	colp/o	8
valve	valv/o	10
valve	valvul/o	10
vein	phleb/o	10
vein	ven/o	10
ventricle	ventricul/o	10
vertebra	vertebr/o	14
vertebral column	rachi/o	14
vessel	angi/o	10

Definition	Combining Form	Chapter
vessel, duct	vas/o	7
vestibule	vestibul/o	13
vision	opt/o	12
vulva	vulv/o	8
vulva	episi/o	8
W		
water	hydr/o	6
white	leuk/o	2
woman	gyn/o	8
woman	gynec/o	8
wrinkles	rhytid/o	4
Y		
yellow	xanth/o	2
yellowish, fatty plaque	ather/o	10

Definition	Prefix	Chapter
above	supra-	14
above, excessive	hyper-	2
after	post-	9
after, beyond, change	meta-	2
all, total	pan-	5
before	ante-, pre-	9
before	pro-	2
below, incomplete, deficient	hypo-	2
beside, beyond, around, abnormal	para-	4
between	inter-	14
difficult, labored, painful, abnormal	dys-	2
fast, rapid	tachy-	10
four	quadri-	14
half	hemi-	11
many	multi-	9
many, much	poly-	5
new	neo-	2
none	nulli-	9
normal, good	eu-	5
on, upon, over	epi-	4
one	uni-	3
slow	brady-	10
small	micro-	9
surrounding (outer)	peri-	8
through, complete	per-	4
through	dia-	2
through, across, beyond	trans-	4
together, joined	sym-	14
together, joined	syn-	14
two	bin-	14
two	bi-	2, 14
under, below	sub-	4
within	intra-	4
within	endo-	5
without, absence of	a-, an-	5

Definition	Suffix	Chapter
abnormal condition (means increase when used with blood cell word roots)	-osis	2
abnormal fear of or aversion to specific things	-phobia	12
abnormal reduction (in number)	-penia	10
absence of a normal opening, occlusion, closure	-atresia	8
amnion, amniotic fluid	-amnios	9

Definition	Suffix	Chapter
berry-shaped (a form of bacterium)	-coccus (pl. -cocci)	4
birth, labor	-tocia	9
blood condition	-emia	5
break	-clasis	14
break	-clasia	14
break	-clast	14
breathing	-pnea	5
cell	-cyte	2
chest	-thorax	5
childbirth	-partum	9
condition	-iasis	6
condition	-esis	6
condition of formation, development, growth	-plasia	2
constriction, narrowing	-stenosis	5
control, stop, standing	-stasis	2
creation of an artificial opening	-stomy	5
cut into or incision	-tomy	5
digestion	-pepsia	11
disease	-pathy	2
diseased or abnormal state, condition of	-ia	4
drooping, sagging, prolapse	-ptosis	6
eating, swallowing	-phagia	4
enlargement	-megaly	6
excision, surgical removal	-ectomy	4
flow, discharge	-rrhea	4
formation	-poiesis	10
growth	-phycic	14
growth, substance, formation	-plasm	2
hardening	-sclerosis	10
hernia, protrusion	-cele	5
inflammation	-itis	4
instrument used for visual examination	-scope	5
instrument used to measure	-meter	5
instrument used to cut	-tome	4
instrument used to record; record	-graph	10
labor	-partum	9
loosening, dissolution, separating	-lysis	6
malignant tumor	-sarcoma	2
measurement	-metry	5
nourishment, development	-trophy	6
one who studies and treats (specialist, physician)	-logist	2
pain	-algia	5
paralysis	-plegia	12
pertaining to	-ac	10
pertaining to	-ous	2, 6
pertaining to	-ar	5
pertaining to	-ic	2
pertaining to	-ior	3
pertaining to	-eal	5
pertaining to	-ary	5
pertaining to	-al	2
pertaining to visual examination	-scopic	5
physician, specialist	-iatrist	15
pregnancy	-cyesis	9
process of recording, radiographic imaging	-graphy	5
producing, originating, causing	-genic	2
rapid flow of blood	-rrhagia	5
record, radiographic image	-gram	5
removal	-apheresis	10

Definition	Suffix	Chapter
resembling	-oid	2
run, running	-drome	16
rupture	-rrhexis	9
seizure, attack	-ictal	15
slight paralysis	-paresis	15
softening	-malacia	4
split, fissure	-schisis	14
state of	-ism	7
state of	-sis	2
stretching out, dilation, expansion	-ectasis	5
study of	-logy	2
substance or agent that produces or causes	-gen	2
sudden, involuntary muscle contraction	-spasm	5
surgical crushing	-tripsy	6
surgical fixation, fusion	-desis	14
surgical fixation, suspension	-pexy	5
surgical puncture to aspirate fluid	-centesis	5
surgical repair	-plasty	4
suturing, repairing	-rrhaphy	6
toward	-ad	3
treatment, specialty	-iatry	15
tumor, swelling	-oma	2
urine, urination	-uria	6
uterine (fallopian) tube	-salpinx	8
view of, viewing	-opsy	4
vision (condition)	-opia	12
visual examination	-scopy	5
weakness	-asthenia	14

APPENDIX C

Abbreviations

Topics include:

Common Medical Abbreviations, p. 805
Institute for Safe Medication Practices' (List of Error-Prone Abbreviations, Symbols and Dose Designations, includes The Joint Commission's "do not use" list), p. 810

Abbreviations are written as they appear most commonly in the medical and health care environment. Some may also appear in both capital and small letters and with or without periods.

Common Medical Abbreviations	Definitions
ab	abortion
abd	abdomen
ABE	acute bacterial endocarditis
ABGs	arterial blood gases
a.c.	before meals
ACS	acute cardiac syndrome
ACTH	adrenocorticotropic hormone
AD	Alzheimer disease
ADH	antidiuretic hormone
ADL	activities of daily living
ad lib	as desired
Adm.	admission
AFB	acid-fast bacillus
AFib	atrial fibrillation
AHD	arteriosclerotic heart disease
AI	aortic insufficiency
AICD	automatic implantable cardioverter defibrillator
AIDS	acquired immune deficiency syndrome
AKA	above-knee amputation
ALB	albumin
alk phos	alkaline phosphatase
ALL	acute lymphocytic leukemia
ALS	amyotrophic lateral sclerosis
AM	between midnight and noon
AMA	against medical advice; American Medical Association
amb	ambulate, ambulatory
AMI	acute myocardial infarction
AML	acute myelocytic leukemia
amp	ampule
amt	amount
ant.	anterior
AODM	adult-onset diabetes mellitus
AOM	acute otitis media
AP	anteroposterior; angina pectoris
A&P	auscultation and percussion; anterior and posterior colporrhaphy
ARDS	adult respiratory distress syndrome
ARF	acute renal failure
ARM	artificial rupture of membranes
ARMD	age-related macular degeneration
ART	assisted reproductive technology
ASA	aspirin
ASCVD	arteriosclerotic cardiovascular disease
ASD	atrial septal defect
ASHD	arteriosclerotic heart disease
Ast.	astigmatism
as tol	as tolerated
AUL	acute undifferentiated leukemia
AV	arteriovenous
AVR	aortic valve replacement
ax	axillary
BA	bronchial asthma
BBB	bundle branch block
BE	barium enema
b.i.d.	twice a day
BK	below knee
BKA	below-knee amputation
BM	bowel movement
BOM	bilateral otitis media
BP	blood pressure
BPH	benign prostatic hyperplasia
BR	bedrest
BRP	bathroom privileges
BS	blood sugar; bowel sounds; breath sounds
BSO	bilateral salpingo-oophorectomy
BUN	blood urea nitrogen
Bx	biopsy
c̄	with
C	Celsius
C_1-C_7	cervical vertebrae
Ca	calcium
CA	cancer; carcinoma
CABG	coronary artery bypass graft
CAD	coronary artery disease
CAL	calorie
CA-MRSA	community-associated MRSA infection
CAP	capsule
CAPD	continuous ambulatory peritoneal dialysis
cath	catheterization

Common Medical Abbreviations	Definitions
CBC	complete blood count
CBR	complete bed rest
CBS	chronic brain syndrome
CC	chief complaint or colony count
CCU	coronary care unit
CDH	congenital dislocation of the hip
CEA	carcinoembryonic antigen
CF	cystic fibrosis
CHB	complete heart block
CHD	coronary heart disease
CHF	congestive heart failure
CHO	carbohydrate
chemo	chemotherapy
chol	cholesterol
CI.	coronary insufficiency
circ	circumcision
CIS	carcinoma in situ
Cl.	chloride
CLD	chronic liver disease
CLL	chronic lymphocytic leukemia
cl liq	clear liquid
cm	centimeter
CML	chronic myelogenous leukemia
CNS	central nervous system
c/o	complains of
CO	carbon monoxide
CO_2	carbon dioxide
COB	coordination of benefits
COLD	chronic obstructive lung disease
comp	compound
cond	condition
COPD	chronic obstructive pulmonary disease
CP	cerebral palsy
CPAP	continuous positive airway pressure
CPD	cephalopelvic disproportion
CPK	creatine phosphokinase
CPN	chronic pyelonephritis
CPR	cardiopulmonary resuscitation
CRD	chronic respiratory disease
creat	creatinine
CRF	chronic renal failure
CRP	C-reactive protein
C&S	culture and sensitivity
C/S, CS, C-section	cesarean section
CSF	cerebrospinal fluid
CT	computed tomography
CTS	carpal tunnel syndrome
Cu	copper
CVA	cerebrovascular accident
CVP	central venous pressure
Cx	cervix
CXR	chest radiograph (x-ray)
DAT	diet as tolerated
D&C	dilation and curettage
del	delivery
derm	dermatology
DI	diabetes insipidus
DIC	diffuse intravascular coagulation
diff.	differential (part of complete blood count)
disch	discharge
DLE	discoid lupus erythematosus
DM	diabetes mellitus
DNA	deoxyribonucleic acid
DND	died natural death
DOA	dead on arrival
DOB	date of birth
DOD	date of death
Dr	dram
DRG	diagnosis-related group
DSA	digital subtraction angiography
DVT	deep vein thrombosis
DW	distilled water
D/W	dextrose in water
Dx	diagnosis
E	enema
EBL	estimated blood loss
ECG	electrocardiogram
echo	echocardiogram
ECT	electroconvulsive therapy
ED	emergency department
EDD	estimated date of delivery
EEG	electroencephalogram
EENT	eyes, ears, nose, and throat
EGD	esophagogastroduodenoscopy
EKG	electrocardiogram
Elix	elixir
EM	emmetropia
EMG	electromyogram
ENG	electronystagmography
ENT	ears, nose, and throat
EP	ectopic pregnancy
EP studies	evoked potential studies
ERCP	endoscopic retrograde cholangiopancreatography
ERT	estrogen replacement therapy
ESR	erythrocyte sedimentation rate
ESRD	end-stage renal disease
ESWL	extracorporeal shock-wave lithotripsy
etio	etiology
exam	examination
ext	extract; external
F	Fahrenheit
FAS	fetal alcohol syndrome
FBD	fibrocystic breast disease
FBS	fasting blood sugar
Fe	iron
FHT	fetal heart tones
flu	influenza
FOBT	fecal occult blood test
Fr	French (catheter size)
FS	frozen section
FSH	follicle-stimulating hormone
FTT	failure to thrive
FUO	fever of undetermined origin

Common Medical Abbreviations	Definitions
Fx	fracture
g	gram
GC	gonorrhea
GERD	gastroesophageal reflux disease
GH	growth hormone
GI	gastrointestinal
GSW	gunshot wound
gtt	drops
GTT	glucose tolerance test
GU	genitourinary
Gyn	gynecology
h	hour
H	hypodermic
HAART	highly active antiretroviral therapy
HA-MRSA	healthcare associated MRSA infection
HB	heart block
HCVD	hypertensive cardiovascular disease
HD	hemodialysis
HHD	hypertensive heart disease
H&H	hemoglobin and hematocrit
HCl	hydrochloric acid
HCO_3	bicarbonate
Hct	hematocrit
Hg	mercury
Hgb	hemoglobin
HIV	human immunodeficiency virus
HMD	hyaline membrane disease
HME	Heat/moisture exchanger
HNP	herniated nucleus pulposus
H_2O	water
H_2O_2	hydrogen peroxide (hydrogen dioxide)
HOB	head of bed
H&P	history and physical examination
H. pylori	*Helicobacter pylori*
HRT	hormone replacement therapy
ht.	height
HTN	hypertension
Hx	history
hypo	hypodermic
IBS	irritable bowel syndrome
ICD	implantable cardiac defibrillator
ICU	intensive care unit
ID	intradermal
IDDM	insulin-dependent diabetes mellitus
I&D	incision and drainage
IHD	ischemic heart disease
IM	intramuscular
inf	inferior
INR	international normalized ratio
I&O	intake and output
IOL	intraocular lens
IOP	intraocular pressure
IPG	impedance plethysmography
IPPB	intermittent positive pressure breathing
irrig	irrigation
isol	isolation
IUD	intrauterine device
IV	intravenous
IVC	intravenous cholangiogram
IVF	in vitro fertilization
IVP	intravenous pyelogram
K	potassium
KCl	potassium chloride
kg	kilogram
KO	keep open
KUB	kidney, ureter, bladder (radiograph)
KVO	keep vein open
L	liter
L_1-L_5	lumbar vertebrae
lab	laboratory
lac	laceration
LAP	laparotomy
lat	lateral
L&D	labor and delivery
LDH	lactic dehydrogenase
LE	lupus erythematosus
lg.	large
LH	luteinizing hormone
LLL	left lower lobe
LLQ	left lower quadrant
LMP	last menstrual period
LOC	loss of consciousness, level of consciousness
LP	lumbar puncture
LPN	licensed practical nurse
LR	lactated Ringer (IV solution)
lt	left
LTB	laryngotracheobronchitis
LUL	left upper lobe
LUQ	left upper quadrant
mcg	microgram
MCH	mean corpuscular hemoglobin
MCV	mean corpuscular volume
MD	muscular dystrophy
mEq	milliequivalent
mets	metastasis
mg	milligram
MG	myasthenia gravis
MI	myocardial infarction
mL	milliliter
mm	millimeter
MM	multiple myeloma
MOM	milk of magnesia
MR	mitral regurgitation
MRI	magnetic resonance imaging
MRCP	magnetic resonance cholangiopancreatography
MRSA	methicillin-resistant *Staphylococcus aureus*
MS	multiple sclerosis
MVP	mitral valve prolapse
Na	sodium
NaCl	sodium chloride (salt)
NAS	no added salt

Common Medical Abbreviations	Definitions
NB	newborn
neg	negative
neuro	neurology
NG	nasogastric
NICU	neurological intensive care unit; neonatal intensive care unit
NIDDM	non-insulin-dependent diabetes mellitus
NIVA	noninvasive vascular assessment
noc	night
noct	night
NPO	nothing by mouth
NPPV	Noninvasive positive-pressure ventilator
NS	normal saline
NSR	normal sinus rhythm
N&V	nausea and vomiting
NVS	neurologic signs
O_2	oxygen
OAB	overactive bladder
OB	obstetrics
OCD	obsessive-compulsive disorder
OD	overdose
oint	ointment
OM	otitis media
OOB	out of bed
OP	outpatient
Ophth	ophthalmic
OR	operating room
Ortho	orthopedics
OSA	obstructive sleep apnea
OT	occupational therapy
OTC	over-the-counter drugs
oto	otology
oz	ounce
p̄	after
P	phosphorus
P	pulse
PA	physician's assistant or posteroanterior
PAC	premature atrial complex
PAD	peripheral arterial disease
PAT	paroxysmal atrial tachycardia
pc	after meals
PCP	*Pneumocystis carinii* pneumonia
PCU	progressive care unit
PCV	packed cell volume
PD	Parkinson disease
PDA	patent ductus arteriosus
PDR	*Physicians' Desk Reference*
PE	pulmonary embolism
Peds	pediatrics
PEEP	positive end expiratory pressure
PEG	percutaneous endoscopic gastrostomy
per	by
PERRLA	pupils equal, round, reactive to light and accommodation
PET scan	positron emission tomography scan
PFM	peak flow meter
PFTs	pulmonary function tests
PHACO	Phacoemulsification
PICC	peripherally inserted central catheter
PICU	pediatric intensive care unit
PID	pelvic inflammatory disease
PKU	phenylketonuria
PM	between noon and midnight
PMS	premenstrual syndrome
PNS	peripheral nervous system
po	orally; postoperative; phone order
post-op	postoperatively
PP	postpartum or postprandial (after meals)
PPD	purified protein derivative
pr	per rectum
PRBC	packed red blood cells
pre-op	preoperatively
PRH	prolactin-releasing hormone
primip	primipara
PRN	as needed
PSA	prostate-specific antigen
pt.	patient; pint
PT	physical therapy
PT	prothrombin time
PTCA	percutaneous transluminal coronary angioplasty
PT/INR	prothrombin time/international normalized ratio
PTT	partial thromboplastin time
PUL	percutaneous ultrasound lithotripsy
PVC	premature ventricular complex
PVD	peripheral vascular disease
Px	prognosis
q	every
q_h	every (number) hour (e.g., q2h)
qt.	quart
R	rectal
RA	rheumatoid arthritis
RAD	reactive airway disease
RAIU	radioactive iodine uptake
RBC	red blood cell count
RDS	respiratory distress syndrome
reg.	regular
REM	rapid eye movement
resp	respirations
RHD	rheumatic heart disease
RLL	right lower lobe
RLQ	right lower quadrant
RN	registered nurse
R/O	rule out
ROM	range of motion
ROM	rupture of membranes
RP	radical prostatectomy
RR	recovery room
rt	right; routine
RT	respiratory therapy
RUL	right upper lobe
Rx	prescription
s̄	without

Common Medical Abbreviations	Definitions	Common Medical Abbreviations	Definitions
SAB	spontaneous abortion	TIA	transient ischemic attack
SARS	severe acute respiratory syndrome	tid	three times per day
SBE	subacute bacterial endocarditis; self-breast examination	tinct	tincture
		TKA	total knee arthroplasty
SHG	sonohysterography	TPN	total parenteral nutrition
SICU	surgical intensive care unit	tr	tincture
SIDS	sudden infant death syndrome	trach	tracheostomy
SLE	systemic lupus erythematosus	TRUS	transrectal ultrasound
SMAC	sequential multiple analysis computer	TSH	thyroid-stimulating hormone
SMR	submucous resection	TSS	toxic shock syndrome
SO	salpingo-oophorectomy	TUIP	transurethral incision of the prostate
SOB	shortness of breath	TULIP	transurethral laser incision of the prostate
SPECT	single-photon emission computed tomography	TUMT	transurethral microwave thermotherapy
ss	one half		
SSE	soapsuds enema	TURP	transurethral resection of the prostate
STAPH or staph	staphylococcus	TVH	total vaginal hysterectomy
stat	immediately	TVS	transvaginal sonography
STD	sexually transmitted disease	TWE	tap water enema
STREP or strep	streptococcus	Tx	treatment
subcut	subcutaneous	UA	urinalysis
subling	sublingual	UAE	uterine artery embolization
sup	superior	UGI	upper gastrointestinal
supp	suppository	UGISBFT	upper gastrointestinal, small bowel follow through
surg	surgical		
SVD	spontaneous vaginal delivery	UNG	ointment
SVN	small-volume nebulizer	UPPP	uvulopalatopharyngoplasty
SWL	shock wave lithotripsy	URI	upper respiratory infection
T_1-T_{12}	thoracic vertebrae	US	ultrasound
T4	thyroxine	UTI	urinary tract infection
tab	tablet	UV	ultraviolet
TAB	therapeutic abortion	UVR	ultraviolet radiation
T&A	tonsillectomy and adenoidectomy	vag	vaginal
TAH	total abdominal hysterectomy	VATS	video-assisted thoracic surgery
TAH-BSO	total abdominal hysterectomy-bilateral salpingo-oophorectomy	VBAC	vaginal birth after cesarean section
		VCUG	voiding cystourethrogram
TAT	tetanus antitoxin	VD	venereal disease
TB	tuberculosis	VDRL	Venereal Disease Research Laboratory
TCDB	turn, cough, deep breathe	VLAP	visual ablation of the prostate
TCT	thrombin clotting time	VPS	ventilation/perfusion scanning
TD	transdermal	VS	vital signs
TEE	transesophageal echocardiogram	WA	while awake
temp	temperature	WBC	white blood cell count
TENS	transcutaneous electrical nerve stimulation	W/C	wheelchair
		wt	weight
THA	total hip arthroplasty	XRT	radiotherapy; radiation therapy
THR	total hip replacement		

Institute for Safe Medication Practices' List of Error-Prone Abbreviations, Symbols, and Dose Designations

The abbreviations, symbols, and dose designations found in this table have been reported to ISMP through the USP-ISMP Medication Error Reporting Program as being frequently misinterpreted and involved in harmful medication errors. They should NEVER be used when communicating medical information. This includes internal communications, telephone/verbal prescriptions, computer-generated labels, labels for drug storage bins, medication administration records, as well as pharmacy and prescriber computer order entry screens.

The Joint Commission (TJC; formerly the Joint Commission on Accreditation of Healthcare Organizations [JCAHO]) has established a National Patient Safety Goal **that specifies that certain abbreviations must appear on an accredited organization's "do not use" list; we have highlighted these items with a double asterisk (**).** However, we hope that you will consider others beyond the minimum TJC requirements. By using and promoting safe practices and by educating one another about hazards, we can better protect our patients.

Abbreviations	Intended Meaning	Misinterpretation	Correction
µg	Microgram	Mistaken as "mg"	Use "mcg"
AD, AS, AU	Right ear, left ear, each ear	Mistaken as OD, OS, OU (right eye, left eye, each eye)	Use "right ear," "left ear," or "each ear"
OD, OS, OU	Right eye, left eye, each eye	Mistaken as AD, AS, AU (right ear, left ear, each ear)	Use "right eye," "left eye," or "each eye"
BT	Bedtime	Mistaken as "BID" (twice daily)	Use "bedtime"
cc	Cubic centimeters	Mistaken as "u" (units)	Use "mL"
D/C	Discharge or discontinue	Premature discontinuation of medications if D/C (intended to mean "discharge") has been misinterpreted as "discontinued" when followed by a list of discharge medications	Use "discharge" and "discontinue"
IJ	Injection	Mistaken as "IV" or "intrajugular"	Use "injection"
IN	Intranasal	Mistaken as "IM" or "IV"	Use "intranasal" or "NAS"
HS	Half strength	Mistaken as bedtime	Use "half strength" or "bedtime"
hs	At bedtime, hours of sleep	Mistaken as half strength	
IU**	International unit	Mistaken as IV (intravenous) or 10 (ten)	Use "units"
o.d. or OD	Once daily	Mistaken as "right eye" (OD-oculus dexter), leading to oral liquid medications administered in the eye	Use "daily"
OJ	Orange juice	Mistaken as OD or OS (right or left eye); drugs meant to be diluted in orange juice may be given in the eye	Use "orange juice"
Per os	By mouth, orally	The "os" can be mistaken as "left eye" (OS-oculus sinister)	Use "PO," "by mouth," or "orally"
q.d. or QD**	Every day	Mistaken as q.i.d., especially if the period after the "q" or the tail of the "q" is misunderstood as an "i"	Use "daily"
qhs	Nightly at bedtime	Mistaken as "qhr" or every hour	Use "nightly"
qn	Nightly or at bedtime	Mistaken as "qh" (every hour)	Use "nightly" or "at bedtime"
q.o.d. or QOD**	Every other day	Mistaken as "q.d." (daily) or "q.i.d." (four times daily) if the "o" is poorly written	Use "every other day"
q1d	Daily	Mistaken as q.i.d. (four times daily)	Use "daily"
q6PM, etc.	Every evening at 6 PM	Mistaken as every 6 hours	Use "6 PM nightly" or "6 PM daily"
SC, SQ, sub q	Subcutaneous	SC mistaken as SL (sublingual); SQ mistaken as "5 every;" the "q" in "sub q" has been mistaken as "every" (e.g., a heparin dose ordered "sub q 2 hours before surgery" misunderstood as every 2 hours before surgery)	Use "subcut" or "subcutaneously"
ss	Sliding scale (insulin) or $^{1}/_{2}$ (apothecary)	Mistaken as "55"	Spell out "sliding scale;" use "one half" or "$^{1}/_{2}$"
SSRI	Sliding scale regular insulin	Mistaken as selective serotonin reuptake inhibitor	Spell out "sliding scale (insulin)"
SSI	Sliding scale insulin	Mistaken as strong solution of iodine (Lugol's)	
i/d	Once daily	Mistaken as "tid"	Use "1 daily"
TIW or tiw	3 times a week	Mistaken as "3 times a day" or "twice in a week"	Use "3 times weekly"

Abbreviations	Intended Meaning	Misinterpretation	Correction
U or u**	Unit	Mistaken as the number 0 or 4, causing a tenfold overdose or greater (e.g., 4U seen as "40" or 4u seen as "44"); mistaken as "cc" so dose given in volume instead of units (e.g., 4u seen as 4cc)	Use "unit"
Dose Designations and Other Information	*Intended Meaning*	*Misinterpretation*	*Correction*
Trailing zero after decimal point (e.g., 1.0 mg)**	1 mg	Mistaken as 10 mg if the decimal point is not seen	Do not use trailing zeros for doses expressed in whole numbers
"Naked" decimal point (e.g., .5 mg)**	0.5 mg	Mistaken as 5 mg if the decimal point is not seen	Use zero before a decimal point when the dose is less than a whole unit
Drug name and dose run together (especially problematic for drug names that end in "l" such as Inderal 40 mg; Tegretol 300 mg)	Inderal 40 mg Tegretol 300 mg	Mistaken as Inderal 140 mg Mistaken as Tegretol 1300 mg	Place adequate space between the drug name, dose, and unit of measure
Numerical dose and unit of measure run together (e.g., 10 mg, 100 mL)	10 mg 100 mL	The "m" is sometimes mistaken as a zero or two zeros, risking a 10- to 100-fold overdose	Place adequate space between the dose and unit of measure
Abbreviations such as mg. or mL. with a period following the abbreviation	mg mL	The period is unnecessary and could be mistaken as the number 1 if written poorly	Use mg, mL, etc., without a terminal period
Large doses without properly placed commas (e.g., 100000 units; 1000000 units)	100,000 units 1,000,000 units	100000 has been mistaken as 10,000 or 1,000,000; 1000000 has been mistaken as 100,000	Use commas for dosing units at or above 1,000, or use words such as 100 "thousand" or 1 "million" to improve readability
Drug Name Abbreviations	*Intended Meaning*	*Misinterpretation*	*Correction*
ARA A	vidarabine	Mistaken as cytarabine (ARA C)	Use complete drug name
AZT	zidovudine (Retrovir)	Mistaken as azathioprine or aztreonam	Use complete drug name
CPZ	Compazine (prochlorperazine)	Mistaken as chlorpromazine	Use complete drug name
DPT	Demerol-Phenergan-Thorazine	Mistaken as diphtheria-pertussis-tetanus (vaccine)	Use complete drug name
DTO	Diluted tincture of opium, or deodorized tincture of opium (Paregoric)	Mistaken as tincture of opium	Use complete drug name
HCl	hydrochloric acid or hydrochloride	Mistaken as potassium chloride (the "H" is misinterpreted as "K")	Use complete drug name unless expressed as a salt of a drug
HCT	hydrocortisone	Mistaken as hydrochlorothiazide	Use complete drug name
HCTZ	hydrochlorothiazide	Mistaken as hydrocortisone (seen as HCT250 mg)	Use complete drug name

Abbreviations	Intended Meaning	Misinterpretation	Correction
Drug Name Abbreviations	*Intended Meaning*	*Misinterpretation*	*Correction*
MgS04**	magnesium sulfate	Mistaken as morphine sulfate	Use complete drug name
MS, MS04**	morphine sulfate	Mistaken as magnesium sulfate	Use complete drug name
MTX	methotrexate	Mistaken as mitoxantrone	Use complete drug name
PCA	procainamide	Mistaken as patient controlled analgesia	Use complete drug name
PTU	propylthiouracil	Mistaken as mercaptopurine	Use complete drug name
T3	Tylenol with codeine No. 3	Mistaken as lithothyronine	Use complete drug name
TAC	triamcinolone	Mistaken as tetracaine, Adrenalin, cocaine	Use complete drug name
TNK	TN Kase	Mistaken as "TPA"	Use complete drug name
ZnS04	zinc sulfate	Mistaken as morphine sulfate	Use complete drug name
Stemmed Drug Names	*Intended Meaning*	*Misinterpretation*	*Correction*
"Nitro" drip	nitroglycerin infusion	Mistaken as sodium nitroprusside infusion	Use complete drug name
"Norflox"	norfloxacin	Mistaken as Norflex	Use complete drug name
"IV Vanc"	intravenous vancomycin	Mistaken as Invanz	Use complete drug name
Symbols	*Intended Meaning*	*Misinterpretation*	*Correction*
ʒ	Dram	Symbol for dram mistaken as "3"	Use metric system
♍	Minim	Symbol for minim mistaken as "mL"	
X3D	For three days	Mistaken as "3 doses"	Use "for three days"
> and <	Greater than and less than	Mistaken as opposite of intended; mistakenly use incorrect symbol; "< 10" mistaken as "40"	Use "greater than" or "less than"
/ (slash mark)	Separates two doses or indicates "per"	Mistaken as the number 1 (e.g., "25 units/10 units" misread as "25 units and 110" units)	Use "per" rather than a slash mark to separate doses
@	At	Mistaken as "2"	Use "at"
&	And	Mistaken as "2"	Use "and"
+	Plus or and	Mistaken as "4"	Use "and
°	Hour	Mistaken as a zero (e.g., q2° seen as q 20)	Use "hr," "h," or "hour"

**These abbreviations are included on the TJC's "minimum list" of dangerous abbreviations, acronyms, and symbols that must be included on an organization's "do not use" list, effective Jan. 1, 2004. Visit www.jointcommission.org for more information about this TJC requirement.

 Unless noted, reports were received through the USP-ISMP Medication Errors Reporting Program (MERP). Report actual and potential medication errors to the MERP via the web at www.ismp.org or by calling 1-800-FAIL-SAF(E). ISMP guarantees confidentiality of information received and respects reporters' wishes as to the level of detail included in publications.

APPENDIX D

Pharmacology Terms

Topics include:

General Drug Categories

antibacterial	a drug that targets bacteria to kill or halt growth or replication
antibiotic	a drug that targets bacteria, fungi, or protozoa to kill or halt growth or replication
antifungal	a drug that targets fungi to kill or halt growth or replication
antihistamine	a drug that treats allergic and hypersensitivity reactions by blocking histamine-1 receptors
antiinflammatory	a drug that reduces inflammation
antimicrobial	a drug that targets microorganisms to kill or halt growth or replication
antineoplastic agent	a drug used to destroy or slow the rapid replication of cancer cells
antiretroviral	a drug that suppresses the replication of HIV; highly active antiretroviral therapy (HAART) is the combination of three or more of these drugs to treat HIV infection
antiviral	a drug that targets viruses to kill or halt growth or replication
antiadrenergic agent	a drug that blocks adrenergic receptors to reduce sympathetic nervous system activity in the body
bactericidal	the designation for an antimicrobial agent that kills or destroys bacteria
bacteriostatic	the designation for an antimicrobial agent that halts the growth or replication of bacteria but does not destroy them
cytotoxic	an agent that causes cell death
disinfectant	a chemical agent that can be applied to inanimate objects to destroy microorganisms
herbal supplement	a naturally derived dietary product that may have some therapeutic effect; rigorous proof of safety and effectiveness is not required because it is not regulated as a drug
immunosuppressant (also called **immunomodulator**)	a drug that reduces the response of the immune system; used in autoimmune diseases and to prepare a patient for an organ transplant
narcotic	a type of drug that has opium-like effects to cause drowsiness, pain relief, and sedation; can be habit-forming and is considered a controlled substance
nonsteroidal antiinflammatory drug (NSAID)	a drug that reduces pain, inflammation, and fever
parasympatholytic	an agent that blocks the actions of the parasympathetic nervous system
parasympathomimetic	an agent that enhances the actions of the parasympathetic nervous system

radiopharmaceutical	a drug with a radioactive component; used for diagnosis or treatment
smoking cessation agent	a drug that helps a patient quit smoking; may be a behavioral deterrent or a nicotine substitute
sympatholytic	an agent that blocks the actions of the sympathetic nervous system
sympathomimetic	an agent that enhances the actions of the sympathetic nervous system
vaccine (also called **immunization**)	a preparation of microbial antigen that will confer a degree of immunity to a future infection by that microbial
vitamin	an organic compound essential in small quantities for normal physiologic and metabolic functioning

General Pharmacy Terms

absorption	the process in which a drug is taken up into the body, organ, tissue, or cell
adverse drug reaction (ADR)	any harmful or unintended reaction to a drug administered at a normal dose
ampoule (or ampule)	a small, sterile glass or plastic container that usually holds a single dose of a solution to be administered parenterally
aseptic technique	the method used to minimize the microbial contamination of compounded sterile drugs
bioavailability	the percentage of administered drug available to affect the body and target site(s) after absorption, metabolism, and other factors
capsule (cap)	a small, digestible container (usually made of gelatin) used to hold a dose of medication for oral administration
chemical name	the exact designation of the chemical structure of a drug
chemotherapy (also called **chemo**)	the treatment of cancer with chemical agents
compounding	the act of combining drug ingredients to prepare a customized prescription or drug order for a patient
contraindication	factor that prohibits administration of a drug
controlled substance	a drug that has been identified as having the potential for abuse or addiction; designated as schedule I, II, III, IV, or V under the Controlled Substance Act
cream	a water-based, semisolid preparation that usually contains a drug and is applied topically to external parts of the body
distribution	the uptake pattern of drug molecules by various tissues throughout the body
dose	the amount of a drug or other substance to be administered at one time
drug	any substance taken by mouth; injected into a muscle, the skin, a blood vessel, or a cavity of the body; or applied topically to treat, cure, prevent, or diagnose a disease or condition
drug-drug interaction (DDI)	a modification of the effect of a drug when administered with another drug; food can also interact with a drug to cause a modification of the drug's effect
elimination	the removal of a substance from the body by any route, including the kidneys, liver, lungs, and sweat glands
elixir	a liquid containing sweeteners, flavorings, water, and/or alcohol in which an oral medication may be dispersed
emulsion	a stable mixture that contains one component suspended within another component that it cannot normally dissolve in or mix with
Food and Drug Administration (FDA)	the U.S. federal agency responsible for the enforcement of federal regulations regarding the manufacturing and distribution of food, drugs, and cosmetics as protection against the sale of impure or dangerous substances

formulary	a listing of drugs and drug information used by health practitioners within an institution to prescribe treatment that is medically appropriate
generic name	the official, established nonproprietary name assigned to a drug
inhaler	a device containing a drug to be breathed in nasally or by mouth
mechanism of action (MOA)	the means by which a drug exerts a desired effect
metabolism	the chemical changes that a drug or other substance undergoes in the body
ointment	an oil-based, semisolid preparation that usually contains a drug and is applied topically to external parts of the body
over-the-counter (OTC) drug (also called **nonprescription drug**)	a drug that may be purchased without a prescription
pharmaceutical	a drug used for medicinal purposes
pharmacist	a person formally trained to formulate and dispense medications
pharmacodynamics	the study of the actions of a drug on the body
pharmacogenomics	the study of the correlation between genetics and response to a drug
pharmacokinetics	the study of the actions of the body on a drug
pharmacology	the study of the preparation, properties, uses, and actions of drugs
pharmacy	a place for preparing and dispensing drugs
placebo	an inactive substance, prescribed as if it were an effective dose of a needed medication
prescription	an order for medication, therapy, or a therapeutic device given by a properly authorized person to a person properly authorized to dispense or perform the order for the specified patient
preservative	a substance included in some parenteral and topical medications used to prevent the growth of microorganisms in the product
route of administration	the method in which a drug or agent is given to a patient
side effect	any reaction or result from a medication other than what was intended
solution	a homogenous mixture of one or more substances dissolved into another substance
state board of pharmacy	the agency responsible for regulating the practice of pharmacy within the state
suppository	a topical form of drug that is inserted into the rectum, vagina, or penis
suspension	a liquid in which particles of a solid are dispersed, but not dissolved, and in which the dispersal is maintained by stirring or shaking
tablet	a small, solid dose form of a medication
toxicity	the level at which a drug's concentration within the body produces serious adverse effects
trade name (also called **brand name**)	a proprietary name assigned to a drug by its manufacturer that is registered as part of the drug's identity
United States Pharmacopeia (USP)	a compendium, recognized officially by the federal Food and Drug Administration that contains descriptions, uses, strengths, and standards of purity for selected drugs and for all their dosage forms

Routes of Administration

enteral	the use of oral ingestion as a mode of drug administration
epidural	injection of a drug into the epidural space of the spine
infusion	the prolonged administration of a fluid substance directly into a vein, artery, or under the skin in which the flow rate is driven by gravity or a mechanical pump

inhalation	a method of drug administration that involves the breathing in of a spray, vapor, or powder via the nose or mouth
injection	the introduction of a substance into the body by using a needle
intramuscular (IM)	the administration of a medication into a muscle
intrathecal	the administration of a drug into the subarachnoid space of the meninges in the spine
intravenous (IV)	the administration of a medication directly into a vein
oral	the administration of a medication by mouth
parenteral	a drug or agent that is administered into the body by an injection, thereby bypassing the digestive tract
subcutaneous	the introduction of a medication into the tissue just beneath the skin
sublingual	a form of drug that dissolves under the tongue
topical	a dosage form of a medication that is applied directly to an external area of the body
transdermal	a method of applying a drug to unbroken skin so that it is continuously absorbed through the skin to produce a systemic effect; a transdermal patch is a drug delivery system that controls the rate of absorption through the skin

Chapter 4: Integumentary System

antibacterial	a drug used to combat an infection caused by bacteria
antifungal	a drug used to combat an infection caused by fungi
antihistamine	a drug used to minimize allergy symptoms by blocking histamine-1 receptors
antipruritic	an agent that reduces itching
antiseptic	a chemical agent that can safely be applied to external tissues to halt the growth of microorganisms
antipsoriatic	a drug that treats psoriasis
astringent	an agent that reduces inflammation and irritation and provides a protective barrier on mucosa and skin by contracting the surface tissue
emollient	an external agent that softens or soothes the skin
keratolytic	an agent that augments the shedding of the top layer of dead skin
pediculicide	an agent that kills lice
retinoid	a derivative of vitamin A that regulates the growth of epithelial cells; often used to treat acne
scabicide	an agent that kills scabies

Chapter 5: Respiratory System

antitussive	a drug that suppresses coughing
bronchodilator	a drug that expands the airways by relaxing smooth muscle in the lungs
decongestant	a drug that relieves nasal congestion by reducing swelling of mucous membranes
expectorant	a drug that promotes expulsion of mucus from the lungs
leukotriene receptor antagonist (LTRA)	a drug that blocks late-stage regulators of allergic and hypersensitivity reactions to treat allergy-induced asthma
mucolytic	a drug that thins out mucus in the lungs so that it can be expelled more easily

Chapter 6: Urinary System

aldosterone receptor antagonist (ARA)	a drug that prevents reabsorption of water and sodium; used in chronic heart failure to minimize edema
angiotensin-converting enzyme inhibitor (ACEI or ACE inhibitor)	a drug that prevents the formation of angiotensin-II, which is a strong vasoconstrictor and major contributor to high blood pressure

angiotensin receptor blocker (ARB) (also called **angiotensin II antagonist**)	a drug that blocks the angiotensin-II molecule from binding to its receptors throughout the body to prevent its effects and to reduce high blood pressure
antispasmodic	a drug that prevents or relieves bladder muscle spasms associated with incontinence
diuretic	a drug that promotes the formation and excretion of urine to reduce the volume of extracellular fluid; used to reduce high blood pressure or edema; commonly referred to as a "water pill"
muscle relaxant	a drug that reduces bladder muscle contractility to relieve spasm-induced pain or uncontrolled urination
renin inhibitor	a drug that blocks renin activity to reduce high blood pressure; renin is the first step in the renin-angiotensin-aldosterone system (RAAS), which is a common contributor to chronic high blood pressure
urinary alkalinizer	an agent that increases the urine pH to make it more basic to treat acidosis
vasopressin (also called **antidiuretic hormone** or **ADH**)	a drug that increases water retention by the kidneys

Chapter 7: Male Reproductive System

androgen	a natural or synthetic hormone involved in male reproduction and secondary gender attributes
antiandrogen	a drug that blocks the effects of androgen hormones in the body
phosphodiesterase-5 inhibitor (PDE5 inhibitor)	a drug that blocks the inactivation of cyclic guanosine monophosphate either to increase vasodilation in the penis or to increase cardiac output
spermicide	an agent that kills sperm

Chapter 8: Female Reproductive System

antiestrogen	a drug used to block the action of estrogen hormones in the body
birth control (BC)	exogenous hormones to prevent pregnancy
contraceptive	an agent (drug or barrier) used to prevent conception or pregnancy
estrogen	a natural or synthetic hormone involved in female reproduction and secondary gender characteristics
hormone replacement therapy	a regimen that mimics the body's normal levels of female hormones when they are no longer produced; typically used during menopause
intrauterine device (IUD)	a hormone-containing or metal-based device that is inserted directly in the uterus to prevent pregnancy long-term
oral contraceptive	exogenous hormones taken by mouth to prevent pregnancy
ovulation stimulant	a drug that enhances the release of an egg from the ovary to promote pregnancy
progestin	a synthetic or natural hormone involved in female reproduction and secondary sex characteristics
vaginal ring	a device containing estrogen and progestin hormones that is inserted in the vagina to prevent pregnancy

Chapter 9: Obstetrics and Neonatology

abortifacient	a drug that causes uterine muscles to contract with subsequent abortion of the fetus
oxytocic	a hormone that stimulates the uterine muscles to contract, thereby inducing labor in a pregnant woman
pregnancy category	a level of risk the Food and Drug Administration assigns a drug based on documented problems with the use of that drug during pregnancy; risk categories from safest to most harmful are A, B, C, D, and X
tocolytic	an agent that suppresses labor contractions

Chapter 10: Cardiovascular, Immune, and Lymphatic Systems and Blood

antianginal	a drug that relieves the chest pain paroxysms caused by lack of oxygen delivery to the heart; typically involves vasodilation
antiarrhythmic	a drug that treats abnormal heart rhythm
anticoagulant	a drug that prevents blood clotting and coagulation
antihypertensive	a drug that lowers blood pressure
antiplatelet agent	a drug that prevents platelet formation or causes platelet destruction
beta-blocker (BB)	a drug that inhibits beta-adrenergic receptors; mostly used to lower blood pressure
calcium channel blocker (CCB)	a drug that regulates the entry of calcium into muscle cells of the heart and blood vessels to lower blood pressure
colony-stimulating factor (CSF)	an agent that aids in the replication of blood cells in the bone marrow
direct thrombin inhibitor (DTI)	a drug that blocks the action of thrombin, thereby reducing blood coagulation
erythropoiesis stimulating agent (ESA)	an agent that stimulates red blood cell production from the bone marrow
hemostatic	a drug that stops bleeding or hemorrhaging
nitrate	a drug that dilates the blood vessels
platelet aggregation inhibitor	a drug that stops platelets from bonding together
thrombolytic	a drug that dissolves blood clots
vasodilator	a drug that expands blood vessels to lower blood pressure
vasopressor (also called **vasoconstrictor**)	a drug that contracts blood vessels to raise blood pressure

Chapter 11: Digestive System

antacid	a drug that neutralizes acid in the stomach
antidiarrheal	a drug that treats diarrhea by increasing water absorption, decreasing muscle contraction of the intestines, altering electrolyte exchange, or absorbing toxins or microorganisms
antiemetic	a drug that reduces or prevents nausea and vomiting
antihyperlipidemic agent (also called hypolipidemic agent)	a drug used to treat high cholesterol by affecting levels of low-density lipoproteins, high-density lipoproteins, total cholesterol, and/or triglycerides, which are collectively called lipids
bile acid sequestrant	a type of antihyperlipidemic drug used to lower high cholesterol levels by increasing the excretion of bile acids
enema	a liquid agent administered rectally to clear the contents of the bowel
fibrate	a type of antihyperlipidemic drug that affects lipid levels by facilitating lipid metabolism
histamine H_2 receptor antagonist (H2RA) (also called **H_2 blocker**)	a drug that reduces production of stomach acid
laxative	a drug that aids the evacuation of the bowel
proton pump inhibitor (PPI)	a drug that blocks acid production in the stomach
statin	a type of antihyperlipidemic drug that treats dyslipidemia by inhibiting 3-hydroxy-3-methylglutaryl coenzyme A reductase

Chapter 12: Eye

antiglaucoma agent	a drug that treats glaucoma of the eye
miotic	an agent that contracts the pupil
mydriatic	an agent that dilates the pupil
ophthalmic	an agent that is intended to be used in the eye

Chapter 13: Ear

ceruminolytic	an agent that breaks down ear wax
otic	an agent intended to be used in the ear

Chapter 14: Musculoskeletal System

antiarthritic agent	a drug used in the treatment of arthritis
antigout agent	a drug that opposes the buildup of uric acid crystals in the joints to prevent and treat gout attacks
antispasmodic	a drug that prevents or relieves muscle spasms
bisphosphonate	a drug that binds to bone matrix to treat osteoporosis
disease-modifying antirheumatic drug (DMARD)	a drug that slows the progression of rheumatoid arthritis
muscle relaxant	a drug that reduces muscle contractility to relieve tension- or spasm-induced pain
neuromuscular blocking agent (NMBA)	a drug that blocks all nerve stimulation of the skeletal muscles to cause paralysis

Chapter 15: Nervous System and Behavioral Health

adrenergic agonist	a drug that stimulates aspects of the sympathetic nervous system
amphetamine	a drug that stimulates the central nervous system
anticonvulsant (also called antiepileptic drug)	a drug that reduces the incidence and severity of seizures and convulsions
analgesic	a drug that relieves pain; a *narcotic analgesic* is used for severe pain but can result in dependence and tolerance; a *nonnarcotic analgesic* is used for mild to moderate pain and is less likely to cause dependence and tolerance
anesthetic	a drug that causes numbness or a loss of feeling that can be used locally or systemically; often used systemically to put a patient "to sleep" during extensive procedures
anticholinergic	a drug that blocks the action of acetylcholine and therefore suppresses the parasympathetic nervous system
anticholinesterase	a drug that prevents the breakdown of acetylcholine to yield a cholinergic or parasympathetic effect
antidepressant	a drug used to treat depression
antiparkinsonian agent	a drug that treats Parkinson disease and parkinsonism by affecting levels of dopamine or acetylcholine in the brain
antipsychotic (also called **neuroleptic**)	a drug that treats psychosis disorders by inducing a calming or tranquilizing effect and/or by adjusting neurotransmitter levels in the brain
antipyretic	a drug that reduces fever
anxiolytic	a drug that relieves anxiety
barbiturate	a drug used to produce relaxation and sleep
benzodiazepine (BZD)	a drug that binds to receptors in the brain to calm and sedate the central nervous system
central nervous system stimulant	a drug that excites the central nervous system; can be used for many brain disorders
cholinergic	an agent that acts like acetylcholine to activate the parasympathetic nervous system
dopaminergic	a drug that acts like dopamine; mostly used to treat Parkinson disease by increasing dopamine-dependent activity in the brain
hypnotic	a drug used to induce sleep; may also be used as a sedative
mood stabilizer	a drug that balances neurotransmitters in the brain to prevent periods of mania or depression
monoamine oxidase inhibitor (MAOI)	a type of antidepressant that prevents the breakdown of many active neurotransmitters in the brain
nonsteroidal antiinflammatory drug (NSAID)	a drug that reduces pain, inflammation, and fever

sedative	a drug that depresses the central nervous system to calm a patient
selective serotonin reuptake inhibitor (SSRI)	a type of antidepressant that maintains a higher level of serotonin in the synapse
serotonin-norepinephrine reuptake inhibitor (SNRI)	a type of antidepressant that maintains a higher level of serotonin and norepinephrine in the synapse
tranquilizer	a drug that reduces anxiety or agitation
tricyclic antidepressant (TCA)	a type of antidepressant that maintains a higher level of various neurotransmitters in the synapse

Chapter 16: Endocrine System

antidiabetic agent	a drug that treats diabetes by controlling blood sugar levels
antithyroid agent	a drug that counters hyperthyroidism by reducing the production of thyroid hormones
corticosteroid	a drug that mimics hormones produced by the adrenal glands and has antiinflammatory and immunosuppressive effects
hypoglycemic agent	a drug that lowers blood sugar levels
thyroid hormone	a replacement hormone to regulate metabolism and endocrine functions

BIBLIOGRAPHY

2009 Conn's current therapy, Philadelphia, 2009, Saunders

American Journal of Nursing, 2008-2010, Lippincott Williams & Wilkins

Applegate EJ: *The anatomy and physiology learning system*, ed 3, St. Louis, 2006, Saunders

Ballinger PW, Frank ED: *Merrill's atlas of radiographic positions and radiologic procedures*, ed 10, St. Louis, 2003, Mosby

Bontrager KL: *Textbook of radiographic positioning and related anatomy*, ed 6, St. Louis, 2005, Mosby

Chabner D: *The language of medicine*, ed 8, Philadelphia, 2007, Saunders

Diehl M: *Medical transcription guide: do's and don'ts*, ed 3, St. Louis, 2005, Saunders

Diehl M: *Diehl and Fordney's medical transcription, techniques and procedures*, ed 5, 2002, Saunders

Dorland's illustrated medical dictionary, ed 31. Philadelphia, 2007, Saunders

Fitzpatrick JE, Aeling JL: *Dermatology secrets in color*, ed 2, Philadelphia, 2001, Hanley and Belfus

Frazier M, Drzymkowski JW: *Essentials of human diseases and conditions*, ed 3, Philadelphia, 2004, Elsevier

Habif T: *A color guide to diagnosis and therapy, clincial dermatology*, ed 4, Philadelphia, 2004, Mosby

Haubrich WS: *Medical meanings: a glossary of word origins*, Philadelphia, 1997, American College of Physicians

Herlihy B, Maebius N: *The human body in health and illness*, ed 3, Philadelphia, 2007, Saunders

Hockenberry MJ, Wilson D: *Wong's nursing care of infants and children*, ed 8, St. Louis, 2007, Mosby

Ignatavicius DD et al: *Medical-surgical nursing: a nursing process approach*, ed 6, Philadelphia, 2010, Saunders

Jarvis C: *Physical examination & health assessment*, ed 5, Philadelphia, 2008, Saunders

LaFleur Brooks M, Gillingham EA: *Health unit coordinating*, ed 5, Philadelphia, 2004, Saunders

LaFleur Brooks M, LaFleur Brooks D: *Basic medical language*, ed 3, St. Louis, 2010, Mosby

Lewis SM et al: *Medical-surgical nursing*, ed 6, St. Louis, 2004, Mosby

Littleton LY, Engebretson JC: *Maternal, neonatal, and women's health nursing*, Albany, 2002, Delmar

Lowdermilk DL, Perry SE: *Maternity & women's health care*, St. Louis, 2007, Mosby

Mayo Clinic Health Letter, Rochester, 2008-2010, Mayo Foundation for Medical Education and Research

Mayo Clinic Women's Health Source, Rochester, 2008-2010, Mayo Foundation for Medical Education and Research

Medline Plus, http://www.nlm.nih.gov/medlineplus, 2008-2010, National Library of Medicine and the National Institutes of Health

Mosby's medical, nursing, and allied health dictionary, ed 8, St. Louis, 2009, Mosby

Masters RM, Gylys BA: *Medical terminology simplified*, ed 3, Philadelphia, 2005, FA Davis

Medicine in quotations, Philadelphia, 2000, American College of Physicians

Nath JL: *Using medical terminology, a practical approach*, Baltimore, 2006, Lippincott Williams & Wilkins

National Cancer Institute, http://www.cancer.gov/, 2008-2010, National Institutes of Health

New England Journal of Medicine, 2008-2010, Massachusetts Medical Society

Novey D: *Clinicians' complete reference to complementary and alternative medicine*, St. Louis, 2000, Mosby

Pagana KD, Pagana TJ: *Mosby's manual of diagnostic and laboratory test reference*, ed 3, St. Louis, 2006, Mosby

Phillips N: *Berry & Kohn's operating room technique*, ed 11, St. Louis, 2007, Mosby

Rakel D: *Integrative medicine*, Philadelphia, 2003, Saunders

Shiland B: *Mastering healthcare terminology*, ed 2, St Louis, 2006, Mosby

Spencer JW, Jacobs JJ: *Complementary and alternative medicine: an evidence-based approach*, St Louis, 2003, Mosby

Stedman's abbreviations, acronyms, and symbols, ed 3, Baltimore, 2003, Lippincott Williams & Wilkins

Thibodeau GA, Patton KT: *Anthony's textbook of anatomy and physiology*, ed 18, St. Louis, 2007, Mosby

Thierer N, Breitbard L: *Medical terminology, language for health care*, ed 2, Boston, 2006, McGraw-Hill

Torpy JM: The metabolic syndrome, *JAMA*, *295*(7):850, 2006

UpToDate, http://www.uptodate.com, 2008-2010

Waldman SD: *Atlas of common pain syndromes*, ed 2, Philadelphia, 2008, Saunders

Whiteside MM et al: Sensory impairment in older adults: part 2, vision loss, *Consultant*, *106*(11):52-62, 2006

ILLUSTRATION CREDITS

Chapter 1

Figure 1-2 reprinted by permission of Tribune Media Services.

Chapter 2

Figure 2-3 from Kamal A, Brockelhurst JC: *Color atlas of geriatric medicine*, ed 2, St. Louis, 1991, Mosby.

Figure 2-5 from Kumar VK: *Basic pathology*, ed 7, Philadelphia, 2003, Saunders.

Figure 2-7 from National Cancer Institute (NCI). Courtesy Rhoda Baer (Photographer).

Figure 2-8 from Damjanov I: *Pathology, A color atlas*, ed 2, St. Louis, 2000, Mosby.

Figure 2-9 from Ballinger PW, Frank ED: *Merrill's atlas of radiographic positions and radiologic procedures*, ed 10, St. Louis, 2003, Mosby.

Exercise Figure C from (1) Mace JD: *Radiography pathology*, ed 4, St. Louis, 2004, Elsevier Mosby; (2) Habif TP: *Clinical dermatology*, ed 4, St. Louis, 2004, Elsevier Mosby; (3) Stevens A: *Pathology*, ed 2, London, 2000, Mosby; (4) Damjanov I, Linder J: *Anderson's pathology*, ed 10, St. Louis, 1996, Mosby.

Chapter 3

Table 3-1 figures and Exercise Figure C from Bontrager KL: *Radiographic positioning and related anatomy*, ed 5, St. Louis, 2002, Mosby.

Exercise Figures E, F(2), G from Bontrager KL, Lampignano JP: *Radiographic positioning and related anatomy*, ed 7, St. Louis, 2010, Mosby.

Exercise Figure F(1) from Chapleau W, Pons P: *Emergency medical technician*, ed 1, St. Louis, 2007, Mosby/JEMS.

Chapter 4

Figure 4-2 from Frazier M: *Essentials of human disease and conditions*, ed 3, St. Louis, 2004, Elsevier Mosby.

Dermatology poem courtesy Julia Frank, MD.

Exercise Figure C (1), Figures 4-3 (A), 4-12, 4-13, 4-14 and 4-16 and Unn Fig 4 from Bork K, Brauninger W: *Skin diseases in clinical practice*, ed 2, Philadelphia, 1998, WB Saunders.

Figure 4-4 (B), 4-5 from Callen JP: *Color atlas of dermatology*, ed 2, Philadelphia, 2000, Saunders.

Figure 4-4 (C) from Wilson S, Giddens J: *Health assessment for nursing practice*, ed 4, St. Louis, 2009, Mosby. Courtesy Gary Monheit, MD, University of Alabama at Birmingham School of Medicine.

Figure 4-6 from *Dorland's illustrated medical dictionary*, ed 31, Philadelphia, 2007, Saunders.

Figure 4-7 from Cohen BA: *Pediatric dermatology*, ed 3, St. Louis, 2005, Mosby.

Table 4-1 figures from Frazier M: *Essentials of human disease and conditions*, ed 3, St. Louis, 2004, Elsevier Mosby.

Figure 4-15 and Exercise Figure D (1 and 2) from Shiland B: *Mastering healthcare terminology*, ed 2, St. Louis, 2006, Elsevier Mosby.

Figure 4-4 (D, E), 4-9, 4-11, and Table 4-1 figures from Habif TP: *Clinical dermatology*, ed 4, St. Louis, 2004, Elsevier Mosby.

Chapter 5

Figure 5-3 from Eisenberg RL, Johnson NM: *Comprehensive radiographic pathology*, ed 3, St. Louis, 2003, Mosby.

Figure 5-5 from Mettler F: *Essentials of radiology*, ed 2, Philadelphia, 2005, Saunders.

Figure 5-7 from Kumar V et al: *Robbins' basic pathology*, ed 7, Philadelphia, 2003, Saunders.

Figure 5-12 from Potter PA, Perry AG: *Fundamentals of nursing: concepts, process, and practice*, ed 5, St. Louis, 2001, Mosby.

Figure 5-13 from Pryor J, Prasad A: *Physiotherapy for respiratory and cardiac problems*, ed 4, Edinburgh, 2009, Churchill Livingstone.

Figure 5-15 from Nelcor Puritan Bennett.

Table 5-1 figures from Ruppel GL: *Manual pulmonary function testing*, ed 7, St. Louis, 1998, Mosby; Siemens Medical Systems, Inc., New Jersey; Ballinger PW, Frank ED: *Merrill's atlas of radiographic positions and radiologic procedures*, ed 10, St. Louis, 2003, Mosby; GE Medical Systems, Waukesha, Wis; Pagana KD, Pagana TJ: *Mosby's manual of diagnostic and laboratory test reference*, ed 7, St. Louis, 2004, Elsevier Mosby. Shiland B: *Mastering healthcare terminology*, ed 2, St. Louis, 2006, Elsevier Mosby.

Chapter 6

Figure 6-5 (A), 6-6 from Damjanov I: *Pathology, a color atlas*, ed 2, St. Louis, 2000, Mosby.

Figure 6-8 from Shiland B: *Mastering healthcare terminology*, ed 2, St. Louis, 2006, Elsevier Mosby.

Figures 6-12 and 6-13 from Ballinger PW, Frank ED: *Merrill's atlas of radiographic positions and radiologic procedures*, ed 10, St. Louis, 2003, Mosby.

Figures 6-14 and 6-15 from Bontrager KL: *Textbook of radiographic positioning and related anatomy*, ed 6, St. Louis, 2002, Mosby.

Figure 6-18 courtesy Baxter Healthcare Corp, Deerfield, Ill.

Exercise Figure E courtesy Dornier Medical Systems, Kennesaw, Ga.

Chapter 7

Figure 7-10 courtesy EDAP Technomed, Inc., Vaulx-en-Velin, France.

Figure 7-11 (A, B) from Habif TP: *Clinical dermatology*, ed 4, St. Louis, 2004, Elsevier Mosby.

Figure 7-11 (C) from Callen JP: *Color atlas of dermatology*, ed 2, Philadelphia, 2000, Saunders.

Exercise Figure C (1) from Zitelli BJ, David HW: *Atlas of pediatric physical diagnosis*, ed 2, St. Louis, 1992, Mosby.

Exercise Figure B from Bork K, Brauninger W: *Skin diseases in clinical practice*, ed 2, Philadelphia, 1998, WB Saunders.

Chapter 8

Figure 8-8 from Black J, Hawks J: *Medical-surgical nursing*, ed 8, St. Louis, 2009, Elsevier.

Figure 8-12 (A) courtesy Biopsys Medical, Inc, Irvine, Calif.

Figure 8-12 (B, C) from Pagana KD, Pagana TJ: *Mosby's manual of diagnostic and laboratory test reference*, ed 7, St. Louis, 2004, Elsevier Mosby.

Figure 8-14 from Bontrager KL, Lampignano JP: *Radiographic positioning and related anatomy*, ed 6, St. Louis, 2005, Mosby.

Figure 8-17 courtesy Richard Wolf Medical Instruments Corp., Vernon Hills, Ill.

Chapter 9

Figure 9-2 from Dickason EJ, Schultz MO, Silverman BL: *Maternal-infant nursing care*, ed 3, St. Louis, 1998, Mosby.

Figure 9-6, 9-7 and 9-9 from Zitelli BJ, David HW: *Atlas of pediatric physical diagnosis*, ed 4, St. Louis, 2002, Mosby.

Figure 9-10 (B) from Hockenberry M, Wilson D: *Wong's essentials of pediatric nursing*, ed 8, St. Louis, 2009, Elsevier.

Figure 9-12 from Bontrager KL, Lampignano JP: *Radiographic positioning and related anatomy*, ed 6, St. Louis, 2005, Mosby.

Exercise Figure B from Lowdermilk DL: *Maternity and women's health care*, ed 8, St. Louis, 2004, Elsevier Mosby.

Exercise Figure C from Lowdermilk DL, Perry S: *Maternity and women's health care*, ed 9, St. Louis, 2007, Elsevier Mosby.

Chapter 10

Figures 10-1 and 10-5 from LaFleur Brooks M, LaFleur Brooks D: *Basic medical language*, ed 3, St. Louis, 2010, Elsevier.

Figure 10-12 (A) from Thibodeau GA, Patton KT: *Anatomy and physiology*, ed 4, St. Louis, 2001, Mosby.

Figure 10-12 (B) from Bork K, Brauninger W: *Skin diseases in clinical practice*, ed 2, Philadelphia, 1998, WB Saunders.

Figures 10-14 (B), 10-19 (B, C), 10-21, 10-22, 10-23, and 10-25 (B) from Ballinger PW, Frank ED: *Merrill's atlas of radiographic positions and radiologic procedures*, ed 10, St. Louis, 2003, Mosby.

Figure 10-25 (A) courtesy GE Medical Systems, Inc, Waukesha, Wis.

Exercise Figure D from LaFleur Brooks M: *Exploring medical language*, ed 5, St. Louis, 2002, Mosby.

Chapter 11

Figure 11-11 from Shiland B: *Mastering healthcare terminology*, ed 2, St. Louis, 2006, Elsevier Mosby.

Figure 11-12 from Anderson KN: *Mosby's medical, nursing and allied health dictionary*, St. Louis, 2003, Mosby.

Figure 11-17 from White RA, Klein SR: *Endoscopic surgery*, St. Louis, 1991, Mosby.

Figure 11-19 from Ballinger PW, Frank ED: *Merrill's atlas of radiographic positions and radiologic procedures*, ed 10, St. Louis, 2003, Mosby.

Figure 11-21 from Lewis SM: *Medical-surgical nursing,* ed 7, St. Louis, 2007, Mosby.

Unnumbered Figure 4 from Hagen-Ansert S: *Textbook of diagnostic ultrasonography,* ed 5, St. Louis, 2001, Mosby.

Chapter 12

Figure 12-3 and Exercise Figures B and D from Zitelli BJ, David HW: *Atlas of pediatric physical diagnosis,* ed 4, St. Louis, 2002, Mosby.

Figure 12-5 (A, B) from Seidel H et al: *Mosby's guide to physical examination,* ed 5, St. Louis, 2003, Mosby.

Exercise Figure C from Stein HA, Slatt BJ, Stein RM: *The ophthalmic assistant: fundamentals and clinical practice,* ed 5, St. Louis, 1998, Mosby.

Figure 12-6 from Newell FW: *Ophthalmology,* ed 7, St. Louis, 1992, Mosby.

Figure 12-7 from Apple DJ, Robb MF: *Ocular pathology,* ed 5, St. Louis, 1998, Mosby.

Figure 12-9 from Bedford MA: *Ophthalmological diagnosis,* London, 1986, Wolfe.

Figure 12-10 from Black J, Hawks J: *Medical-surgical nursing,* ed 7, Philadelphia, 2005, Saunders. Courtesy of Ophthalmic Photography at the University of Michigan, WK Kellogg Center, Ann Arbor.

Figure 12-11 courtesy Nidek, Inc., Fremont, Calif.

Figure 12-13 from Thompson J, Wilson S: *Health assessment for nursing practice,* St. Louis, 1996, Mosby.

Chapter 13

Figure 13-4 courtesy Richard A. Buckingham, MD, University of Illinois, Chicago.

Figure 13-3 from Zitelli BJ, David HW: *Atlas of pediatric physical diagnosis,* ed 4, St. Louis, 2002, Mosby.

Exercise Figure C from Jarvis C: *Physical examination and health assessment,* ed 5, Philadelphia, 2008, Saunders.

Chapter 14

Figure 14-6 from Thibodeau GA, Patton KT: *Anatomy and physiology,* ed 5, St. Louis, 2003, Mosby.

Figures 14-12 and 14-23 from Mercier LR: *Practical orthopedics,* ed 4, St. Louis, 1995, Mosby.

Figure 14-16 from Stone D: *Atlas of infectious diseases,* St. Louis, 1999, WB Saunders.

Figure 14-20 from Pagana KD, Pagana TJ: *Mosby's manual of diagnostic and laboratory test reference,* ed 7, St. Louis, 2004, Elsevier Mosby.

Figure 14-21 courtesy Marconi Medical Systems, Cleveland, Ohio.

Figure 14-22 from Ballinger PW, Frank ED: *Merrill's atlas of radiographic positions and radiologic procedures,* ed 10, St. Louis, 2003, Mosby.

Chapter 15

Figure 15-1 and 15-2 from Thibodeau GA, Patton KT: *Anatomy and physiology,* ed 5, St. Louis, 2003, Mosby.

Figure 15-5 from Waldman S: *Atlas of common pain syndromes*, ed 2, Philadelphia, 2008, Saunders.

Figure 15-8 from Shiland B: *Mastering healthcare terminology*, ed 2, St. Louis, 2006, Elsevier Mosby.

Figure 15-9 from Perkin GD, Hotchberg FH, Miller D: *The atlas of clinical neurology*, St. Louis, 1986, Mosby.

Figure 15-11 from Habif TP: *Clinical dermatology*, ed 4, St. Louis, 2004, Elsevier Mosby.

Figures 15-14 (B), 15-15, and Exercise Figure D from Ballinger PW, Frank ED: *Merrill's atlas of radiographic positions and radiologic procedures*, ed 10, St. Louis, 2003, Mosby.

Chapter 16

Figure 16-5 and Exercise C from Shiland B: *Mastering healthcare terminology*, ed 2, St. Louis, 2006, Elsevier Mosby.

Figure 16-6 courtesy CD Forbes and WF Jackson.

Figure 16-7 from Seidel H et al: *Mosby's guide to physical examination*, ed 5, St. Louis, 2003, Mosby.

Figure 16-8 courtesy Paul W. Ladenson, MD, The Johns Hopkins University and Hospital, Baltimore, Md.

INDEX

Page numbers followed by b indicate boxes; f, figures; t, tables.

H

J

K